Diagnostic and Clinical Pathology

Diagnostic and Clinical Pathology

Edited by **Hans Affleck**

hayle medical

New York

Published by Hayle Medical,
30 West, 37th Street, Suite 612,
New York, NY 10018, USA
www.haylemedical.com

Diagnostic and Clinical Pathology
Edited by Hans Affleck

International Standard Book Number: 978-1-63241-425-0 (Hardback)

Printed in China.

Contents

Preface

This book aims to highlight the current researches and provides a platform to further the scope of innovations in this area. This book is a product of the combined efforts of many researchers and scientists from different parts of the world. The objective of this book is to provide the readers with the latest information in the field.

Diagnostic and clinical pathology refers to that branch of medical science which deals with diagnosing and treating diseases by using laboratory tests of urine, blood and other body fluids. It uses the elements of chemistry, hematology, microbiology, etc. to identify the disorders. Clinical pathologists use different techniques of examination like microscopical examination, analyzers, macroscopic examination, cultures, etc. This book outlines the processes and applications of this topic in detail. It elucidates new techniques in a multidisciplinary approach. Some of the diverse topics covered in this book address the varied branches that fall under pathology. It is compiled in such a manner, that it will provide in-depth knowledge about the theory and practice related to the field of pathology. Students, researchers, pathologists, experts and all associated with this subject will benefit alike form this book.

I would like to express my sincere thanks to the authors for their dedicated efforts in the completion of this book. I acknowledge the efforts of the publisher for providing constant support. Lastly, I would like to thank my family for their support in all academic endeavors.

Editor

1

Eumycetoma Osteomyelitis of the Calcaneus in a Child: A Radiologic-Pathologic Correlation following Total Calcanectomy

Tamer Ahmed EL-Sobky, John Fathy Haleem, and Shady Samir

Orthopedic Surgery Department, Faculty of Medicine, Ain Shams University, 38 Abbasia Square, Masjed Alnoor, Cairo, Egypt

Correspondence should be addressed to Tamer Ahmed EL-Sobky; tamer.ahmed@med.asu.edu.eg

Academic Editor: Marco Mazzocchi

Fungi are unusual causes of pedal osteomyelitis in children and adolescents. Eumycetoma is a chronic cutaneous and subcutaneous infection caused by various genera of fungi. A provisional diagnosis of foot mycetoma is made after clinical assessment. Radiologic-pathologic correlation is an essential supplement for the accurate diagnosis of osteoarticular infections. This paper aims to sensitize orthopedic surgeons, radiologists, and pathologists to the importance of correlative imaging findings in relation to surgical and microscopic pathology in osteoarticular infections, specifically eumycetoma osteomyelitis of the foot. From our review of the published data, the present case is the first report of radiologic-pathologic correlation in eumycetoma osteomyelitis of the calcaneus. This paper describes a case of eumycetoma osteomyelitis of the calcaneus in a child in which diagnostic X-rays and magnetic resonance imaging (MRI) were correlated with the surgical and microscopic pathologic features, for establishing an appropriate diagnosis and treatment. We conclude that there is a significant agreement between radiologic and pathologic evaluation for assessment of eumycetoma osteomyelitis of the calcaneus. Radiologic-pathologic correlation amplified our interpretation of imaging information available on plain radiographs and MRI and augmented diagnostic confidence. Similarly, anatomic-histopathological correlations consolidated diagnostic accuracy.

1. Introduction

Eumycetoma is an unusual chronic cutaneous and subcutaneous infection caused by various genera of fungi. Approximately 40% of mycetomas worldwide are eumycotic rather than actinomycotic (i.e., caused by bacterial actinomycetes). The disease is characterized by marked progressive destruction of soft tissue and bones causing functional disability. The most common site of occurrence is the foot [1]. A provisional diagnosis of foot mycetoma is made after clinical assessment. Some causal agents of mycetoma are difficult to identify by culture methods alone. Besides, clinical and histopathological examinations alone do not detect the spread of disease along the different tissue planes and bone and are not specific enough to identify the causative agent to the species level. Imaging techniques such as X-rays and MRI can aid in the early diagnosis of the lesion and can be used to determine the extent of lesions [2–4].

We assume that radiologic-pathologic correlation is an essential supplement for the accurate diagnosis and management of osteoarticular infections. From our review of the published data, the present case is the first report of radiologic-pathologic correlation in eumycetoma osteomyelitis of the calcaneus. The purpose of this review is to demonstrate why performing this correlation is an essential part of the diagnostic process of osteoarticular infections. This paper aims to sensitize orthopedic surgeons, radiologists, and pathologists to the importance of correlative imaging findings in relation to surgical and microscopic pathology in eumycetoma osteomyelitis of the foot. Our patient was informed that data concerning the case would be submitted for publication.

2. Case Report

A 14-and-a-half-year-old boy from Fayoum Governorate in rural Egypt complained of an initially painless right foot swelling for the past six years. Multiple sinus tracts developed with an initial purulent discharge and an eventual extensive black granular discharge. He was previously subjected to multiple bony debridement procedures in other institutions

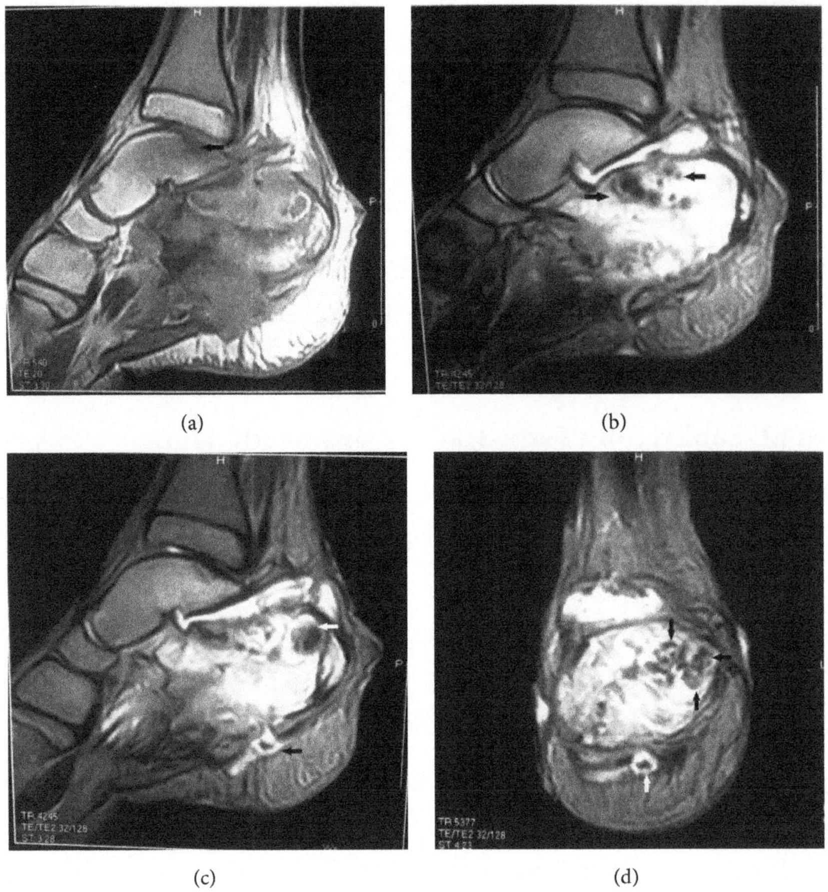

FIGURE 1: (a) T1-weighted sagittal MRI of the right foot. Note the altered marrow signals seen almost totally replacing the marrow texture of the calcaneus and to a lesser extent the opposing posteromedial aspect of the talus (black arrow) eliciting an abnormal low signal. (b) T2-weighted sagittal MRI of the right foot. Note the abnormal high signals replacing the marrow texture of the calcaneus. Note the multiple low-intensity lesions (black arrows) that may represent a conglomerate of grains in the background of diffuse high-intensity inflammatory bone changes. These low-intensity lesions are known as dot in circle. (c) T2-weighted sagittal MRI of the right foot. Note the low-intensity cavitary lesion of the posterior calcaneus (white arrow) that was found to correlate well to a conglomerate of black grains noticed in the gross pathologic specimen of the calcaneus. Note the same low-intensity lesion (black arrow) in the background of diffuse hyperintense inflammatory soft tissue changes (dot in circle). (d) T2-weighted coronal MRI of the right foot. Note the multiple small low-intensity lesions (black arrows) that may represent a conglomerate of grains in the background of diffuse hyperintense inflammatory bone changes. The same lesion is depicted in the soft tissue (white arrow).

to which the he did not respond. Based on the clinical/radiologic suspicion and results of culture and sensitivity from discharging sinuses that revealed Gram positive *Staphylococcus aureus*, the patient was diagnosed with nonspecific bacterial calcaneal osteomyelitis. The patient was treated with multiple courses of oral and intravenous antibiotics over the following six years, to which he did not respond. The patient walked with painful limp that deteriorated over the past years till he finally used crutches permanently and became a household ambulatory. The patient was nonimmunosuppressed and had no systemic manifestations or other skeletal complaints. Blood and serum chemistry were also unremarkable.

By examination, there was diffuse right foot oedema and tenderness especially over the hind foot. Two discharging sinuses were observed in relation to the hind foot. There was painful passive motion of the subtalar and ankle joints.

2.1. Radiologic-Pathologic Examination. X-ray findings of the foot and ankle revealed massive bony destruction of the calcaneus consistent with chronic osteomyelitis. MRI of the right ankle and foot was performed to characterize and evaluate the extent of the disease. Technique of examination included sagittal T1-, STIR, and T2-weighted images, axial T1- and T2-weighted images, and coronal T2-weighted images. The salient abnormality was the markedly altered marrow signals seen almost totally replacing the marrow texture of the calcaneus and to a lesser extent involving the opposing posteromedial aspect of the talus eliciting abnormal low T1, high T2, and iso-to-high STIR signals with evident cortical breaching and associated large soft tissue component eliciting low T1 and high T2 and STIR signals (Figures 1(a), 1(b), 1(c), and 1(d)).

In march 2015, we performed total calcanectomy through a heel splitting approach. Under general anesthesia, a high

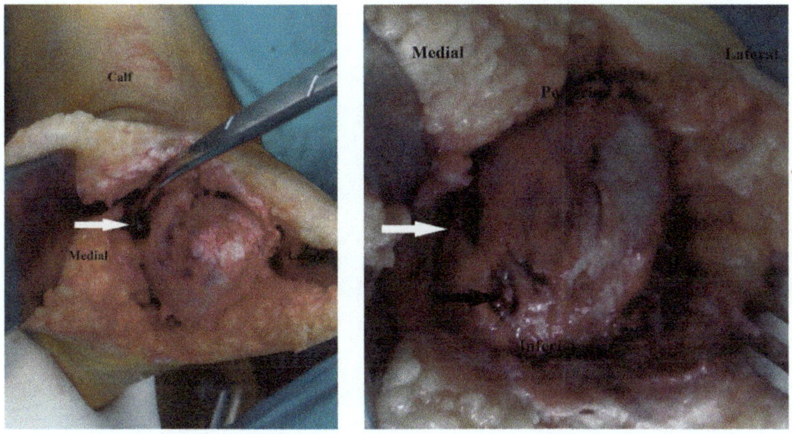

(a) (b)

FIGURE 2: (a) Intraoperative images of calcaneus employing the heel splitting approach. Note the conglomerate of black grains arising from the cavity on the medial surface of calcaneus (white arrow). (b) Intraoperative images of calcaneus employing the heel splitting approach. Note the large medial cavity (white arrow) and cortical erosion covered by minute black grains (black arrow).

tourniquet was employed in the prone position. Anatomic pathology of the excised calcaneus is depicted in Figures 2(a), 2(b), 3(a), 3(b), and 3(c). The histopathological features were consistent with eumycetoma (Figure 3(d)). The patient was put on oral Itraconazole therapy for 8 weeks. Oral clindamycin therapy was used to treat secondary bacterial infection. Significant clinical improvement was observed at regular followup intervals. The discharging sinuses and the surgical wound demonstrated sound healing.

3. Discussion

The concept of radiologic-pathologic correlation was born in 1947 with the establishment of the Radiologic Pathology Department and Registry at the Armed Forces Institute of Pathology in Washington, DC. This method has become a key teaching tool to understand the radiological manifestations of disease, initially on plain films and later with cross-sectional techniques [5]. Obviously, the most suitable candidate for radiologic-pathologic correlation is the study of neoplasms, since they are resected ideally in toto and therefore offer excellent imaging-gross pathologic comparisons.

Musculoskeletal infection is common in clinical practice. Osteomyelitis refers to infection of the bone and marrow usually by pus producing organisms. It is commonly caused by bacteria, but fungi are also considered. Usually, the diagnosis of fungal osteomyelitis is challenging. The clinical and radiological findings of osteoarticular infection may be conflicting and confusing. Even with the advancement of imaging technology, findings may remain inconclusive. There are a wide variety of presentations seen on imaging reflecting the balance between host and organism, disease duration, and institution of antimicrobial treatment. A good understanding of various stages of osteoarticular infection is essential to augment the interpretation of the vast amount of imaging information available to arrive at an accurate diagnosis and thereby institute timely and effective treatment to prevent destructive sequelae in the immature skeleton [5].

In eumycetoma fungal osteomyelitis bones are almost always attacked from outside, in contrast to bacterial osteomyelitis, and periosteal reaction, cortical erosions, and bone texture abnormalities may then be seen. It is important to detect whether bone is infected as nonsurgical cure is uncertain in such cases. Conventional radiographs are used to determine whether bone is affected and to identify the limits of lesions in eumycetoma. Multiple radiographic changes can be detected [3]. Abd El Bagi suggested a radiographic classification of mycetoma to determine the extent of lesions based on radiographic records of 516 patients seen in the Mycetoma Research Centre, Khartoum, Sudan [3]. Radiographs of our patient depicted soft tissue involvement, cortical erosion, and central cavitation of the calcaneus with minimal involvement of the talus and are classified as stage IV. These findings indicate the extent and severity of infection in our patient.

Several authors found that MRI is useful for visualizing soft tissue involvement and bone destruction; with MRI, multiple small spherical hyperintense lesions separated by tissue of low signal intensity appear. Some of these lesions show a central tiny hypointense focus. These hypointense foci were named "dot in circle" and were seen in 80% of patients, which made this appearance highly indicative of mycetoma [2, 4, 6, 7]. We were able to demonstrate similar MRI findings in all image sequences in our case. We were also able to clearly correlate the hypointense foci with the massive black fungal grains noticed on growth pathological examination of the calcaneus following total calcanectomy. In addition, we suggest that these characteristic (dot-in-circle) lesions may differentiate mycetoma from other infections and tumorous lesions.

The MRI of our patient revealed thickening of the overlying skin with multiple defects, ulceration, and sinus tracts breaching the posterior and plantar posterior skin, subcutaneous fat, and plantar fascia. These findings clearly correlated with the intraoperative multiple small cavities and black grain discharge observed on the plantar surface of the calcaneus following calcanectomy. There was a significant

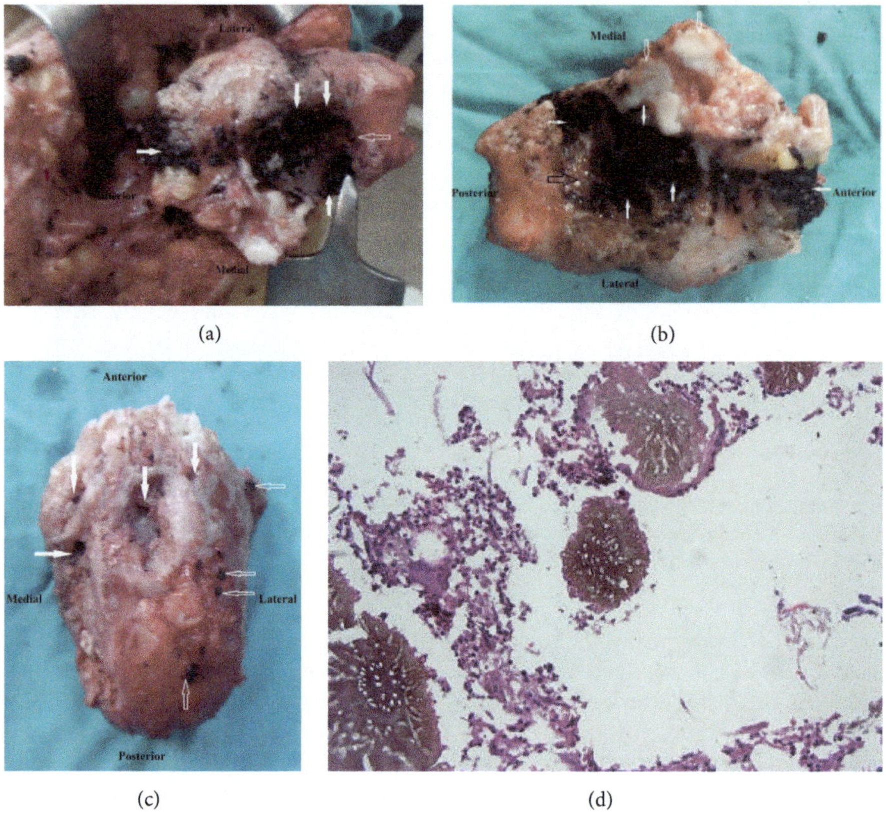

FIGURE 3: (a) Intraoperative images of superior surface of calcaneus employing the heel splitting approach. Note the extensive conglomerates of black grains scattered over that surface (solid arrows). Note the complete destruction of the articular cartilage of the posterior facet of the subtalar joint (hollow arrows). (b) Operative images of superior surface of calcaneus following total resection, employing the heel splitting approach. Note the extensive conglomerates of black grains scattered over that surface (white solid arrows) and the articular cartilage erosions of the anterior and middle facets of the subtalar joint (hollow white arrows). Complete destruction of the articular cartilage of the posterior facet of the subtalar joint with gross deformation is depicted (hollow black arrow). (c) Operative images of inferior surface of the calcaneus following total resection, employing the heel splitting approach. Note the presence of multiple bony cavities of various sizes (white arrows). Foci of black granular discharge are depicted (hollow arrows). (d) Brown fungal colonies with surrounding inflammatory cells and fibrosis (H and E, ×400).

correlation between the previous radiologic-pathologic findings and the black grain discharging sinuses observed on clinical examination.

The MRI findings of our patient revealed markedly abnormal signal intensity involving the sinus tarsi and the subtalar articulation. The gross pathologic findings of the calcaneus revealed complete destruction of the articular cartilage of posterior subtalar joint, joint depression, and partial destruction of the middle facet. There was a significant correlation between the previous radiologic-pathologic findings and the preoperative painful passive range of motion of the subtalar joint.

In 2012, El Shamy and colleagues reported a new grading system for MRI diagnosis of mycetoma. They found that actinomycetoma more often showed soft tissue microabscesses, bony periosteal reaction, and reactive sclerosis, while eumycetoma frequently exhibited soft tissue macroabscesses with bone cavitation; such differences were not statistically significant [8]. The MRI findings of eumycetoma in our patient typically correlated with the eumycetoma findings presented by the previous authors. Additionally, there was a correlation between MRI findings in our patient and both the gross and histopathological findings that revealed bone cavitation and intervening abscesses full of brown fungal colonies (eumycetoma).

3.1. Anatomic-Histopathological Correlation. Since both actinomycetes and fungi are implicated as causative agents, it is important to distinguish them in order to ensure that correct treatments are given [9]. Mycetoma is characterized by the development of discharging sinuses. Within the discharged material, the causative organism is located both in and outside the grains. The colours of the grains can often be indicative of the aetiological agent: fungal grains are usually black or pale, while those of actinomycetes are white, yellow, or red [9].

Culture methods are still considered to be the gold standard in species identification of the causal agents of mycetoma. However, some agents are difficult to identify by morphology alone. Furthermore, most cultures methods are time consuming, contamination is common, and experience is needed to read results accurately [10]. Histology and cytology appeared to be not specific enough to identify the causative agent to the species level [10]. In the current study, black granular discharge was demonstrable on the surface of and inside cavities of the gross specimen of the calcaneus. These findings are consistent with eumycetoma.

The granules of actinomycetoma consist of fine, branching filaments, only about 1 micron thick, whereas the granules of eumycetoma are composed of septate hyphae 4-5 microns thick [11]. This histopathological description of eumycetoma conforms to that reported in our histograms. Furthermore, eumycetoma grains can be divided into black and pale grains. In histology sections, two types of grains of this agent are seen: filamentous and vesicular. The filamentous type is the most common and consists of brown septate and branched hyphae [10]. The histograms of our patient correlated to the detailed description of the filamentous type.

In our patient, all of the above mentioned histopathological findings clearly correlated to the anatomic pathology aiding definitive species diagnosis.

4. Conclusion

Agreement between radiology and pathology was recognizable. The radiologic-pathologic correlation may be used in explaining the role of plain radiographs and MRI in identifying eumycetoma osteomyelitis of the calcaneus in children. Establishment of a clear correlation between radiology and pathology may help differentiate eumycetoma from other infections and tumorous lesions. Radiologic-pathologic correlation augmented diagnostic confidence. Similarly, anatomic-histopathological correlations consolidated diagnostic accuracy.

Conflict of Interests

The authors declare that there is no conflict of interests regarding the publication of this paper.

Acknowledgment

The authors thank Dr. Shady Elia Anis, Lecturer of pathology, Cairo University, for providing the histograms.

References

[1] M. Develoux, M. T. Dieng, A. Kane, and B. Ndiaye, "Management of mycetoma in West-Africa," *Bulletin de la Societe de Pathologie Exotique*, vol. 96, no. 5, pp. 376–382, 2004.

[2] J. Kumar, A. Kumar, P. Sethy, and S. Gupta, "The dot-in-circle sign of mycetoma on MRI," *Diagnostic and Interventional Radiology*, vol. 13, no. 4, pp. 193–195, 2007.

[3] M. E. Abd El Bagi, "New radiographic classification of bone involvement in pedal mycetoma," *American Journal of Roentgenology*, vol. 180, no. 3, pp. 665–668, 2003.

[4] R. S. Cherian, M. Betty, M. T. Manipadam et al., "The "dot-in-circle" sign: a characteristic MRI finding in mycetoma foot: a report of three cases," *British Journal of Radiology*, vol. 82, no. 980, pp. 662–665, 2009.

[5] S. H. M. Khan and J. L. Bloem, "Radiologic-pathologic correlations of bone infections," in *Radiologic-Pathologic Correlations from Head to Toe: Understanding the Manifestations of Disease*, N. C. Gourtsoyiannis and P. R. Ros, Eds., pp. 647–659, Springer, Berlin, Germany, 2005.

[6] A. Sen and R. S. Pillay, "Case report: dot-in-circle sign—an MRI and USG sign for 'Madura foot'," *Indian Journal of Radiology and Imaging*, vol. 21, no. 4, pp. 264–266, 2011.

[7] V. Jain, G. E. Makwana, M. Mathur, and N. Bahri, "The 'dot in circle' sign on MRI in maduramycosis: a characteristic finding," *Journal of Clinical Imaging Science*, vol. 2, article 66, 2012.

[8] M. E. El Shamy, A. H. Fahal, M. Y. Shakir, and M. M. Homeida, "New MRI grading system for the diagnosis and management of mycetoma," *Transactions of the Royal Society of Tropical Medicine and Hygiene*, vol. 106, no. 12, pp. 738–742, 2012.

[9] A. A. O. Ahmed, W. W. J. van de Sande, A. Fahal, I. Bakker-Woudenberg, H. Verbrugh, and A. V. Belkum, "Management of mycetoma: major challenge in tropical mycoses with limited international recognition," *Current Opinion in Infectious Diseases*, vol. 20, no. 2, pp. 146–151, 2007.

[10] W. W. J. van de Sande, A. H. Fahal, M. Goodfellow, E. S. Mahgoub, O. Welsh, and E. E. Zijlstra, "Merits and pitfalls of currently used diagnostic tools in mycetoma," *PLoS Neglected Tropical Diseases*, vol. 8, no. 7, article e2918, 2014.

[11] V. V. Taralakshmi, V. V. Pankajalakshmi, S. Arumugam, and S. Subramanian, "Mycetoma caused by Madurella mycetomii in Madras," *Australasian Journal of Dermatology*, vol. 19, no. 3, pp. 125–129, 1978.

2

Tumor-to-Tumor Metastasis: Lung Carcinoma Metastasizing to Thyroid Neoplasms

Shiuan-Li Wey and Kuo-Ming Chang

Department of Pathology, Mackay Memorial Hospital, Hsinchu 30071, Taiwan

Correspondence should be addressed to Shiuan-Li Wey; shiuanliwey@gmail.com

Academic Editor: Prashant Bavi

Tumor-to-tumor metastasis is extremely rare in the thyroid glands, and only seven cases of lung carcinoma metastasizing to thyroid tumors have been reported in the literature. We report another two cases of lung carcinoma metastasizing to thyroid neoplasms and review of the literature. The first case was a 64-year-old man presenting with neck mass, hoarseness, and easy choking for 2 months. Image studies showed several nodular lesions within bilateral thyroid glands. A histological examination after radical thyroidectomy revealed lung small cell carcinoma metastasizing to a thyroid follicular adenoma. The second case was a 71-year-old woman with a history of lung adenosquamous carcinoma. The PET/CT scan showed left lower lung cancer and a hypermetabolic area in the right thyroid lobe, highly suspicious for malignancy. Radical thyroidectomy and left lung lobectomy were performed, and the thyroid gland revealed lung adenosquamous carcinoma metastasizing to a papillary thyroid carcinoma.

1. Introduction

The thyroid gland is an uncommon site for metastatic tumors, and most thyroid gland tumors are primary. The overall incidence of metastatic thyroid gland tumors is ranging from 1.4 to 3% [1]. Tumor-to-tumor metastasis is exceedingly rare, which is defined as the recipient tumor being a true neoplasm and the donor neoplasm being a true metastasis [2, 3]. To our knowledge, only seven cases of lung carcinoma metastasis to thyroid gland tumors have been reported in the literature [2–8]. Among histological types of lung carcinoma metastasizing to thyroid neoplasms, adenocarcinoma was the most commonly reported, followed by poorly differentiated carcinoma and small cell carcinoma. We present one case of lung small cell carcinoma metastasizing to thyroid follicular adenoma and another case of lung adenosquamous carcinoma metastasizing to papillary thyroid carcinoma.

2. Case Presentation

2.1. Case 1. A 64-year-old man, who had no past history of major disease, presented with neck mass, hoarseness, and easy choking. Fine needle aspiration of bilateral thyroid glands was performed and cytology showed plenty of single or cohesive tumor cells, and anaplastic carcinoma was suspected. Image studies revealed several nodular lesions with strong heterogeneous enhancement within bilateral thyroid glands. The patient received a radical thyroidectomy. On gross examination, the left thyroid gland was $7.3 \times 4 \times 3.5$ cm in size with one major well-defined nodule, and the right thyroid gland was $5.5 \times 4 \times 3$ cm in size with several nodules. The major well-defined nodule in the left thyroid gland measured $4.5 \times 3.5 \times 3$ cm in size, which appeared tan and partially white in color. It was solid and soft to mildly firm in consistency. Histological exam of thyroid glands revealed follicular adenoma with thick to thin capsule in left side and adenomatoid nodules in right side. Within follicular adenoma and adenomatoid nodules were multifocal areas showing an abrupt transition to a morphologically distinct neoplasm comprised of cells with hyperchromatic nuclei and scanty cytoplasm arranged in large sheets and broad ribbons (Figures 1(a) and 1(b)). The immunohistochemical stains of those neoplastic cells with hyperchromatic nuclei were positive for synaptophysin, chromogranin-A, TTF-1, and cytokeratin, while being negative for calcitonin and thyroglobulin (Figures 1(c) and 1(d)). The surrounding nonneoplastic gland

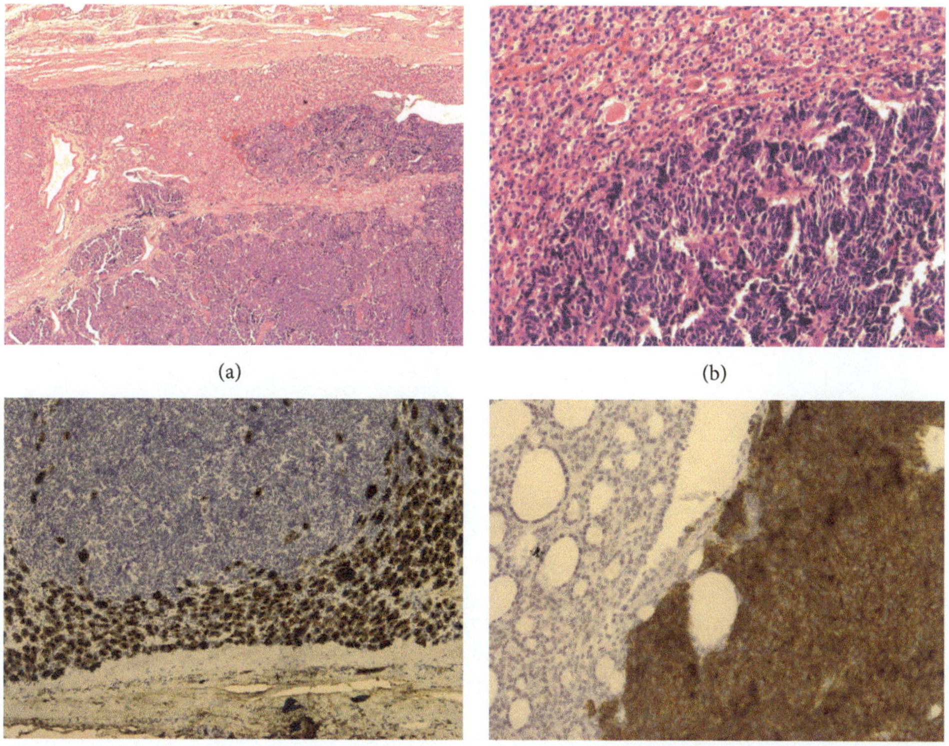

(a) (b) (c) (d)

Figure 1: (a) Within the encapsulated follicular adenoma is an abrupt transition to a morphologically distinct neoplasm (magnification ×40). (b) Metastatic carcinoma is arranged in sheets with hyperchromatic nuclei and scanty cytoplasm infiltrating the follicular adenoma (magnification ×200). (c) The metastatic carcinoma is negative for thyroglobulin, while the adenoma is strongly positive (magnification ×100). (d) Synaptophysin is strongly positive in the metastatic carcinoma (magnification ×200).

was not involved by the carcinoma. The features suggest metastatic small cell carcinoma of lung origin. Postoperative computed tomography revealed a 4.7 cm tumor mass in the left upper lobe of lung with mediastinal lymphadenopathy. A mediastinum lymph node biopsy was performed. There were many metastatic neoplastic cells present in the lymph node which cytomorphologically and immunohistochemically was identical to metastatic small cell carcinoma in thyroid glands. Small cell carcinoma of lung metastasizing to follicular adenoma and adenomatoid nodules of thyroid glands was diagnosed.

2.2. Case 2. A 71-year-old woman presented with a pulmonary mass diagnosed as adenosquamous carcinoma based on biopsy and received adjuvant chemotherapy. Three months later, PET/CT scan revealed left lower lung cancer and a hypermetabolic area in the right thyroid lobe, highly suspicious for malignancy. Fine needle aspiration of right thyroid gland was performed and cytology showed groups of follicular cells with features of papillary thyroid carcinoma. The patient received a radical thyroidectomy and left lung lobectomy. On gross examination, there was a tumor measuring 5.6 × 4.5 × 3 cm in size in the left lower lobe of lung, and the histological exam revealed adenosquamous carcinoma. The right thyroid gland was 4.4 × 2.3 × 1.8 cm in size with one major nodule and several small nodules. Histological exam of the major nodule revealed papillary thyroid carcinoma. Within the nodule was a focal area showing an abrupt transition to a morphologically distinct neoplasm comprised of cells with large nuclei, distinctive nucleoli, and abundant eosinophilic cytoplasm arranged in solid nests and few glandular pattern (Figures 2(a) and 2(b)). The mucicarmine stain reveals cytoplasmic positive in those large neoplastic cells. The immunohistochemical stains of large neoplastic cells were also positive for TTF-1 and napsin-A, while being negative for thyroglobulin (Figures 2(c) and 2(d)). A part of adenocarcinoma of primary lung adenosquamous carcinoma metastasizing to a papillary thyroid carcinoma was diagnosed.

3. Discussion

Metastatic disease to thyroid gland is uncommon, with reported incidence ranging from 1.4 to 3% of all patients who undergo surgery for suspected cancer in the thyroid gland [1]. The pathogenesis of metastasis is either through lymphovascular spread or extension from adjacent tissue [9]. Although the thyroid glands are rich in blood supply, few metastatic tumors occur. Fast arterial flow, high oxygen saturation, and iodine content of the thyroid glands are inhibiting the growth of malignant cells [1]. The most common metastatic tumors in thyroid were from the kidney, lung, gastrointestinal tract,

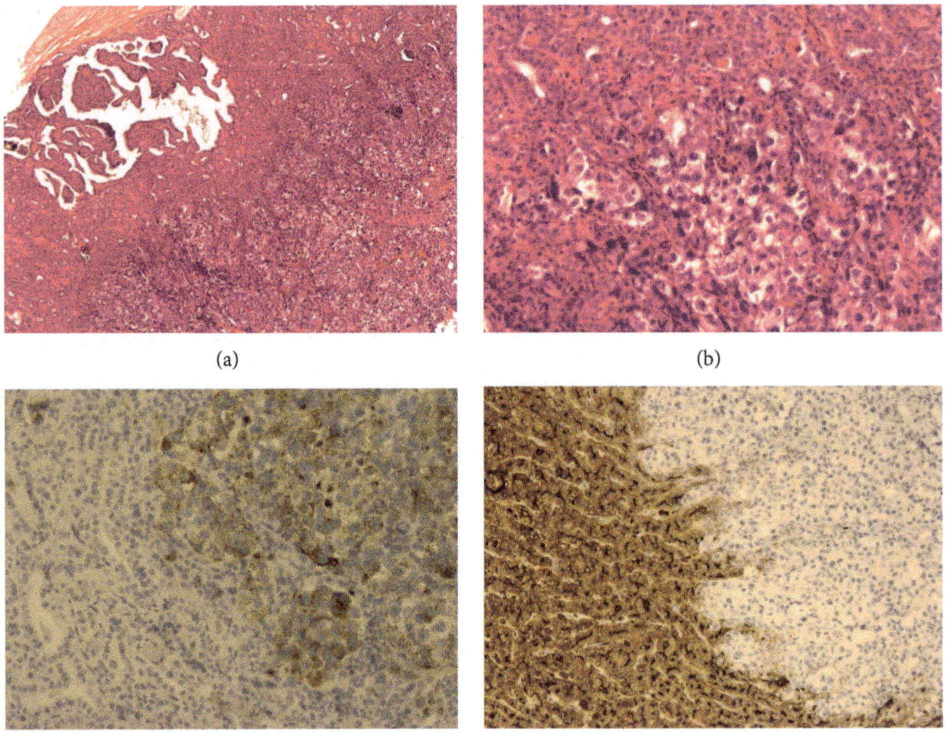

(a) (b) (c) (d)

Figure 2: (a) Within the papillary carcinoma is an abrupt transition to a morphologically distinct neoplasm (magnification ×40). (b) Metastatic carcinoma is arranged in nests with large nuclei, nucleoli, and abundant clear-to-eosinophilic cytoplasm (magnification ×200). (c) Napsin-A is shown to be positive in the metastatic carcinoma (magnification ×200). (d) Thyroglobulin is negative in the metastatic carcinoma, while being strongly positive in papillary carcinoma (magnification ×100).

and breast [1, 9]. Lung carcinoma was the second common neoplasm to metastasize to the thyroid gland. Among histological types of lung carcinoma, adenocarcinoma was the most commonly reported tumor, followed by squamous cell carcinoma, large cell carcinoma, and small cell carcinoma [10]. In the study of Chung et al., 44.2% metastatic tumors to the thyroid gland occurred in glands with abnormalities, such as neoplasm or benign conditions [1]. The abnormal thyroid gland may have decreased blood supply resulting in decreased oxygen content and iodine content and thus is more vulnerable to metastatic malignancy [1, 3, 11].

Metastasis to a thyroid neoplasm—tumor-to-tumor metastasis—is extremely rare, and only about 31 cases have been reported in the literature [3, 5, 7, 11]. Tumor-to-tumor metastasis is defined as the recipient tumor being a true neoplasm and the donor neoplasm being a true metastasis [3]. Renal cell carcinoma was the most common primary tumor metastasizing to a thyroid neoplasm (10 cases), followed by lung carcinoma (7 cases), breast carcinoma (5 cases), colon carcinoma (3 cases), and others [3, 5, 8, 11]. We presented 2 cases of lung carcinoma metastasizing to thyroid tumors.

In the 9 cases of lung carcinoma metastasizing to thyroid tumor (including our 2 cases, Table 1), the recipient tumor was follicular adenoma in 5 cases, follicular variant of papillary thyroid carcinoma in 3 cases, and papillary carcinoma in 1 case [2–8]. The donor tumor was adenocarcinoma in 4 cases [4–6, 8], poorly differentiated carcinoma in 2 cases [3, 7], small cell carcinoma in 2 cases [2], and adenosquamous carcinoma in 1 case. The mean age of these patients was 63 (46–75) years old, and the male to female ratio was 4 : 5. Diagnosis of primary tumor and its metastasis into a thyroid neoplasm were synchronous in two case, metachronous in four cases (2 months–2 years), and autopsy in three cases. We presented the first case of metastatic lung adenosquamous carcinoma in papillary thyroid carcinoma and another case of metastatic small cell carcinoma in thyroid follicular adenoma.

Tumor-to-tumor metastasis should be considered when a distinct histological pattern is encountered in a tumor or in a patient with previous history of malignancy. Preoperative diagnosis of a primary thyroid tumor versus metastatic disease is difficult because of similar radiological findings and clinical presentations [11]. The history of previous lung carcinoma may be helpful, and fine needle aspiration cytology of tumor is also useful. However, two of our cases were misinterpreted as a primary thyroid tumor in fine needle aspiration cytology due to lack of clinical history and sampling error. Hence, the diagnosis of metastatic lung carcinoma was made with histological examination and immunohistochemical studies after thyroidectomy. To distinguish metastatic malignancy from a primary thyroid neoplasm on histology or cytology, this may require further immunohistochemical or molecular studies [9]. The thyroid tumors are usually reactive for immunohistochemical markers of thyroglobulin

Table 1: Lung carcinoma metastasizing to thyroid tumor: the cases reported in the literature.

Authors	Age	Gender	Receiving thyroid neoplasm	Lung carcinoma	Interval
Akamatsu et al. [4]	46	Female	Follicular adenoma	Well-differentiated adenocarcinoma	4 months
Hashimoto et al. [5]	60	Female	Follicular variant of papillary thyroid carcinoma	Adenocarcinoma	Synchronous
Kameyama et al. [6]	51	Male	Follicular adenoma	Moderately differentiated adenocarcinoma	Autopsy
Mori et al. [8]	54	Male	Follicular variant of papillary thyroid carcinoma	Poorly differentiated adenocarcinoma	Autopsy
Stevens et al. [3]	65	Male	Follicular adenoma	Poorly differentiated carcinoma	2 months
Mizukami et al. [7]	75	Female	Follicular adenoma	Poorly differentiated carcinoma	Autopsy
Baloch and LiVolsi [2]	75	Female	Follicular variant of papillary thyroid carcinoma	Small cell carcinoma	2 years
Wey (present case 1)	66	Male	Follicular adenoma	Small cell carcinoma	Synchronous
Wey (present case 2)	72	Female	Papillary thyroid carcinoma	Adenosquamous carcinoma	3 months

and thyroid transcription factor-1 (TTF-1). However, most of the lung adenocarcinomas and small cell carcinomas are also positive for TTF-1, making the distinction even more challenging. More specific markers are needed for differential diagnosis, such as neuroendocrine markers and mucicarmine stain. Molecular studies and a dual-probe "break-apart" fluorescence *in situ* hybridization (FISH) assay are also helpful in the diagnosis of thyroid papillary carcinoma and lung carcinomas. *RET/PTC* rearrangements, *BRAF* mutations, and *RAS* mutations are frequently identified in thyroid papillary carcinoma, while *EGFR* mutations and *ALK* rearrangements are usually found in lung carcinoma [12].

The treatment of metastatic disease is dependent on the stage and grade of the primary tumor, extension of the thyroid lesion, and the general condition of the patient [13]. Thyroidectomy is generally performed in the patients with minimal disease in the thyroid and no evidence of metastasis in other sites. In these patients, the prognosis is good. Surgery is also palliative for relieving compressive symptoms in patients with disseminated disease [11, 13]. The extent of surgery should depend on the ability to completely remove the metastatic tumor.

In conclusion, tumor-to-tumor metastasis in thyroid gland is exceedingly rare, and it should be considered in patients with a thyroid mass and previous history of malignancy. The abnormal thyroid glands with goiter or tumors might be more susceptible to metastatic malignancies because of a decrease in oxygen and iodine content. Lung carcinoma is the second common primary tumor metastasizing to a thyroid neoplasm, and only about 7 cases have been reported in the literature. We present another two cases of lung carcinoma metastasizing to thyroid tumors. The distinction between primary and metastatic tumors is difficult in some cases. Careful histological examination and molecular and immunohistochemical studies are helpful for differential diagnosis.

Consent

An informed consent was provided by the patients.

Conflict of Interests

The authors declare that there is no conflict of interests regarding the publication of this paper.

References

[1] A. Y. Chung, T. B. Tran, K. T. Brumund, R. A. Weisman, and M. Bouvet, "Metastases to the thyroid: a review of the literature from the last decade," *Thyroid*, vol. 22, no. 3, pp. 258–268, 2012.

[2] Z. W. Baloch and V. A. LiVolsi, "Tumor-to-tumor metastasis to follicular variant of papillary carcinoma of thyroid," *Archives of Pathology & Laboratory Medicine*, vol. 123, no. 8, pp. 703–706, 1999.

[3] T. M. Stevens, A. T. Richards, C. Bewtra, and P. Sharma, "Tumors metastatic to thyroid neoplasms: a case report and review of the literature," *Pathology Research International*, vol. 2011, Article ID 238693, 5 pages, 2011.

[4] H. Akamatsu, J. Amano, A. Suzuki, and Y. Kikushima, "A case of micro-metastatic lung adenocarcinoma into adenoma of the thyroid," *Kyobu Geka*, vol. 47, no. 4, pp. 319–321, 1994.

[5] K. Hashimoto, H. Yamamoto, T. Nakano et al., "Tumor-to-tumor metastasis: lung adenocarcinoma metastasizing to a follicular variant of papillary thyroid carcinoma," *Pathology International*, vol. 61, no. 7, pp. 435–441, 2011.

[6] K. Kameyama, N. Kamio, H. Okita, and J.-I. Hata, "Metastatic carcinoma in follicular adenoma of the thyroid gland," *Pathology—Research and Practice*, vol. 196, no. 5, pp. 333–336, 2000.

[7] Y. Mizukami, K. Saito, A. Nonomura et al., "Lung carcinoma metastatic to microfollicular adenoma of the thyroid. A case report," *Acta Pathologica Japonica*, vol. 40, no. 8, pp. 602–608, 1990.

[8] K. Mori, R. Kitazawa, T. Kondo, and S. Kitazawa, "Lung adenocarcinoma with micropapillary component presenting with metastatic scrotum tumor and cancer-to-cancer metastasis: a case report," *Cases Journal*, vol. 1, no. 1, p. 162, 2008.

[9] P. A. Moghaddam, K. M. Cornejo, and A. Khan, "Metastatic carcinoma to the thyroid gland: a single institution 20-year experience and review of the literature," *Endocrine Pathology*, vol. 24, no. 3, pp. 116–124, 2013.

[10] G. Papi, G. Fadda, S. M. Corsello et al., "Metastases to the thyroid gland: prevalence, clinicopathological aspects and prognosis: a 10-year experience," *Clinical Endocrinology*, vol. 66, no. 4, pp. 565–571, 2007.

[11] F. Medas, P. G. Calò, M. L. Lai, M. Tuveri, G. Pisano, and A. Nicolosi, "Renal cell carcinoma metastasis to thyroid tumor: a case report and review of the literature," *Journal of Medical Case Reports*, vol. 7, article 265, 2013.

[12] E. T. Kimura, M. N. Nikiforova, Z. Zhu, J. A. Knauf, Y. E. Nikiforov, and J. A. Fagin, "High prevalence of BRAF mutations in thyroid cancer: genetic evidence for constitutive activation of the RET/PTC-RAS-BRAF signaling pathway in papillary thyroid carcinoma," *Cancer Research*, vol. 63, no. 7, pp. 1454–1457, 2003.

[13] P. H. Montero, T. Ibrahimpasic, I. J. Nixon, and A. R. Shaha, "Thyroid metastasectomy," *Journal of Surgical Oncology*, vol. 109, no. 1, pp. 36–41, 2014.

3

Primary Invasive Squamous Cell Carcinoma of the Nipple

Avani A. Pendse and Siobhan M. O'Connor

Department of Pathology, University of North Carolina, Chapel Hill, NC 27599-7525, USA

Correspondence should be addressed to Siobhan M. O'Connor; siobhan_oconnor@med.unc.edu

Academic Editor: Yoji Nagashima

Squamous cell carcinoma is one of the most common cutaneous cancers; however, primary squamous cell carcinoma of the nipple is extremely rare. Among the few reported cases, the majority have occurred in older women with rare cases seen in younger women and male patients. Our patient presented with an exophytic mass of the right nipple while pregnant. A superficial biopsy was reviewed at an outside institution and then at our institution and diagnosed as squamous papilloma and then as hyperkeratosis of the nipple, respectively. The subsequent excisional biopsy revealed multiple nests of tumor cells extending into the dermis with associated chronic inflammatory infiltrate, and the lesion was diagnosed as a primary invasive squamous cell carcinoma of the nipple. Following that, a wide local excision of the excision site and sampling of the regional lymph nodes were negative for carcinoma. Due to the rarity of this diagnosis, it is not known whether prognosis and response to therapy differ from cutaneous squamous cell carcinoma at other sites. Therefore, risk stratification and therapy have been based on those for cutaneous squamous cell carcinoma.

1. Introduction

Primary squamous cell carcinoma of the nipple is an extremely rare condition, with only nine cases reported in the English literature [1–8]. The majority of the previously reported cases have been in older women with an age range of 62 to 87 years with rare occurrences in younger individuals. Of the younger patients, one was male and positive for human immunodeficiency virus (HIV) [7] and the other was female with no known risk factors [1]. Here, we report a well-differentiated primary invasive squamous cell carcinoma of the nipple occurring in a young pregnant woman.

2. Case Presentation

The patient is a 29-year-old pregnant female, who originally presented with a small nodule on the tip of her right nipple, at approximately 28 weeks of gestation. The lesion increased in size over the next few weeks and showed no improvement with a 2-week course of antibiotic treatment (Keflex). Due to the progressive increase in the size of the lesion, the patient was referred to a general surgeon and underwent an incisional biopsy. As seen in Figures 1 and 2, the biopsy showed fragments of squamous epithelium with hyperkeratosis, keratotic plugging, and filiform acanthosis. These features were interpreted as consistent with a squamous papilloma. On review at our institution, we agreed with the originating pathologist's description of the lesion. However, due to the patient's clinical history and the degree of hyperkeratosis and keratotic plugging, in our opinion, findings were more consistent with hyperkeratosis of the nipple.

The patient delivered a healthy infant but was unable to nurse on the right side due to sloughing of the nipple skin and pain. In addition, the lesion continued to increase in size. On physical examination at our institution, a soft, exophytic mass of the right nipple was noted. The areola was uninvolved. No other abnormalities in either breast and no axillary lymphadenopathy were detected. A mammogram was performed and revealed no masses, calcifications, or sites of architectural distortion within the breast parenchyma. The radiologist noted that, due to the heterogeneously dense breast composition, small masses could be obscured and a targeted ultrasound was performed. The ultrasound revealed an enlarged right nipple, approximately 1.7 cm in diameter with a hypervascular nipple mass. The subareolar ducts were normal in size, without evidence of an intraductal

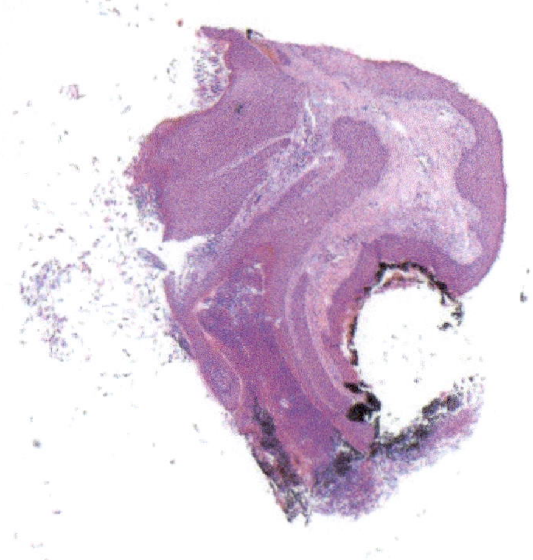

FIGURE 1: Low power view of the initial biopsy (HE, 4x).

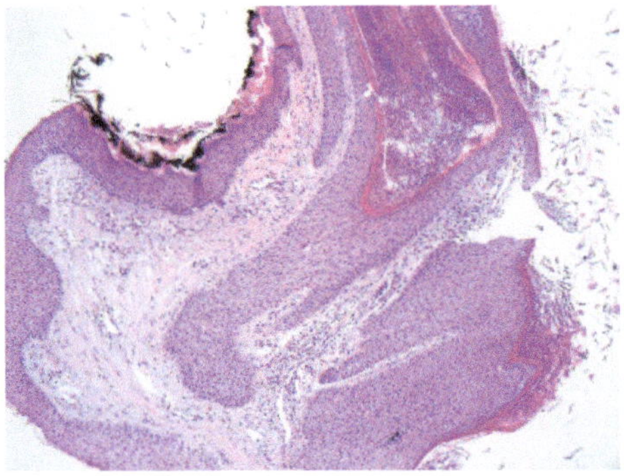

FIGURE 2: Initial biopsy showing acanthosis, hyperkeratosis, and keratotic plugging (HE, 10x).

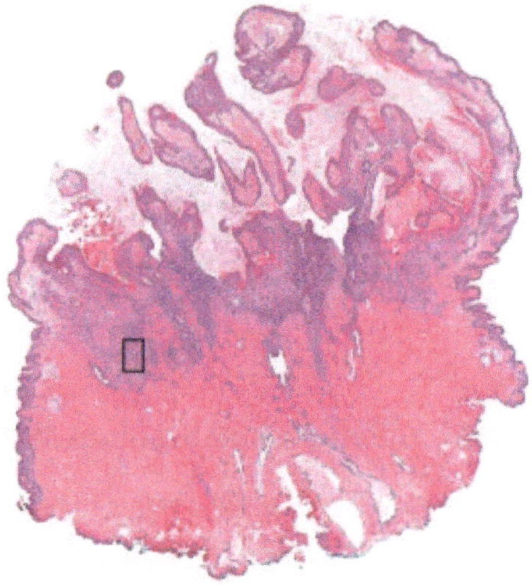

FIGURE 3: Whole slide image of the squamous cell carcinoma showing the keratoacanthoma-like features (HE). The box indicates the area shown in Figure 4.

mass. Although the previous sample had been interpreted as benign, the biopsy was superficial, and, given the progressive increase in size, excision of the lesion was recommended. The patient underwent excisional biopsy of the right nipple lesion and, on gross examination, the nipple showed an ill-defined soft yellow/white friable verrucous mass measuring 2.4 × 1.6 × 1.1 cm. Histology revealed an exuberant squamous proliferation with exophytic growth pattern, marked hyperkeratosis, acanthosis, and collarettes at the periphery, all features suggestive of a keratoacanthoma (Figure 3). Multiple irregular nests of tumor extended into the dermis along with rare infiltrating single cells (Figure 4). Maximum tumor thickness was 1.4 cm with depth of invasion 4 mm.

The distinction between keratoacanthoma and squamous cell carcinoma remains difficult and controversial. Features of our lesion that favor invasive squamous cell carcinoma include prominent nuclear atypia, mitotic figures (Figure 5), and desmoplastic stromal response [9] (Figure 6). In addition, keratoacanthoma does not typically extend beyond the level of the sweat glands [9]. There are no sweat glands present in our specimen, but Figure 7 shows extension of the tumor deep to the sebaceous glands and a lactiferous duct. The infiltrating nests were positive for p16 immunohistochemical stain, but in situ hybridization for high risk HPV was negative. Immunostain for p53 was diffusely positive in the infiltrating nests (Figure 8). One study showed a significant trend in the proportion of p53 reactivity from keratoacanthomas to poorly differentiated squamous cell carcinomas, although p53 reactivity could not reliably distinguish between keratoacanthoma and well-differentiated squamous cell carcinoma [10]. Another series showed more frequent p53 expression in squamous cell carcinomas with keratoacanthoma like features versus well-differentiated squamous cell carcinomas and keratoacanthomas, but the differences did not reach statistical significance [11]. Taken all together, features supported the diagnosis of squamous cell carcinoma with a keratoacanthoma-like growth pattern rather than a keratoacanthoma.

Subsequently, the patient underwent a wide local excision with regional lymph node dissection. The entire excision specimen was submitted for histopathologic evaluation and was negative for carcinoma. Regional lymph nodes were also negative for metastatic disease. The patient has no evidence of recurrence after 15 months.

3. Discussion

Squamous cell carcinoma is one of the most common cutaneous cancers and causes significant morbidity, particularly in elderly patients [12]. Exposure to ultraviolet radiation and lighter skin color are well-established risk factors for cutaneous squamous cell carcinoma, along with an emerging role for human papillomavirus infection [13]. Primary squamous cell carcinoma of the nipple is rare, possibly due to less exposure of this area to sunlight.

The previous case reports are summarized in Table 1. Of the nine reported cases, three were in situ [4, 7, 8] and one showed <1 mm of invasion [5]. Six carcinomas (in situ or

TABLE 1: Case reports, squamous cell carcinoma of the nipple and areola.

	Patient	Risk factors	Carcinoma	Therapy	Outcome
Venkataseshan et al. [4]	84 y.o. F	Not known	In situ	WLE	DF × 30 months
Sharma and Iyer [7]	41 y.o. M	HIV disease	In situ Negative LNs	Mastectomy, SLN	DF × 3 years
Brookes et al. [8]	71 y.o. F	XRT	In situ	Photodynamic	Residual × 2, cryotherapy DF × 9 months
	69 y.o. F	Not known	Invasive	WLE	Recurrence at 3 months, repeat excision DF × 6 months
Loveland-Jones et al. [3]	66 y.o. F	XRT	Invasive	WLE	Not reported
Hosaka et al. [5]	73 y.o. F	Not known	Superficially invasive (<1 mm) Negative LNs	Mastectomy, ALND	DF × 5 years
Upasham et al. [6]	87 y.o. F	Not known	Invasive Positive LN 1/11	Mod. rad. mastectomy	Not reported
Sofos et al. [1]	34 y.o. F	Not known	Invasive	WLE	DF × 12 months
King and Kremer [2]	62 y.o. M	Sun exposure × 10 years	Invasive with NE differentiation	WLE	Not reported

XRT = radiation therapy; LN = lymph node; SLN = sentinel lymph node; ALND = axillary lymph node dissection; WLE = wide local excision; DF = disease-free.

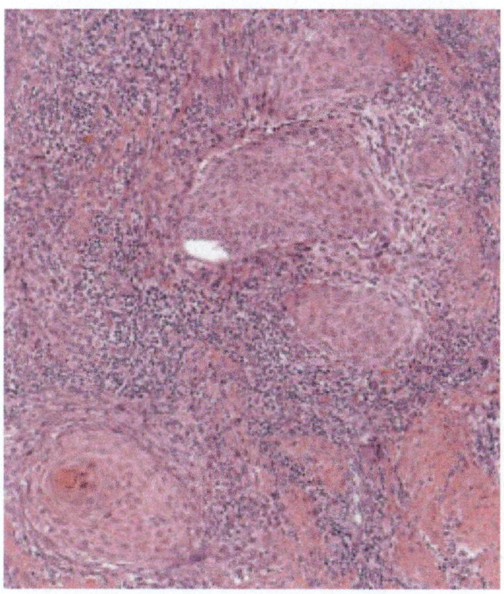

FIGURE 4: Area extracted from the whole slide image showing nests of invasion and surrounding inflammation (HE).

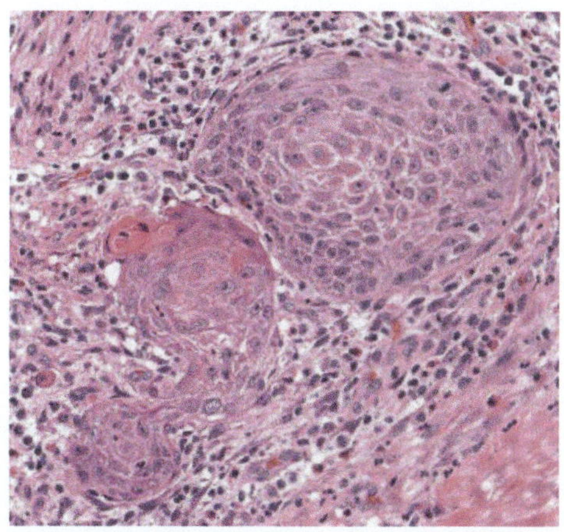

FIGURE 5: Area extracted from the whole slide image showing cytologic detail and mitotic figure (HE).

invasive) occurred in postmenopausal women ranging in age from 62 to 87 years [3–6, 8] and one invasive carcinoma was found in a 62-year-old male [2]. Of the two cases reported in younger patients, one was in a 41-year-old male who was HIV positive (in situ) [7] and one was in a 34-year-old female (invasive) [1]. Given the rarity of primary squamous cell carcinoma of the nipple and areola, firm causative or correlative relationships with genetic and environmental risk factors have not been established. Similarly, the natural history of this disease is largely unknown. Our patient has a history of hormonal contraceptive use, although no exposure to other hormones was reported. Family history was also negative for skin and breast malignancy. Known risk factors were identified in four of the nine previous patients, a male with HIV [7], a male with work associated sun exposure over a 10-year period [2], and two women who had previously undergone radiation therapy for breast carcinoma [3, 8].

In the previously reported cases of squamous cell carcinoma of the nipple, two patients presented with an exophytic mass [5, 6]. In the remaining patients, physical examination revealed scaling, erythema, and/or ulceration, which raised the possibility of Paget disease of the nipple, a much more common entity [1–4, 7, 8]. The exophytic nature of the lesion in our patient made Paget disease less likely but instead was suggestive of hyperkeratotic processes such as nevoid hyperkeratosis and, particularly in our patient, pregnancy

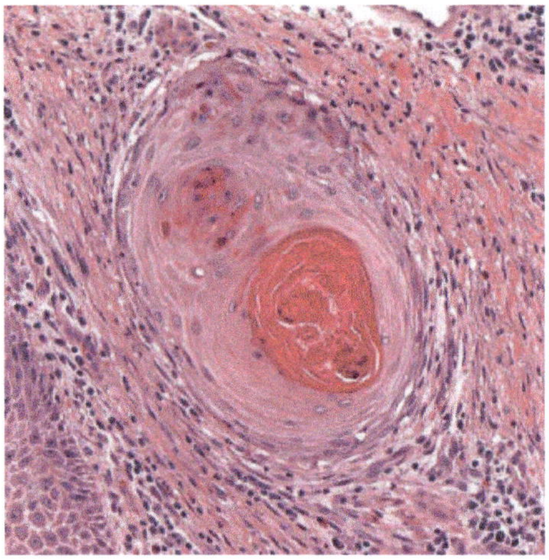

Figure 6: Area extracted from the whole slide image showing desmoplastic response (HE).

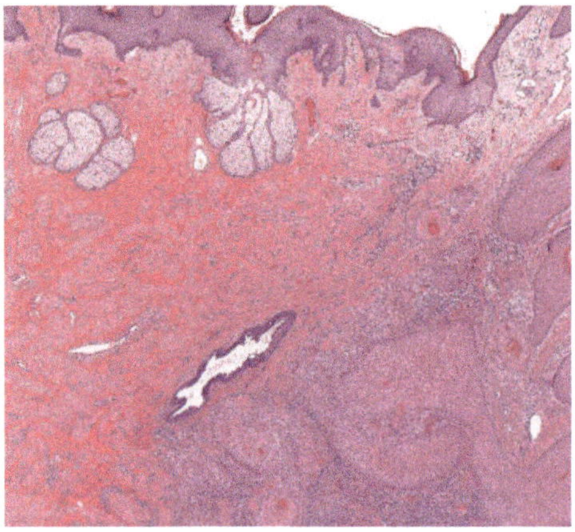

Figure 7: Area extracted from the whole slide image showing extension of tumor deep to the sebaceous glands and a lactiferous duct (HE).

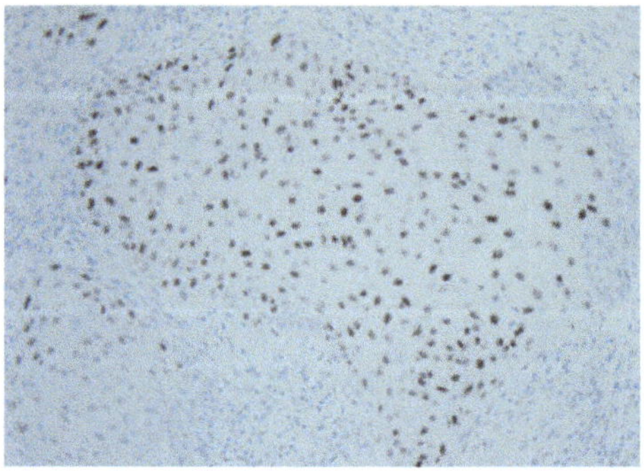

Figure 8: Positive nuclear immunostaining for p53 in invasive nests (p53, 20x).

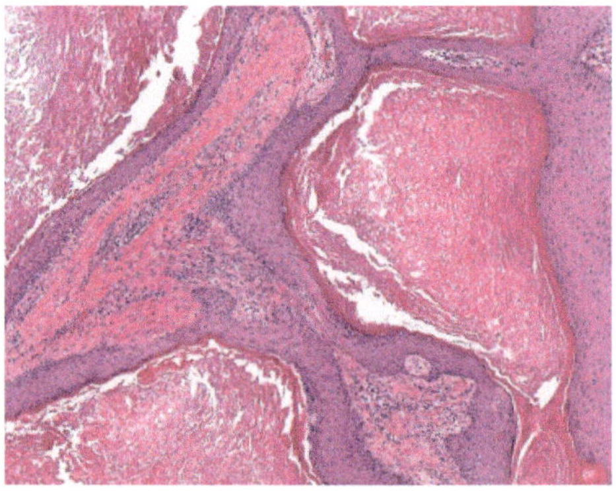

Figure 9: Superficial aspect of resected specimen (HE, 20x).

associated hyperkeratosis. In fact, our patient's initial biopsy was interpreted as changes consistent with hyperkeratosis but was not subcategorized since clinical presentation and histology did not fit neatly into a specific subtype.

Nevoid hyperkeratosis is a rare lesion and, in one small series [14], presented as a pigmented hyperkeratotic plaque diffusely involving the nipple and/or areola. Typical findings on histologic examination include orthokeratotic hyperkeratosis, filiform acanthosis, papillomatosis, and occasional keratotic plugging. It is a benign lesion most commonly occurring in women in the second or third decade, essentially asymptomatic, and tends to persist if not treated. Two patients in this series showed improvement with topical retinoic acid but recurred when the treatment was discontinued [14].

In the context of our case, pregnancy associated hyperkeratosis was a consideration based on the initial biopsy. In one case series of pregnancy associated hyperkeratosis, most of the lesions were yellow to tan or mildly pigmented, hyperkeratotic, and/or warty papules on clinical examination [15]. All patients had bilateral involvement, and most lesions were located at the top of the nipple. In contrast to nevoid hyperkeratosis, the majority of patients were symptomatic with complaints including mild tenderness, sensitivity to touch, or mild pruritus. Lesions persisted in the postpartum period in the majority of patients. Histologically, orthokeratotic hyperkeratosis was the most typical feature of pregnancy associated hyperkeratosis with papillomatosis and acanthosis being mild to absent [15].

In general, invasive squamous cell carcinoma of the nipple is easily distinguishable from hyperkeratosis of the nipple. In this case, the initial diagnosis of a hyperkeratotic rather than invasive entity was due to the superficial nature of the biopsy. As is evident in comparing Figures 2 and 9, the features seen in the initial biopsy (Figure 2) are identical to those seen in the superficial aspect of the resected lesion (Figure 9). Once the entire lesion was available for review, it became clear that it was invasive, and benign hyperkeratotic lesions were no longer included in the differential diagnosis. The contrast between the initial biopsy and the subsequent resection specimen dramatically emphasizes the impact that sampling may have on diagnostic accuracy.

In our patient, histologic examination failed to reveal lymphovascular or perineural invasion and the carcinoma was staged based on the American Joint Committee on Cancer (AJCC) staging for cutaneous squamous cell carcinoma [16]. However, it is unknown whether these staging criteria have the same prognostic value in this unique location. Likewise, it is unclear whether standard treatment recommendations are applicable to squamous cell carcinoma of the nipple. Depending on the risk category, the primary treatment options included in the National Comprehensive Cancer Network (NCCN) Guidelines include curettage and electrodissection, surgical excision with 4 to 6 mm margins, or excision with wider surgical margins [17].

Eight of the previously reported patients with squamous cell carcinoma were treated with surgery [1–8], either wide local excision or mastectomy and one patient with in situ disease underwent photodynamic therapy with 5-aminolevulinic acid as a photosensitizer [8]. The latter patient had small areas of residual carcinoma, which were treated with cryotherapy, and she was recurrence-free at 9 months. Of the five patients who underwent wide local excision, one recurred three months postoperatively. The patient underwent repeat wide excision and was free of recurrence at 6 months [8]. Two patients who were treated with mastectomy were free of tumor at 3 and 5 years, respectively [5, 7].

4. Conclusion

Primary squamous cell carcinoma of the nipple is a very rare diagnosis. Occurrence of this lesion in a young pregnant woman with no known risk factors for cutaneous cancer made this case all the more challenging. This example highlights the importance of considering rare entities in the differential diagnosis of a hyperkeratotic lesion of the nipple. We hope that our report of a primary squamous cell carcinoma of the nipple in a young pregnant woman will help further understanding of this rare entity.

Conflict of Interests

The authors declare that there is no conflict of interests regarding the publication of this paper.

References

[1] S. S. Sofos, H. Tehrani, N. Lymperopoulos, J. Constantinides, and M. I. James, "Primary squamous cell carcinoma of the nipple: a diagnosis of suspicion," *Journal of Plastic, Reconstructive and Aesthetic Surgery*, vol. 66, no. 11, pp. e315–e317, 2013.

[2] J. King and H. Kremer, "Squamous cell carcinoma of the nipple: an unusual location in a male patient," *American Surgeon*, vol. 78, no. 2, pp. E101–E102, 2012.

[3] C. E. Loveland-Jones, F. Wang, R. R. Bankhead, Y. Huang, and K. J. Reilly, "Squamous cell carcinoma of the nipple following radiation therapy for ductal carcinoma in situ: a case report," *Journal of Medical Case Reports*, vol. 4, article 186, 2010.

[4] V. S. Venkataseshan, D. C. Budd, D. U. Kim, and R. V. P. Hutter, "Intraepidermal squamous carcinoma (Bowen's disease) of the nipple," *Human Pathology*, vol. 25, no. 12, pp. 1371–1374, 1994.

[5] N. Hosaka, K. Uesaka, T. Takaki, Y. Zhang, K. Takasu, and S. Ikehara, "Poorly differentiated squamous cell carcinoma of the nipple: a unique case for marked exophytic growth, but little invasion with neuroendocrine differentiation," *Medical Molecular Morphology*, vol. 44, no. 3, pp. 174–178, 2011.

[6] S. P. Upasham, M. Vinodkiri, and S. Sudhamani, "One more common tumor in an uncommon location: squamous cell carcinoma on nipple areola complex," *Indian Journal of Cancer*, vol. 51, no. 3, pp. 376–377, 2014.

[7] R. Sharma and M. Iyer, "Bowen's disease of the nipple in a young man with AIDS: a case report," *Clinical Breast Cancer*, vol. 9, no. 1, pp. 53–55, 2009.

[8] P. T. Brookes, S. Jhawar, C. P. Hinton, S. Murdoch, and T. Usman, "Bowen's disease of the nipple—a new method of treatment," *Breast*, vol. 14, no. 1, pp. 65–67, 2005.

[9] D. Weedon, *Weedon's Skin Pathology*, vol. 1, Churchill Livingstone, Elsevier, Edinburgh, UK, 3rd edition, 2010.

[10] T. J. Stephenson, J. Royds, P. B. Silcocks, and S. S. Bleehen, "Mutant p53 oncogene expression in keratoacanthoma and squamous cell carcinoma," *British Journal of Dermatology*, vol. 127, no. 6, pp. 566–570, 1992.

[11] C. T. Cain, T. H. Niemann, and Z. B. Argenyi, "Keratoacanthoma versus squamous cell carcinoma. An immunohistochemical reappraisal of p53 protein and proliferating cell nuclear antigen expression in keratoacanthoma-like tumors," *The American Journal of Dermatopathology*, vol. 17, no. 4, pp. 324–331, 1995.

[12] M. Alam and D. Ratner, "Cutaneous squamous-cell carcinoma," *The New England Journal of Medicine*, vol. 344, no. 13, pp. 975–983, 2001.

[13] J. M. McGregor and C. M. Proby, "The role of papillomaviruses in human non-melanoma skin cancer," *Cancer Surveys*, vol. 26, pp. 219–236, 1996.

[14] C. Baykal, N. Büyükbabani, A. Kavak, and M. Alper, "Nevoid hyperkeratosis of the nipple and areola: a distinct entity," *Journal of the American Academy of Dermatology*, vol. 46, no. 3, pp. 414–418, 2002.

[15] H. W. Higgins, J. Jenkins, T. D. Horn, and G. Kroumpouzos, "Pregnancy-associated hyperkeratosis of the nipple: a report of 25 cases," *JAMA Dermatology*, vol. 149, no. 6, pp. 722–726, 2013.

[16] "Cutaneous squamous cell carcinoma and other cutaneous carcinomas," in *AJCC Cancer Staging Manual*, S. B. Edge, D. R. Byrd, C. C. Compton, A. G. Fritz, F. L. Greene, and A. Trotti, Eds., pp. 301–314, Springer Science+Business Media, New York, NY, USA, 2010.

[17] NCCN Guidelines for Squamous Cell Carcinoma Version 1.2015 Squamous Cell Skin Cancer, 2015.

4

Importance of *NAB2-STAT6* Fusion in the Diagnosis of Pancreatic Solitary Fibrous Tumor with Hamartoma-Like Features: A Case Report and Review of the Literature

Kei Tanaka,[1,2] Takashi Kishimoto,[3] Masayuki Ohtsuka,[2] Yukio Nakatani,[4] and Masaru Miyazaki[2]

[1]*Department of Surgery, Kensei General Hospital, 604 Kuwata, Sakuragawa, Ibaraki 309-1223, Japan*
[2]*General Surgery, Chiba University Graduate School of Medicine, 1-8-1 Inohana, Chuo-ku, Chiba 260-8670, Japan*
[3]*Department of Molecular Pathology, Chiba University Graduate School of Medicine, 1-8-1 Inohana, Chuo-ku, Chiba 260-8670, Japan*
[4]*Diagnostic Pathology, Chiba University Graduate School of Medicine, 1-8-1 Inohana, Chuo-ku, Chiba 260-8670, Japan*

Correspondence should be addressed to Takashi Kishimoto; tkishi@faculty.chiba-u.jp

Academic Editor: Zsuzsa Schaff

We report a case of pancreatic hamartoma-like solitary fibrous tumor which was differentiated from pancreatic hamartoma with the detection of *NAB2-STAT6* fusion, a specific mutation for solitary fibrous tumors. A pancreatic well-demarcated solid nodule, 21×17 mm, of 82-year-old man was surgically enucleated. Microscopic findings were close to a pancreatic hamartoma that consisted of sparsely distributed pancreatic ducts and acini in heavily collagenized fibrous stroma. Neither islet nor peripheral nerve existed in the tumor. The fibroblastic cells in the stroma were immune-positive for CD34, CD99, and bcl-2. But these expressions were not decisive in the differentiation between solitary fibrous tumor and pancreatic hamartoma, because CD34 was positive for both tumors, and CD99 and bcl-2 expressions were not elucidated in the previous cases of pancreatic hamartomas. Thus, we evaluated *NAB2-STAT6* fusion. The fibroblastic cells were positive for STAT6 and sequencing analysis revealed the gene fusion between *NAB2* exon 4 and *STAT6* exon 2, with which the final diagnos is of solitary fibrous tumor was achieved. In conclusion, detection of *NAB2-STAT6* fusion has a great diagnostic value for pancreatic solitary fibrous tumors with hamartoma-like features.

1. Introduction

Solitary fibrous tumors (SFTs) are mesenchymal neoplasms, most of which are benign although a part of cases are aggressive with local or distant recurrence. Tumor cells were initially thought to be of mesothelial-cell origin since first report of pleural SFTs was described as localized fibrous mesotheliomas in 1931 [1]. But a series of studies has indicated the fibroblastic or myofibroblastic phenotype of the tumor cells [2–4]. It is now known that SFT can develop in a variety of extrapleural tissues. Among the cases of extrapleural SFT, pancreatic SFT is exceedingly rare; review of the literature yielded 11 prior cases [5–15].

The neoplastic cells in SFTs are spindle or ovoid, and they proliferate in a patternless arrangement characterized by a combination of hyper- and hypocellular areas with varying amounts of collagenized stroma. Hemangiopericytomatous pattern with stag-horn shaped vessels is often observed. Immunohistochemical detection of CD34, CD99, and bcl-2 expressions is commonly employed for the accurate diagnosis of SFT [5]. However, diagnosis is actually challenging in some cases for a wide histological spectrum of this tumor and exceptional immune-phenotype. Recently, *NAB2-STAT6* fusion was discovered in SFTs by means of whole-genome and transcriptome sequencing analysis, and following studies have confirmed that *NAB2-STAT6* fusion is highly sensitive and specific for SFTs [16, 17]. The *NAB2-STAT6* fusion is associated with high nuclear expression of STAT6, so that the STAT6 immunohistochemistry has become a powerful tool in the diagnosis of SFTs [18–20]. *NAB2* codes a transcriptional repressor of the early growth response (EGR) zinc-finger transcription factor, which regulates cell differentiation and

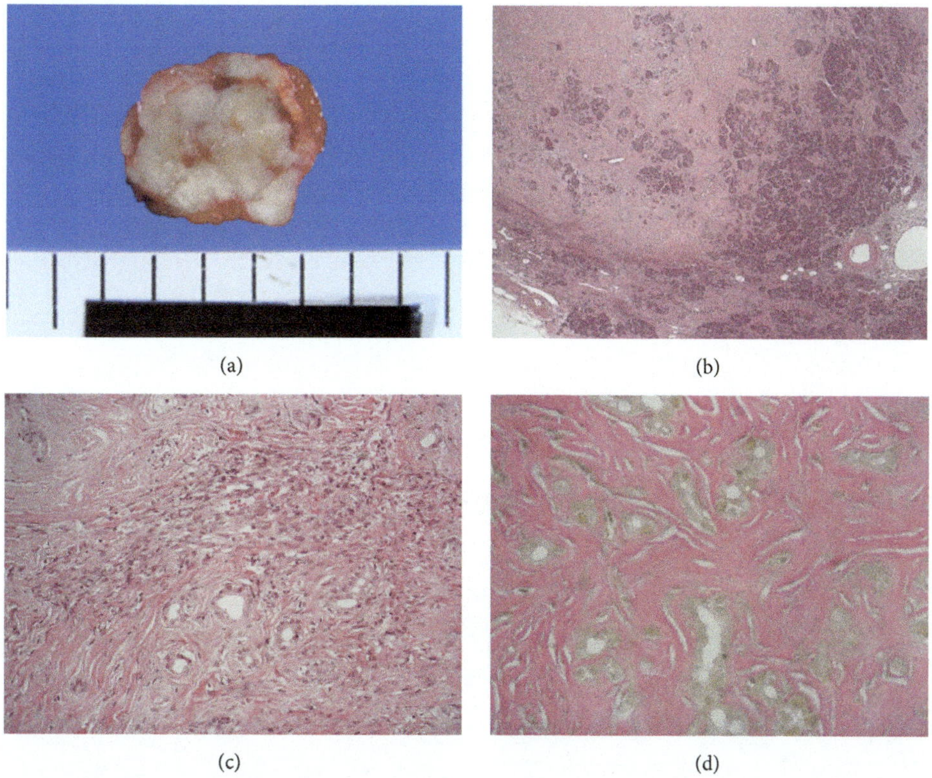

FIGURE 1: (a) Gross appearance of the surgical specimen showing a well-demarcated and vaguely lobulated ivory-white tumor. (b) Pancreatic parenchyma was haphazardly distributed in the tumor. (c) Spindle cells proliferated in heavily collagenized fibrous stroma. (d) Concentric elastic fibers in the duct walls were not evident with Elastica van Gieson staining.

proliferation. Fusion of activation domain of *STAT6* converts *NAB2* into a transcriptional activator for EGR families and drives tumorigenic effect [16, 21, 22].

Pancreatic hamartoma is a rare benign tumor-like nodule. Microscopically, the distorted epithelial components are distributed in fibrous stroma. Hamartomatous properties are supported by those features of cystic dilation of the ducts, lack of both peripheral nerves and well-formed islets of Langerhans, and lack of concentric elastic fibers in the duct wall. Stromal spindle cells are immune-positive for CD34 as well as those in SFTs [23]. The expressions of CD99 and bcl-2 are unknown, because these expressions were not elucidated in the previously reported pancreatic hamartomas [23–39].

We report a case of pancreatic hamartoma-like SFT. The final diagnosis of SFT was dependent on a validation of *NAB2-STAT6* fusion, because the features were indistinguishable from the pancreatic hamartoma by microscopic examination with conventional immunohistochemical study.

2. Case Presentation

An 82-year-old man was referred to our hospital for further evaluation of a pancreatic and a liver nodule that had been found on abdominal CT in the previous hospital. On admission, the patient had no symptoms. PIVKA-2 was elevated (84 mAU/mL), but other tumor markers, that is, CEA, CA19-9, and alpha-fetoprotein, were within normal limits. Abdominal CT revealed a mass, 18 mm in diameter, protruding from the pancreatic tail. The pancreatic mass showed progressive enhancement from the arterial phase to the venous phase on dynamic CT and was hypointense on T2-weighted and diffusion-weighted MR images, which suggested a fibrous tumor. An endoscopic ultrasound with fine-needle aspiration from the pancreatic mass was performed, but paucity of the specimen precluded a diagnosis. At a distance from this nodule, the branch-duct type intraductal papillary-mucinous neoplasm (IPMN) was detected in the preoperative workup. The patient underwent extraction of the pancreatic mass and subsegmentectomy of S8 of the liver. IPMN got a follow-up examination, because it was assessed to be benign on the imaging study. Pathological examination of the surgical specimen of the liver revealed that the liver mass was hepatocellular carcinoma. Eleven months postoperatively, the patient is disease-free and well.

The specimen resected from the pancreas contained a white, well-demarcated solid nodule, measuring 21 × 17 mm, with a homogeneous appearance on its cut surface (Figure 1(a)). Microscopically, pancreatic acini and ductal tissues were sparsely distributed in the heavily collagenized fibrous stroma with fibroblast-like spindle cells. The cellularity of the spindle cells was low in most areas, but there were a few hypercellular areas where the spindle cells haphazardly proliferated (Figures 1(b) and 1(c)). Mitotic figures, necrosis, and vascular invasion were not identified. Neither islet of

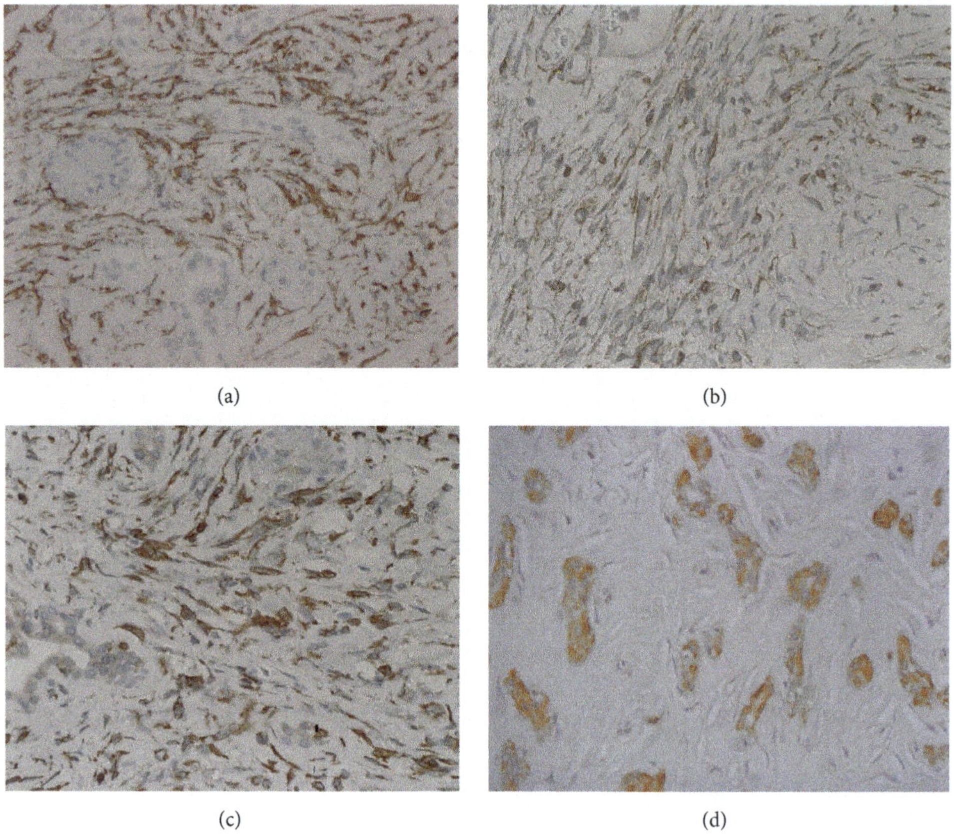

FIGURE 2: Spindle cells were immune-positive for (a) CD34, (b) CD99, and (c) bcl-2. (d) Ductal epithelia were immune-positive for S-100.

Langerhans nor peripheral nerves existed in the whole area. The stroma was hypovascular and the stag-horn-like vessel was not found. Concentric elastic fibers in the duct walls were not evident with Elastica van Gieson staining (Figure 1(d)). Immunohistochemically, the spindle cells were positive for CD34, CD99, and bcl-2 (Figures 2(a)–2(c)) but negative for α-SMA, c-kit, DOG1, desmin, S-100, and calretinin. The ductal epithelia were positive for cytokeratin 7 and S-100 protein (Figure 2(d)). These histological and immunohistochemical findings closely resembled pancreatic hamartomas. For the precise diagnosis, we examined the existence of *NAB2-STAT6* fusion in the spindle cells. Immunohistochemical study revealed that STAT6 was highly expressed in the nuclei of the spindle cells (Figure 3(a)). Next, total RNA was extracted from formalin-fixed paraffin embedded tissues with RNeasy FFPE kit (Qiagen, Tokyo, Japan), and RT-PCR was performed to detect *NAB2-STAT6* using two forward primers in *NAB2*, 5′-CAAGTAGCCCGAGAGAGCAC-3′ (exon 3) and 5′-CTGTGTGCCTGCGAAGCC-3′ (exon 6), and two reverse primers in *STAT6*, 5′-GGGAAAGTCGACATAGAGCC-3′ (exon 3) and 5′-TTCCACGGTCATCTTGATGG-3′ (exon 18) [40]. The condition of PCR was initial denaturing at 95°C for 10 min, followed by 40 cycles of denaturing at 95°C for 30 s, annealing at 55°C for 30 s, and extension at 72°C for 60 s. The primer set of *NAB2* exon 3 and *STAT6* exon 3 was only able to amplify the product (Figure 3(b)). The direct sequence of the product (PRISM 3730 DNA Analyzer, Hokkaido System Science Co., Ltd., Sapporo, Japan) revealed the gene fusion between *NAB2* exon 4 and *STAT6* exon 2 (Figure 3(c)). Based on these results, SFT was finally diagnosed for the pancreatic nodule.

3. Discussion

We presented a case of hamartoma-like SFT of the pancreas where the final diagnosis was achieved with *NAB2-STAT6* fusion. Solitary fibrous tumor is one of the mesenchymal neoplasms where pathological diagnosis is difficult because of broad spectrum of histological appearance. For example, cellular variants of SFTs were previously termed hemangiopericytoma as a different histological entity but hemangiopericytoma is now defined as an obsolete synonym in the latest edition of WHO classification [41]. In the SFT in our patient, components of pancreatic parenchyma were haphazardly entrapped in the tumor, which gave rise to a different diagnosis of pancreatic hamartoma. Yamaguchi and colleagues have studied 9 cases of pancreatic hamartomas and noted that distinct characteristic of pancreatic hamartoma is lack of three components: concentric elastic fibers in duct walls, peripheral nerves, and well-formed islets of Langerhans [23]. They also demonstrated the expression of S-100 protein in ductal epithelia in their cases of pancreatic hamartomas [23]. Our presented pancreatic nodule had these characteristics, although the cystic dilated duct that was observed

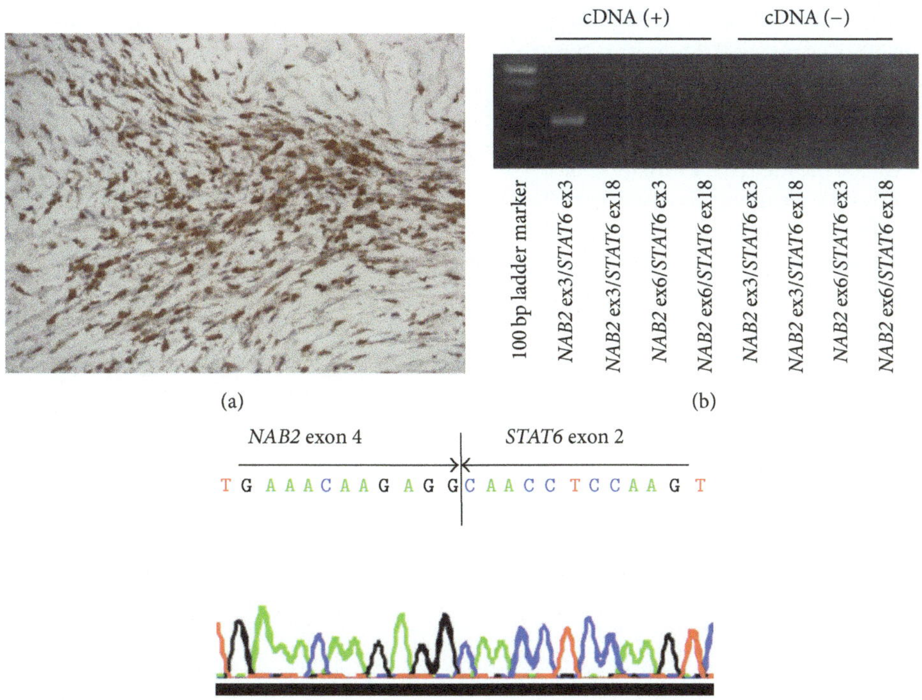

(a) (b) (c)

Figure 3: (a) Immunohistochemically, STAT6 was highly expressed in the nuclei of the spindle cells. The results of (b) RT-PCR and (c) sequencing analysis indicated that *NAB2* exon 4 fused to *STAT6* exon 2.

in some previous cases of pancreatic hamartomas was not evident.

We reviewed the previous cases of pancreatic SFTs (11 cases) and pancreatic hamartomas (29 cases) [23–39] and compared histological features of each disease to get knowledge for the differentiation. As per the result summarized in Table 1, some SFTs had hamartoma-like characters resembling our case, such as entrapped acini (6/7, no description in 4 cases) and lack of islet (2/4, no description in 7 cases). On the other hand, several cases of pancreatic hamartomas lack the characteristics of pancreatic hamartomas, although entrapped acini were observed in all cases; cystic dilation of duct was not observed in 5/26 cases (no description in 3 cases), and islets existed in 6/21 cases (no description in 8 cases).

Most of pancreatic SFTs were diagnosed with the immunohistochemical detection of CD34, CD99, and bcl-2 expressions that have been considered valuable for the pathological diagnosis of SFTs. On the other hand, the diagnosis of the pancreatic hamartoma has been mainly achieved by the microscopic appearance. The most examined molecule was CD34, which was examined in 16/29 cases and was positive in 15/16 cases. The expression of bcl-2 was examined only in 5/29 cases and was positive in 2/5 cases. There was no previous case of pancreatic hamartomas in which CD99 expression was examined. Thus, immunohistochemical detection of CD34, CD99, and bcl-2 is inefficient in differentiation of hamartoma-like SFTs from pancreatic hamartomas.

Since Robinson and colleagues discovered that *NAB2-STAT6* gene fusion is the driver mutation of SFTs in 2013, the existence of *NAB2-STAT6* fusion became a diagnostic hallmark of SFTs [16]. The following studies based on this discovery have elucidated the usefulness of immunohistochemical detection of nuclear localization of STAT6 as reliable marker for the diagnosis of SFTs [18–20]. Several variants of *NAB2-STAT6* have been detected; exon 2, 4, 6, or 7 of *NAB2* is fused to exon 2, 3, 5, 6, 17, or 18 of *STAT6* [16, 42]. The presented case had the *NAB2* exon 4-*STAT6* exon 2 fusion. Akaike and colleagues have studied the variation of *NAB2-STAT6* fusion compared with clinicopathologic

Table 1: Clinicopathological comparison between solitary fibrous tumors and pancreatic hamartomas.

	SFT (n = 11)	Hamartoma (N = 29)	Present case
Age (mean)	41–78 (51.8)	0–78 (45.8)	82
Male/female	2/9	15/14	M
Size (cm) (mean)	2.0–18.5 (8.0)	1.0–14 (4.5)	2.1
Cystic change	0/4 (NE 7)	21/26 (NE 3)	(−)
Entrapped acini	6/7 (NE 4)	26/26 (NE 3)	(+)
Lack of islet	2/4 (NE 7)	15/21 (NE 8)	(+)
CD34	11/11	15/16 (NE 13)	(+)
CD99	6/7 (NE 4)	NE 29	(+)
bcl-2	8/8 (NE 3)	2/5 (NE 24)	(+)

SFT: pancreatic solitary fibrous tumor; NE: not examined.

features and showed that the *NAB2* exon 4-*STAT6* exon 2 genotype is significantly associated with less aggressive phenotype [42]. Although the existence of *NAB2-STAT6* fusion in pancreatic hamartomas is unknown, proliferation of cells with driver gene mutation highly indicates the neoplastic property. Thus, we advocate the idea that evaluation of *NAB2-STAT6* fusion is most informative in the diagnosis of SFTs and is indispensable for differentiation of hamartoma-like SFTs from true pancreatic hamartomas.

In summary, we described a case of pancreatic SFT with hamartoma-like feature. The evaluation of *NAB2-STAT6* fusion was of great importance in the diagnosis, especially in the differentiation of a pancreatic hamartoma.

Conflict of Interests

The authors declare that there is no conflict of interests regarding the publication of this paper.

References

[1] P. Klemperer and B. R. Caleman, "Primary neoplasms of the pleura: a report of five cases," *Archives of Pathology*, vol. 11, pp. 385–412, 1931.

[2] S. H. Sung, J.-W. Chang, J. Kim, K. S. Lee, J. Han, and S. I. Park, "Solitary fibrous tumors of the pleura: surgical outcome and clinical course," *Annals of Thoracic Surgery*, vol. 79, no. 1, pp. 303–307, 2005.

[3] F. J. Hernandez and B. B. Fernandez, "Localized fibrous tumors of pleura: a light and electron microscopic study," *Cancer*, vol. 34, no. 5, pp. 1667–1674, 1974.

[4] M. Al-Izzi, N. P. Thurlow, and B. Corrin, "Pleural mesothelioma of connective tissue type, localized fibrous tumour of the pleura, and reactive submesothelial hyperplasia. An immunohistochemical comparison," *Journal of Pathology*, vol. 158, no. 1, pp. 41–44, 1989.

[5] J. Lüttges, T. Mentzel, G. Hübner, and G. Klöppel, "Solitary fibrous tumour of the pancreas: a new member of the small group of mesenchymal pancreatic tumours," *Virchows Archiv*, vol. 435, no. 1, pp. 37–42, 1999.

[6] H. Miyamoto, D. A. Molena, L. O. Schoeniger, and H. Xu, "Solitary fibrous tumor of the pancreas: a case report," *International Journal of Surgical Pathology*, vol. 15, no. 3, pp. 311–314, 2007.

[7] H.-J. Kwon, J. H. Byun, J. Kang, H. P. Seong, and M.-G. Lee, "Solitary fibrous tumor of the pancreas: imaging findings," *Korean Journal of Radiology*, vol. 9, pp. S48–S51, 2008.

[8] V. D. Srinivasan, J. D. Wayne, M. S. Rao, and D. L. Zynger, "Solitary fibrous tumor of the pancreas: case report with cytologic and surgical pathology correlation and review of the literature," *Journal of the Pancreas*, vol. 9, no. 4, pp. 526–530, 2008.

[9] K. Chatti, K. Nouira, M. Ben Reguigua et al., "Solitary fibrous tumour of the pancreas. À case report," *Gastroentérologie Clinique et Biologique*, vol. 30, no. 2, pp. 317–319, 2006.

[10] H. Ishiwatari, T. Hayashi, M. Yoshida et al., "A case of solitary fibrous tumor of the pancreas," *Nippon Shokakibyo Gakkai Zasshi*, vol. 106, no. 7, pp. 1078–1085, 2009.

[11] Y. Sugawara, S. Sakai, S. Aono et al., "Solitary fibrous tumor of the pancreas," *Japanese Journal of Radiology*, vol. 28, no. 6, pp. 479–482, 2010.

[12] L. A. M. Santos, V. M. Santos, O. C. G. Oliveira, and M. de Marco, "Solitary fibrous tumour of the pancreas: a case report," *Anales del Sistema Sanitario de Navarra*, vol. 35, no. 1, pp. 133–136, 2012.

[13] A. Tasdemir, I. Soyuer, A. Yurci, I. Karahanli, and H. Akyildiz, "A huge solitary fibrous tumor localized in the pancreas: a young women," *Journal of the Pancreas*, vol. 13, no. 3, pp. 304–307, 2012.

[14] J.-W. Chen, T. Lü, H.-B. Liu et al., "A solitary fibrous tumor in the pancreas," *Chinese Medical Journal*, vol. 126, no. 7, pp. 1388–1389, 2013.

[15] A. Gardini, A. Dubini, L. Saragoni, F. Padovani, and D. Garcea, "Benign solitary fibrous tumor of the pancreas: a rare location of extra-pleural fibrous tumor. Single case report and review of the literature," *Pathologica*, vol. 99, no. 1, pp. 15–18, 2007.

[16] D. R. Robinson, Y.-M. Wu, S. Kalyana-Sundaram et al., "Identification of recurrent NAB2-STAT6 gene fusions in solitary fibrous tumor by integrative sequencing," *Nature Genetics*, vol. 45, no. 2, pp. 180–185, 2013.

[17] J. Chmielecki, A. M. Crago, M. Rosenberg et al., "Whole-exome sequencing identifies a recurrent NAB2-STAT6 fusion in solitary fibrous tumors," *Nature Genetics*, vol. 45, no. 2, pp. 131–132, 2013.

[18] A. Yoshida, K. Tsuta, M. Ohno et al., "STAT6 immunohistochemistry is helpful in the diagnosis of solitary fibrous tumors," *American Journal of Surgical Pathology*, vol. 38, no. 4, pp. 552–559, 2014.

[19] C. Koelsche, L. Schweizer, M. Renner et al., "Nuclear relocation of STAT6 reliably predicts *NAB2-STAT6* fusion for the diagnosis of solitary fibrous tumour," *Histopathology*, vol. 65, no. 5, pp. 613–622, 1991.

[20] L. A. Doyle, M. Vivero, C. D. M. Fletcher, F. Mertens, and J. L. Hornick, "Nuclear expression of STAT6 distinguishes solitary fibrous tumor from histologic mimics," *Modern Pathology*, vol. 27, no. 3, pp. 390–395, 2014.

[21] R. Srinivasan, G. M. Mager, R. M. Ward, J. Mayer, and J. Svaren, "NAB2 represses transcription by interacting with the CHD4 subunit of the nucleosome remodeling and deacetylase (NuRD) complex," *The Journal of Biological Chemistry*, vol. 281, no. 22, pp. 15129–15137, 2006.

[22] J. Svaren, B. R. Sevetson, E. D. Apel, D. B. Zimonjic, N. C. Popescu, and J. Milbrandt, "NAB2, a corepressor of NGFI-A (Egr-1) and Krox20, is induced by proliferative and differentiative stimuli," *Molecular and Cellular Biology*, vol. 16, no. 7, pp. 3545–3553, 1996.

[23] H. Yamaguchi, S. Aishima, Y. Oda et al., "Distinctive histopathologic findings of pancreatic hamartomas suggesting their 'hamartomatous' nature: a study of 9 cases," *American Journal of Surgical Pathology*, vol. 37, no. 7, pp. 1006–1013, 2013.

[24] P. P. Anthony, R. G. Faber, and R. C. G. Russell, "Pseudotumours of the pancreas," *British Medical Journal*, vol. 1, article 814, 1977.

[25] T. B. Burt, V. R. Condon, and M. E. Matlak, "Fetal pancreatic hamartoma," *Pediatric Radiology*, vol. 13, no. 5, pp. 287–289, 1983.

[26] M. J. Flaherty and D. R. Benjamin, "Multicystic pancreatic hamartoma: a distinctive lesion with immunohistochemical and ultrastructural study," *Human Pathology*, vol. 23, no. 11, pp. 1309–1312, 1992.

[27] J. R. Izbicki, W. T. Knoefel, J. Muller-Hocker, and H. K. Mandelkow, "Pancreatic hamartoma: a benign tumor of the pancreas," *The American Journal of Gastroenterology*, vol. 89, no. 8, pp. 1261–1262, 1994.

[28] S. S. Wu, H. I. Vargas, and S. W. French, "Pancreatic hamartoma with Langerhans cell histiocytosis in a draining lymph node," *Histopathology*, vol. 33, no. 5, pp. 485–487, 1998.

[29] C. D. McFaul, L. J. Vitone, F. Campbell et al., "Pancreatic hamartoma," *Pancreatology*, vol. 4, no. 6, pp. 533–537, 2004.

[30] U. Pauser, M. T. S. da Silva, J. Placke, D. S. Klimstra, and G. Klöppel, "Cellular hamartoma resembling gastrointestinal stromal tumor: a solid tumor of the pancreas expressing c-kit (CD117)," *Modern Pathology*, vol. 18, no. 9, pp. 1211–1216, 2005.

[31] U. Pauser, M. Kosmahl, B. Krušlin, D. S. Klimstra, and G. Klöppel, "Pancreatic solid and cystic hamartoma in adults: characterization of a new tumorous lesion," *American Journal of Surgical Pathology*, vol. 29, no. 6, pp. 797–800, 2005.

[32] S. Nagata, K. Yamaguchi, T. Inoue et al., "Solid pancreatic hamartoma," *Pathology International*, vol. 57, no. 5, pp. 276–280, 2007.

[33] M. Thrall, J. Jessurun, E. B. Stelow et al., "Multicystic adenomatoid hamartoma of the pancreas: a hitherto undescribed pancreatic tumor occurring in a 3-year-old boy," *Pediatric and Developmental Pathology*, vol. 11, no. 4, pp. 314–320, 2008.

[34] D. Sampelean, M. Adam, V. Muntean, B. Hanescu, and I. Domsa, "Pancreatic hamartoma and SAPHO syndrome: a case report," *Journal of Gastrointestinal and Liver Diseases*, vol. 18, no. 4, pp. 483–486, 2009.

[35] F. Kawakami, M. Shimizu, H. Yamaguchi et al., "Multiple solid pancreatic hamartomas: a case report and review of the literature," *World Journal of Gastrointestinal Oncology*, vol. 4, pp. 202–206, 2012.

[36] H.-H. Kim, C.-K. Cho, Y.-H. Hur et al., "Pancreatic hamartoma diagnosed after surgical resection," *Journal of the Korean Surgical Society*, vol. 83, no. 5, pp. 330–334, 2012.

[37] R. Sueyoshi, T. Okazaki, G. J. Lane, A. Arakawa, T. Yao, and A. Yamataka, "Multicystic adenomatoid pancreatic hamartoma in a child: case report and literature review," *International Journal of Surgery Case Reports*, vol. 4, no. 1, pp. 1–3, 2013.

[38] P. Addeo, G. Tudor, E. Oussoultzoglou, G. Averous, and P. Bachellier, "Pancreatic hamartoma," *Surgery*, vol. 156, no. 5, pp. 1284–1285, 2014.

[39] H. Inoue, M. Tameda, R. Yamada et al., "Pancreatic hamartoma: a rare cause of obstructive jaundice," *Endoscopy*, vol. 46, no. 1, pp. E157–E158, 2014.

[40] R. Vogels, M. Vlenterie, Y. Versleijen-Jonkers et al., "Solitary fibrous tumor—clinicopathologic, immunohistochemical and molecular analysis of 28 cases," *Diagnostic Pathology*, vol. 9, no. 1, article 224, 2014.

[41] C. D. M. Fletcher, J. A. Bridge, P. C. W. Hogendoom et al., *WHO Classification of Tumours of Soft Tissue and Bone*, IARC, Lyon, France, 2013.

[42] K. Akaike, A. Kurisaki-Arakawa, K. Hara et al., "Distinct clinicopathological features of NAB2-STAT6 fusion gene variants in solitary fibrous tumor with emphasis on the acquisition of highly malignant potential," *Human Pathology*, vol. 46, no. 3, pp. 347–356, 2015.

5

Unusual Initial Presentation of Herpes Simplex Virus as Inguinal Lymphadenopathy

Sarah A. Fleming and John G. Strickler

Hospital Pathology Associates, 2800 10th Avenue South Suite 2200, Minneapolis, MN 55407, USA

Correspondence should be addressed to Sarah A. Fleming; flemi361@umn.edu

Academic Editor: Katsuyuki Aozasa

Genital herpes simplex virus (HSV) infections are a common cause of inguinal lymphadenopathy. However, surgical excision of enlarged inguinal nodes is almost never performed to initially diagnose genital herpes simplex virus, due to the distinct external presentation of genital herpetic vesicles that usually occur with the first symptoms of infection. Therefore, the histologic and immunophenotypic features of HSV-associated inguinal lymphadenopathy are unfamiliar to most pathologists. The current report describes the lymph node pathology of two immunocompetent patients, whose initial HSV diagnosis was established through surgical excision of enlarged inguinal lymph nodes. Histologic examination showed features consistent with viral lymphadenopathy, including florid follicular hyperplasia, monocytoid B-cell hyperplasia, and paracortical hyperplasia without extensive necrosis. Immunohistochemical stains for HSV antigens, using polyclonal anti-HSV I and II antibodies, demonstrate strong immunoreactivity for HSV in a small number of cells in the subcapsular sinuses, especially in areas with monocytoid B-cell hyperplasia. Rare scattered HSV-positive cells also are identified in paracortical areas and germinal centers. We conclude that an initial diagnosis of genital HSV infection may be established by inguinal lymph node biopsy.

1. Introduction

Surgical excision of enlarged inguinal lymph nodes is often performed to exclude hematologic malignancies. These lymph node biopsy specimens often show lymphoid hyperplasia, which may be due to a wide variety of reactive conditions including various sexually transmitted infections [1]. However, it is unusual for genital herpes simplex virus (HSV) to present initially as inguinal lymphadenopathy, which is significant enough to warrant nodal excision, unless the patient also has a known underlying lymphoma [2]. Although the initial histologic diagnosis of genital HSV by inguinal lymph node biopsy is rare [3], we now describe two immunocompetent patients with active genital herpes diagnosed by inguinal lymph node biopsy.

2. Materials and Methods

Formalin-fixed, paraffin-embedded tissue and hematoxylin and eosin-stained slides were studied in both cases. Immunohistochemical studies on paraffin-embedded material were performed, using antibodies for herpes simplex virus (HSV) I and II following fixation in 10% neutral buffered formalin. The rabbit polyclonal HSV I and II antibodies from Cell Marque (CMC36111031, CMC36211031, Rocklin, California) were used at a dilution of 1:200 for HSV I and 1:50 for HSV 2. Immunostaining was performed using the Leica Bond-Max automation system and Leica Refine detection kit (Leica Biosystems, Bannockburn, IL). The approximately 3-hour protocol included online deparaffinization and low-pH epitope retrieval for 10 minutes, incubation with primary antibodies for 15 minutes, postprimary IgG linker reagent (rabbit anti-mouse IgG) for 8 minutes, polymer anti-rabbit HRP IgG for 8 minutes, and DAB as the chromogen for 10 minutes, followed by 5-minute hematoxylin counterstaining. A positive control was run with each sample.

3. Case Presentation

Both patients presented clinically with enlarged and tender inguinal lymph nodes. CT scans confirmed enlarged inguinal

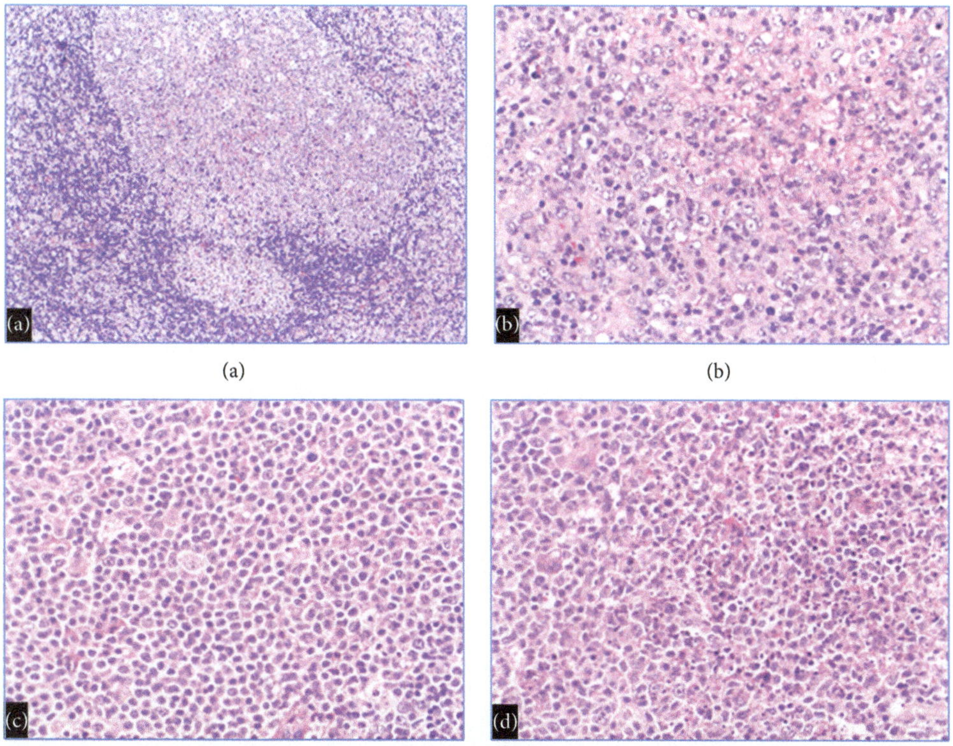

(a) (b) (c) (d)

FIGURE 1: Histologic sections show (a) follicular hyperplasia with attenuated mantle zones and adjacent monocytoid B-cell hyperplasia (Case 1) 100x magnification, (b) paracortical hyperplasia with a moderate number of immunoblasts (Case 1) 200x magnification, (c) monocytoid B-cell hyperplasia (Case 1) 200x magnification, and (d) monocytoid B-cell hyperplasia with focal necrosis (Case 2) 200x magnification.

nodes (both measuring greater than 3 cm in diameter), without evidence of systemic lymphadenopathy. Lymph node biopsies in both patients were performed to exclude lymphoma and other malignancies. Biopsy specimens from the inguinal lymph nodes showed similar histologic features (Figure 1).

3.1. Case 1. The patient is a 16-year-old female, who had a 3.7 × 3.5 × 1.7 cm inguinal lymph node removed. Histologic examination showed florid follicular hyperplasia including some follicles with attenuated mantle zones. Subsequent HIV serology studies were negative. Monocytoid B-cell hyperplasia was prominent. Extranodal marginal zone lymphoma, which occasionally is difficult to distinguish from monocytoid B-cell hyperplasia, was excluded by absence of diffuse architectural effacement and by absence of a monoclonal B-cell population by flow cytometry. The lymph node also showed paracortical hyperplasia, including a moderate number of immunoblasts with prominent nucleoli, but absence of Reed-Sternberg cells/variants excluded Hodgkin lymphoma.

3.2. Case 2. The patient is a 43-year-old male who had a 3 × 2 × 1 cm inguinal lymph node removed. Histologic examination shows florid follicular hyperplasia with minimal paracortical hyperplasia. Some of the sinusoidal areas show monocytoid B-cell hyperplasia, focally associated with necrosis. Histologic examination revealed no evidence of hematologic malignancy, and flow cytometry confirmed the absence of lymphoma.

Immunohistochemical stains (Figure 2) of both cases show small numbers of HSV-I/HSV-II positive cells in the lymph node sinuses, predominantly in the subcapsular sinus. The viral inclusions were found mainly in sinuses containing monocytoid B-cell hyperplasia, with rare scattered HSV-positive cells in the paracortex, and rare weak HSV-positive cells in germinal centers. The HSV-infected cells appear to be mainly macrophages (CD68-positive) rather than B-lymphocytes (CD20-positive). The significance of these findings in the HSV-associated immune response is not clear.

Immunostains for CMV, cat scratch disease, and toxoplasmosis were negative. A small number of EBV positive lymphoid cells were present in Case 1, indicative of a prior EBV infection rather than acute EBV associated infectious mononucleosis.

4. Discussion

An initial diagnosis of HSV-associated lymphadenopathy was established by inguinal lymph node biopsy in both of our patients. The patients were immunocompetent, presented with palpable tender inguinal nodes, and did not have current or prior genital herpes infection or hematologic malignancy. Localized lymphadenopathy has been reported in up to 80% of patients who have an active genital HSV infection [4].

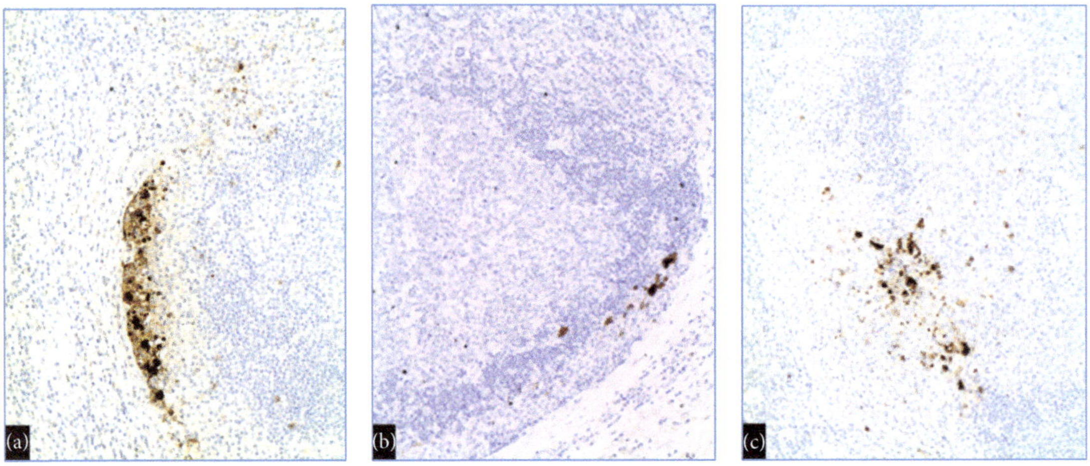

(a) (b) (c)

FIGURE 2: Immunohistochemical stains show small numbers of HSV-I/HSV-II positive cells in (a) subcapsular sinus (Case 2) 40x magnification, (b) subcapsular sinus (Case 1) 100x magnification, and (c) areas of monocytoid B-cell hyperplasia (Case 2) 100x magnification.

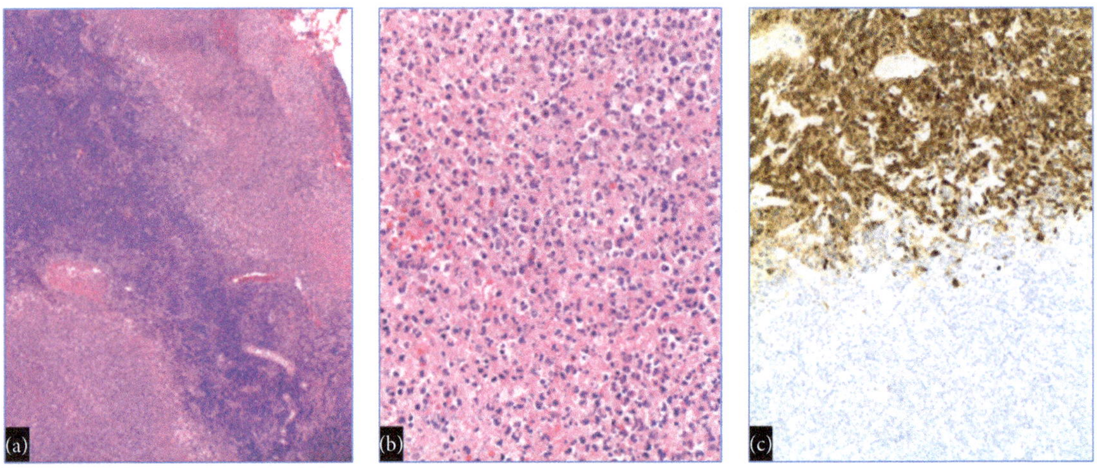

(a) (b) (c)

FIGURE 3: HSV infections when superimposed on low grade B-cell lymphomas show (a) well-demarcated areas of necrosis (Reference case) 40x magnification, (b) necrosis containing HSV viral inclusions (Reference case) 200x magnification, and (c) numerous viral inclusions only in the necrotic areas by HSV immunohistochemistry (Reference case) 100x magnification.

However, lymph node biopsy is very rarely performed for initial diagnostic purposes, as genital HSV infections usually present with predominant local symptoms such as pain, itching, dysuria, vaginal or urethral discharge, or lesions before tender lymphadenopathy develops [4].

Our patients were both young sexually active individuals, suggesting that both had recent exposure to HSV, which presented initially as inguinal lymphadenopathy. In an autopsy review study of disseminated herpes disease, HSV was never found as an incidental finding in lymphoid tissues, except in patients with an underlying hematologic malignancy [5]. In addition, previous studies have shown a correlation between HSV derived inguinal lymphadenopathy and subsequent development of genital HSV-related lesions [6, 7].

Previous reports of biopsy-proven HSV-associated lymphadenopathy indicate that many patients are immunocompromised and/or have underlying low-grade B-cell lymphomas [6, 8, 9]. Neither of our patients showed histologic or immunologic evidence of concurrent lymphoma. Simultaneous nodal involvement by HSV and low-grade B-cell lymphoma (Figure 3) is characterized by diffuse effacement of nodal architecture, with well-demarcated foci of necrosis containing numerous HSV-I/HSV-II infected cells.

The histologic appearance in our two patients (florid follicular hyperplasia, monocytoid B-cell hyperplasia, and paracortical hyperplasia) overlaps with lymphadenopathy associated with other viral-associated lymphadenopathy, and HSV immunohistochemistry is essential for establishing the correct diagnosis. Note that monocytoid B-cell hyperplasia may be related to memory B-cell reactivation, although this histologic pattern also is commonly associated with acute viral lymphadenopathy. Cytomegalovirus (CMV) lymphadenopathy has similar histologic features, including prominent follicular hyperplasia and monocytoid B-cell hyperplasia. Cytomegalovirus inclusions (typically within the monocytoid B-cell hyperplasia) can be identified histologically and confirmed by immunohistochemistry. The lymphadenopathy associated with acute EBV-associated infectious mononucleosis has more prominent paracortical hyperplasia than HSV-associated lymphadenopathy. EBV in situ hybridization studies (on tissue sections) or serologic studies are required for confirmation. The follicular hyperplasia associated with human immunodeficiency virus (HIV) infections is typically characterized by absent mantle zones and follicle lysis. The mantle zones in our first patient were somewhat attenuated, but HIV serologic studies excluded concurrent HIV-associated lymphadenopathy.

Although rare, HSV can initially present as inguinal lymphadenopathy without other associated symptoms. We conclude that HSV-associated lymphadenopathy should be considered whenever enlarged inguinal lymph nodes show a viral histologic appearance, especially when encountered in young, sexually active adults.

Conflict of Interests

The authors disclose that they have no significant relationships with or financial interest in any commercial companies pertaining to this paper.

Acknowledgments

The authors thank Milton W. Datta, M.D., for guidance with the IRB approval process. They also thank Joesph Hodapp, B.S., for his help in the submission process.

References

[1] I. Bogoch, J. Andrews, E. Nagami, A. Rivera, R. Gandhi, and D. Stone, "Clinical predictors for the aetiology of peripheral lymphadenopathy in HIV-infected adults," *HIV Medicine*, vol. 14, no. 3, pp. 182–186, 2013.

[2] M. J. Gaffey, J. M. Ben-Ezra, and L. M. Weiss, "Herpes simplex lymphadenitis," *The American Journal of Clinical Pathology*, vol. 95, no. 5, pp. 709–714, 1991.

[3] J. B. Taxy, I. Tillawi, and P. M. Goldman, "Herpes simplex lymphadenitis. An unusual presentation with necrosis and viral particles," *Archives of Pathology and Laboratory Medicine*, vol. 109, no. 11, pp. 1043–1044, 1985.

[4] L. Corey, H. G. Adams, Z. A. Brown, and K. K. Holmes, "Genital herpes simplex virus infections: clinical manifestations, course, and complications," *Annals of Internal Medicine*, vol. 98, no. 6, pp. 958–972, 1983.

[5] D. H. Buss and M. Scharyj, "Herpesvirus infection of the esophagus and other visceral organs in adults. Incidence and clinical significance," *The American Journal of Medicine*, vol. 66, no. 3, pp. 457–462, 1979.

[6] M. D. Witt, M. S. Torno, N. Sun, and T. Stein, "Herpes simplex virus lymphadenitis: case report and review of the literature," *Clinical Infectious Diseases*, vol. 34, no. 1, pp. 1–6, 2002.

[7] J. R. Miliauskas and A. S.-Y. Leong, "Localized herpes simplex lymphadenitis: report of three cases and review of the literature," *Histopathology*, vol. 19, no. 4, pp. 355–360, 1991.

[8] M. E. Pilichowska, J. H. Smouse, and D. M. Dorfman, "Concurrent herpes simplex viral lymphadenitis and mantle cell lymphoma: a case report and review of the literature," *Archives of Pathology and Laboratory Medicine*, vol. 130, no. 4, pp. 536–539, 2006.

[9] J. I. Epstein, R. F. Ambinder, F. P. Kuhajda, S. H. Pearlman, V. E. Reuter, and R. B. Mann, "Localized herpes simplex lymphadenitis," *American Journal of Clinical Pathology*, vol. 86, no. 4, pp. 444–448, 1986.

6

MYC Amplification in Angiosarcoma Arising from an Arteriovenous Graft Site

Kristen M. Paral,[1] Gordana Raca,[2] and Thomas Krausz[3]

[1]*Department of Medicine, Section of Dermatology, University of Chicago, 5841 S Maryland Avenue, MC 5067, Chicago, IL 60637, USA*
[2]*Department of Medicine, Section of Hematology/Oncology, University of Chicago, 5841 S Maryland Avenue, MC 6092, Chicago, IL 60637, USA*
[3]*Department of Pathology, University of Chicago, 5841 S Maryland Avenue, MC 6161, Chicago, IL 60637, USA*

Correspondence should be addressed to Kristen M. Paral; kristen.paral@uchospitals.edu

Academic Editor: Khin Thway

Angiosarcoma arising in association with an arteriovenous graft (AVG) or fistula is a unique clinicopathologic scenario that appears to be gaining recognition in the literature. Among reported cases, none has described high-level *MYC* gene amplification, a genetic aberration that is increasingly unifying the various clinicopathologic subdivisions of angiosarcoma. We therefore report the *MYC* gene status in a case of angiosarcoma arising at an AVG site.

1. Introduction

Certain predisposing conditions have been clearly associated with angiosarcoma, including (i) radiation exposure, such as ultraviolet light in skin cases and therapeutic irradiation in breast cases; (ii) longstanding lymphedema (i.e., Stewart-Treves syndrome); and (iii) exogenous toxins (e.g., vinyl chloride, thorotrast, and arsenic) in liver cases [1]. Angiosarcoma associated with AVG, however, has not yet achieved the same level of recognition as the aforementioned scenarios. Despite a steady trickle of such cases into the literature over the recent decades [2–11], few authoritative sources acknowledge its existence [12].

An AVG or fistula is an artificial connection between an artery and a vein created with synthetic materials such as polytetrafluoroethylene (PTFE) or Dacron [13]. Implanted foreign material has been linked to the development of sarcoma for many decades [14]. Most cases of angiosarcoma associated with an AVG have been linked to immunosuppression, although other etiological factors have been suggested, such as the alteration of blood flow [2, 11]. Minimal attention has been devoted to the role of genetic aberrations in these cases.

Recent findings of frequent high-level *MYC* gene amplification in angiosarcomas suggest a genetic basis for the disease [15]. The *MYC* gene is a potent oncogene that is amplified in various clinicopathologic subdivisions of angiosarcoma, including secondary (postirradiation and lymphedema-associated) and a subset of primary angiosarcomas (breast, skin, and bone) [15–19]. *MYC* amplification status has not yet been described in the unusual setting of AVG-associated angiosarcoma; we therefore report *MYC* amplification status in one such case.

2. Case Report

A 63-year-old Hispanic man presented in 2013 for evaluation of left arm pain in an area where an AVG had been placed 15 years previously (a brachiocephalic "loop graft" with PTFE). The AVG had not been in use for eight years owing to a kidney transplant in 2005. Prior to the transplant, the patient required regular hemodialysis due to end-stage renal disease from chronic hypertension and diabetes.

Physical examination revealed swelling and tenderness of the AVG site, which was attributed to probable thrombosis. This was pursued by angiogram, which was interpreted as a thrombosed pseudoaneurysm at the site. The angiogram also disclosed an unexpected finding: a destructive mass involving the elbow. Further imaging with MRI studies revealed a 20 cm mass encircling the elbow and tracking distally into

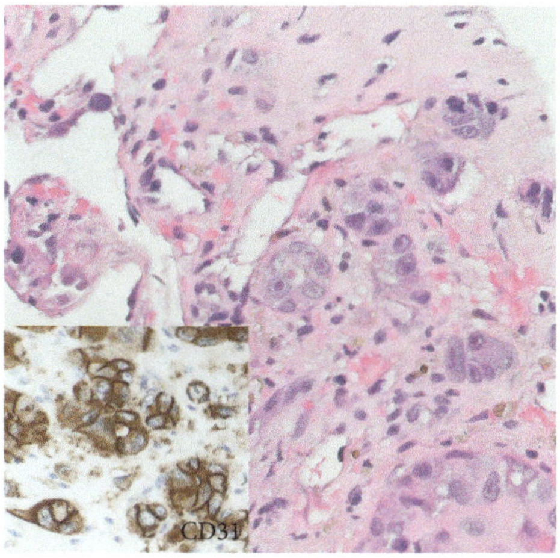

Figure 1: Microscopic examination, biopsy material. The conspicuous clusters of malignant epithelioid cells dominate the picture and could give rise to a broad differential diagnosis that includes carcinoma and melanoma. The poorly formed vascular channels in the background could easily be overlooked. Immunohistochemistry was key (inset).

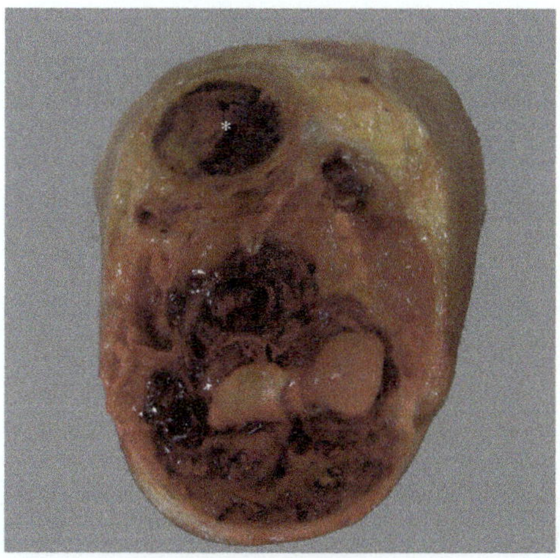

Figure 2: Gross examination, amputation specimen. The AVG site (asterisk) in the antecubital region exhibits a dilated space distended with tumor, which radiologically was thought to be thrombus within a pseudoaneurysm. Tumor envelopes the elbow and tracks distally into the forearm.

the forearm. The mass was biopsied to show angiosarcoma, resulting in transhumeral amputation. Six months after the amputation, the patient is alive without evidence of sarcoma.

2.1. Pathology. Initial biopsy of the mass disclosed clusters of malignant epithelioid cells adjacent to poorly formed vascular spaces that showed strong, diffuse expression of vascular markers by immunohistochemistry (Figure 1). Patchy cytokeratin expression paralleled the epithelioid morphology (CK AE1/AE3, CK7, and CK8/18). The subsequent amputation specimen showed tumor at the AVG site (Figure 2). Microscopic examination showed predominantly epithelioid cells with minimal spindle cell morphology and near-absent vasoformation; therefore, a final diagnosis of epithelioid angiosarcoma was rendered. Among the most interesting findings were (1) the presence of tumor juxtaposed to foreign graft material and (2) the finding of tumor tracking along a vessel wall. Two lymph nodes recovered near the resection margin showed metastatic angiosarcoma. The salient histopathologic findings are shown in Figure 3.

2.2. Molecular Findings. FISH analysis for the quantitation of *MYC* was performed on formalin-fixed, paraffin-embedded tissue sections cut at 5 mm using commercially available break-apart FISH probe-set for the *MYC* locus (8q24), with the 5′ probe labeled with Spectrum Red and the 3′ probe labeled with Spectrum Green (Abbott Molecular, Des Plaines, IL, USA). With this probe-set a yellow fusion signal is produced by the juxtaposition of the 5′ and the 3′ probe when the *MYC* locus has a normal configuration. Standard laboratory protocols and quality control measures were followed for this study. In each case, 100 interphase nuclei were analyzed in a blinded manner by two technicians (200 total nuclei). Amplification of the *MYC* locus was defined as the presence of increased number of *MYC* signals (more than 6) in tumor cells. Clear high-level *MYC* amplification was seen in large areas, with an average of more than 20 signals per cell (Figure 4).

3. Discussion

The finding of *MYC* amplification in this case of AVG-associated angiosarcoma expands the spectrum of recognized clinicopathologic subtypes of angiosarcoma bearing this aberration and suggests they share similar pathogenesis. The present case exhibited large regions of clear signal amplification by FISH, consistent with the most commonly observed pattern described in the literature for angiosarcoma [15]. One of the many effects of *MYC* gene amplification is augmentation of a cell's preexisting gene expression program [20] and promotion of angiogenesis [15]. The presence of *MYC* amplification in this case does not necessarily exclude a pathogenic role for the synthetic graft material. There is evidence to suggest that the fibrous capsule that develops around foreign material may stimulate carcinogenesis by providing a home-base for macrophages, which secrete cytokines, growth factors, and free radicals that can induce genetic damage, even after fibrosis is complete [14]. Perhaps this mechanism can account for *MYC* gene aberration in foreign body-associated angiosarcoma. Although the fibrous capsule in this case was fully appreciated, documentation of fibrous encapsulation tends to be inconsistently reported [21].

Alternatively, the graft material may itself directly provoke angiogenesis and subsequent tumorigenesis. Indeed, newer-generation "biopolymers" seek to incorporate bioactive molecules that directly stimulate vascular regeneration [13]. Further studies will be necessary to investigate this and other possible contributing factors, such as immunosuppression. A link to immunosuppression in this case could not be established because the patient was partially managed by an external institution. In any event, the true underlying

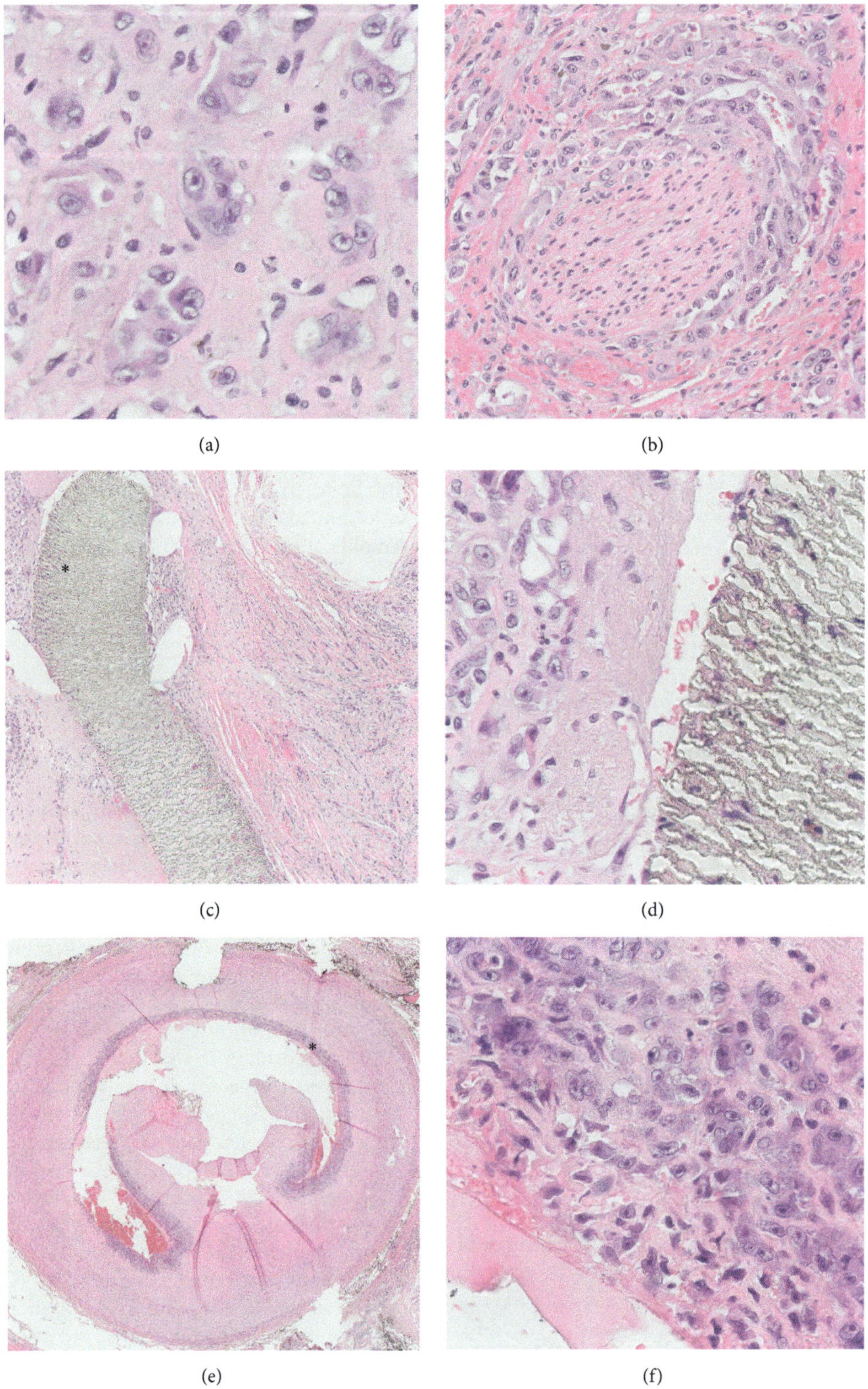

Figure 3: Microscopic examination, amputation specimen. (a) Clusters of malignant epithelioid cells, similar to those seen in the biopsy specimen, are noted (original magnification ×400). (b) Perineural invasion can explain the patient's pain symptoms (original magnification ×200). (c) Tumor clusters are embedded within the dense fibrous sheath around the graft material; the region marked by the asterisk is shown at higher power in (d) (original magnification ×50, ×400). (e) Tumor cells are seen tracking along the intimal layer of a large artery; the region marked by the asterisk is shown at higher power in (f) (original magnification ×10, ×400).

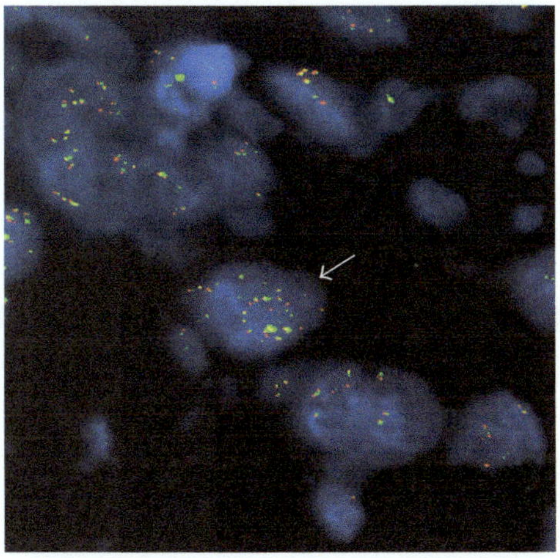

FIGURE 4: FISH results using a *MYC* break-apart probe. Representative tumor cell (indicated by arrow) is showing an increased number of fusion signals (more than 20), indicative of high-level amplification of the *MYC* locus.

mechanism for tumorigenesis in this case and in many cases of angiosarcoma likely involves a tangled web of interactions between genetic changes and microenvironment alterations.

Conflict of Interests

The authors declare that there are no financial disclosures for this study.

References

[1] R. J. Young, N. J. Brown, M. W. Reed, D. Hughes, and P. J. Woll, "Angiosarcoma," *The Lancet Oncology*, vol. 11, no. 10, pp. 983–991, 2010.

[2] Y. A. Qureshi, D. C. Strauss, K. Thway, C. Fisher, and J. M. Thomas, "Angiosarcoma developing in a non-functioning arteriovenous fistula post-renal transplant," *Journal of Surgical Oncology*, vol. 101, no. 6, pp. 520–523, 2010.

[3] K. Demey, L.-M. Reyns, and S. Schepers, "Angiosarcoma arising in an arteriovenous fistula in a patient without kidney transplant," *Acta Chirurgica Belgica*, vol. 114, no. 1, pp. 75–78, 2014.

[4] M. M. Keane and D. N. Carney, "Angiosarcoma arising from a defunctionalized arteriovenous fistula," *Journal of Urology*, vol. 149, no. 2, pp. 364–365, 1993.

[5] N. R. Parrott, P. D. Scott, A. J. Freemont, and R. W. G. Johnson, "Angiosarcoma in an arteriovenous fistula following successful renal transplantation—a case report," *Transplantation*, vol. 55, no. 3, pp. 676–677, 1993.

[6] P. J. Conlon Jr., T. Daly, G. Doyle, and M. Carmody, "Angiosarcoma at the site of a ligated arteriovenous fistula in a renal transplant recipient," *Nephrology Dialysis Transplantation*, vol. 8, no. 3, pp. 259–262, 1993.

[7] B. M. Wehrli, D. L. Janzen, O. Shokeir, B. A. Masri, S. K. Byrne, and J. X. O'Connell, "Epithelioid angiosarcoma arising in a surgically constructed arteriovenous fistula: a rare complication of chronic immunosuppression in the setting of renal transplantation," *The American Journal of Surgical Pathology*, vol. 22, no. 9, pp. 1154–1159, 1998.

[8] D. Bessis, A. Sotto, P. Roubert, P.-E. Chabrier, G. Mourad, and J.-J. Guilhou, "Endothelin-secreting angiosarcoma occurring at the site of an arteriovenous fistula for haemodialysis in a renal transplant recipient," *British Journal of Dermatology*, vol. 138, no. 2, pp. 361–363, 1998.

[9] R. Farag, J. A. Schulak, F. W. Abdul-Karim, and J. K. Wasman, "Angiosarcoma arising in an arteriovenous fistula site in a renal transplant patient: a case report and literature review," *Clinical Nephrology*, vol. 63, no. 5, pp. 408–412, 2005.

[10] J. Chanyaputhipong, D. L. T. Hock, and M. G. Sebastian, "Disseminated angiosarcoma of the dialysis fistula in 2 patients without kidney transplants," *American Journal of Kidney Diseases*, vol. 57, no. 6, pp. 917–920, 2011.

[11] P. Webster, L. Wujanto, C. Fisher et al., "Malignancies confined to disused arteriovenous fistulae in renal transplant patients: an important differential diagnosis," *American Journal of Nephrology*, vol. 34, no. 1, pp. 42–48, 2011.

[12] C. D. M. Fletcher, J. A. Bridge, P. C. W. Hogendoorn, and F. Mertens, Eds., *WHO Classification of Tumours of Soft Tissue and Bone*, IARC, Lyon, France, 2013.

[13] S. Ravi and E. L. Chaikof, "Biomaterials for vascular tissue engineering," *Regenerative Medicine*, vol. 5, no. 1, pp. 107–120, 2010.

[14] T. G. Moizhess, "Carcinogenesis induced by foreign bodies," *Biochemistry*, vol. 73, no. 7, pp. 763–775, 2008.

[15] C. Antonescu, "Malignant vascular tumors—an update," *Modern Pathology*, vol. 27, supplement 1, pp. S30–S38, 2014.

[16] T. Guo, L. Zhang, N.-E. Chang, S. Singer, R. G. Maki, and C. R. Antonescu, "Consistent MYC and FLT4 gene amplification in radiation-induced angiosarcoma but not in other radiation-associated atypical vascular lesions," *Genes Chromosomes and Cancer*, vol. 50, no. 1, pp. 25–33, 2011.

[17] J. Manner, B. Radlwimmer, P. Hohenberger et al., "MYC high level gene amplification is a distinctive feature of angiosarcomas after irradiation or chronic lymphedema," *The American Journal of Pathology*, vol. 176, no. 1, pp. 34–39, 2010.

[18] S. L. J. Verbeke, D. de Jong, F. Bertoni et al., "Array CGH analysis identifies two distinct subgroups of primary angiosarcoma of bone," *Genes Chromosomes and Cancer*, vol. 54, no. 2, pp. 72–81, 2014.

[19] W. Shon, W. R. Sukov, S. M. Jenkins, and A. L. Folpe, "MYC amplification and overexpression in primary cutaneous angiosarcoma: a fluorescence in-situ hybridization and immunohistochemical study," *Modern Pathology*, vol. 27, no. 4, pp. 509–515, 2014.

[20] C. Y. Lin, J. Lovén, P. B. Rahl et al., "Transcriptional amplification in tumor cells with elevated c-Myc," *Cell*, vol. 151, no. 1, pp. 56–67, 2012.

[21] T. A. Jennings, L. Peterson, C. A. Axiotis, G. E. Friedlaender, R. A. Cooke, and J. Rosai, "Angiosarcoma associated with foreign body material: a report of three cases," *Cancer*, vol. 62, no. 11, pp. 2436–2444, 1988.

Massive Localized Lymphedema Arising from Abdominal Wall: A Case Report and Review of the Literature

Teodóra Tóth, Yi-Che Chang Chien, Sándor Kollár, and Ilona Kovács

Department of Pathology, Kenézy Gyula County Hospital, Bartók Béla út 2-26, Debrecen 4031, Hungary

Correspondence should be addressed to Yi-Che Chang Chien; ccwilly@hotmail.com

Academic Editor: Khin Thway

Massive localized lymphedema (MLL) is a rare pseudosarcomatous lesion due to localized lymphatic obstruction from variable causes. It is most common on medial aspect of thigh and inguinal region. Abdominal localization is rare and may cause clinical diagnostic confusion with other malignant tumors due to its large size. We report a case of abdominal wall MLL of a 56-year-old male patient under clinical suspicion of well differentiated liposarcoma. The literature search and differential diagnosis will be addressed. In doubt cases, immunohistochemical stain or fluorescent in situ hybridization can help to separate this entity from the other mimickers.

1. Introduction

Massive localized lymphedema (MLL) is a rare pseudosarcomatous lesion that usually develops in morbidly obese individual. The underlying pathophysiology is a lymphatic flow disturbance that may be due to the massive amount of adipose tissue [1]. Lymphatic disruption due to previous surgery, trauma, and hypothyroidism also serve as possible causes [2]. The overlying skin usually shows induration and "peau d'orange" appearance consistent with chronic lymphedema and the dermal layer also exhibits stasis dermatitis morphology. It may clinically mimic well-differentiated liposarcoma or other lipogenic tumors which may lead to error in diagnosis.

MLL most commonly occurs in the medial aspect of proximal thigh. Abdominal wall, scrotum, and upper extremity, although rare, are the other possible areas of occurrence. We present an abdominal MLL clinically mimicking well-differentiated liposarcoma from an obese patient which can be excluded by histological and immunohistochemical characteristics. The literature search and differential diagnosis from other mimickers will also be discussed.

2. Materials and Methods

2.1. Clinical Data. A fifty-six-year-old obese male patient (155 kg), with previous medical history of type II diabetes, hypertension, and dilative cardiomyopathy, presented to our surgery department with a $26 \times 22 \times 9.5$ cm sized, polypoid subcutaneous mass below his umbilicus over 4 years. It was soft in consistency and painless. The overlying skin was thicker with "peau d'orange-" like appearance. Neither previous operation nor history of hypothyroidism was claimed. No sign of hypothyroidism was identified during the clinical examination. Due to the large size of the tumor, the patient underwent surgical excision under the impression of sarcoma.

2.2. Immunohistochemistry. After sectioning of 4 μm slides from the formalin-fixed, paraffin-embedded blocks, deparaffinization in xylene and rehydration in a series of decreasing concentration of ethanol were done. Antigen retrieval using either the Bond Epitope Retrieval Solution 1 (pH 6) or the Bond Epitope Retrieval Solution 2 (pH 9) (Leica Microsystems, Wetzlar, Germany) at 99-100°C for 20–30 min was performed. The slides were treated with S-100 (1 : 300, clone S-100, DAKO, Carpinteria, California, USA, incubation time: 30 min in room temperature), vimentin (prediluted, clone V91, DAKO, incubation time: 30 min in room temperature), CD31 (1 : 30, clone JC70A, DAKO, incubation time: 30 min in room temperature), MDM2 (1 : 200, clone IB10, Novocastra, Wetzlar, Germany, incubation time: 45 min in room temperature), and p16 (1 : 10, clone G175-405, DAKO, incubation

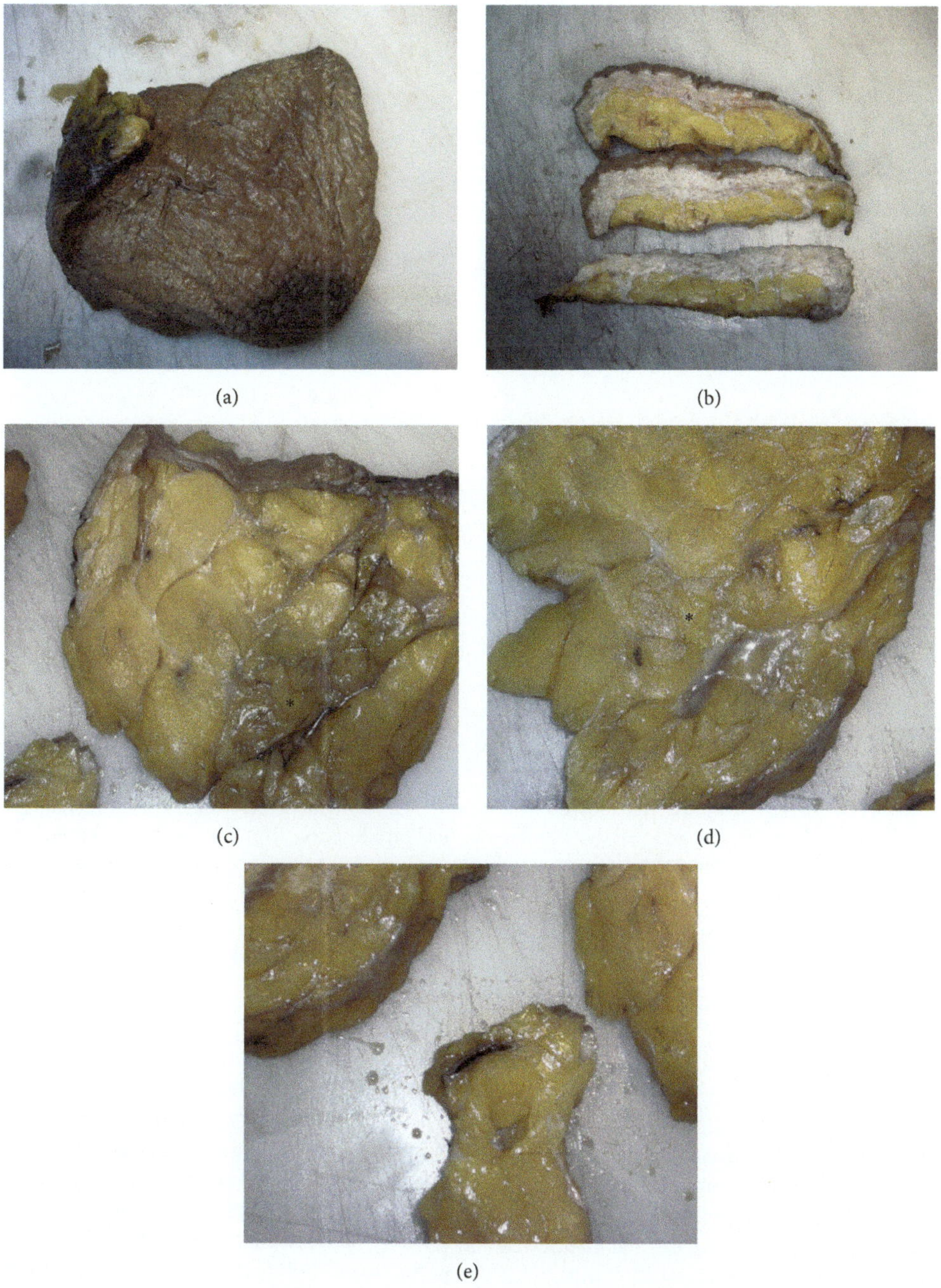

FIGURE 1: Macroscopic characteristics of MLL. The skin is indurated and hyperpigmented with classical "peau d'orange" appearance (a). The cut surface revealed the thickened skin (b). The subcutaneous tissue cut surface showed serous fluid (indicated by "∗") and also lobulated proliferation of fatty tissue (c) partially surround by thickened fibrous bands ((d), indicated by "∗"). Focal dilated, thrombotised vessels were also noted (e).

time: 30 min in room temperature), separately. Immunostaining was performed on Leica BOND-MAX autostainer (Leica Microsystems) and we used peroxidase/DAB Bond Polymer Refine Detection System (Leica Microsystems) for visualization. Cytoplasmic staining for vimentin and CD31 and nuclear staining for MDM2 are regarded as positive stain whereas, for S-100 and p16, both nuclear and cytoplasmic stains are required.

3. Results

3.1. Gross Findings. During pathological examination, a polypoid skin-covering subcutaneous lesion was received measured 26 × 22 × 9.5 cm in size. The skin was indurated and hyperpigmented with classical "peau d'orange" appearance (Figure 1(a)). On cut surface revealed the thickened skin (Figure 1(b)). The subcutaneous tissue cut surface revealed

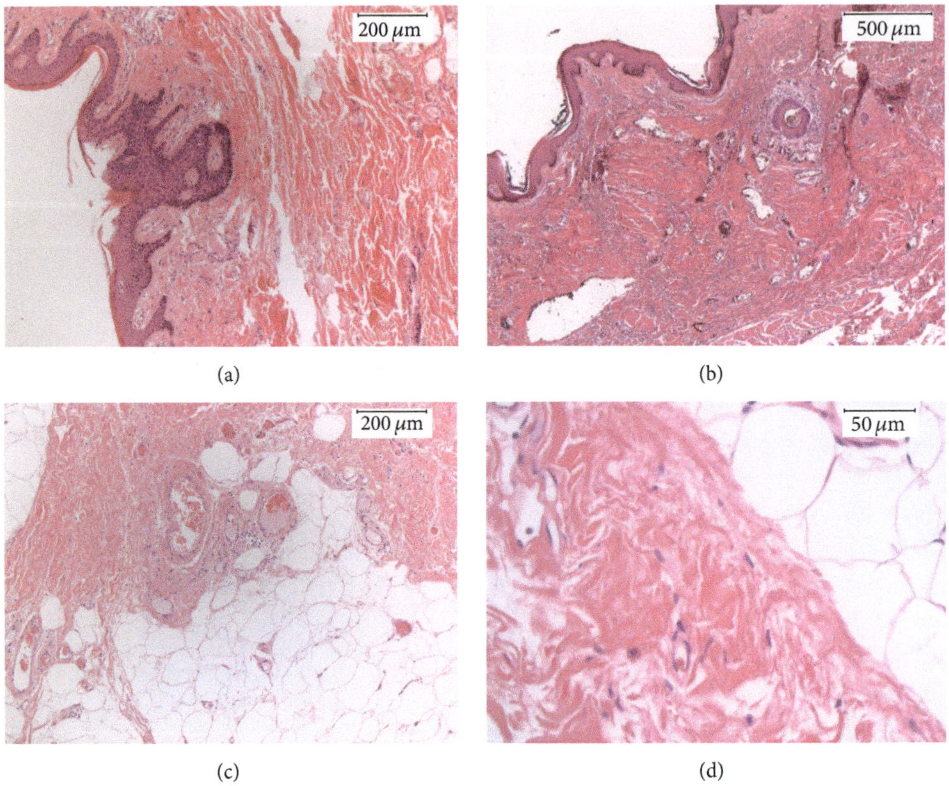

FIGURE 2: Histomorphology of MLL. The epidermis showed mild acanthosis, elongated rete ridges, basal melanocytic proliferation, and hyperpigmentation ((a), 20x). The dermis revealed reactive lobular vascular proliferation with congestion and mild lymphocytic infiltration similar to stasis dermatitis ((b), 10x). The subcutaneous areas show adipose tissue and reactive vascular proliferation ((c), 20x) and reactive fibroblasts ((d), 40x).

clear, serous-like fluid and also massive amount of fat tissue partially surrounded and traversed by thickened fibrous bands (Figures 1(c)-1(d)). Focal dilated, thrombotised vessels were also noted (Figure 1(e)).

3.2. Histopathological Findings. Microscopically, the epidermis showed mild acanthosis, elongated rete ridges, basal melanocytic proliferation, and hyperpigmentation (Figure 2(a)). The dermis revealed reactive lobular congested vascular proliferation (Figure 2(b)) with mild lymphocyte filtration and fibrosis similar to stasis dermatitis. Subcutaneous tissue showed lobulated adipose tissue proliferation traversed by expanded, edematous subcutaneous septa. Scattered reactive fibroblasts are seen; however, the atypical, hyperchromatic stromal cells and lipoblasts, typically seen in well-differentiated liposarcomas, are not identified. Reactive fibroblast and vascular proliferation surrounded the fatty lobules (Figures 2(c) and 2(d)); the latter was also highlighted by CD31 (Figure 3(a)). Mitosis and necrosis were not seen.

Immunohistochemically, the reactive fibroblast cells were stained for vimentin (Figure 3(b)) and they were negative for S-100, MDM2, and p16 (Figures 3(c)–3(e)).

3.3. Clinical Follow-Up Data. The patient underwent follow-up control for 8 months since the operation. No recurrence of the lesion was found and plastic surgery was advised.

4. Discussion

MLL is a rare clinical entity that has relatively few literature published [1, 3, 4]. It is usually associated with lymphedema from variable causes which may lead to lymphatic obstruction and lymphedema. It usually occurs in morbidly obese patient by the weight of large amount of fat which may create an ischemic microenvironment and stimulate a wound-like process that recruits growth factors to the area [2]. The association between MLL and hypothyroidism had been reported as well [2]. Women are more commonly affected than men. The average size of the lesion is 28.5 cm ranging from 19.5 to 61.5 cm [1]. MLL are frequently present for a considerable time before resection and may only reach clinical attention when they interfere with daily activities or are secondarily inflamed. The radiological study usually revealed expanded subcutaneous tissue with soft tissue bands but without a discrete mass lesion which may indicate its adipose tissue nature. The most common location is around the medial aspect of thigh. Recently several reports have documented that MLL can also occur in other areas such as vulva, mons pubis, scrotum, and upper extremity [5–9]. Abdominal localization is relatively rare and clinically is usually underdiagnosed as malignant tumor, particularly well differentiated liposarcoma (WDLPS), based on clinical and radiological impressions [10].

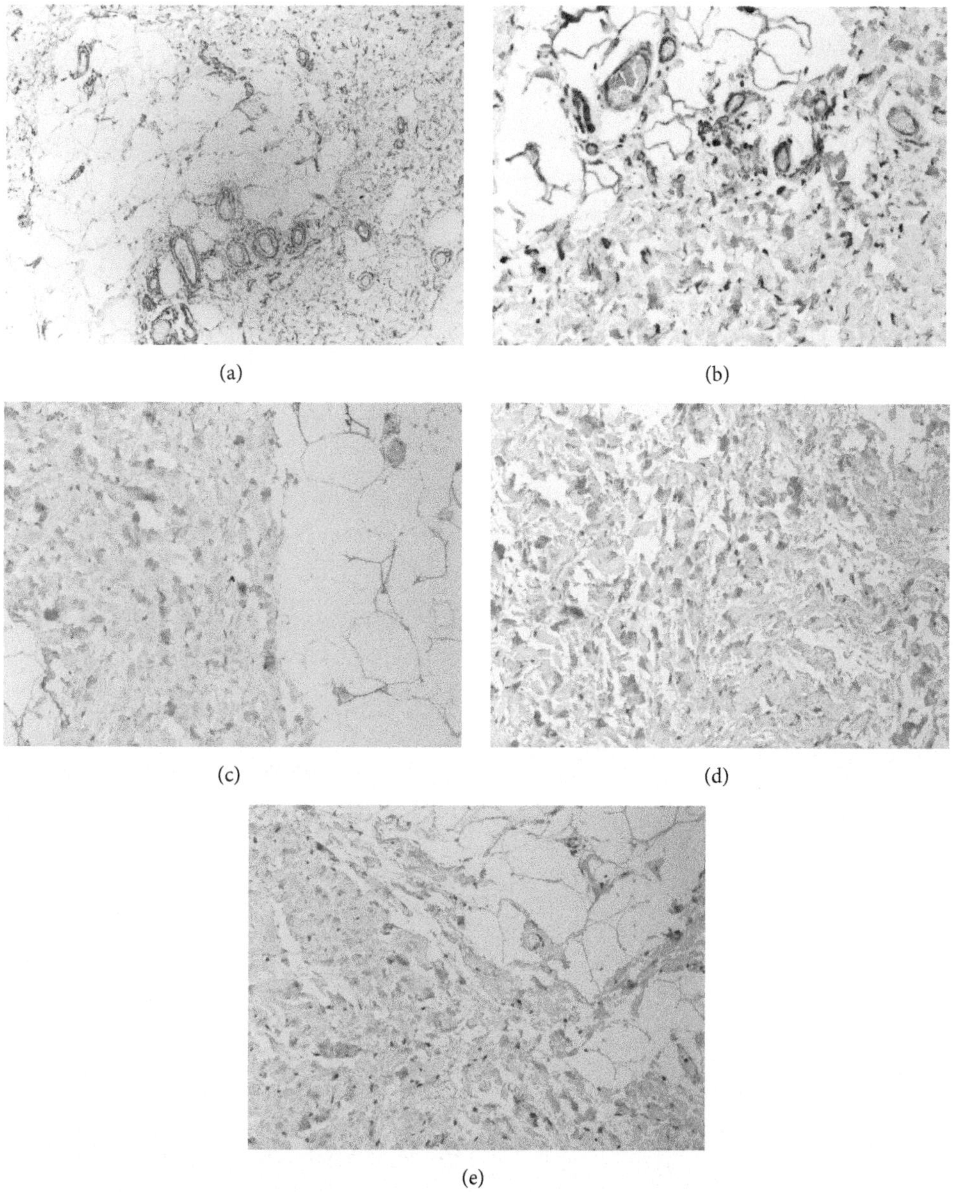

Figure 3: Reactive lobular vascular proliferation, highlighted by CD31 ((a), 10x). The stromal cells are positive for vimentin ((b), 20x) and negative for S-100, MDM2, and p16 ((c)–(e), all 20x).

Indeed, clinical pictures and histologically expanded interlobular septae and massive amount of adipose tissue may mimic WDLPS; nevertheless, lymphedema is a superficial process that involves mainly skin and dermo-/epidermochanges related to chronic lymphedema without rapid growth imply a benign process. WDLPS usually forms a discrete lesion, as opposed to the diffuse changes seen in MLL. In microscopic levels, the presence of widened, edematous fibrous septa together with reactive fibroblasts may mimic WDLP.

In MLL, the adipocytes are evenly sized and lack the characteristic hyperchromatic stromal cells, thick-walled blood vessels containing similar hyperchromatic cells within their walls, and lipoblasts. In challenge cases, immunohistochemical stain for MDM2, CDK4, and p16 [11] or fluorescent in situ hybridization to detect MDM2 gene amplification can confidently separate MLL from WDLPS. Lack of plexiform-type capillaries, myxoid stroma, and lipoblast/round cell can also rule out myxoid liposarcoma. On demand, fluorescent in situ hybridization to detect t(12;16) (*FUS*;*CHOP*) translocation can be used as a confirmation test.

Desmoid-type fibromatosis may also be one of differential diagnoses due to the reactive fibroblasts and fibroedematous stroma. However, similar to WDLPS, desmoid-type fibromatosis usually presents as a discrete fibrous lesion within the soft tissues with long, sweeping fascicles of bland (myo)fibroblasts together with thin-walled, dilated vasculature and perivascular oedema and peripheral chronic inflammatory cell infiltration which cannot be found in MLL. Negative nuclear stain of β-catenin of fibroblast in MLL can also serve as a great diagnostic clue.

Low grade myxofibrosarcoma occurs usually in elderly patient's extremities. It can be differentiated from MLL by its relatively localized nature, atypical hyperchromatic spindle cells, myxoid stroma, and well-developed arcing vasculature.

Since the underlying cause of MLL is lymphatic obstruction possibly due to morbid obesity, persistence or even recurrence of these lesions is expected after the surgical resection although recurrence with an aggressive manner has not been documented [1]. Recently, cases of squamous cell carcinoma and cutaneous angiosarcoma arising from long-standing MLL have been reported [12, 13] probably through similar pathomechanism as Stewart–Treves syndrome. Hence long term follow-up is still recommended.

In conclusion, we present a case of MLL arising from abdominal wall from a morbidly obese patient which is a rare pseudosarcomatous lesion and diagnosis can be challenging for pathologists. Awareness of this rare entity and detailed clinical and radiological information and correlation are required. Differential diagnosis of WDLPS, the most common mimicker, can be ruled out by immunohistochemical stains and fluorescent in situ hybridization. Although rare, secondary sarcomatous transformation had been documented; frequent follow-up is recommended.

Abbreviations

ALT: Atypical lipomatous tumor
IHC: Immunohistochemistry
MLL: Massive localized lymphoedema
WDLPS: Well differentiated liposarcoma.

Consent

Written informed consent was obtained from the patient for publication of this case report and accompanying images.

Conflict of Interests

The authors declare they have no conflict of interests.

Authors' Contribution

Teodóra Tóth and Yi-Che Chang Chien contributed equally. Teodóra Tóth designed and wrote the paper. Yi-Che Chang Chien conceived and designed the paper, helped in performing immunohistochemical stains and interpretation, and also carried out coordination and helped in drafting the paper. Ilona Kovács and Sándor Kollár helped in drafting the paper. All authors read and approved the final paper.

References

[1] M. Manduch, A. M. Oliveira, A. G. Nascimento, and A. L. Folpe, "Massive localised lymphoedema: a clinicopathological study of 22 cases and review of the literature," *Journal of Clinical Pathology*, vol. 62, no. 9, pp. 808–811, 2009.

[2] D. Wu, J. Gibbs, D. Corral, M. Intengan, and J. J. Brooks, "Massive localized lymphedema: additional locations and association with hypothyroidism," *Human Pathology*, vol. 31, no. 9, pp. 1162–1168, 2000.

[3] R. J. Evans and C. Scilley, "Massive localized lymphedema: a case series and literature review," *Canadian Journal of Plastic Surgery*, vol. 19, no. 3, pp. e30–e31, 2011.

[4] G. Farshid and S. W. Weiss, "Massive localized lymphedema in the morbidly obese: a histologically distinct reactive lesion simulating liposarcoma," *The American Journal of Surgical Pathology*, vol. 22, no. 10, pp. 1277–1283, 1998.

[5] G. Bognár, A. Novák, and G. István, "Massive localized lymphoedema (MLL) in the mons pubis," *Magyar Sebészet*, vol. 67, no. 4, pp. 265–267, 2014.

[6] C. Fife, "Massive localized lymphedema, a disease unique to the morbidly obese: a case study," *Ostomy Wound Management*, vol. 60, no. 1, pp. 30–35, 2014.

[7] D. S. Heller, V. A. Fitzhugh, B. Cracchiolo, T. Barrett Jr., and R. S. Suidan, "Massive localized lymphedema of the vulva: report of a case and review of the literature," *Journal of Lower Genital Tract Disease*, vol. 18, no. 2, pp. E46–E49, 2014.

[8] M. Jones, D. Marshall, and D. Mason, "Massive localized lymphoedema," *ANZ Journal of Surgery*, vol. 81, no. 1-2, pp. 103–104, 2011.

[9] S. Lee, J. S. Han, H. M. Ross, and J. I. Epstein, "Massive localized lymphedema of the male external genitalia: a clinicopathologic study of 6 cases," *Human Pathology*, vol. 44, no. 2, pp. 277–281, 2013.

[10] M. S. El-Sharkawy, A. C. Al-Rikabi, N. Alarfaj, and F. M. Al Mugaren, "Localized massive lymphedema masquerading as an anterior abdominal mass mimicking a liposarcoma," *The American Journal of the Medical Sciences*, vol. 347, no. 1, pp. 84–85, 2014.

[11] K. Thway, R. Flora, C. Shah, D. Olmos, and C. Fisher, "Diagnostic utility of p16, CDK4, and MDM2 as an immunohistochemical panel in distinguishing well-differentiated and dedifferentiated liposarcomas from other adipocytic tumors," *The American Journal of Surgical Pathology*, vol. 36, no. 3, pp. 462–469, 2012.

[12] W. Shon, C. M. Ida, J. M. Boland-Froemming, P. S. Rose, and A. Folpe, "Cutaneous angiosarcoma arising in massive localized lymphedema of the morbidly obese: a report of five cases and review of the literature," *Journal of Cutaneous Pathology*, vol. 38, no. 7, pp. 560–564, 2011.

[13] T. Su, H. Lee, H. Gao, S. Nieh, and C. Lin, "Squamous cell carcinoma arising from massive localized lymphedema of scrotum mimicking scrotal smooth muscle hamartoma of darto: a case report," *The American Journal of Dermatopathology*, vol. 37, no. 7, pp. 551–554, 2015.

Congenital Oligodendroglioma: Clinicopathologic and Molecular Assessment with Review of the Literature

Hope Richard,[1] Kimberly Stogner-Underwood,[1,2] and Christine Fuller[1]

[1]*Department of Pathology, Virginia Commonwealth University Health System, 1101 E. Marshall Street, P.O. Box 980662, Richmond, VA 23298, USA*
[2]*Department of Pathology, Wake Forest Baptist Medical Center, Medical Center Boulevard, Winston-Salem, NC 27157, USA*

Correspondence should be addressed to Hope Richard; hrichard@mcvh-vcu.edu

Academic Editor: Hiroko Kuwabara

Oligodendroglioma is an infiltrating glial neoplasm frequently seen in adults. Pediatric oligodendrogliomas are rare, with very few cases presenting in infancy and only rare congenital examples. In contrast to adult oligodendrogliomas, pediatric cases typically lack 1p/19q codeletion. Herein we report a case of WHO grade II oligodendroglioma diagnosed in a 7-month-old male infant. The patient initially presented at 3 months of age with symptoms suspicious for seizure. Initial workup including electroencephalography (EEG), electrocardiogram (EKG), and computed tomography (CT) of the head was negative. His symptoms persisted, and subsequent magnetic resonance imaging (MRI) performed at age of 7 months revealed a 2 cm contrast-enhancing left temporal lobe mass. The mass was excised and the microscopic appearance was that of a classic low grade oligodendroglioma composed of cells with uniformly round nuclei, perinuclear halos, delicate branching capillaries, and an absence of high grade features. Mutant specific (R132H) isocitrate dehydrogenase-1 (IDH1) immunohistochemistry was negative, and the tumor lacked detectable 1p or 19q deletions by fluorescent in situ hybridization (FISH). The onset of neurological symptoms in early infancy followed by the positive MRI findings suggests that this case represents a rare example of congenital oligodendroglioma.

1. Introduction

As a group, gliomas are the most common primary central nervous system (CNS) neoplasms in both adult and pediatric populations, whereas infiltrative gliomas, in particular glioblastoma, make up the bulk of adult glial tumors, pilocytic astrocytoma, and ependymoma predominate in children. Oligodendrogliomas may be encountered at any age; however, they are generally infrequent in the pediatric population. Congenital examples, those presenting at or shortly after birth, are even rarer. Here we describe a case we believe to represent a congenital oligodendroglioma, the patient initially presenting with seizure-like activity at three months of age.

2. Case Report

A 3-month-old male infant was brought to the Emergency Department (ED) for evaluation of multiple episodes of presumed seizure activity. The episodes, which lasted 20–25 seconds, were described as staring spells accompanied by apnea and perioral cyanosis. A period of deep sleep followed, and upon waking the infant returned to baseline activity. No seizure activity was identified on electroencephalogram (EEG), and computed tomography (CT) of the head was negative for the presence of an intracranial abnormality. He was diagnosed with reflux and started on an antacid and specific feeding regimen. Seizure-like activity continued and follow-up magnetic resonance imaging (MRI) performed at 7 months of age revealed a 2 cm left temporal lobe lesion which was hyperintense on both T2-weighted (Figure 1(d)) and FLAIR images and isointense on T1 sequences (Figure 1(a)). The lesion enhanced heterogeneously with contrast (Figures 1(b) and 1(c)); however, no definite cysts or calcifications were detected. Gross total surgical resection of the mass was accomplished.

Histologically, tumor consisted of a monomorphous population of cells with round, regular nuclei surrounded by clear

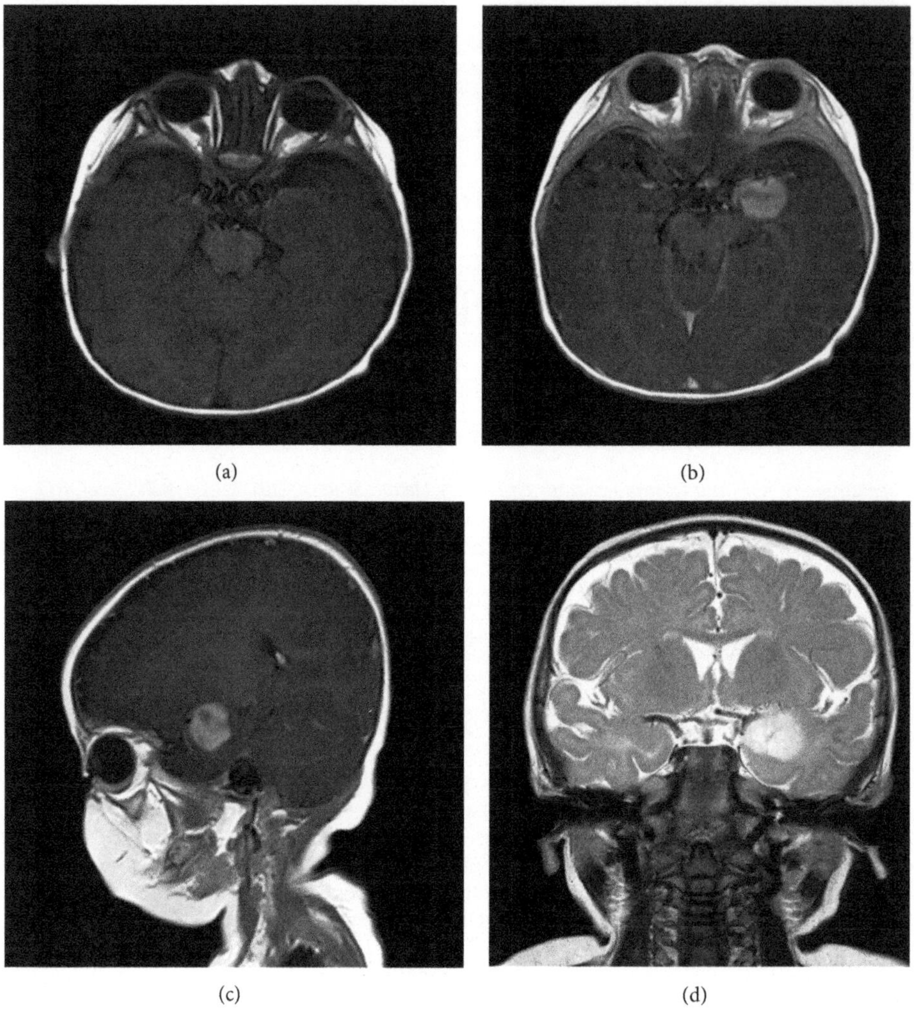

Figure 1: (a) Axial T1 precontrast, (b) axial T1 postcontrast, (c) sagittal T1 postcontrast, and (d) coronal T2 magnetic resonance imaging show a heterogeneously enhancing mass in the left temporal lobe.

perinuclear halos. Delicate, branching capillaries were interspersed throughout the tumor and calcifications were present focally. High grade features such as necrosis, microvascular proliferation, frequent mitoses, and nuclear pleomorphism were absent. The morphologic appearance was that of a classic low grade oligodendroglioma (Figures 2(a) and 2(b)). By immunohistochemistry, the tumor cells showed nuclear labeling for S100, with diffuse background staining for both S100 and glial fibrillary acidic protein (GFAP). Synaptophysin and mutant-specific isocitrate dehydrogenase-1 (R132H) immunohistochemistry were negative (Figures 2(c) and 2(d)). The Ki-67 labeling index was low (<1%) (Figure 2(e)). Fluorescent in situ hybridization (FISH) testing confirmed the absence of deletion of either chromosome 1p or 19q (Figure 2(f)).

Follow-up revealed that at five years of age the patient is clinically stable. A small focus of enhancement was identified on MRI at his one-year follow-up; however, this lesion has remained stable to date.

3. Discussion

As a group, glial neoplasms are by far the most common CNS tumors arising in the pediatric population, with astrocytomas and ependymomas representing the majority of these tumors. Oligodendrogliomas account for less than 3% of primary CNS tumors in children [1]. Congenital brain tumors are quite rare, the most common being teratoma, astrocytoma, medulloblastoma, choroid plexus papilloma, and ependymoma [2, 3]. Congenital oligodendroglial tumors are even rarer. Reported cases of congenital oligodendroglioma range from cases identified in utero [3] or within the first few days of life [2] to cases presumed to be congenital, with a tumor diagnosed in the first few months of life [4, 5]. Presenting signs and symptoms of these patients have included decreased fetal movement [3], seizure, headache, visual field defects, weakness, cranial nerve palsy [6], irritability [2], and apnea [4]. The report of one case noted an initial presentation of jaundice [2], thought to be secondary to hemorrhage within the tumor.

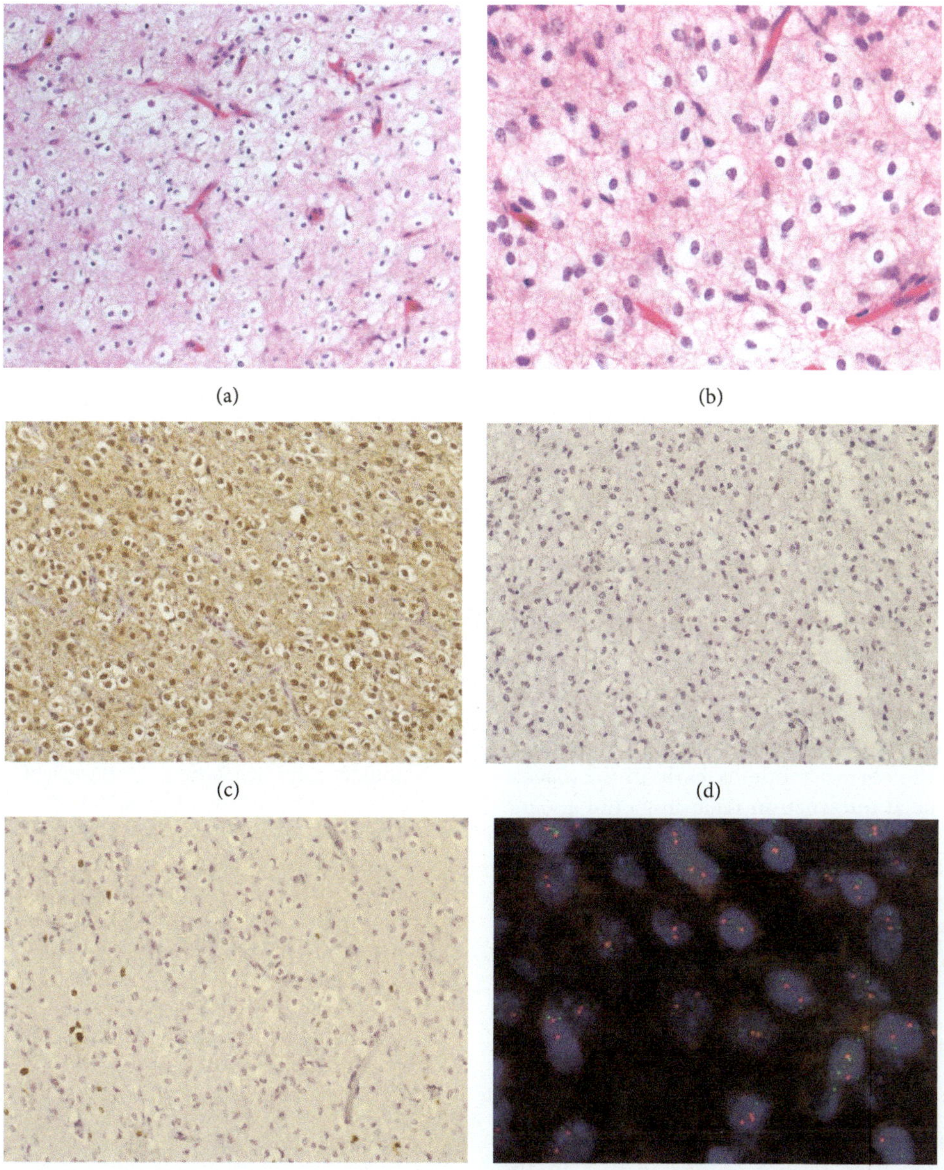

(a) (b) (c) (d) (e) (f)

FIGURE 2: H&E stained sections at 20x (a) and 40x (b). Cytoplasmic and nuclear staining with S100 (c). Negative staining for mutant specific (R132H) IDH-1 (d). Low proliferation index (<1%) by Ki67 immunohistochemistry (e). Intact 1p and 19q by FISH (f).

The early onset of neurologic symptoms in the current case is most consistent with a congenital oligodendroglioma.

A number of alternate diagnoses should be considered when an oligodendroglial-like lesion is encountered in a child. These include neurocytoma, other gliomas such as astrocytoma and clear cell ependymoma, and dysembryoplastic neuroepithelial tumor (DNET). In the current case, S-100 positivity confirms a neuroectodermal origin. The lack of synaptophysin positivity makes a diagnosis of neurocytoma unlikely. Other glial neoplasms are made less likely by the classic oligodendroglial morphology seen in this tumor, including round, regular nuclei surrounded by perinuclear halos and interspersed fine, branching capillaries; there was likewise a lack of astrocytic morphology or classic features of ependymoma, such as perivascular pseudorosettes or ependymal canals. Pilocytic astrocytomas may contain areas with oligodendroglioma-like morphology; however, the current tumor lacks the typical piloid processes and biphasic architecture of a pilocytic astrocytoma, and no Rosenthal fibers or eosinophilic granular bodies were identified. DNETs can contain areas resembling oligodendroglial morphology, with small, round cells with perinuclear halos, but these lesions also have patterned nodules and a neuronal component not seen in the present tumor. Another rare entity that should be considered is leptomeningeal oligodenrogliomatosis. The histologic features are that of a classic oligodendroglioma and can have low or high grade features; however, the radiologic appearance consists predominately of focal or diffuse leptomeningeal enhancement as opposed to a mass forming lesion within the cortex [7, 8].

Codeletion of 1p and 19q is a frequent finding in oligodendroglial neoplasms in the adult population but is much less common in pediatric oligodendrogliomas, especially in children less than 10 years old [1, 5, 9, 10]. Recently, Rodriguez et al. examined a group of 50 pediatric patients with oligodendrogliomas; they found that, with rare exception, patients with 1p/19q codeleted tumors were older than 16 at the time of diagnosis. Therefore, the lack of the 1p/19q codeletion in the present case is not unexpected and does not conflict with the diagnosis of congenital oligodendroglioma. Likewise, although adult oligodendrogliomas frequently harbor detectable isocitrate dehydrogenase (IDH1) mutations, these mutations are almost always absent in pediatric gliomas [5, 11, 12]. In the series presented by Rodriguez et al., mutant IDH1 (R132H) immunohistochemistry was only positive in a subset of their 1p/19q codeleted pediatric oligodendrogliomas. Based on these previous reports, the expectation is that congenital gliomas (including congenital oligodendroglioma) would similarly be negative for the mutant specific IDH1 immunohistochemical stain, as was exhibited in the current case.

Structural neuroimaging plays an important diagnostic and prognostic role in children presenting with acute onset epilepsy. Choosing the correct modality early in the disease process provides crucial information regarding etiology and allows identification of lesions requiring surgical intervention. Although MRI is the imaging modality of choice in these cases because of superior anatomic resolution [13–15], computed tomography (CT) is advantageous in the resolution of blood and calcification [13]. Additionally, CT scans are cheaper, more widely available and are less likely to require sedation in young children. Coupled with EEG, as was done in the reported case, CT scan is described as an acceptable screening tool but is not definitive for the resolution of mass lesions [13, 16]. The current case underscores the importance of choosing the most appropriate imaging modality as the described lesion may have been identified earlier in the disease course with MRI.

In conclusion, this case of a low grade oligodendroglioma presenting within the first few months of life represents a rare example of congenital oligodendroglioma and underscores the importance of maintaining these tumors in the differential diagnosis of infants presenting with new-onset seizures. Similar to previously reported pediatric oligodendrogliomas, this congenital tumor was negative for 1p/19q codeletion as well as for R132H mutant specific IDH1 by immunohistochemistry. Though as a group pediatric oligodendroglioma patients have demonstrated good overall survival, particularly in those patients with nonanaplastic tumor histology [5], our experience with congenital oligodendrogliomas remains limited, warranting close clinical and radiologic follow-up for these unique patients.

Conflict of Interests

The authors declare that there is no conflict of interests regarding the publication of this paper.

References

[1] C. E. Fuller, *Oligodendrogilal Tumors*, Springer, New York, NY, USA, 1st edition, 2010.

[2] W.-S. Hsieh, R.-I. Lien, T.-N. Lui, C.-R. Wang, and S.-M. Jung, "Congenital oligodendroglioma with initial manifestation of jaundice," *Pediatric Neurology*, vol. 27, no. 3, pp. 230–233, 2002.

[3] T. Narita, H. Kurotaki, T. Hashimoto, and Y. Ogawa, "Congenital oligodendroglioma: a case of a 34th-gestational week fetus with immunohistochemical study and review of the literature," *Human Pathology*, vol. 28, no. 10, pp. 1213–1217, 1997.

[4] A. H. Koeppen and R. J. Cassidy, "Oligodendroglioma of the medulla oblongata in a neonate," *Archives of Neurology*, vol. 38, no. 8, pp. 520–523, 1981.

[5] F. J. Rodriguez, T. Tihan, D. Lin et al., "Clinicopathologic features of pediatric oligodendrogliomas: a series of 50 patients," *The American Journal of Surgical Pathology*, vol. 38, no. 8, pp. 1058–1070, 2014.

[6] N. Razack, J. Baumgartner, and J. Bruner, "Pediatric oligodendrogliomas," *Pediatric Neurosurgery*, vol. 28, no. 3, pp. 121–129, 1998.

[7] F. J. Rodriguez, A. Perry, M. K. Rosenblum et al., "Disseminated oligodendroglial-like leptomeningeal tumor of childhood: a distinctive clinicopathologic entity," *Acta Neuropathologica*, vol. 124, no. 5, pp. 627–641, 2012.

[8] D. M. Armao, J. Stone, M. Castillo, K.-M. Mitchell, T. W. Bouldin, and K. Suzuki, "Diffuse leptomeningeal oligodendrogliomatosis: Radiologic/pathologic correlation," *The American Journal of Neuroradiology*, vol. 21, no. 6, pp. 1122–1126, 2000.

[9] R. Raghavan, J. Balani, A. Perry et al., "Pediatric oligodendrogliomas: a study of molecular alterations on 1p and 19q using fluorescence in situ hybridization," *Journal of Neuropathology and Experimental Neurology*, vol. 62, no. 5, pp. 530–537, 2003.

[10] P. A. Kreiger, Y. Okada, S. Simon, L. B. Rorke, D. N. Louis, and J. A. Golden, "Losses of chromosomes 1p and 19q are rare in pediatric oligodendrogliomas," *Acta Neuropathologica*, vol. 109, no. 4, pp. 387–392, 2005.

[11] H. Yan, D. W. Parsons, G. Jin et al., "IDH1 and IDH2 mutations in gliomas," *The New England Journal of Medicine*, vol. 360, no. 8, pp. 765–773, 2009.

[12] V. Suri, P. Jha, S. Agarwal et al., "Molecular profile of oligodendrogliomas in young patients," *Neuro-Oncology*, vol. 13, no. 10, pp. 1099–1106, 2011.

[13] W. D. Gaillard, C. Chiron, J. Helen Cross et al., "Guidelines for imaging infants and children with recent-onset epilepsy," *Epilepsia*, vol. 50, no. 9, pp. 2147–2153, 2009.

[14] D. T. Hsieh, T. Chang, T. N. Tsuchida et al., "New-onset afebrile seizures in infants: role of neuroimaging," *Neurology*, vol. 74, no. 2, pp. 150–156, 2010.

[15] R. I. Kuzniecky and R. C. Knowlton, "Neuroimaging of epilepsy," *Seminars in Neurology*, vol. 22, no. 3, pp. 279–281, 2002.

[16] J. Maytal, J. M. Krauss, G. Novak, J. Nagelberg, and M. Patel, "The role of brain computed tomography in evaluating children with new onset of seizures in the emergency department," *Epilepsia*, vol. 41, no. 8, pp. 950–954, 2000.

9

Extramedullary Hematopoiesis in a Sentinel Lymph Node as an Early Sign of Chronic Myelomonocytic Leukemia

Joslin M. Bowen,[1] Anamarija M. Perry,[2] Erin Quist,[3] and Mojtaba Akhtari[4]

[1] *Physicians Laboratory, 4840 F Street, Omaha, NE 68117, USA*
[2] *Department of Pathology, University of Manitoba, MS559S Thorlakson Building, 820 Sherbrook Street, Winnipeg, MB, Canada R3A 1R9*
[3] *Department of Pathology and Microbiology, University of Nebraska Medical Center, 985900 Nebraska Medical Center, Omaha, NE 68198, USA*
[4] *Jane Anne Nohl Division of Hematology and Center for the Study of Blood Diseases, University of Southern California (USC) and Norris Cancer Center, USC University Hospital, 1441 Eastlake Avenue, Norris Topping Tower 3463, MC 9172, Los Angeles, CA 90033-9172, USA*

Correspondence should be addressed to Anamarija M. Perry; anamarijamorovic@hotmail.com

Academic Editor: Sami Shousha

Chronic myelomonocytic leukemia (CMML) is a clonal hematopoietic malignancy with features of both a myeloproliferative neoplasm and a myelodysplastic syndrome. Even though extramedullary leukemic infiltration is common in CMML patients, lymph node involvement has rarely been reported in the literature. We present an unusual case of a 72-year-old female who was found to have extramedullary hematopoiesis (EMH) in a sentinel lymph node that was excised during mastectomy for lobular breast carcinoma. One year later bone marrow biopsy was performed due to persistent anemia, thrombocytopenia, and monocytosis and the patient was diagnosed with CMML. Our case illustrates the importance of recognizing EMH in a lymph node during routine histological examination, especially in adults. Proliferation of bone marrow elements in a lymph node, in a patient with no known hematologic disorder, should trigger immediate bone marrow evaluation, as this could be the first clue in diagnosing underlying bone marrow disorder.

1. Introduction

Chronic myelomonocytic leukemia (CMML) is a clonal hematopoietic malignancy characterized by overlapping features of both a myeloproliferative neoplasm and a myelodysplastic syndrome [1, 2]. The 2008 World Health Organization (WHO) classification defines CMML using the following criteria: (1) persistent monocytosis of $>1 \times 10^9$ in the peripheral blood (PB), (2) absence of Philadelphia chromosome and *BCR-ABL1* fusion gene, (3) no rearrangement of *PDGFRA* or *PDGFRB* in the cases with eosinophilia, (4) fewer than 20% blasts and/or promonocytes in the PB and bone marrow (BM), and (5) dysplasia involving one or more myeloid lineages [1]. Clinically, PB and BM are always involved. Extramedullary leukemic infiltration can be seen in CMML, and it is most commonly encountered in spleen and liver [1, 3]. Disease less frequently involves other sites such as skin and genitourinary tract [4–6]. Lymph node enlargement in CMML has been reported in the older literature (i.e., before the advent of 2001 WHO classification [7]) in 14% to 30% of patients [3, 8]; however, there are very few reports in the literature that histologically describe involved lymph nodes [8–11].

Herein, we report an unusual case of a 72-year-old female who was found to have extramedullary hematopoiesis in a sentinel lymph node, excised for lobular carcinoma of the breast, and was diagnosed with CMML one year later. Extramedullary hematopoiesis in a sentinel lymph node can be considered as an early sign of CMML.

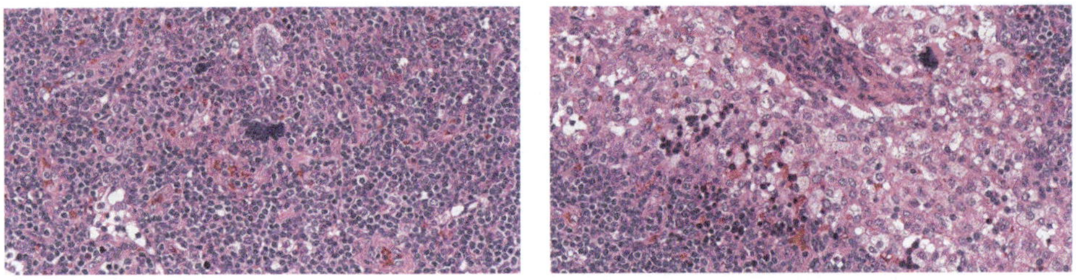

(a) (b)

Figure 1: (a) Paracortical area of the lymph node with extramedullary hematopoiesis (H&E ×200); (b) extramedullary hematopoiesis in the lymph node sinus with prominent red blood cell precursors and megakaryocytes (H&E ×200).

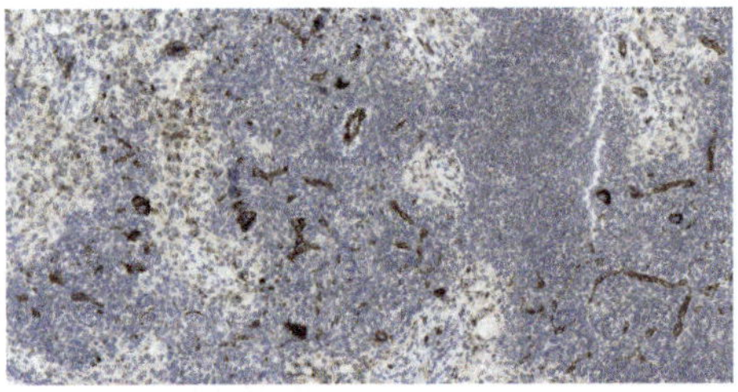

Figure 2: Immunohistochemical stain for Factor VII shows positivity in megakaryocytes (×100).

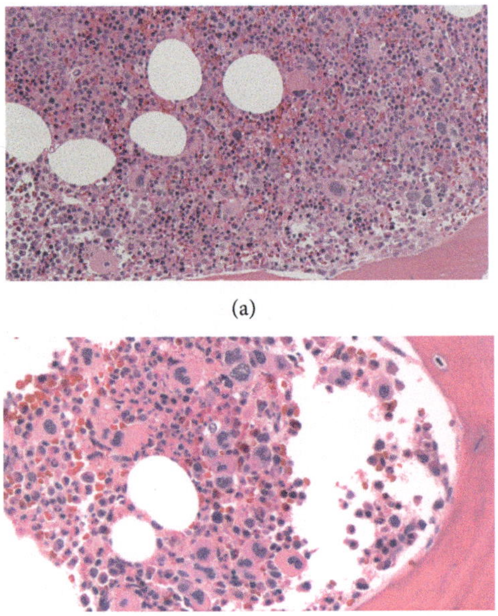

(a)

(b)

Figure 3: (a) Hypercellular bone marrow with increase in all three hematopoietic lineages (H&E ×100); (b) prominent dysplasia and clustering of megakaryocytes (H&E ×200).

2. Case Presentation

A 72-year-old lady was found to have a 1 cm spiculated lesion on screening mammography. She underwent mastectomy and sentinel lymph node excision for a biopsy proven lobular breast carcinoma. Sentinel lymph node showed overall preserved architecture with follicular and paracortical hyperplasia and dilated sinuses. In the paracortical area (Figure 1(a)) and the sinuses (Figure 1(b)) there were small clusters of immature erythroid cells, as well as scattered megakaryocytes, consistent with extramedullary hematopoiesis (EMH). Megakaryocytes showed dyspoietic changes including hyperlobation and hyperchromatic nuclei. There was no significant dyspoiesis in erythroid precursors. Myeloid precursors were not prominent component of the EMH. There was no morphological increase in blasts or promonocytes. Immunohistochemical stain for Factor VIII further highlighted the megakaryocytes (Figure 2). One year later, the patient was referred to a hematologist for worsening anemia (hemoglobin 10.5 g/dL; normal range, 11.5–15.5 g/dL) and thrombocytopenia (platelets ranged from 89,000 to 124,000/μL; normal range, 150,000–400,000/μL), and persistent monocytosis (absolute monocyte count $1.2 \times 10^3/\mu$L; normal range, $0.1\text{–}1.0 \times 10^3/\mu$L). Of note, absolute monocyte count at the time of the sentinel lymph node biopsy one year prior was $1.5 \times 10^3/\mu$L. The patient underwent a bone marrow biopsy which showed markedly hypercellular marrow for patient's age (80% cellularity; Figure 3(a)). Dyspoiesis was present in all three hematopoietic lineages but most prominent in megakaryocytes that showed clustering with numerous small and hypolobated forms (Figure 3(b)). There was prominent monocytosis with 18% monocytes by differential count. Blasts (including promonocytes) were not significantly increased and by differential counts were <5% in the PB and <10% in the BM. There was moderate (grade 2/3) diffuse reticulin fibrosis. Conventional cytogenetic studies showed the following karyotype: 46,XX,del(20)(q11.2q13.3)[20]. Fluorescence in situ hybridization studies showed del20q12 and del20q13. Molecular studies were negative for *JAK2* V617F mutation and for *BCL-ABL1* fusion gene. The patient was diagnosed with CMML-1. She became symptomatic due to progressive anemia and was initially treated with 6 cycles of azacitidine, to which she responded; however, she lost her response after 8 cycles. Her regimen was then switched to decitabine, to which she had a fair response. Her general condition started deteriorating; she had prolonged neutropenia and passed away due to septic shock.

3. Discussion

Extramedullary hematopoiesis is a result of conditions that disrupt the bone marrow microenvironment, facilitating the egress of precursor cell, with an increase in circulating mature and immature marrow elements. After birth, there is normally very little proliferation of hematopoietic elements outside the marrow. Extramedullary hematopoiesis occurs in a number of conditions, including benign hematologic disorders (e.g., thalassemia, hereditary spherocytosis, sickle cell anemia, and congenital dyserythroblastic anemia), hematopoietic neoplasms, stromal disorders of the marrow (e.g., osteopetrosis), nonhematopoietic tumors, infectious, and storage diseases, as well as disorders of the circulation [12, 13]. In a case of hematopoietic neoplasm that involves extramedullary site, better term to use is neoplastic myeloid proliferation (NMP), to differentiate it from EMH that occurs as a consequence of benign disorders. Neoplastic myeloid proliferation can be seen in association with myeloproliferative neoplasms, myelodysplastic syndromes, myelodysplastic/myeloproliferative neoplasms, and other myeloid derived malignancies [13]. Extramedullary hematopoiesis has been reported in almost all body sites, including lymph nodes [12–14].

In the case of our patient, EMH was an incidental finding in a sentinel lymph node that was excised due to lobular carcinoma of the breast. Proliferation of bone marrow elements in a lymph node is not considered normal in an adult and should prompt an immediate search for an underlying bone marrow disorder [13]. However, our patient was not evaluated for hematologic neoplasm until a year later when she was referred to a hematologist for worsening cytopenias and was diagnosed with CMML. Median survival of CMML patients is 20–40 months and multiple drugs are being used in treatment of this disease [1, 2]. Delay in diagnosis and treatment could potentially shorten patient's survival. In children, the presence of EMH in lymph nodes could indicate undiagnosed benign hematologic disorder, and lymphadenopathy with EMH may be an initial manifestation [13]. Even though lymph node involvement, detected by imaging studies, is not uncommon in patients with myeloproliferative/myelodysplastic neoplasms, routine lymph node biopsies are not performed in these patients [3, 8, 14]. Sudden appearance of lymphadenopathy can also indicate transformation to acute myeloid leukemia/myeloid sarcoma [11].

Several authors have reported EMH in axillary lymph nodes following neoadjuvant therapy for breast cancer [15–17]. This finding is likely related to use of bone marrow suppressing chemotherapeutic agents along with granulocyte colony stimulating factors in these patients [16]. Extramedullary hematopoiesis in a lymph node is a potential diagnostic pitfall in these cases as it could be mistaken for metastatic carcinoma. Furthermore, presence of EMH can be especially problematic when evaluating lymph nodes during frozen section where morphology is frequently less than optimal [15, 16]. Our patient did not receive neoadjuvant chemotherapy prior to lymph node sampling, but it is important to keep this "phenomenon" in differential diagnosis in patients with a history of chemotherapy.

In conclusion, our case illustrates the importance of recognizing EMH in a lymph node during routine histological examination, especially in adults, since it can be an early sign of an underlying hematological malignancy. Proliferation of bone marrow elements in a lymph node, in a patient with no known hematologic disorder, should trigger immediate bone marrow evaluation, as this could be the first clue in diagnosing underlying bone marrow disorder.

Conflict of Interests

The authors declare that there is no conflict of interests regarding the publication of this paper.

References

[1] A. Orazi, J. M. Bennett, U. Germing, R. D. Brunning, B. J. Bain, and J. Thiele, "Chronic myelomonocytic leukemia," in *WHO Classification of Tumours of Haematopoietic and Lymphoid Tissues*, S. H. Swerdlow, E. Campo, N. L. Harris et al., Eds., pp. 76–79, IARC, Lyon, France, 2008.

[2] M. M. Patnaik, S. A. Parikh, C. A. Hanson, and A. Tefferi, "Chronic myelomonocytic leukaemia: a concise clinical and pathophysiological review," *British Journal of Haematology*, vol. 165, no. 3, pp. 273–286, 2014.

[3] Groupe Français de Cytogénétique Hématologique, "Chronic myelomonocytic leukemia: single entity or heterogeneous disorder?: a prospective multicenter study of 100 patients," *Cancer Genetics and Cytogenetics*, vol. 55, no. 1, pp. 57–65, 1991.

[4] N. M. Corcoran, A. Tsui, A. J. Costello, and D. Bouchier-Hayes, "Unilateral testicular mass in man with chronic myelomonocytic leukemia: unusual presentation of chronic myelomonocytic leukemia sequela," *Urology*, vol. 65, no. 5, p. 1001, 2005.

[5] E. S. Hyams, R. Gupta, J. Melamed, S. S. Taneja, and O. Shah, "Renal involvement by chronic myelomonocytic leukemia requiring nephroureterectomy," *Reviews in Urology*, vol. 11, no. 1, pp. 33–37, 2009.

[6] R. A. Mathew, J. M. Bennett, J. J. Liu et al., "Cutaneous manifestations in CMML: indication of disease acceleration or transformation to AML and review of the literature," *Leukemia Research*, vol. 36, no. 1, pp. 72–80, 2012.

[7] E. S. Jaffe, N. L. Harris, H. Stein et al., Eds., *World Health Organization Classification of Tumours: Pathology and Genetics of Tumours of Haematopoietic and Lymphoid Tissues*, IARC Press, Lyon, France, 2001.

[8] A. E. Hunter, N. H. Russell, and I. Ellis, "Extramedullary haemopoiesis as a cause of mediastinal lymphadenopathy in chronic myelomonocytic leukaemia," *Clinical and Laboratory Haematology*, vol. 12, no. 4, pp. 465–469, 1990.

[9] A. Manoharan, "Malignant pleural effusion in chronic myelomonocytic leukaemia," *Thorax*, vol. 46, no. 6, pp. 461–462, 1991.

[10] X. Gong, X. Lu, Y. Fu et al., "Cytological features of chronic myelomonocytic leukaemia in pleural effusion and lymph node fine needle aspiration," *Cytopathology*, vol. 21, no. 6, pp. 411–413, 2010.

[11] T. Derlin, T. S. Clauditz, and P. Bannas, "18F-FDG PET/CT for staging and detection of extramedullary organ involvement in chronic myelomonocytic leukemia," *Clinical Nuclear Medicine*, vol. 39, no. 9, pp. 811–812, 2014.

[12] D. P. O'Malley, Y. S. Kim, S. L. Perkins, L. Baldridge, B. E. Juliar, and A. Orazi, "Morphologic and immunohistochemical evaluation of splenic hematopoietic proliferations in neoplastic

and benign disorders," *Modern Pathology*, vol. 18, no. 12, pp. 1550–1561, 2005.

[13] D. P. O'Malley, "Benign extramedullary myeloid proliferations," *Modern Pathology*, vol. 20, no. 4, pp. 405–415, 2007.

[14] D. Sohawon, K. K. Lau, T. Lau, and D. K. Bowden, "Extramedullary haematopoiesis: a pictorial review of its typical and atypical locations," *Journal of Medical Imaging and Radiation Oncology*, vol. 56, no. 5, pp. 538–544, 2012.

[15] E. K. A. Millar, S. Inder, and J. Lynch, "Extramedullary haematopoiesis in axillary lymph nodes following neoadjuvant chemotherapy for locally advanced breast cancer—a potential diagnostic pitfall," *Histopathology*, vol. 54, no. 5, pp. 622–623, 2009.

[16] C. Prieto-Granada, N. Setia, and C. N. Otis, "Lymph node extramedullary hematopoiesis in breast cancer patients receiving neoadjuvant therapy: a potential diagnostic pitfall," *International Journal of Surgical Pathology*, vol. 21, no. 3, pp. 264–266, 2013.

[17] A. S. Takhar, A. Ney, M. Patel, and A. Sharma, "Extramedullary haematopoiesis in axillary lymph nodes following neoadjuvant chemotherapy for locally advanced breast cancer," *BMJ Case Reports*, 2013.

10

Cytological Features of a Variant NUT Midline Carcinoma of the Lung Harboring the *NSD3-NUT* Fusion Gene: A Case Report and Literature Review

Shiho Kuroda,[1] Shioto Suzuki,[1] Akira Kurita,[1] Mari Muraki,[1] Yoichiro Aoshima,[2] Fumihiko Tanioka,[1] and Haruhiko Sugimura[3]

[1] *Division of Pathology, Iwata City Hospital, 512-3 Ookubo, Iwata, Shizuoka 438-8550, Japan*
[2] *Division of Respiratory Medicine, Iwata City Hospital, 512-3 Ookubo, Iwata, Shizuoka 438-8550, Japan*
[3] *Department of Tumor Pathology, Hamamatsu University School of Medicine, 1-20-1 Handayama, Higashi-ku, Hamamatsu, Shizuoka 431-3192, Japan*

Correspondence should be addressed to Shioto Suzuki; shiosuzuki-path@umin.net

Academic Editor: Imtiaz A. Chaudhry

Background. Nuclear protein in testis (NUT) midline carcinoma (NMC) is a very rare and aggressive malignancy. In more than two-thirds of these NMC cases, a fusion between *NUT* and *BRD4* or *BRD3* has been documented; other variants are rare. The cytology of NMC itself has been sparsely documented and that of variant NMC has never been reported. *Case Presentation.* A 36-year-old woman was admitted because of a rapidly progressing lung tumor with metastases to the breast and bone. We recently reported this patient as the first case of a variant NMC of the lung harboring an *NSD3-NUT* fusion, based on immunohistochemical and genetic analyses. Cytological material was available for the present review. A highly cellular smear contained a predominantly noncohesive pattern of monomorphic cells with diameters 2–2.5 times greater than those of small lymphocytes, with a round-to-oval nucleus, slightly irregular nuclear contours, variably prominent nucleoli, scant cytoplasm, and identifiable mitotic figures. Foci of stratification and overt pearl formation, including a dyskeratocyte, were occasionally observed. The necrotic background contained naked nuclei, karyorrhectic debris, apoptotic cells, and macrophages phagocytizing karyorrhectic debris; nuclear crushing was noted. *Conclusion.* The cytological features of a variant NMC of the lung are described for the first time.

1. Introduction

Nuclear protein in testis (NUT) midline carcinoma (NMC) is a recently recognized entity that is characterized by undifferentiated morphological features and immunoreactivity to NUT [1]. This disease is a very rare [2–4] and aggressive [3, 4] malignancy that most often occurs in the midline of the body, including the head and neck and the mediastinum [2, 4]. Currently, the diagnosis of NMC depends on the identification of a rearrangement involving the *NUT* locus at 15q14 that generates a specific fusion transcript with a member of the bromodomain-containing protein (BRD) family, such as *BRD4* located on chromosome 19p13.1. In more than two-thirds of NMC cases, a gene fusion between *NUT* and *BRD4* or *BRD3* has been documented [2, 5–7]; other variant fusions are rare [6]. Recently, we described a variant NMC in which an *NSD3- (nuclear receptor binding SET domain 3-) NUT* rearrangement was identified in the primary tissue using 5′-rapid amplification of the cDNA end (RACE); the fusion was validated using fluorescence *in situ* hybridization (FISH) [8].

Little information is available on the cytological features of NMC. Three reports have described the cytological features of 4 common NMC cases [9, 10] and another NMC case in which the gene rearrangement was not analyzed [11], and no information on the cytology of variant NMC is presently available. We herein describe, for the first time, the cytological features of a variant NMC of the lung harboring an *NSD3-NUT* fusion gene.

2. Clinical Summary

A 36-year-old woman sought medical advice because of a cough accompanied by wheezing with a 2-month duration. An enhanced computed tomography scan performed at the time of hospitalization revealed a mass (75 × 38 × 35 mm in size) in the left lung that extended to the middle mediastinum; metastatic lesions in the liver, breast, bones, and lymph nodes were also detected [8]. A transbronchial biopsy (TBB) of the lung tumor and an endobronchial ultrasound-guided transbronchial needle aspiration (EBUS-TBNA) of a lower mediastinal lymph node with lung tumor involvement were performed.

3. Materials and Methods

The aspiration material obtained from the lymph node was separated into two parts; its small portion was available for cytological investigation. The specimen was air-dried and Hemacolor-stained (MERCK, Darmstadt, Germany) at bedside according to the manufacturer's instructions and a portion was fixed in 95% ethanol and stained with Papanicolaou as ordinary methods. The larger part of the aspiration material obtained from the lymph node and the biopsy material taken from the lung tumor were immediately immersed in 20% buffered neutral formalin, fixed overnight, and embedded in paraffin. These specimens were then sectioned and used for hematoxylin-eosin staining, immunohistochemistry with antibodies for EMA (DAKO, Glostrup, Denmark), p63 (Santa Cruz Biotechnology, Dallas, TX, USA), cytokeratin AE1/AE3 (DAKO), cytokeratin CAM 5.2 (Becton, Dickinson and Company, CA, USA), CD138 (DAKO), vimentin (DAKO), and others, and FISH, as reported previously [8].

3.1. Cytological Findings. An overview of the Papanicolaou-stained smear showed the specimen to be highly cellular with loosely cohesive cells and/or isolated cells (Figure 1). The cells were 2–2.5 times greater in diameter than that of a small lymphocyte. The nuclei were round to oval in shape and had slightly irregular contours, with one or more prominent nucleoli (Figure 1). The chromatin was hyperchromatic and finely granular in most of the cells or vesicular in occasional cells. The main cells, which had scant cytoplasm and an indistinct cell border, often formed loosely cohesive clusters (Figure 2). These clusters were in contact with foci of stratification (Figure 2), which consisted of occasional cells with a clear cell border and moderately delicate cytoplasm, often with cytoplasmic coarse vacuoles (Figure 3, arrowhead) that were negative for epithelial mucin. In addition, a few cells showed an overt pearl formation, including a dyskeratocyte (Figure 3, arrow), whereas occasional small apoptotic cells with orange G-colored cytoplasm were scattered throughout the specimen. A glandular structure was not observed.

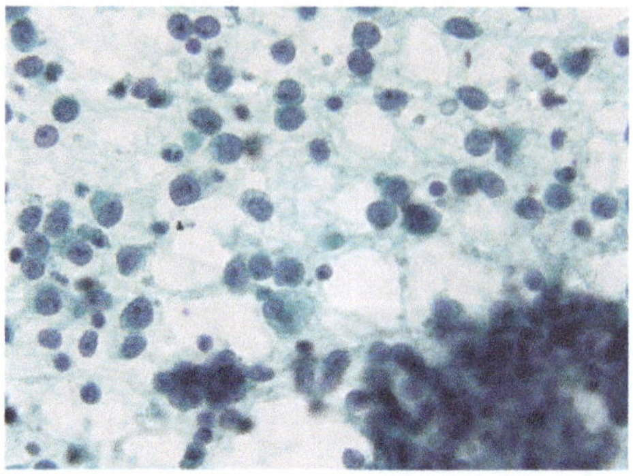

FIGURE 1: Papanicolaou-stained smear showing a high cellularity with loosely cohesive cells or isolated cells. The cells were 2–2.5 times greater in diameter than that of a small lymphocyte. The nuclei were round to oval in shape with slightly irregular contours and contained one or more prominent nucleoli. The chromatin was hyperchromatic and finely granular.

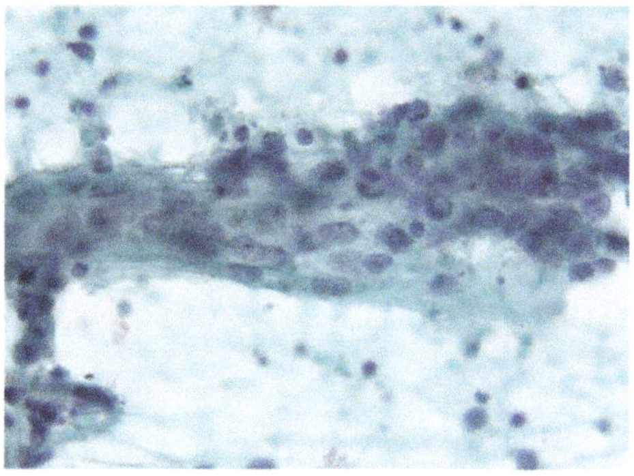

FIGURE 2: Papanicolaou-stained smear showing loosely cohesive clusters and stratification. The main cells exhibited scant cytoplasm and an indistinct cell border, forming loosely cohesive clusters (right side) that were in contact with foci of stratification (center-left side), which consisted of occasional cells with a clear cell border and moderately delicate cytoplasm.

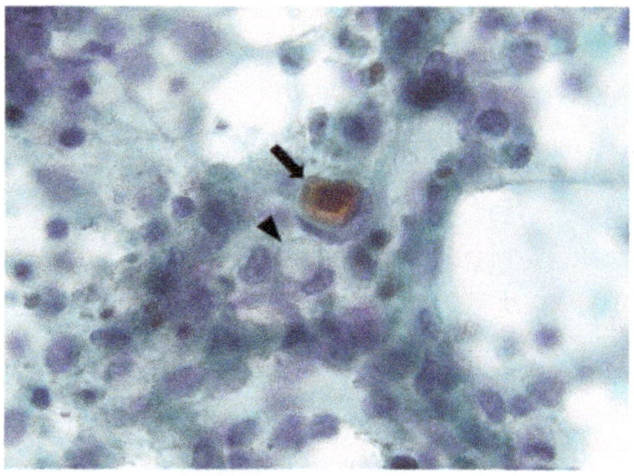

FIGURE 3: Papanicolaou-stained smear showing pearl formation. A few cells showed overt pearl formation, including a dyskeratocyte (arrow), implying keratinization. Occasional cells with moderately delicate cytoplasm and cytoplasmic coarse vacuoles (arrow head) are visible.

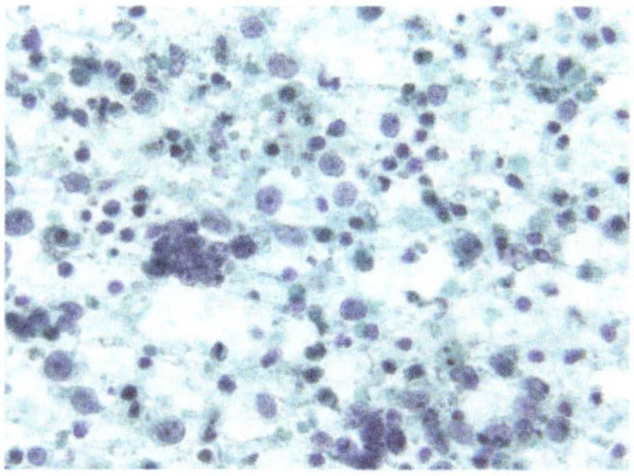

FIGURE 4: Papanicolaou-stained smear showing a necrotic background containing naked nuclei, karyorrhectic debris, apoptotic cells, and macrophages phagocytizing karyorrhectic debris.

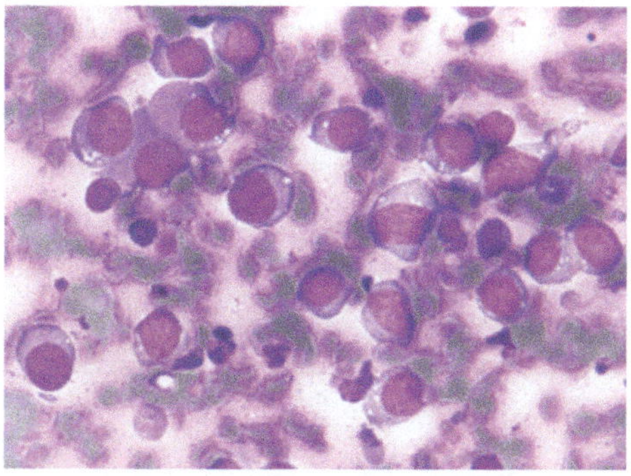

FIGURE 5: Hemacolor-stained smear showing cells bearing basophilic cytoplasm focally with several cytoplasmic fine vacuoles.

Pleomorphism of the cells was not prominent. Mitotic figures were often identified. The necrotic background contained naked nuclei, karyorrhectic debris, apoptotic cells, and macrophages phagocytizing karyorrhectic debris (Figure 4); nuclear crushing was noted.

On the other hand, the Hemacolor-stained smear showed occasional cells bearing delicate basophilic cytoplasm focally with several cytoplasmic fine vacuoles (Figure 5), whereas these cytoplasmic fine vacuoles were not identified in the Papanicolaou-stained smear material.

3.2. Histological, Immunohistological, and FISH Findings. Details of the histological and molecular features of this case have been previously reported [8]. Briefly, only a small amount of biopsy was available for histological investigation, and it revealed an undifferentiated neoplasm with necrosis (Figure 6). In this material, squamous differentiation, which is a possible characteristic of variant NMC, was not apparent.

Immunohistochemical staining demonstrated focal positivity for EMA, p63, cytokeratin AE1/AE3, cytokeratin CAM 5.2, CD138, and vimentin. In addition, a nuclear staining pattern for NUT was evident (Figure 7). Furthermore, FISH analyses revealed an *NSD3-NUT* rearrangement (Figure 8), whereas *BRD3/4-NUT* fusion genes were not identified.

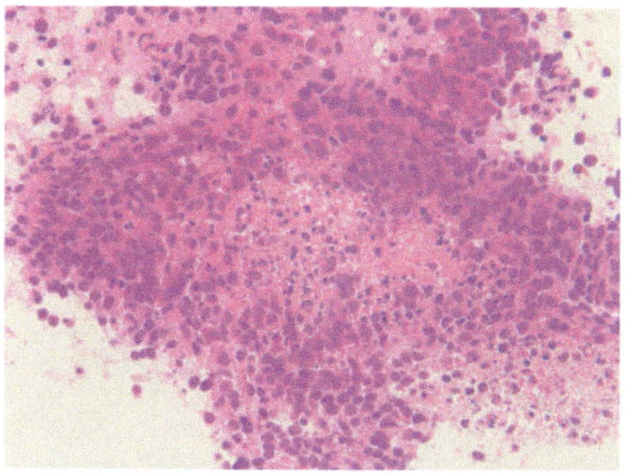

FIGURE 6: Representative histological image showing sheets of undifferentiated malignant cells with focal necrosis.

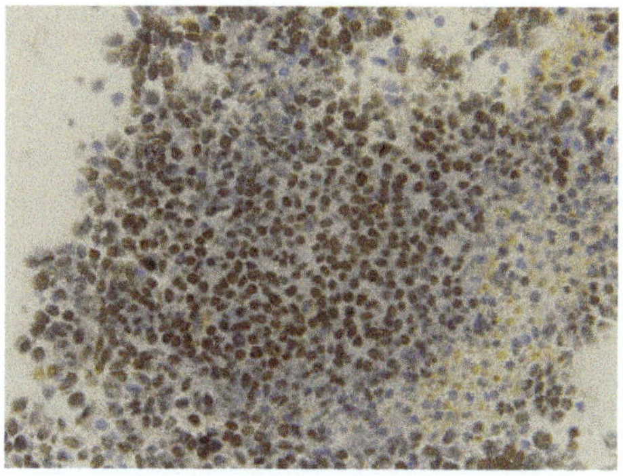

FIGURE 7: Immunohistochemistry showing a nuclear staining pattern for NUT.

3.3. Treatment and Follow-Up. The patient received chemoradiation therapy for 10 months after her diagnosis. However, the patient died with disease progression at 10 months after the diagnosis. Autopsy was not permitted.

4. Discussion

The histological features of NMCs range from entirely undifferentiated carcinomas to carcinomas with prominent squamous differentiation [2, 7, 12–15]. Thus, a diagnosis of NMC based solely on morphology can be difficult. Previous studies have described the cytological features of 4 common NMCs harboring a *BRD3/4-NUT* fusion gene [9, 10] and another NMC case in which the gene rearrangement was not analyzed [11]; the cytological characteristics of these NMCs showed a highly cellular, predominantly noncohesive pattern of relatively small cells with a round nucleus, scant cytoplasm, irregular nuclear contours, variably prominent nucleoli, and identifiable mitotic figures. These findings were also observed in the present variant NMC case. Thus, the previously reported findings imply that the cytological characteristics of NMC are nonspecific and similar to those of undifferentiated carcinoma.

Keratinization has not been identified in previous studies examining the cytology of NMCs [9–11]. In theory, overt keratinization is very important and sometimes pathognomonic for a scrutinized diagnosis of NMC; that is, it is assumed

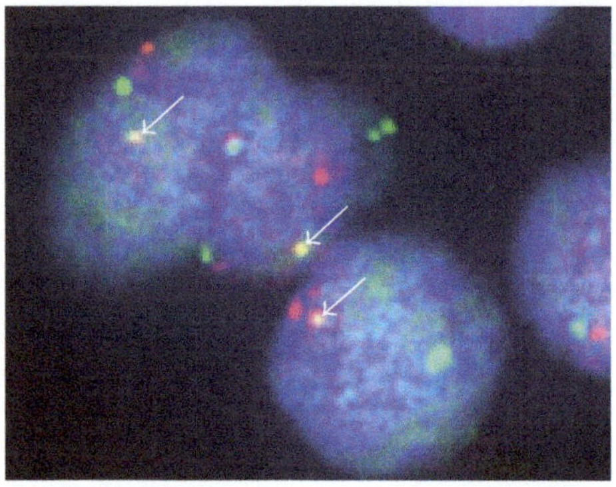

FIGURE 8: A dual-color FISH analysis showing the fusion gene as a single yellow (overlapping) signal (arrows), including a green (*NSD3*) and an orange (*NUT*) signal.

to be a relatively characteristic finding of NMC harboring a *NUT* gene rearrangement involving a gene other than *BRD4* [16]. Keratinization in surgical material, however, is notorious for evading observation because its distribution is often very focal [6, 16], and sampling biases often occur. The cytology of the present NMC variant showed overt pearl formation, including a dyskeratocyte, and the stratification in contact with loosely cohesive clusters; we believe that this finding corresponds to abrupt keratinization, which has been reported as a peculiar characteristic of variant NMC [16] but was not recognized in our corresponding histology specimen [8]. Thus, the combination of cytological and histological findings may help to reveal keratinization concurrent with stratification in undifferentiated carcinoma, which is one clue for a diagnosis of NMC, especially variant NMC, rather than other tumors.

The Hemacolor-stained smear showed occasional cells possessing delicate basophilic cytoplasm with several fine vacuoles, which were not observed in our Papanicolaou-stained smear. In a previous NMC case harboring a *BRD3-NUT* fusion gene, the cells were described as possessing delicate to finely vacuolated cytoplasm, although we could not observe the cytoplasm in detail because of the low magnification of the published figures [10]. On the other hand, these cytoplasmic fine vacuoles were not observed in NMC cases harboring a *BRD4-NUT* fusion gene [9]. Further studies are needed to clarify whether these cytoplasmic fine vacuoles are specific for NMC harboring a fusion gene involving *NUT* and a gene other than *BRD4*.

In conclusion, although the distinction of NMC from other poorly differentiated carcinomas based solely on morphology is difficult, cytological investigation is helpful, especially for identifying abrupt keratinization, which histopathological investigations can miss because of sampling biases. Our experience has shown that the identification of the following clues may suggest a diagnosis of NMC; overt pearl formation including a dyskeratocyte, stratification, and cytoplasmic fine vacuoles, especially in cases where the initial suspected diagnosis was "undifferentiated or poorly differentiated carcinoma with little pleomorphism." Furthermore, the identification of this entity is critical, and immunohistochemistry or FISH studies should be considered for the identification of *NUT* gene rearrangements.

Conflict of Interests

The authors have no conflicts of interest to declare.

Acknowledgments

The authors appreciate the technical assistance of all the clinical and technical staff members of the Pathology Division of Iwata City Hospital. This contribution was supported, in part, by Grants-in-Aid for the US-Japan Cooperative Medical Science Program; the National Cancer Center Research and Development Fund; a grant for priority areas from the Japanese Ministry of Education, Culture, Sports, Science and Technology (221S0001); and Grants-in-Aid for Cancer Research from the Japanese Ministry of Health, Labour and Welfare (23120201 and 10103838), the Smoking Research Foundation, and the Princess Takamatsu Cancer Research Fund.

References

[1] H. Haack, L. A. Johnson, C. J. Fry et al., "Diagnosis of NUT midline carcinoma using a NUT-specific monoclonal antibody," *The American Journal of Surgical Pathology*, vol. 33, no. 7, pp. 984–991, 2009.

[2] C. A. French, "NUT midline carcinoma," *Cancer Genetics and Cytogenetics*, vol. 203, no. 1, pp. 16–20, 2010.

[3] D. E. Bauer, C. M. Mitchell, K. M. Strait et al., "Clinicopathologic features and long-term outcomes of NUT midline carcinoma," *Clinical Cancer Research*, vol. 18, no. 20, pp. 5773–5779, 2012.

[4] E. B. Stelow, "A review of NUT midline carcinoma," *Head and Neck Pathology*, vol. 5, no. 1, pp. 31–35, 2011.

[5] C. A. French, I. Miyoshi, I. Kubonishi, H. E. Grier, A. R. Perez-Atayde, and J. A. Fletcher, "BRD4-NUT fusion oncogene: a novel mechanism in aggressive carcinoma," *Cancer Research*, vol. 63, no. 2, pp. 304–307, 2003.

[6] C. A. French, "Pathogenesis of NUT midline carcinoma," *Annual Review of Pathology: Mechanisms of Disease*, vol. 7, pp. 247–265, 2012.

[7] S. Suzuki, N. Kurabe, H. Minato et al., "A rare Japanese case with a NUT midline carcinoma in the nasal cavity: a case report with immunohistochemical and genetic analyses," *Pathology Research and Practice*, vol. 210, no. 6, pp. 383–388, 2014.

[8] S. Suzuki, N. Kurabe, I. Ohnishi et al., "NSD3-NUT-expressing midline carcinoma of the lung: first characterization of primary cancer tissue," *Pathology—Research and Practice*. In press.

[9] A. M. Bellizzi, C. Bruzzi, C. A. French, and E. B. Stelow, "The cytologic features of NUT midline carcinoma," *Cancer Cytopathology*, vol. 117, no. 6, pp. 508–515, 2009.

[10] B. Zhu, W. Laskin, Y. Chen et al., "NUT midline carcinoma: a neoplasm with diagnostic challenges in cytology," *Cytopathology*, vol. 22, no. 6, pp. 414–417, 2011.

[11] H. S. Park, Y. S. Bae, S. O. Yoon et al., "Usefulness of nuclear protein in testis (NUT) immunohistochemistry in the cytodiagnosis of NUT midline carcinoma: a brief case report," *The Korean Journal of Pathology*, vol. 48, no. 4, pp. 335–338, 2014.

[12] A. G. Evans, C. A. French, M. J. Cameron et al., "Pathologic characteristics of NUT midline carcinoma arising in the mediastinum," *American Journal of Surgical Pathology*, vol. 36, no. 8, pp. 1222–1227, 2012.

[13] J. A. Bishop and W. H. Westra, "NUT midline carcinomas of the sinonasal tract," *American Journal of Surgical Pathology*, vol. 36, no. 8, pp. 1216–1221, 2012.

[14] B. N. Davis, R. G. Karabakhtsian, A. L. Pettigrew, S. M. Arnold, C. A. French, and Y. M. Brill, "Nuclear protein in testis midline carcinomas: a lethal and underrecognized entity," *Archives of Pathology and Laboratory Medicine*, vol. 135, no. 11, pp. 1494–1498, 2011.

[15] E. B. Stelow, A. M. Bellizzi, K. Taneja et al., "NUT rearrangement in undifferentiated carcinomas of the upper aerodigestive tract," *The American Journal of Surgical Pathology*, vol. 32, no. 6, pp. 828–834, 2008.

[16] C. A. French, J. L. Kutok, W. C. Faquin et al., "Midline carcinoma of children and young adults with NUT rearrangement," *Journal of Clinical Oncology*, vol. 22, no. 20, pp. 4135–4139, 2004.

11

Ameloblastic Fibrosarcoma of the Mandible: A Case Report and Brief Review of the Literature

Abelardo Loya-Solis,[1] Karla Judith González-Colunga,[1] Cynthia M. Pérez-Rodríguez,[2] Natalie Sofía Ramírez-Ochoa,[2] Luis Ceceñas-Falcón,[1] and Oralia Barboza-Quintana[1]

[1] *Pathology Department, University Hospital "Dr. Jose E. Gonzalez" and Medical School of the Autonomous University of Nuevo Leon, Francisco I. Madero and Gonzalitos, 64460 Monterrey, NL, Mexico*
[2] *Otolaryngology-Head and Neck Surgery Department, University Hospital "Dr. Jose E. Gonzalez" and Medical School of the Autonomous University of Nuevo Leon, Francisco I. Madero and Gonzalitos, 64460 Monterrey, NL, Mexico*

Correspondence should be addressed to Abelardo Loya-Solis; a_loya_solis@hotmail.com

Academic Editor: Khin Thway

Ameloblastic fibrosarcoma is an uncommon odontogenic tumor composed of a benign epithelial component and a malignant ectomesenchymal component most frequently seen in the third and fourth decades of life. It mainly presents as a painful maxillary or mandibular swelling. Radiographs show a radiolucent mass with ill-defined borders. Radical surgical excision and long-term follow-up are the suggested treatment. We report the case of a 22-year-old female with a 2-month history of an asymptomatic swelling in her left mandible. Examination revealed an exophytic growth measuring 3×3 cm extending from the mandibular left first premolar to the second molar. The patient underwent a left hemimandibular resection. Histopathological examination revealed a biphasic tumor composed of inconspicuous islands of benign odontogenic epithelium and an abundant malignant mesenchymal component with marked cellularity, nuclear pleomorphism, hyperchromatism, and moderate mitotic figures with clear margins; one year after the surgical procedure, the patient is clinically and radiologically disease-free.

1. Introduction

Odontogenic tumors and tumor-like lesions constitute a rare group of heterogeneous diseases that range from nonneoplastic tissue proliferations to malignant tumors with metastatic potential. They are derived from epithelial, ectomesenchymal, and mesenchymal elements of the tooth-forming apparatus. Malignant odontogenic tumors are classified as odontogenic carcinomas and odontogenic sarcomas [1]. Ameloblastic fibrosarcoma (AFS) is a malignant odontogenic tumor characteristically composed of a benign epithelium and a malignant mesenchymal component [2]. Clinically, patients present with pain and swelling [3] and the mandible is the most commonly affected site [1]. The prognosis associated with AFS is good when treated with surgical resection [4].

2. Case Report

A 22-year-old female presented with a 2-month history of an asymptomatic swelling in her left mandible. Extraoral evaluation revealed a gross swelling over the left mandible (Figure 1). Upon intraoral examination, an exophytic growth measuring roughly 3×3 cm extending from the mandibular left first premolar to the second molar with buccolingual expansion and ulceration of the overlying mucosa was identified. Radiographic examination showed an extensive ill-defined unilocular radiolucent lesion around an impacted mandibular left first molar. An odontogenic lesion was the clinical impression and an incisional biopsy was performed. Histopathological examination revealed a biphasic tumor composed of inconspicuous islands of benign odontogenic

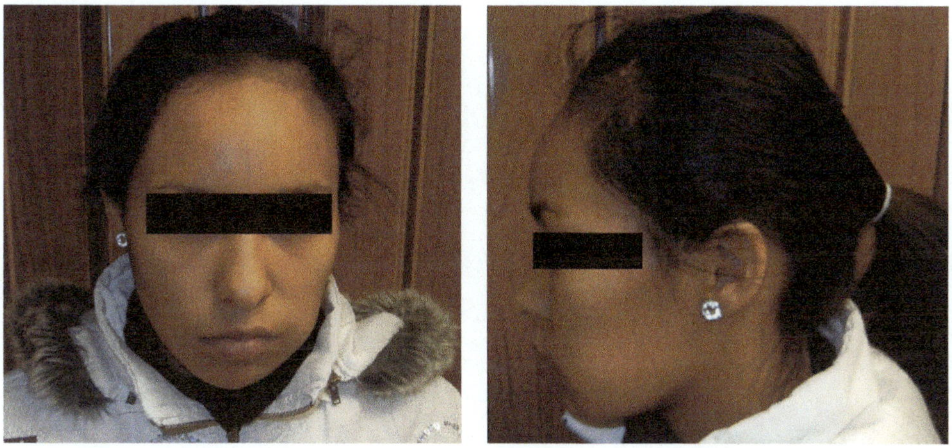

(a) (b)

FIGURE 1: ((a) and (b)) Extraoral evaluation revealed a gross swelling over the left mandible.

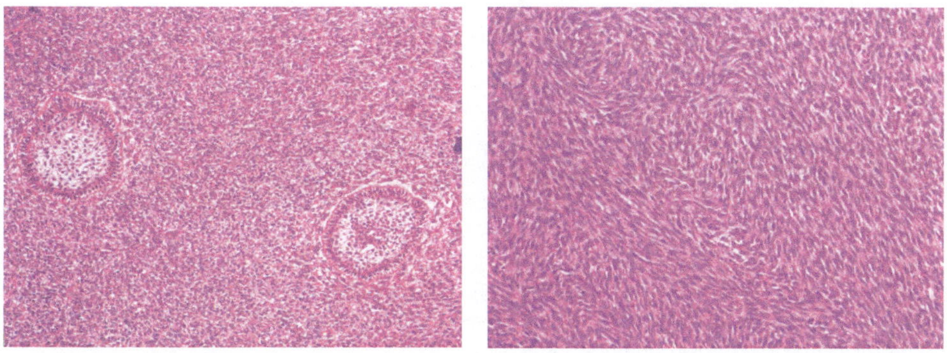

(a) (b)

FIGURE 2: (a) Biphasic tumor composed of islands of benign odontogenic epithelium and an abundant malignant mesenchymal component. H&E stain, ×50. (b) The malignant mesenchymal component consists of plump and spindle stromal cells which show mild to moderate cytologic atypia and numerous mitotic figures arranged in storiform and herringbone fashion. H&E stain, ×100.

epithelium and an abundant malignant mesenchymal component with marked cellularity, nuclear pleomorphism, hyperchromatism, and moderate mitotic figures (Figure 2). Immunohistochemistry was performed using Cytokeratin AE1/AE3, Vimentin, and Ki67 (Figure 3). CK was strongly positive in the odontogenic epithelium and negative in the mesenchymal component, while Vimentin was strongly positive in the mesenchymal component and negative in the odontogenic epithelium. Ki67 was expressed by 30% of the mesenchymal cells. In view of these histopathological and immunohistochemistry findings, an AFS was diagnosed.

Four months later a panoramic radiograph and CT scan of head and neck were performed disregarding locoregional and distant metastases while also revealing again the same ill-defined radiolucent lesion around an impacted mandibular left first molar (Figure 4). The patient underwent a left hemimandibular resection and immediate fibular free flap reconstruction. The excised specimen consisted of the left half of the body and ramus of the mandible measuring 5 × 4.2 × 3 cm with a gray solid tumor mass of 1.8 cm with widely clear margins (Figure 5). Histopathological examination showed the same biphasic tumor previously described. Additional immunohistochemistry was performed using PCNA and p53 (Figure 6). PCNA was strongly positive in both components, while p53 was strongly positive only in the mesenchymal component. The final histopathological diagnosis was identical to that of the incisional biopsy and an AFS was confirmed. Currently, one year after the surgical procedure, the patient is clinically and radiologically disease-free (Figure 7).

3. Discussion

AFS was first reported by Heath in 1887 describing it as a spindle cell sarcoma that also had epithelial cells resembling the cells of the enamel organ [5]. To the best of our knowledge, less than 100 documented cases have been reported in the English language literature [6]. The usual clinical presentation consists of a patient who complains of a painful but occasionally painless facial mass with accompanying paresthesia or dysesthesia. The duration of symptoms varies widely from a few weeks up to 2 years [7]. The mean age of

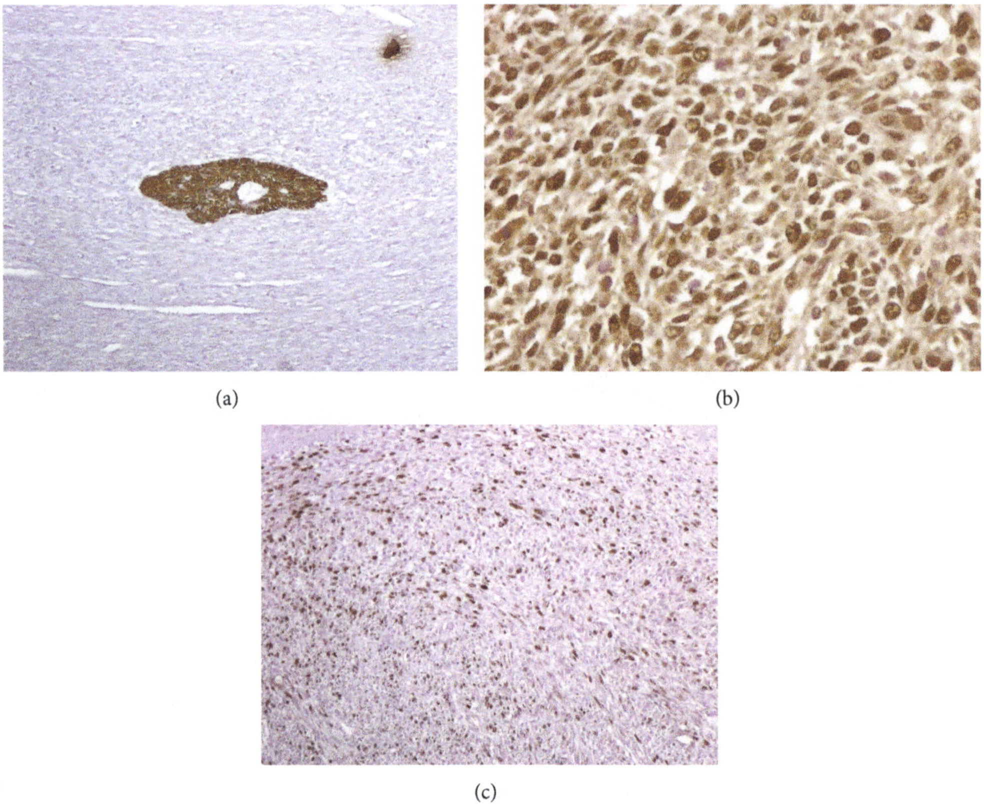

FIGURE 3: (a) Reactivity to Cytokeratin AE1/AE3 in the epithelial component, lack of reactivity in the mesenchymal component. Immunohistochemical stain with anti-Cytokeratin AE1/AE3 antibody, ×50. (b) Reactivity to Vimentin in the mesenchymal component. Immunohistochemical stain with anti-Vimentin antibody, ×400. (c) Reactivity to Ki67 in the mesenchymal component with a labeling index of 30%. Immunohistochemical stain with anti-Ki67 antibody, ×50.

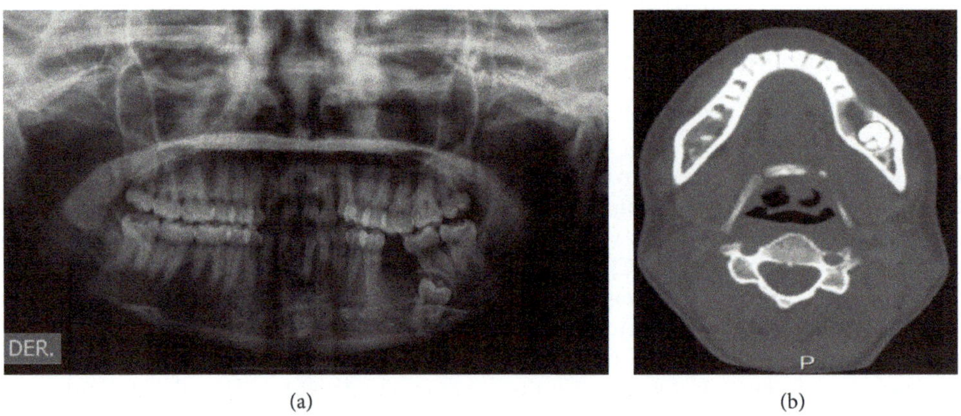

FIGURE 4: Panoramic radiograph (a) and axial CT scan (b) revealing an ill-defined radiolucent lesion around an impacted mandibular left first molar.

presentation is 28.3 years with a wide age range from 3 to 89 years and a male-to-female ratio of 1.6 : 1 [8].

AFS can arise de novo or from a previous ameloblastic fibroma (AF). Kobayashi et al. suggest that up to one-third of AFSs arise from transformation of an AF [9], while Lai et al. found in their review of the literature that 51% of AFS had previously documented AF at the same site [8]. Those lesions arising from an AF tend to occur in patients aged approximately a decade older than those arising de novo [10]. The posterior mandible is the most commonly affected site [8]. Radiologically, AFS presents as a radiolucent mass with ill-defined borders. Grossly the tumor may be cystic or solid with a fleshy whitish to yellow appearance [7]. The histological architecture of AFS is characterized by benign epithelial islands that are composed of columnar or cuboidal peripheral cells arranged in a palisading pattern.

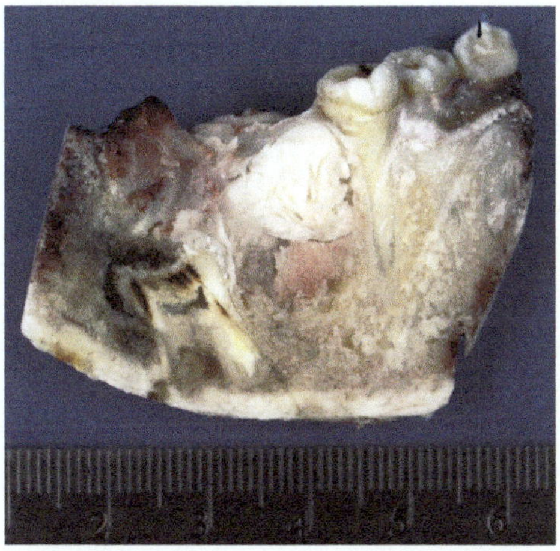

Figure 5: Gross photograph of the cut surface of the left half of the mandible showing a solid gray tumor mass.

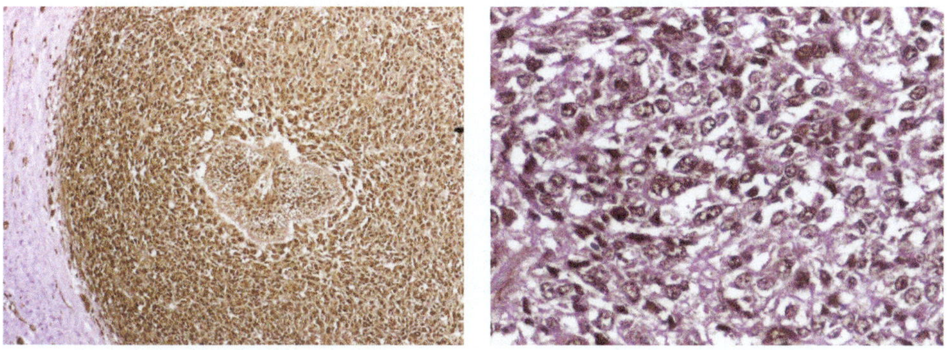

(a) (b)

Figure 6: (a) Reactivity to PCNA in both components. Immunohistochemical stain with anti-PCNA antibody, ×50. (b) Reactivity to p53 only in the mesenchymal component. Immunohistochemical stain with anti-p53 antibody, ×400.

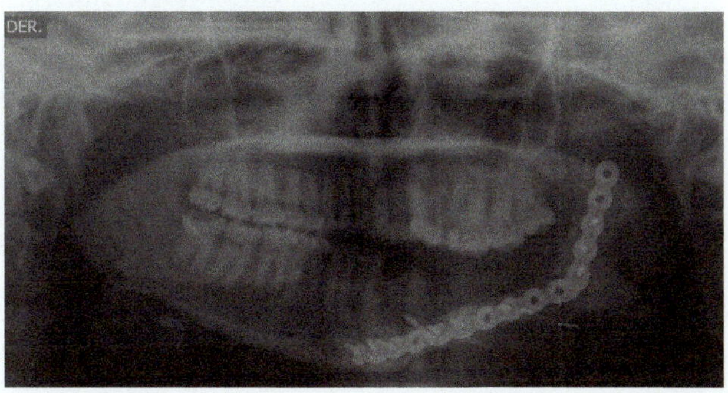

Figure 7: Panoramic radiograph showing area of mandibular resection with no evidence of recurrence 1 year after surgery.

At the center of these islands is polyhedral cell reminiscent of stellate reticulum. The mesenchymal component consists of plump and spindle stromal cells which show mild to moderate cytologic atypia and numerous mitotic figures [11].

AF is the main differential diagnosis of AFS. Both neoplasms have a biphasic nature; however, AF has no malignant component, unlike AFS in which the mesenchymal component presents marked cellularity, nuclear pleomorphism, hyperchromatism, and a moderate to high number of mitotic figures. Immunohistochemical markers can be helpful to distinguish AFS and AF, and the mesenchymal component of AFS is positive for p53 and PCNA unlike the negativity for these stains in AF [12, 13]. Regarding its Ki67 expression, AFS usually shows higher labeling indices than AF [13, 14].

AFS has a reported recurrence rate of 37% and a mortality rate of 19% [4]. Only 2 cases of metastasis have been reported [15, 16]. Due to lack of experience, there is no consensus on the treatment yet. In general, the treatment of choice is surgical excision with clear margins and long-term follow-up. Adjuvant radiotherapy has been used with no evidence of recurrence [9]. Adjuvant chemotherapy has also been used with moderate success [17], although no specific chemotherapy protocols have been established yet.

Our patient presented an AFS in the posterior mandible. Such location is the most frequent affected site reported in the literature. Her age at presentation was 22 years old, a little younger than the mean age of presentation, but still in the third decade of life, like most patients from previous reports. Her tumor was considered a de novo AFS since she did not have a history of previous AF. The origin of our patients AFS and her age are two important features to consider since they seem to further support the observation made by Noordhoek et al., claiming that de novo AFS tends to occur in younger patients than AFS arising from an AF. Histologically our case had very few islands of odontogenic epithelium compared to the extensive malignant mesenchymal component, a feature commonly seen. Although the immunohistochemical profile of this neoplasm was identical to the one described in the literature and helped to establish the diagnosis, we agree with Kobayashi and most authors, and believe the diagnosis is essentially made by histology.

In summary, AFS is a rare malignant odontogenic tumor characterized by a benign odontogenic epithelium and a malignant mesenchymal component that can arise from a previous AF or de novo. Resection with a wide margin is the optimal treatment strategy and close follow-up is advised due to its relatively high recurrence rate.

Consent

Written informed consent was obtained from the patient for publication of this case report and the accompanying images. A copy of the written consent is available upon request for review.

Conflict of Interests

The authors have no conflict of interests to declare.

References

[1] L. Barnes, J. W. Eveson, P. Reichart, and D. Sidransky, *World Health Organization Classification of Tumours: Pathology and Genetics of Head and Neck Tumours*, IARC Press, Lyon, France, 2005.

[2] P. Dallera, F. Bertoni, C. Marchetti, P. Bacchini, and A. Campobassi, "Ameloblastic fibrosarcoma of the jaw: report of five cases," *Journal of Cranio-Maxillo-Facial Surgery*, vol. 22, no. 6, pp. 349–354, 1994.

[3] R. C. Bregni, A. M. Taylor, and A. M. García, "Ameloblastic fibrosarcoma of the mandible: report of two cases and review of the literature," *Journal of Oral Pathology & Medicine*, vol. 30, no. 5, pp. 316–320, 2001.

[4] R. E. Marx and D. Stern, *Oral and Maxillofacial Pathology: A Rationale for Diagnosis and Treatment*, 2nd edition, 2012.

[5] C. Heath, "Lectures on certain diseases of the jaws," *British Medical Journal*, vol. 2, no. 1383, pp. 5–13, 1887.

[6] Y.-Y. Hu, M.-H. Deng, L.-L. Yuan, and Y.-M. Niu, "Ameloblastic fibrosarcoma of the mandible: a case report and mini review," *Experimental and Therapeutic Medicine*, vol. 8, no. 5, pp. 1463–1466, 2014.

[7] S. M. Gilani, A. Raza, and B. M. Al-Khafaji, "Ameloblastic fibrosarcoma: a rare malignant odontogenic tumor," *European Annals of Otorhinolaryngology, Head and Neck Diseases*, vol. 131, no. 1, pp. 53–56, 2014.

[8] J. Lai, N. Blanas, K. Higgins, and H. Klieb, "Ameloblastic fibrosarcoma: report of a case, study of immunophenotype, and comprehensive review of the literature," *Journal of Oral and Maxillofacial Surgery*, vol. 70, no. 8, pp. 2007–2012, 2012.

[9] K. Kobayashi, R. Murakami, T. Fujii, and A. Hirano, "Malignant transformation of ameloblastic fibroma to ameloblastic fibrosarcoma: case report and review of the literature," *Journal of Cranio-Maxillofacial Surgery*, vol. 33, no. 5, pp. 352–355, 2005.

[10] R. Noordhoek, M. E. Pizer, and D. M. Laskin, "Ameloblastic fibrosarcoma of the mandible: treatment, long-term follow-up, and subsequent reconstruction of a case," *Journal of Oral and Maxillofacial Surgery*, vol. 70, no. 12, pp. 2930–2935, 2012.

[11] P. A. Reichar and H. P. Philipsen, *Odontogenic Tumors and Allied Lesions*, Quintessence Publishing, London, UK, 2004.

[12] P. Huguet, J. Castellví, M. Ávila et al., "Ameloblastic fibrosarcoma: report of a case. Immunohistochemical study and review of the literature," *Medicina Oral*, vol. 6, no. 3, pp. 173–179, 2001.

[13] H. A. R. Pontes, F. S. C. Pontes, B. S. de Freitas Silva et al., "Immunoexpression of Ki67, proliferative cell nuclear antigen, and Bcl-2 proteins in a case of ameloblastic fibrosarcoma," *Annals of Diagnostic Pathology*, vol. 14, no. 6, pp. 447–452, 2010.

[14] K. Sano, S.-I. Yoshida, H. Ninomiya et al., "Assessment of growth potential by MIB-1 immunohistochemistry in ameloblastic fibroma and related lesions of the jaws compared with ameloblastic fibrosarcoma," *Journal of Oral Pathology and Medicine*, vol. 27, no. 2, pp. 59–63, 1998.

[15] A. Kousar, M. M. Hosein, Z. Ahmed, and K. Minhas, "Rapid sarcomatous transformation of an ameloblastic fibroma of the mandible: case report and literature review," *Oral Surgery, Oral Medicine, Oral Pathology, Oral Radiology and Endodontology*, vol. 108, no. 3, pp. e80–e85, 2009.

[16] G. Chomette, M. Auriol, F. Guilbert, and A. Delcourt, "Ameloblastic fibrosarcoma of the jaws - report of three cases. Clinicopathologic, histoenzymological and ultrastructural study," *Pathology Research and Practice*, vol. 178, no. 1, pp. 40–47, 1983.

[17] C. Demoor-Goldschmidt, V. Minard-Colin, E. Cassagneau et al., "Ameloblastic fibrosarcoma of the mandible: report of 2 chemosensitive pediatric cases," *Journal of Pediatric Hematology/Oncology*, vol. 34, no. 2, pp. e72–e76, 2012.

12

Invasive Aspergillosis Associated with a Foreign Body

Akifuddin Syed,[1] Prashanth Panta,[2] Imran Shahid,[2] and David H. Felix[3]

[1]*Princess DurruShehvar Children's and General Hospital, Purani Haveli, Hyderabad, Telangana 500002, India*
[2]*Department of Oral Medicine and Radiology, MNR Dental College and Hospital, Narsapur Road, Sangareddy, Medak District, Telangana 502294, India*
[3]*NHS Education for Scotland, Westport 102, WestPort, Edinburgh EH3 9DN, UK*

Correspondence should be addressed to Prashanth Panta; maithreya.prashanth@gmail.com

Academic Editor: Hiroko Kuwabara

Invasive aspergillosis is a serious complication in immunocompromised individuals. It is associated with a high mortality rate, which demands a combined approach involving radical surgery and antifungal therapy. Here, we describe a patient who presented with nonspecific fever, refractory to antimicrobial agents. Though it primarily involved the nasal cavity and sinuses, it perforated into the oral cavity causing palatal changes. Surprisingly, a foreign body was found in the involved tissues that might have acted as a nidus of infection. A sufficient dose (3 mg/kg/day) of liposomal amphotericin B was initiated soon after a thorough debridement procedure and the patient survived.

1. Introduction

Aspergillosis is an infection caused by a group of soil dwelling fungal organisms. About 837 *Aspergillus* species are now known of which only a few are implicated in human disease [1]. The conidia of these organisms germinate into hyphae filaments and result in disease. B-glucans present in the cell walls of these hyphae along with other ligands can precipitate a severe inflammatory response. *Aspergillus* species also release enzymes (proteases, peptidases, and phospholipases) and toxins (14 kDa diffusible substance from conidia, fumigaclavin C, aurasperon C, gliotoxin, helvolic acid, fumagillin, hemolysin, and ribotoxin) which mediate invasion and tissue necrosis [2]. The pathogenicity of aspergillosis is dependent on two factors, the involved fungal strain and the immune status of the host.

Patients with hematological malignancies, HIV/AIDS, neutropenia, and multiple myeloma and those who received bone marrow transplantation are at risk of invasive aspergillosis [3]. There is some male predilection and the most frequent sites include lungs, liver, spleen, bone, meninges, sinuses, and oral cavity. Primary intraoral aspergillosis is rare and it usually involves gingiva, palate, and rarely tongue. However, *Aspergillus* infection might spread from the maxillary sinus into the palate. Aspergillosis can broadly be divided into invasive and noninvasive forms. The most frequently isolated strains in invasive aspergillosis are *Aspergillus fumigatus* and *Aspergillus flavus* [4]. In the present case, the culprit organism was *Aspergillus niger*, a species that is less pathogenic to humans, suggesting the role of nonfumigatus organisms in invasive aspergillosis.

2. Case Report

A 51-year-old male farmer initially reported to a general physician with the chief complaint of fever and malaise. Routine blood investigations revealed leukocytosis (15,200/mm^3), but the source of sepsis could not be identified and his condition was refractory to empirical antimicrobial therapy. His medical history included diabetes diagnosed ten years earlier; he was a heavy smoker for the last 20 years. On day 5, the patient complained of acute pain from the upper left central incisor region, so, he was reviewed by a maxillofacial surgeon. Upon extraoral examination, a diffuse swelling (Figure 1) was found on the left and right malar region; there was no cervical lymphadenopathy. Intraorally, the palatal gingiva showed a yellow ulcerated area (3 × 1 cm) in the anterior hard palate and many blackish areas near the soft palate region (Figure 2). The palatal mucosa was

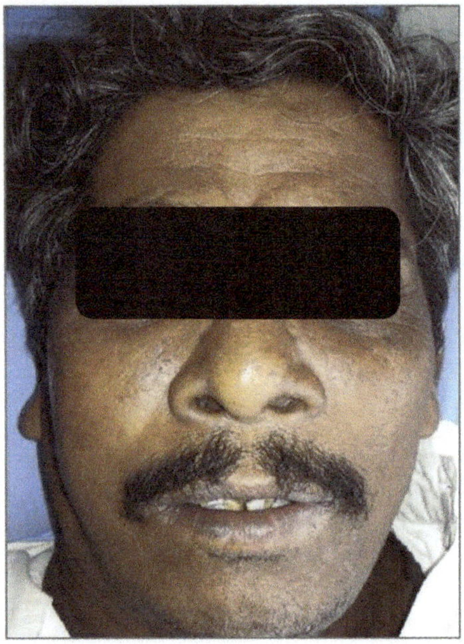

FIGURE 1: Diffuse facial swelling and mild bilateral obliteration of the nasolabial folds.

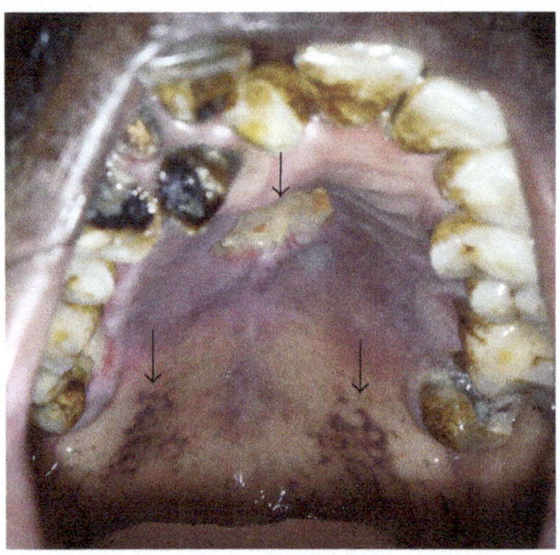

FIGURE 2: Diffuse oedematous swelling of the palatal mucosa with focal ulceration. Note violaceous discolouration with black pigmented areas over soft palate.

grayish-violet, blanched, and oedematous and all his upper teeth showed mobility ranging from grade I to II.

A chairside KOH test from the palatal ulcer showed features suggestive of a fungal aetiology, but the type was in question. A provisional diagnosis of fungal osteomyelitis was proposed. Following this, a decision was taken, to perform a debridement procedure, aiming at improving the patient's condition. A preoperative CT scan showed features, suggestive of erosive sinusitis with nasal involvement (Figure 3). Maxillectomy (Figure 4(a)) was performed, sparing the tuberosity region alone. Several muddy areas were found in the nasal cavity, maxillary sinus, and the alveolar process (Figure 4(b)). In the middle of these muddy areas was

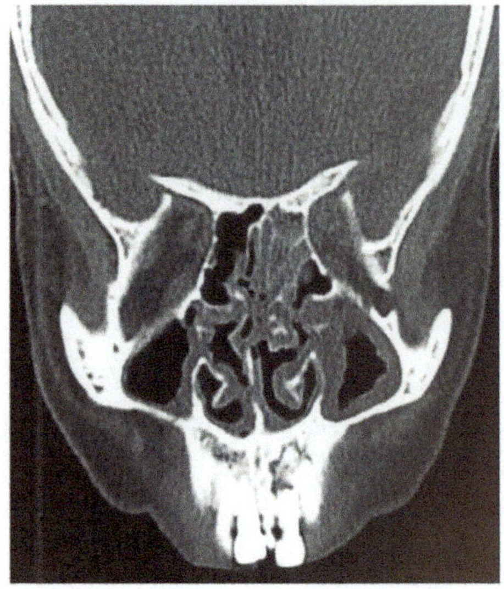

FIGURE 3: CT scan images shows thickening of mucosa and opacification of the sinuses.

a foreign body measuring approximately 2.5 cm in its maximum dimension (Figure 5). Further analysis of the foreign body showed this to be a fragment of a plant leaf. Hematoxylin and eosin stained section (Figure 6(a)) showed fungal elements, and Gomori methanamine silver stained section (Figure 6(b)) showed 45° branching hyphae (pointed by a red arrow), a feature characteristic of *Aspergillus niger*. The histopathological features suggested aspergillosis, caused by niger. *Aspergillus niger* was also grown on Sabaraud's dextrose agar and the colonies were blackish in color (Figure 6(c)). The patient was started on intravenous liposomal amphotericin B (3 mg/kg/day for 5 weeks). He responded very well to this drug and had complete recovery. One month postoperatively, he was provided with an obturator to close off the palatal defect.

3. Discussion

Invasive aspergillosis is a rapidly spreading infection and is more likely to occur in patients with an underlying immune deficiency. *Aspergillus fumigates* (80–90%) is the most common cause of invasive aspergillosis followed by *Aspergillus flavus* (5–10%) and *Aspergillus niger* (1–5%) [5].

The first case of aspergillosis of the paranasal sinus was described by Katzenstein in 1983. Sinonasal aspergillosis can be invasive (chronic indolent and invasive fulminant sinusitis) or noninvasive (aspergilloma and allergic *Aspergillus* sinusitis) [6]. The present case may represent a chronic indolent fungal sinusitis progressing into an invasive fulminant fungal sinusitis. Chronic indolent fungal sinusitis occurs in patients with altered immune responsiveness (e.g., diabetes mellitus) [7]. The invasive form can extend into the oral cavity causing palatal perforation. In such cases, gray-violaceous gingival changes are found that soon transform into necrotic lesions. Proptosis is another important feature of paranasal and orbital aspergillosis.

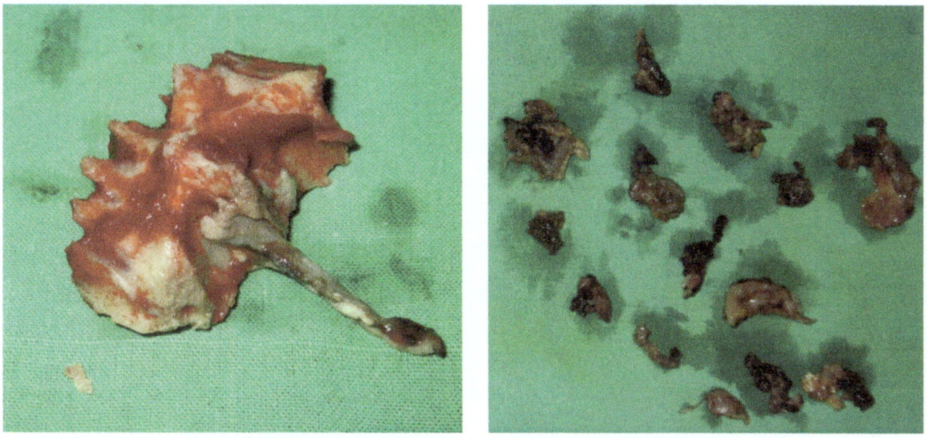

(a) (b)

FIGURE 4: (a) Excised maxilla. (b) Black muddy areas were found in the nasal cavity, alveolar process, and the sinus region.

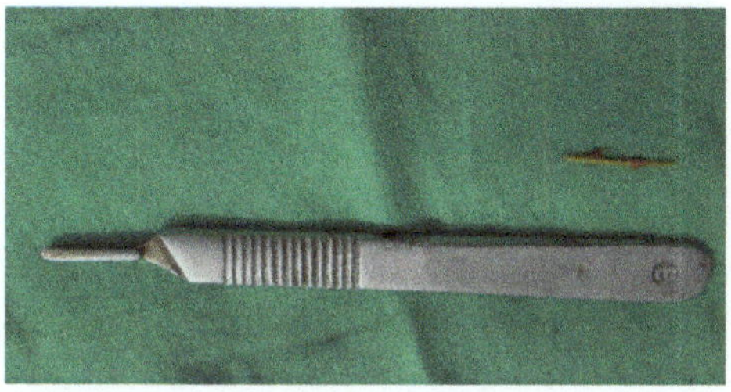

FIGURE 5: Image shows a foreign body that corresponded to a plant leaf.

In the past, foreign bodies were shown as an etiological factor for aspergillosis [8, 9]. Burnham and Bridle reported a case of maxillary sinus aspergilloma which was triggered due to extrusion of an amalgam filling [10]. Liston and Walters presented a case of *Aspergillus* sinusitis where six gutta percha points served as etiological agents after being accidentally introduced into the maxillary sinus [11]. In the present case, a foreign body was discovered in the nasal cavity that corresponded to a "plant leaf." It was found in the middle of necrotic tissues and may have served as a source of contamination. The epicenter of tissue destruction was predominantly in the paranasal sinus region and the nasal cavity. No actual palatal perforation occurred although there was some ulceration. The large size of the foreign body (2.5 cm) and the absence of palatal perforation clearly point at the nasal route, as the probable route of entry. The patient may have accidentally inhaled the foreign body during agricultural activities.

Aspergillus sps. are found in soil, stored grains, litter, and decaying plant leaves [3]. They exist in spore form on dried leaves and derive the necessary nutrients from it. It is possible that spores of *Aspergillus* sp. on the foreign body/plant leaf settled in his nasal cavity. Due to his already immunocompromised and ketoacidic state, the spores may have attained full growth potential.

Aspergillus niger/black aspergilli is a group of black-shaded spore producing organisms that can survive even in hostile environments reflected in their ability to withstand extremes of temperature and humidity [12]. Their ability to withstand extreme temperatures and humidity may be the reason for their colonization in nasal and paranasal areas, a relatively warm and moist environment. A foreign body further complicates the scenario, favouring fungal growth.

Clinically, aspergillosis can mimic mucormycosis, an entity which is relatively common in diabetics. A differentiation between the two is possible microscopically. Special stains such as periodic acid Schiff and methenamine silver along with fungal culture can confirm the diagnosis. Recently, galactomannan assay, B-glucan assays, and polymerase chain reaction have shown high sensitivity and specificity in the detection of invasive aspergillosis [3]. Differential diagnosis of single palatal ulcer such as the one presented in this case includes oral tuberculosis, necrotizing sialometaplasia, syphilis, malignant ulcer, and deep fungal infection. Such ulcers must caution the clinician to consider the possibility of fungal infection, especially when the host is immunecompromised. In this case, there was sinus opacification with erosion of the medial and lateral walls of maxillary sinus, bony nasal septum, and alveolar process of the maxilla. There was severe mucosal thickening of the turbinates bilaterally and also deviation of the nasal septum. Radiological findings of invasive sinus disease include soft tissue mass, opacification, necrosis of multiple sinuses, and bone destruction [13].

Though amphotericin has some toxic side effects, most of the patients usually tolerate this drug well. Emerging antifungal agents such as voriconazole, echinocandins, or caspofungin alone or in combination with amphotericin/voriconazole have shown good clinical results [3]. Future studies should focus on dosage standardization, which is not well established.

4. Conclusion

This paper reports a case of invasive aspergillosis in a male farmer, caused by *Aspergillus niger*, a species that is believed to be less pathogenic than other strains. Invasive aspergillosis involving nasal cavity and sinuses can be expected in farmers

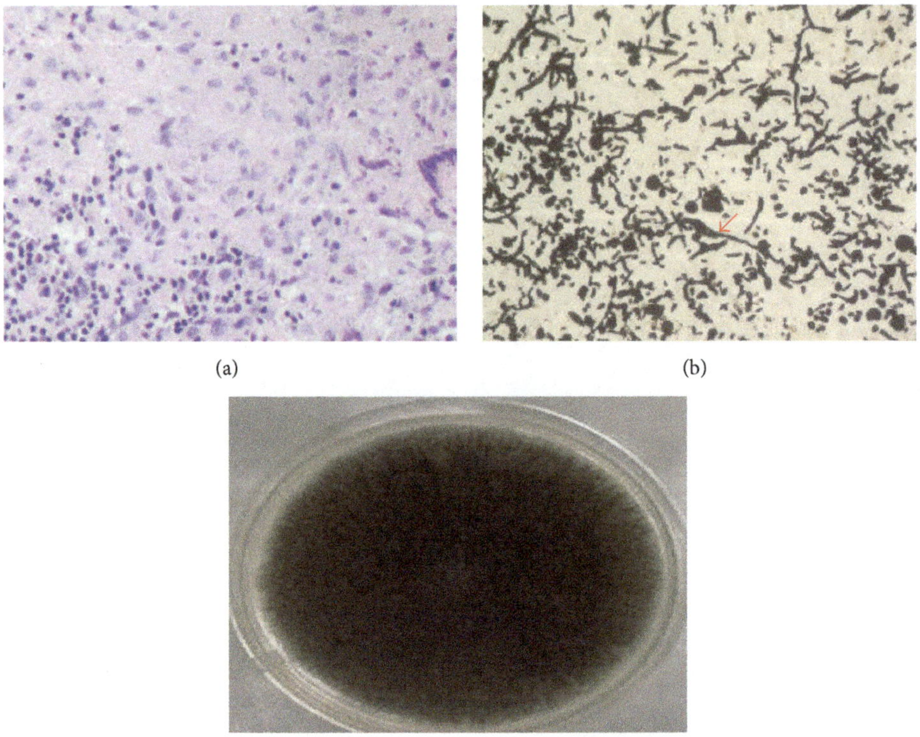

(a) (b) (c)

FIGURE 6: Microbiological features suggested aspergillosis caused by *niger*.

and horticulture workers. Environmental factors may play some role in this disease, so taking a thorough occupational history is crucial for diagnosis. Single palatal ulcers along with gray-violet discolouration of the gingiva may be early indicators of invasive sinonasal aspergillosis. It is important that invasive aspergillosis is considered in patients with an underlying immune deficiency such as diabetes and in patients who present with nonspecific fever, refractory to antimicrobials. In advanced cases, a combination of radical surgical debridement and antifungal therapy should be considered. Systemic dissemination and the high mortality associated with this condition should persuade researchers to work on newer methods of identification and treatment.

Conflict of Interests

The authors declare that they have no conflict of interests.

References

[1] D. L. Hawksworth, "Naming *Aspergillus* species: progress towards one name for each species," *Medical Mycology*, vol. 49, no. 1, pp. S70–S76, 2011.

[2] A. Rementeria, N. López-Molina, A. Ludwig et al., "Genes and molecules involved in *Aspergillus fumigatus* virulence," *Revista Iberoamericana de Micologia*, vol. 22, no. 1, pp. 1–23, 2005.

[3] P. D. Barnes and K. A. Marr, "Aspergillosis: spectrum of disease, diagnosis, and treatment," *Infectious Disease Clinics of North America*, vol. 20, no. 3, pp. 545–561, 2006.

[4] A. Filippi, T. Dreyer, R.-M. Bohle, Y. Pohl, and S. Rosseau, "Sequestration of the alveolar bone by invasive aspergillosis in acute myeloid leukemia," *Journal of Oral Pathology & Medicine*, vol. 26, no. 9, pp. 437–440, 1997.

[5] A. Akhaddar, M. Gazzaz, A. Albouzidi, B. Lmimouni, B. Elmostarchid, and M. Boucetta, "Invasive *Aspergillus terreus* sinusitis with orbitocranial extension: case report," *Surgical Neurology*, vol. 69, no. 5, pp. 490–495, 2008.

[6] R. W. Hartwick and J. G. Batsakis, "Sinus aspergillosis and allergic fungal sinusitis," *Annals of Otology, Rhinology and Laryngology*, vol. 100, no. 5 I, pp. 427–430, 1991.

[7] H. Stammberger, R. Jakse, and F. Beaufort, "Aspergillosis of the paranasal sinuses X-ray diagnosis, histopathology, and clinical aspects," *Annals of Otology, Rhinology & Laryngology*, vol. 93, no. 3, pp. 251–256, 1984.

[8] D. H. Lee and S. C. Lim, "Maxillary fungus ball caused by retained foreign bodies for 25 years," *Journal of Craniofacial Surgery*, vol. 23, no. 3, pp. e176–e177, 2012.

[9] F. Legent, J. Billet, C. Beauvillain, J. Bonnet, and M. Miegeville, "The role of dental canal fillings in the development of *Aspergillus* sinusitis—a report of 85 cases," *Archives of Oto-Rhino-Laryngology*, vol. 246, no. 5, pp. 318–320, 1989.

[10] R. Burnham and C. Bridle, "Aspergillosis of the maxillary sinus secondary to a foreign body (amalgam) in the maxillary antrum," *British Journal of Oral and Maxillofacial Surgery*, vol. 47, no. 4, pp. 313–315, 2009.

[11] P. N. Liston and R. F. Walters, "Foreign bodies in the maxillary antrum: a case report," *Australian Dental Journal*, vol. 47, no. 4, pp. 344–346, 2002.

[12] A. Astoreca, C. Magnoli, M. L. Ramirez, M. Combina, and A. Dalcero, "Water activity and temperature effects on growth of *Aspergillus niger*, *A. awamori* and *A. carbonarius* isolated from different substrates in Argentina," *International Journal of Food Microbiology*, vol. 119, no. 3, pp. 314–318, 2007.

[13] L. A. Al-Bhlal, "Fungal infection of the nasal cavity and paranasal sinuses: review of 26 cases," *Annals of Saudi Medicine*, vol. 16, no. 6, pp. 615–621, 1996.

13

Poorly Differentiated Thyroid Carcinoma Arising in Struma Ovarii

Surapan Khunamornpong,[1] Jongkolnee Settakorn,[1] Kornkanok Sukpan,[1] Prapaporn Suprasert,[2] and Sumalee Siriaunkgul[1]

[1]*Department of Pathology, Faculty of Medicine, Chiang Mai University, Chiang Mai 50200, Thailand*
[2]*Department of Obstetrics and Gynecology, Faculty of Medicine, Chiang Mai University, Chiang Mai 50200, Thailand*

Correspondence should be addressed to Surapan Khunamornpong; skhunamo@yahoo.com

Academic Editor: Sarah M. Bean

Struma ovarii is an uncommon type of ovarian mature teratoma with a predominant thyroid component. The morphological spectrum of the thyroid tissue ranges from that of normal thyroid to proliferative adenoma-like lesions and thyroid-type carcinomas (malignant transformation). The histologic features of ovarian strumal lesions sometimes cause diagnostic problems due to the confusion with other types of ovarian neoplasms and the difficulty in the prediction of their clinical behavior. We report an extremely rare case of poorly differentiated thyroid carcinoma arising in struma ovarii. A 22-year-old woman presented with a 15 cm right ovarian mass. The tumor showed a predominantly tubular pattern which raised a differential diagnosis between endometrioid adenocarcinoma and Sertoli cell tumor. A review of the gross specimen with additional tissue sampling helped identify the teratomatous and strumal nature, with a support by immunohistochemical staining. Despite FIGO stage IA by optimal staging procedure and the absence of identifiable lymphovascular invasion, the patient developed pulmonary metastasis 15 months after surgery and died from the progression of the disease 7 years after the diagnosis. This case emphasizes the importance of macroscopic examination of the specimen and the awareness of this uncommon tumor in the differential diagnosis of ovarian neoplasms.

1. Introduction

Struma ovarii is an uncommon type of ovarian mature teratoma which is composed predominantly (i.e., > 50% of tumor component) or purely of thyroid tissue [1]. The morphological spectrum of the thyroid component ranges from that similar to normal thyroid, cellular or "proliferative" lesions with adenoma-like or hyperplastic features, to thyroid-type carcinomas similar to those of the thyroid (malignant transformation) [2, 3]. The histologic features of the proliferative and malignant spectrum in struma ovarii sometimes cause diagnostic confusion with other types of ovarian neoplasm, particularly sex cord-stromal and epithelial tumors [4, 5].

A malignant transformation of ovarian struma is very rare, with an estimated annual incidence of less than 1 in 10,000,000 women-years [2]. Although it is sometimes referred to as "malignant struma ovarii," this term represents a heterogenous group of tumors. A better diagnosis should include a specific type of thyroid carcinoma that arises in a strumal background as this would provide meaningful prognostic information [6, 7]. Malignancy arising in struma ovarii can pose diagnostic problems for pathologists in the identification of the strumal nature and also in the determination of tumor behavior [2]. A correct diagnosis is very important due to major differences in the therapeutic approaches among tumors which are included in the differential diagnoses.

This report describes an extremely rare case of poorly differentiated thyroid carcinoma arising in struma ovarii. This case emphasizes the importance of macroscopic examination of the specimen and the awareness of this uncommon tumor in the differential diagnosis of ovarian neoplasms.

2. Case Report

2.1. Clinical History. A 22-year-old woman presented with increased abdominal girth which she had experienced for 5 months. Physical examination and pelvic ultrasonography revealed a 15 cm right ovarian solid mass. The patient underwent an exploratory laparotomy. The intraoperative findings were unremarkable except for the right ovarian mass. Peritoneal washing fluid was collected for cytology. A right salpingooophorectomy, right pelvic and para-aortic lymph node and omental biopsies, and appendectomy were performed. The initial diagnosis of the right ovarian mass was FIGO stage IA endometrioid adenocarcinoma grade 2. Postoperatively, the patient was referred to Chiang Mai University Hospital for further management. The review of the histologic slides of the initial tissue samples raised a differential diagnosis of Sertoli cell tumor. Immunohistochemical staining was performed and the residual gross specimen was reviewed with additional tissue sampling. The pathological diagnosis was reported as proliferative struma ovarii with atypical features, and a clinical metastatic work-up was recommended.

The patient underwent a thyroid scan which showed no evidence of a primary thyroid lesion. No clinical evidence of a metastatic lesion was detected in the chest X-ray and abdominal computed tomography (CT) scan. Close surveillance was planned, but the patient was lost to follow-up. Fifteen months after surgery, she presented with a dry cough for 1 month. A chest X-ray and CT scan revealed multiple and bilateral pulmonary nodules, consistent with metastatic lesions. No intra-abdominal disease was identified in the CT scan. The serum thyroglobulin level was 247.3 ng/mL (normal range $\leq$ 40 ng/mL). Recurrence of malignant struma ovarii was clinically considered. A pulmonary biopsy was not performed. The patient underwent a total thyroidectomy, followed by high dose radioactive iodine (I-131) therapy. The resected thyroid specimen was unremarkable. The clinical condition of the patient was stable and there was no progression of the pulmonary nodules seen after 3 episodes of iodine treatment during a 2-year period.

Forty-two months after the surgery, the patient developed hemoptysis and dyspnea. Chemotherapy (cisplatin and Adriamycin) was started and continued for 6 cycles. Five years after surgery, there was a progressive enlargement of the pulmonary nodules, accompanied by weakness of her left arm due to intramedullary spinal cord metastasis. The patient died of the disease 7 years after the initial surgery.

2.2. Pathological Findings. Macroscopically, the right ovarian mass was a solid yellow white mass with areas of necrosis and hemorrhage (Figure 1). The capsule was intact. The review of the residual gross specimen with additional serial sectioning revealed few gelatinous tan foci and a 1 cm focus of gray sebaceous material.

Microscopically, the ovarian mass was composed of relatively uniform cuboidal to columnar cells with round to oval nuclei, predominantly arranged in a tubular pattern (Figures 2(a) and 2(b)). Dilated gland-like spaces with papillary-like infolding lined by elongated columnar cells simulating endometrioid adenocarcinoma were focally observed (Figures 2(c) and 2(d)). Solid tubules, a trabecular arrangement, and solid cell nests or an insular pattern were also present. The insular pattern (Figure 3(a)) accounted for approximately 20% of the tumor tissue. Mitotic activity was variable, ranging from absent or rare in the tubular areas to 11 in 10 high-power fields in the solid areas (Figure 3(b)). Large zones of previous infarction with hyalinized fibrosis were observed in the macroscopically necrotic areas. However, small foci of coagulative tumor cell necrosis were present within the neoplastic cell sheets (Figure 3(c)). Neither true papillary structures with fibrovascular cores nor ground glass/grooved nuclei were observed. Areas of typical thyroid-type tissue (Figure 3(d)) and a focus of mature cystic teratoma (dermoid cyst with cartilage) were identified in the second round of tissue sampling. Neither capsular involvement nor lymphovascular invasion was detected. Immunohistochemical stains showed a diffuse positive reaction for pancytokeratin (AE3/AE3), cytokeratin 7, and thyroglobulin (Figure 4), with focal reactions for epithelial membrane antigen (EMA) and vimentin. The immunostains for calretinin, CD99, chromogranin A, and synaptophysin were negative.

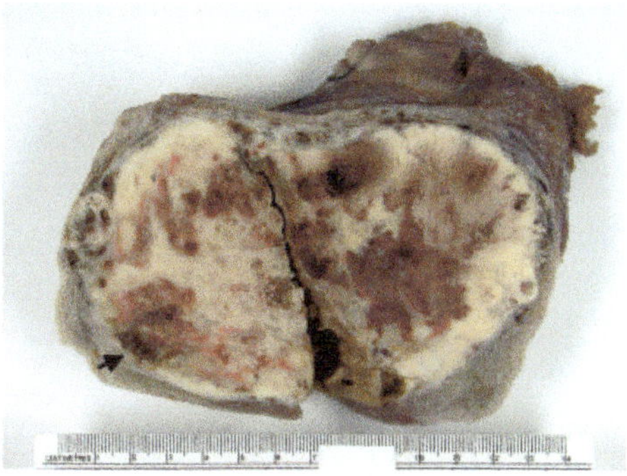

FIGURE 1: The right ovarian mass shows a solid yellow white sectioned surface with areas of necrosis and hemorrhage. A small gelatinous focus is observed (arrow).

3. Discussion

Strumal lesions of the ovary may occasionally be confused with ovarian tumors, particularly when the typical thyroid or teratomatous component is not apparent [4, 5]. Foci of the usual-type teratomatous tissue may be small and sometimes cannot be histologically documented, even with extensive tissue sampling. A rare possibility of metastatic ovarian involvement from primary thyroid cancer should be borne in mind in the examination of an ovarian strumal lesion without an associated teratomatous component, and a correlation with the clinical data is required to rule out this possibility because the clinical history of primary thyroid cancer may be remote [8].

Histologically, the microfollicular pattern commonly present in ovarian strumal lesions tends to raise a differential diagnosis of granulosa cell tumor [2]. In the cases with tubular pattern, differential diagnoses may include Sertoli cell tumor and endometrioid adenocarcinoma (sertoliform variant). In

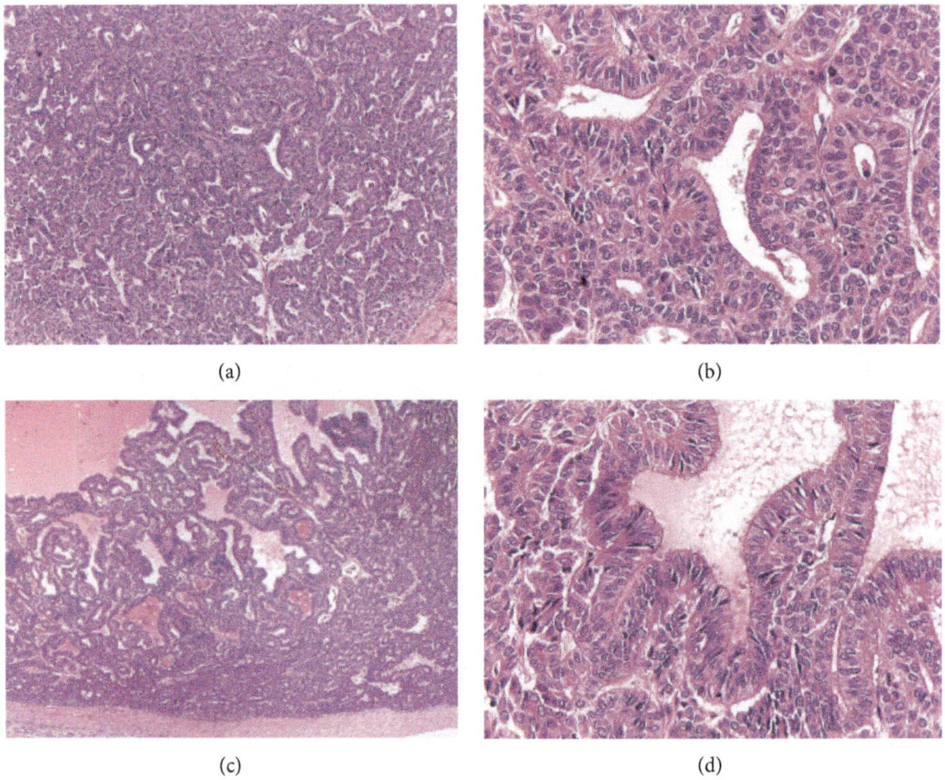

Figure 2: A significant histological appearance of the ovarian tumor. ((a) and (b)) Tubular pattern composed of columnar cells with uniform nuclei. ((c) and (d)) Focal endometrioid-like pattern characterized by dilated gland-like structures with papillary-like infolding.

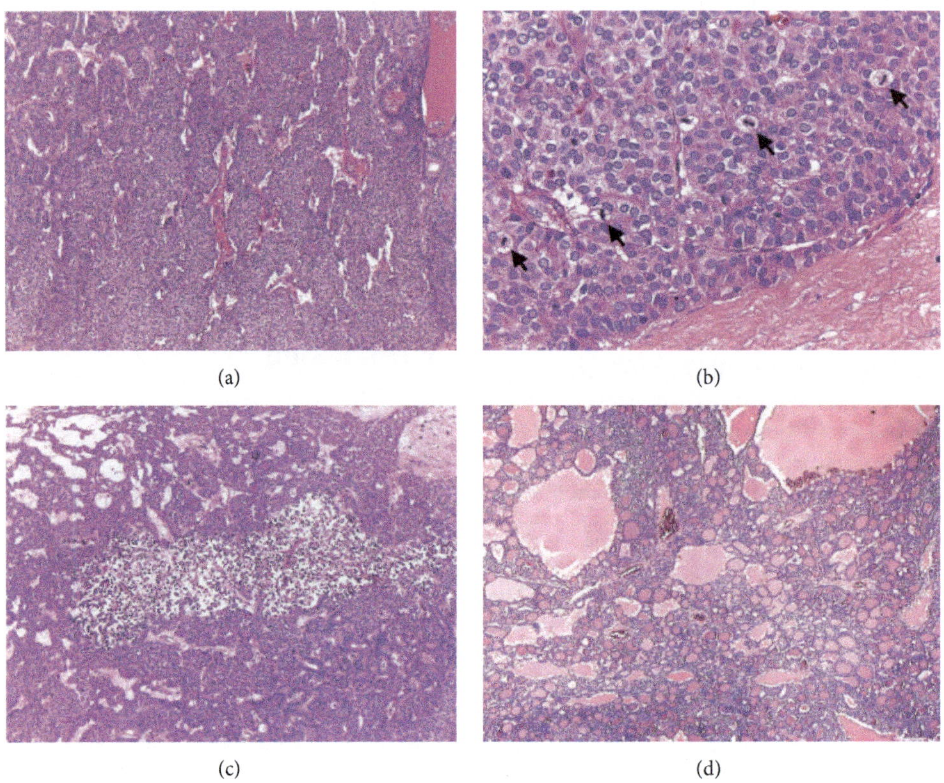

Figure 3: A poorly differentiated thyroid carcinoma component ((a) to (c)) and a typical thyroid area (d) in the ovarian tumor. ((a) and (b)) Insular and solid patterns composed of uniform cells with increased mitotic activity (arrows). (c) A focus of coagulative tumor cell necrosis. (d) Typical thyroid follicles with abundant colloid are identified in additional tissue samples.

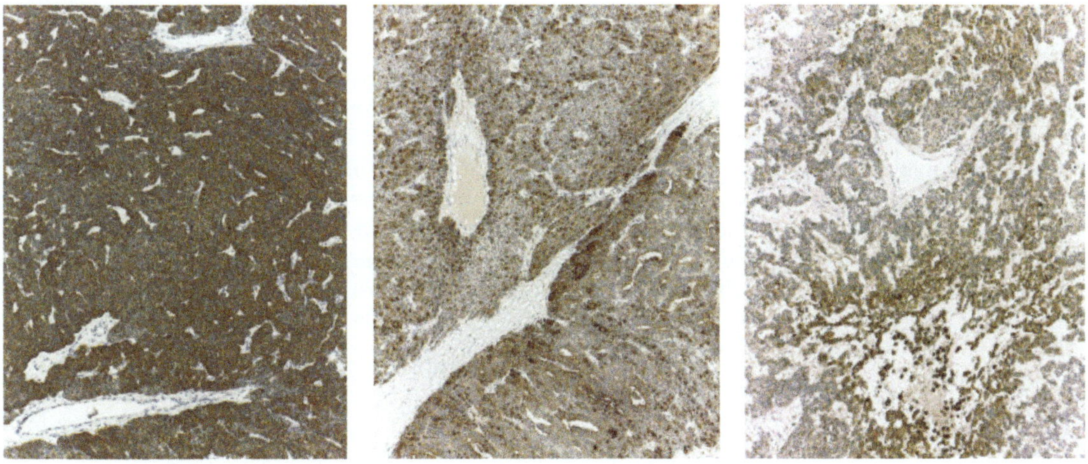

(a) (b) (c)

FIGURE 4: Positive immunohistochemical staining of ovarian tumor. (a) Cytokeratin 7. (b) Thyroglobulin (including an area of insular pattern in the top). (c) Epithelial membrane antigen.

TABLE 1: Comparison of immunohistochemical stain results in the differential diagnoses.

	Ovarian strumal lesions	Endometrioid tumor	Sertoli cell tumor	Carcinoid tumor
Cytokeratin 7	+	+	−	+ or −
Epithelial membrane antigen	+	+	−	+
Calretinin/inhibin	−	−	+	−
Thyroglobulin/TTF-1	+	−	−	−
Chromogranin/synaptophysin	−	−	−	+

addition, cord-like or trabecular arrangement and insular pattern may raise a concern of carcinoid tumor [4].

Sertoli cell tumor is an important differential diagnosis of an ovarian tumor with a tubular pattern in young women [5]. Sertoli cell tumor also shows a cord-like/trabecular arrangement, or a nest-like or solid pattern [5], which overlaps with the histological patterns in poorly differentiated thyroid carcinoma (i.e., trabecular, insular, or solid) as seen in this case. In addition, tumor cell necrosis and increased mitotic activity can be observed in Sertoli cell tumors [5].

Endometrioid adenocarcinoma may have a prominent tubular (sertoliform) pattern. A microglandular pattern in endometrioid adenocarcinoma may be similar to thyroid microfollicles. However, endometrioid tumors are uncommon in young women [9]. An association with endometriosis and/or adenofibroma and the presence of squamous differentiation are helpful features in supporting the diagnosis of an endometrioid tumor [9].

Carcinoid (or neuroendocrine) tumor is classified in the ovarian teratoma category and may occur in admixture with struma ovarii (strumal carcinoid) [1]. Carcinoid tumor may show insular and trabecular patterns and acinar/follicle-like arrangement which overlap with the features of poorly differentiated thyroid carcinoma. Although most ovarian carcinoid tumors have a favorable prognosis, the presence of increased mitotic activity and degree of nuclear atypia signifies the spectrum of atypical carcinoid tumor or neuroendocrine carcinoma which may exhibit aggressive behavior [10].

Immunohistochemical stains are helpful in confirmation of the diagnosis (Table 1). However, immunohistochemical stains can also be a pitfall when the strumal nature is not included in the consideration and the main differential diagnoses are only endometrioid tumor and Sertoli cell tumor. Using the immunohistochemical panel of EMA, CK7, inhibin, and calretinin, the EMA/CK7-positive and inhibin/calretinin-negative profile can lead to a misdiagnosis as an endometrioid tumor.

The diagnostic criteria for malignant struma ovarii were previously based on those applied to the identification of typical thyroid-type carcinomas. Due to the lack of a tumor capsule in struma ovarii, the capsular invasion criterion for thyroid follicular carcinoma was previously omitted in the evaluation of ovarian strumal follicular lesions [3]. Recently, extension of the tumor through the ovarian serosa forming a polypoid or nodular growth on the surface and/or the spread of tumor beyond the ovary at the diagnosis is considered to be a criterion for malignancy regardless of a bland-appearing or highly differentiated histomorphology of thyroid tissue [2, 11]. In addition to surface involvement or an extraovarian spread, a large tumor size (12 cm or more), dense surface adhesion, or ascites can provide a further clue regarding the risk of clinical disease progression [2, 7]. However, there are a minor proportion of cases in which the clinical detection of metastatic lesions during follow-up was the only indicator of malignant behavior [2].

Papillary carcinoma is the most common malignant form of struma ovarii and is promptly diagnosable by the presence of papillary architecture and well-recognized "ground glass" nuclei [2, 7]. Nevertheless, in the absence of true papillary structures, only the focal presence of ground glass nuclei is not sufficient for the diagnosis of papillary carcinoma in struma ovarii [2, 12]. For the diagnosis of follicular carcinoma arising in ovarian struma, vascular invasion is a useful feature but this is rarely observed [2, 7]. Thus, the presence of ovarian serosal invasion is an important diagnostic clue. Anaplastic carcinoma is recognized by marked nuclear atypia which should be distinguished from atypical nuclei in Hürthle cell change [2].

Poorly differentiated thyroid carcinoma represents a rare type of primary thyroid cancer and occurs extremely rarely in ovarian struma [7, 13]. Until recently, the diagnostic criteria of poorly differentiated thyroid carcinomas have been a controversial issue [14]. In recent consensus criteria, poorly differentiated thyroid carcinoma is characterized by a uniform population of small follicular cells arranged in a solid, trabecular, or insular pattern, commonly accompanied by significant mitotic activity (≥3 in 10 high-power fields), tumor necrosis, or convoluted nuclei, in the absence of typical nuclear characteristics of papillary carcinoma [14]. Using these criteria, the minor solid component with increased mitotic activity and focal necrosis in the present case (Figure 3) is qualified for a diagnosis of poorly differentiated thyroid carcinoma arising in struma ovarii. The presence of a poorly differentiated carcinoma component is an adverse prognostic indicator as observed in thyroid cancer. Even a minor poorly differentiated component (10–50%) within usual follicular thyroid carcinoma is associated with a significantly decreased survival [15].

The clinical course of thyroid carcinoma arising in struma ovarii is typically protracted with late recurrence and long survival duration in most cases [2]. In patients with malignant histological features, the 10-year and 25-year survival rates were 81% and 60%, respectively [2]. Among patients who died of disease, the median survival duration was 21 years in those with stage 1A, which was much longer than that of higher stage patients (5 years) [12]. In recent large studies on malignant struma ovarii, the clinical behavior was difficult to predict based on tumor histomorphology alone [2, 12, 16]. However, the presence of a minor component of anaplastic or poorly differentiated carcinoma appears to signify a poor clinical outcome. Patients with anaplastic or poorly differentiated thyroid carcinoma in struma ovarii had a shorter survival duration than those with the differentiated-type (papillary and follicular) carcinoma [2, 7].

Of 4 reported cases of poorly differentiated thyroid carcinoma arising in struma ovarii (including the present case), 3 patients were less than 30 years (22, 24, and 27 years) and at FIGO stage I (2 in stage IA and 1 in stage IC), whereas the remaining patient was 70 years of age and at stage II [7, 13, 17]. In 2 patients with available follow-up data, both received radioactive iodine treatment; the stage II patient died of the disease 3 years after the initial diagnosis [13], while the stage IA patient (the present case) died 7 years after the diagnosis.

In patients with advanced stage thyroid-type carcinoma arising in ovarian struma or those with tumor recurrence, thyroid ablation by surgery and radioactive iodine therapy has been recommended [6, 12]. The treatment in a stage I patient should be determined on an individual basis, with consideration of the risk and benefit to each patient [16]. Due to the poor prognosis of cases with anaplastic or poorly differentiated thyroid carcinoma in struma ovarii, stage IA patients with such component may benefit from an aggressive treatment approach [16].

Conflict of Interests

The authors declare that there is no conflict of interests regarding the publication of this paper.

Acknowledgments

This study was supported by (1) the National Research University Project, under Thailand's Office of the Higher Education Commission, and (2) the Faculty of Medicine, Chiang Mai University.

References

[1] J. Prat, D. Cao, S. G. Carinelli, F. F. Nogales, R. Vang, and C. J. Zaloudek, "Monodermal teratomas and somatic-type tumors arising in a dermoid cyst," in *WHO Classification of Tumors of Female Reproductive Organs*, R. J. Kurman, M. L. Carcangiu, S. Herrington, and R. H. Young, Eds., pp. 63–66, IARC, Lyon, France, 2014.

[2] S. J. Robboy, R. Shaco-Levy, R. Y. Peng et al., "Malignant struma ovarii: an analysis of 88 cases, including 27 with extraovarian spread," *International Journal of Gynecological Pathology*, vol. 28, no. 5, pp. 405–422, 2009.

[3] K. Devaney, R. Snyder, H. J. Norris, and F. A. Tavassoli, "Proliferative and histologically malignant struma ovarii: a clinicopathologic study of 54 cases," *International Journal of Gynecological Pathology*, vol. 12, no. 4, pp. 333–343, 1993.

[4] W. M. Szyfelbein, R. H. Young, and R. E. Scully, "Struma ovarii simulating ovarian tumors of other types: a report of 30 cases," *American Journal of Surgical Pathology*, vol. 19, no. 1, pp. 21–29, 1995.

[5] E. Oliva, T. Alvarez, and R. H. Young, "Sertoli cell tumors of the ovary: a clinicopathologic and immunohistochemical study of 54 cases," *American Journal of Surgical Pathology*, vol. 29, no. 2, pp. 143–156, 2005.

[6] X. Zhang and C. Axiotis, "Thyroid-type carcinoma of struma ovarii," *Archives of Pathology and Laboratory Medicine*, vol. 134, no. 5, pp. 786–791, 2010.

[7] L. M. Roth, A. Talerman, J. Wadsley, and A. I. Karseladze, "Risk factors in thyroid-type carcinoma arising in ovarian struma: a report of 15 cases with comparison to ordinary struma ovarii," *Histopathology*, vol. 57, no. 1, pp. 148–152, 2010.

[8] R. H. Young, A. Jackson, and M. Wells, "Ovarian metastasis from thyroid carcinoma 12 years after partial thyroidectomy mimicking struma ovarii: report of a case," *International Journal of Gynecological Pathology*, vol. 13, no. 2, pp. 181–185, 1994.

[9] W. G. McCluggage and R. H. Young, "Ovarian sertoli-leydig cell tumors with pseudoendometrioid tubules (pseudoendometrioid Sertoli-Leydig cell tumors)," *The American Journal of Surgical Pathology*, vol. 31, no. 4, pp. 592–597, 2007.

[10] T. Kurabayashi, T. Minamikawa, S. Nishijima et al., "Primary strumal carcinoid tumor of the ovary with multiple bone and breast metastases," *Journal of Obstetrics and Gynaecology Research*, vol. 36, no. 3, pp. 567–571, 2010.

[11] L. M. Roth and A. I. Karseladze, "Highly differentiated follicular carcinoma arising from struma ovarii: a report of 3 cases, a review of the literature, and a reassessment of so-called peritoneal strumosis," *International Journal of Gynecological Pathology*, vol. 27, no. 2, pp. 213–222, 2008.

[12] R. Shaco-Levy, S. M. Bean, R. C. Bentley, and S. J. Robboy, "Natural history of biologically malignant struma ovarii: analysis of 27 cases with extraovarian spread," *International Journal of Gynecological Pathology*, vol. 29, no. 3, pp. 212–227, 2010.

[13] L. M. Roth, A. W. Miller III, and A. Talerman, "Typical thyroid-type carcinoma arising in struma ovarii: a report of 4 cases and review of the literature," *International Journal of Gynecological Pathology*, vol. 27, no. 4, pp. 496–506, 2008.

[14] M. Volante, P. Collini, Y. E. Nikiforov et al., "Poorly differentiated thyroid carcinoma: the Turin proposal for the use of uniform diagnostic criteria and an algorithmic diagnostic approach," *American Journal of Surgical Pathology*, vol. 31, no. 8, pp. 1256–1264, 2007.

[15] M. Dettmer, A. Schmitt, H. Steinert et al., "Poorly differentiated thyroid carcinomas: how much poorly differentiated is needed?" *American Journal of Surgical Pathology*, vol. 35, no. 12, pp. 1866–1872, 2011.

[16] R. Shaco-Levy, R. Y. Peng, M. J. Snyder et al., "Malignant struma ovarii: a blinded study of 86 cases assessing which histologic features correlate with aggressive clinical behavior," *Archives of Pathology and Laboratory Medicine*, vol. 136, no. 2, pp. 172–178, 2012.

[17] C. D. Olinici and M. Mera, "Poorly differentiated ('insular') thyroid carcinoma of the ovary," *Morphologie et Embryologie*, vol. 34, no. 2, pp. 135–137, 1988.

14

Colorectal Microcarcinoids in Association with Long-Term Exposure to Urinary Content: A Case Report and Review of the Literature

Grace W. Weyant, Dipti M. Karamchandani, and Negar Rassaei

Department of Pathology, Penn State Milton S. Hershey Medical Center, 500 University Drive, P.O. Box 850, MC H179, Hershey, PA 17033, USA

Correspondence should be addressed to Grace W. Weyant; gweyant@hmc.psu.edu

Academic Editor: Dengfeng Cao

Long-term exposure of colonic mucosa to urinary content and its association with increased risk of infection, mechanical and biochemical irritation, and malignancy have been described in the literature. Existing case reports and studies depict the low but distinct risk of malignancy in gastrointestinal segments which come in contact with urinary content as a result of surgical correction of urinary tract abnormalities. However, these reports are largely limited to colonic adenocarcinoma and urothelial cell carcinoma. Late urointestinal carcinoma in patients with ileal incorporation into the urinary tract has also been reported. To the best of our knowledge, however, there is only one case report documenting neuroendocrine (NE) cell hyperplasia in colonic mucosa after long-term cystoplasty. Our case is the first to describe microcarcinoids and diffuse NE hyperplasia occurring in a patient with congenital anorectal anomalies, resulting in long-term exposure of colonic mucosa to fecal stream and urinary content. This case, in conjunction with the reported cases in the literature, raises the distinct possibility of an association between exposure of colonic mucosa to urine and long-term development of malignancy, including NE neoplasms.

1. Introduction

Gastrointestinal segments are commonly utilized for urinary tract reconstruction when the creation of a conduit or bladder replacement is indicated [1, 2]. Long-term exposure of colonic mucosa to urinary content is associated with risk of infection, mechanical and biochemical irritation, and malignancy [1, 3]. Rare case reports and studies of malignancy, particularly colonic adenocarcinoma and urothelial cell carcinoma, have been reported in the literature in this setting [1, 4, 5]. Rarely, neuroendocrine (NE) cells, which are usually inconspicuous occupants within the colonic mucosa, may become hyperplastic [2, 6]. We herein describe the first case of microcarcinoids with diffuse NE cell hyperplasia occurring in a patient with a history of congenital imperforate anus and colovesicular fistula, which resulted in prolonged exposure of colonic mucosa to urinary content.

2. Case Presentation

A 29-year-old male presented to our tertiary facility with imperforate anus and associated urinary incontinence. The patient had a history of multiple congenital abnormalities detected at birth, including atrial septal defect (ASD), persistent left-sided superior vena cava, cardiac conduction abnormalities, Wolff-Parkinson-White (WPW) syndrome, and vertebral anomalies. The gastrointestinal and genitourinary abnormalities were comprised of malformations including imperforate anus with the rectum terminating to the left and above the sphincteric complex, a connection between the rectum and bladder, and left vesicoureteral reflux.

He underwent open cardiac surgery for repair of the ASD and ablation of the WPW foci. Also, shortly after birth, the patient underwent surgery during which a loop transverse colostomy was created and an anoplasty was

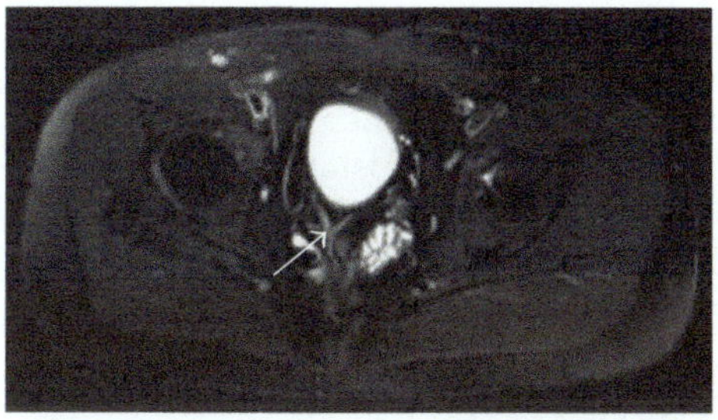

FIGURE 1: MRI of pelvis at the level of the bladder and rectum. Arrow: colovesicular fistula.

attempted unsuccessfully. Subsequently at the age of 26, a posterior sagittal anorectoplasty could not be completed due to technical difficulties. For the past several years, the patient had stool from the proximal portion of his colostomy and urine from the distal nonfunctional limb with persistent exposure of both colostomy limbs to urine and fecal material.

On physical examination, a left upper quadrant colostomy and imperforate anus were confirmed. MRI demonstrated the abnormalities stated above and suggested a mass near the colovesicular fistula (Figure 1). Endoscopic evaluation with colonoscopy and cystoscopy with biopsies did not demonstrate any pathologic alterations. Examination under anesthesia with muscle stimulation demonstrated functional anal sphincter muscles. Thus, the patient underwent takedown of the colovesicular fistula, closure of the bladder neck, reimplantation of the right ureter, small bowel resection with creation of an ileovesicostomy, colostomy takedown, colocolonic anastomosis, low anterior resection, posterior sagittal anorectoplasty, and coloanal anastomosis with a diverting loop ileostomy. He recovered well from the surgery without complications.

The specimen consisted of a segment of rectum containing the colovesicular fistula and a segment of sigmoid colon submitted separately, measuring 8.2 cm and 6.8 cm in length, respectively. Examination of initial representative sections revealed the incidental finding of neuroendocrine cell hyperplasia, after which the entire rectal specimen was submitted for microscopic evaluation. Histologic sections of the rectum and sigmoid demonstrated multiple microscopic foci of neuroendocrine cell hyperplasia with rare foci of microcarcinoids, the largest of which measured 5 mm in greatest dimension. These foci involved the mucosa and submucosa and were composed of small clusters of medium-sized cells with small round to oval nuclei containing fine chromatin with a salt and pepper appearance (Figures 2 and 3). The mitotic rate was 1 per 10 high power fields. Necrosis was absent. By immunohistochemistry, the lesional cells were strongly and diffusely immunoreactive with synaptophysin and chromogranin (Figure 4). The proliferative index, assessed with Ki-67, was less than 2% (Figure 5). Additionally, serum chromogranin A levels were found to be normal.

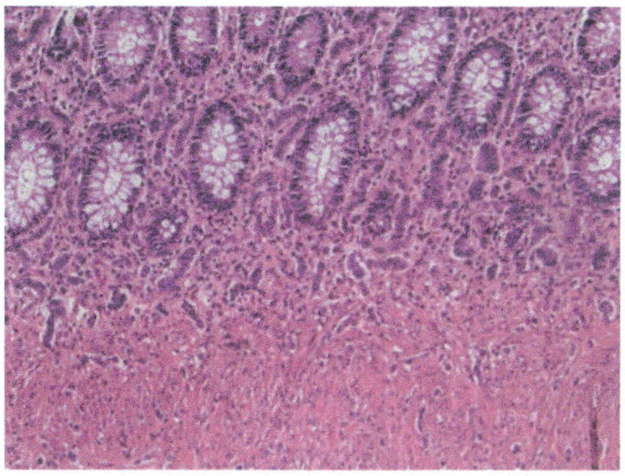

FIGURE 2: Clusters and cords of medium-sized cells with small round to oval nuclei dispersed within the colonic mucosa (H&E, ×200).

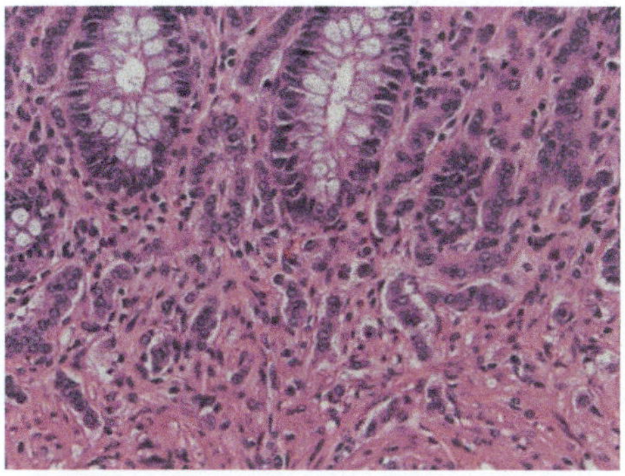

FIGURE 3: At high power, the cells contain fine chromatin. Nucleoli and mitoses are inconspicuous (H&E, ×400).

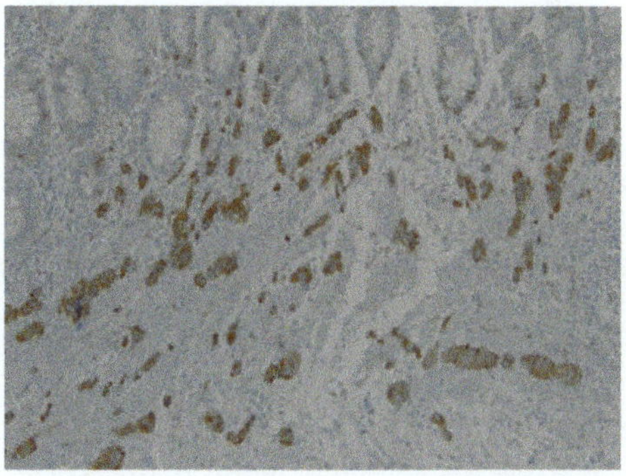

FIGURE 4: Strong and diffuse immunoreactivity with synaptophysin confirms neuroendocrine differentiation (Synaptophysin, ×200).

3. Discussion

Review of the literature demonstrates a risk of malignancy in gastrointestinal segments exposed to urine following surgical correction of urinary tract abnormalities [3–5, 7]. Late occurrence of colonic adenocarcinoma after ureterosigmoidostomy has been reported with an incidence of 5 to 40%, representing a significant increase compared to the age-matched general population [1, 8, 9]. Also, a higher risk of malignancy in bowel segments after cystoplasty or urinary conduit reconstruction has been documented [3, 10, 11]. The most commonly reported cancers include adenocarcinoma and urothelial cell carcinoma; however, rare cases of squamous cell carcinoma have been reported as well [1]. Typically, these tumors develop within a few years to decades after the surgical procedure and are located at the anastomotic site [12].

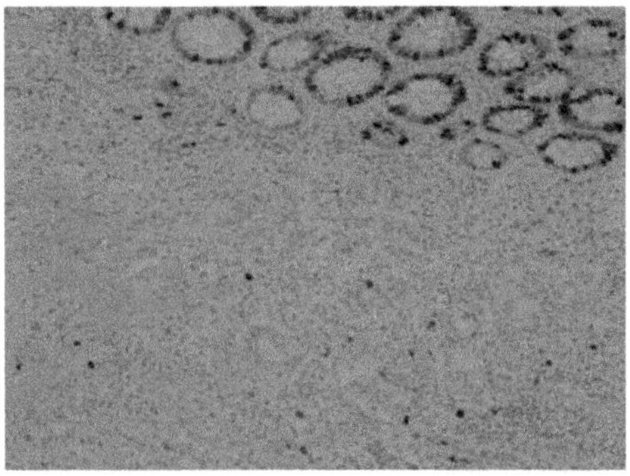

FIGURE 5: The proliferation index was <2% (Ki-67, ×200).

While the physiopathologic mechanism is not well known, it has been postulated that contact among urine, feces, urothelium, and colonic epithelium at the anastomotic site of ureterosigmoidostomies activates fecal carcinogens [8, 13]. Also, bacteriuria and production of N-nitrosamine have been considered responsible factors for tumorigenesis [11, 12].

Neuroendocrine cell hyperplasia (NEH) is a well-established entity in the lung and in the upper gastrointestinal tract, particularly stomach [6] and pancreas. However, there is no such well-defined entity in the colon. NE tumors in the colon represent approximately 1-2% of colorectal neoplasms. In the rectum, this type of tumor typically occurs in the 6th decade of life and has a low propensity for lymph node involvement and distant metastasis [14–16].

While the association of NEH with certain entities such as inflammatory bowel disease and diversion colitis is well documented [2, 17, 18], to the best of our knowledge, there is only one case report describing NEH in colonic tissue used for cystoplasty [2]. Kochevar reports a case of adenocarcinoid tumor arising in an ureteroileal conduit [7]. These studies describe the development of different types of cellular hyperplasia and malignancy in intestinal mucosa in contact with urine after ureterosigmoidostomy or cystoplasty exposing intestinal mucosa to urine with no or low fecal stream. Our case is the first to show microcarcinoids and NEH in colonic mucosa exposed to urinary content due to the type of conduit implemented. Interestingly, in our case NEH was observed not only at the fistula site but also distantly in the sigmoid, suggesting a more diffuse phenomenon. There was no significant inflammation despite long-term exposure of colonic mucosa to urinary content. The biologic mechanism of this finding is not known; however, the possibility of a process akin to that described in patients with ureterosigmoidostomy and cystoplasty who develop carcinoma has been raised.

4. Conclusion

Review of the literature demonstrates that few cases have been reported exhibiting the occurrence of different types of malignancy in association with long-term exposure of colonic mucosa with urinary content. Our case shows development of NEH and microcarcinoids in association with long-term exposure of colonic mucosa to urinary content. While uncommon, the reported cases establish the possibility of development of malignancy including NE neoplasms in the urointestinal tract postoperatively. Thus, one may recommend long-term follow-up of those patients who have undergone a surgical procedure exposing intestinal mucosa to urinary contents with or without fecal stream.

Conflict of Interests

The authors declare that there is no conflict of interests regarding the publication of this paper.

References

[1] A. A. Shokeir, M. Shamaa, M. M. El-Mekresh, M. El-Baz, and M. A. Ghoneim, "Late malignancy in bowel segments exposed to urine without fecal stream," *Urology*, vol. 46, no. 5, pp. 657–661, 1995.

[2] K. Oien, M. Akyol, and G. Lindop, "Neuroendocrine cell hyperplasia in colonic tissue used for long term augmentation cystoplasty," *Journal of Clinical Pathology*, vol. 51, no. 3, pp. 258–261, 1998.

[3] R. B. Filmer and J. R. Spencer, "Malignancies in bladder augmentations and intestinal conduits," *Journal of Urology*, vol. 143, no. 4, pp. 671–678, 1990.

[4] J. Moorcraft, C. E. H. DuBoulay, P. Isaacson, and J. D. Atwell, "Changes in the mucosa of colon conduits with particular reference to the risk of malignant change," *British Journal of Urology*, vol. 55, no. 2, pp. 185–188, 1983.

[5] J. S. Little Jr., L. W. Klee, D. M. Hoover, and R. C. Rink, "Long-term histopathological changes observed in rats subjected to augmentation cystoplasty," *The Journal of Urology*, vol. 152, no. 2, part 2, pp. 720–724, 1994.

[6] Y. Dayal, R. A. DeLellis, and H. J. Wolfe, "Hyperplastic lesions of the gastrointestinal endocrine cells," *The American Journal of Surgical Pathology*, vol. 11, supplement 1, pp. 87–101, 1987.

[7] J. Kochevar, "Adenocarcinoid tumor, goblet cell type, arising in a ureterioleal conduit: a case report," *Journal of Urology*, vol. 131, no. 5, pp. 957–959, 1984.

[8] R. F. Gittes, "Carcinogenesis in ureterosigmoidostomy," *Urologic Clinics of North America*, vol. 13, no. 2, pp. 201–205, 1986.

[9] G. W. Leadbetter Jr., P. Zickerman, and E. Pierce, "Ureterosigmoidostomy and carcinoma of the colon," *The Journal of Urology*, vol. 121, no. 6, pp. 732–735, 1979.

[10] D. A. Husmann and H. M. Spence, "Current status of tumor of the bowel following ureterosigmoidostomy: a review," *The Journal of Urology*, vol. 144, no. 3, pp. 607–610, 1990.

[11] M. S. Chiang, J. P. Minton, K. Clausen, H. W. Clatworthy, and H. A. Wise II, "Carcinoma in a colon conduit urinary diversion," *The Journal of Urology*, vol. 127, no. 6, pp. 1185–1187, 1982.

[12] W. Mansson and R. Willen, "Mucosal morphology and histochemistry of the continent cecal reservoir for urine," *Journal of Urology*, vol. 139, no. 6, pp. 1199–1201, 1988.

[13] N. Daher, R. Gautier, H. Abourachid, C. Decaens, and J. Bara, "Rat colonic carcinogenesis after ureterosigmoidostomy: pathogenesis and immunohistological study," *The Journal of Urology*, vol. 139, no. 6, pp. 1331–1336, 1988.

[14] E. Solcia, R. Fiocca, L. Villani, O. Luinetti, and C. Capella, "Hyperplastic, dysplastic, and neoplastic enterochromaffin-like-cell proliferations of the gastric mucosa. Classification and

histogenesis," *The American Journal of Surgical Pathology*, vol. 19, supplement 1, pp. S1–S7, 1995.

[15] G. Klöppel, M. Anlauf, and A. Perren, "Endocrine precursor lesions of gastroenteropancreatic neuroendocrine tumors," *Endocrine Pathology*, vol. 18, no. 3, pp. 150–155, 2007.

[16] G. Rindi and E. Solcia, "Endocrine hyperplasia and dysplasia in the pathogenesis of gastrointestinal and pancreatic endocrine tumors," *Gastroenterology Clinics of North America*, vol. 36, no. 4, pp. 851–865, 2007.

[17] G. B. M. Lindop, "Enterochromaffin cell hyperplasia and megacolon: report of a case," *Gut*, vol. 24, no. 6, pp. 575–578, 1983.

[18] A. P. Griffiths and M. F. Dixon, "Microcarcinoids and diversion colitis in a colon defunctioned for 18 years—report of a case," *Diseases of the Colon & Rectum*, vol. 35, no. 7, pp. 685–688, 1992.

15

Pediatric Papillary Renal Cell Carcinoma in a Horseshoe Kidney: A Case Report with Review of the Literature

Abelardo Loya-Solis,[1] Lucía Alemán-Meza,[2] Luis Carlos Canales-Martínez,[2] Rodolfo Franco-Márquez,[2] Alim Adriana Rincón-Bahena,[2] Karla María Nuñez-Barragán,[3] Raquel Garza-Guajardo,[2] and Marco Antonio Ponce-Camacho[2]

[1]*Pathology Department, Spanish Hospital of Mexico, Ejercito Nacional 613, 11560 Mexico City, DF, Mexico*
[2]*Pathology Department, University Hospital "Dr. Jose E. Gonzalez" and Medical School of the Autonomous University of Nuevo Leon, Francisco I. Madero and Gonzalitos, 64460 Monterrey, NL, Mexico*
[3]*Medical Imaging Department, University Hospital "Dr. Jose E. Gonzalez" and Medical School of the Autonomous University of Nuevo Leon, Francisco I. Madero and Gonzalitos, 64460 Monterrey, NL, Mexico*

Correspondence should be addressed to Abelardo Loya-Solis; a_loya_solis@hotmail.com

Academic Editor: Yoji Nagashima

Renal cell carcinoma is the most common malignancy of the kidney in adults. In children, however, it only accounts for an estimated 1.8 to 6.3% of all pediatric malignant renal tumors. Papillary renal cell carcinoma is the second most common type of renal cell carcinoma in children. We present the case of a 12-year-old boy with a 2-month history of abdominal pain, unexplained weight loss, and gross hematuria. Computed tomography revealed a horseshoe kidney and a well-defined mass of 4 cm arising from the lower pole of the right kidney. Microscopically the tumor was composed of papillae covered with cells with abundant eosinophilic cytoplasm and high-grade nuclei with prominent nucleoli. Immunohistochemistry was performed; EMA, Vimentin, and AMACR were strongly positive while CK7, CD10, RCC antigen, TFE3, HMB-45, and WT-1 were negative. Currently, 10 months after the surgical procedure, the patient remains clinically and radiologically disease-free.

1. Introduction

Malignant neoplasms of the kidney are a fairly common group of tumors representing up to 2% of the total human cancer burden [1]. Renal cell carcinoma (RCC) is the most common malignancy of the kidney in adults [1]. In children, however, it only accounts for an estimated 1.8 to 6.3% of all pediatric malignant renal tumors [2, 3]. Papillary renal cell carcinoma (PRCC) is a malignant renal parenchymal tumor with a papillary or tubulopapillary architecture. PRCC is the second most common type of RCC in children and accounts for 30% of RCCs [4]. The usual clinical presentation consists of abdominal pain, palpable mass, and gross hematuria, but this classic triad is only found in 6% of cases [5]. No proper therapy has been defined for children with RCC. Surgery constitutes the main treatment and results in cure when the tumor is localized and completely resected [6].

2. Case Report

A 12-year-old boy presented with a 2-month history of abdominal pain, unexplained weight loss, and gross hematuria. Physical examination revealed no abnormalities. Urine examination confirmed gross hematuria and urine culture was sterile. Laboratory blood analyses were within normal limits and urinary excretion of catecholamines was also within the normal range. Upper abdominal computed tomography revealed a horseshoe kidney and a well-defined mass of 4 cm arising from the lower pole of the right kidney (Figure 1). Right nephroureterectomy with division of the isthmus of the horseshoe kidney was performed. The cut surface of the excised specimen showed a solid, circumscribed, heterogeneous tumor (size 4.3 × 3.5 cm), with solid areas alternating with cystic and hemorrhagic areas with widely clear margins (Figure 2). Histopathological examination

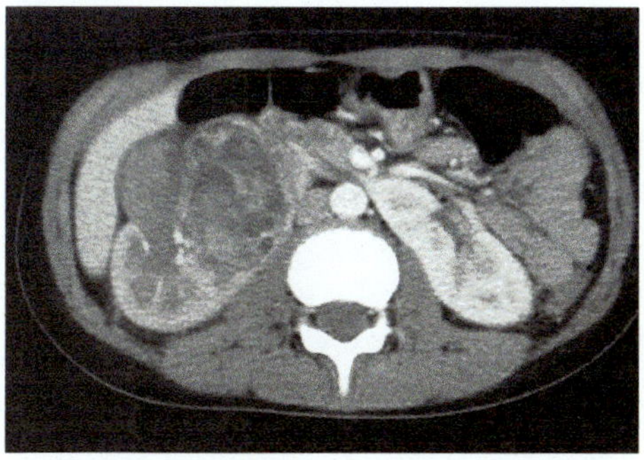

FIGURE 1: Abdominal computed tomography revealed an ill-defined tumor arising from the lower pole of the right kidney.

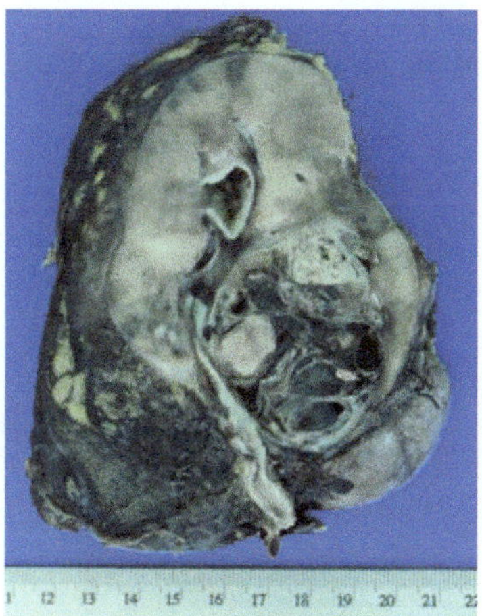

FIGURE 2: Gross photograph of the cut surface of the right kidney showing a heterogeneous tumor mass.

revealed a tumor surrounded by a pseudocapsule, composed of papillae covered with cells with abundant eosinophilic cytoplasm and high-grade nuclei with prominent nucleoli (Figure 3). Immunohistochemistry was performed using cytokeratin 7 (CK7), epithelial membrane antigen (EMA), Vimentin, CD10, RCC antigen, TFE3, HMB-45, WT-1, and alpha-methylacyl coenzyme-A racemase (AMACR). EMA, Vimentin, and AMACR were strongly positive (Figure 4). CK7, CD10, RCC antigen, TFE3, HMB-45, and WT-1 were negative. In view of these histopathological and immunohistochemistry findings a type 2 PRCC was diagnosed. Currently, 10 months after the surgical procedure, the patient remains clinically and radiologically disease-free.

3. Discussion

Horseshoe kidney is the most common type of renal fusion anomaly; it occurs in 1 per 400–600 live births and is twice as common in males as in females [7]. Horseshoe kidney consists of two distinct functioning kidneys on each side of the midline, connected at the lower poles by an isthmus of functioning renal parenchyma or fibrous tissue that crosses the midline of the body [8]. Almost one-third of all patients with horseshoe kidney remain asymptomatic, only being diagnosed incidentally during physical examination or by CT scans [9]. The incidence of neoplasms in a horseshoe kidney is approximately 3 to 4 times greater than in normal population and is possibly the result of chronic obstruction, lithiasis, and infection [3]. RCC is the most common neoplasm described in horseshoe kidneys, accounting for about 50% of cases [10]. The tumor can be localized at any part of the kidney but is most frequently found within the isthmus [11]. There has been only one reported case of a PRCC arising in a horseshoe kidney [9], and this is, to the best of our knowledge, the first reported case in a child.

The differential diagnosis of a renal tumor with tubulopapillary architecture in a child, like in our case, should include translocation-associated RCCs (Xp11.2 translocation RCC and RCC with t(6; 11)), epithelial predominant Wilms tumor (EPWT), metanephric adenoma (MA), and PRCC.

Unlike other types of RCC, Xp11.2 translocation RCC is not defined by its histologic features, although the most common feature is a papillary or nested architecture made up of cells with ample acidophilic cytoplasm. This tumor does not express cytokeratins or EMA, but HMB-45, CD10, and RCC are often expressed [12]. Nuclear immunoreactivity for TFE3 is confirmatory of this entity [12]. RCC with t(6; 11) features a biphasic population of neoplastic cells. The main cell type is epithelioid, with abundance of clear to eosinophilic cytoplasm and round nuclei with small nucleoli. The second population is composed of smaller cells typically clustered around nodules of hyaline basement membrane material [13]. Most cases have been negative for cytokeratins and EMA but positive for HMB-45 and Melan A [14]. Nuclear TFEB expression by immunohistochemistry is the most commonly used technique to establish this diagnosis [15]. Our case presented negativity for HMB-45 and TFE3, allowing us to disregard the possibility of an Xp11.2 translocation RCC. Although we could not perform an immunohistochemical stain for TFEB, the lack of a second population of neoplastic cells and the negativity for HMB-45 allowed us to discard the possibility of a RCC with t(6; 11).

Both EPWT and MA have cells with little cytoplasm and low grade nuclei without nucleoli. EPWTs like PRCC present a pseudocapsule composed of fibrous tissue, while MA does not present it [16]. Both EPWT and MA are characteristically positive to WT-1 [4]. The cytological features and the lack of expression for WT-1 of our case helped us to discard EPWT and MA as possible diagnoses.

Two subtypes of PRCC are recognized based on their histologic features [17]. Type 1 PRCC is the most frequent, accounting for approximately two-thirds of all PRCCs and is composed of papillae covered with a single layer of small cells and scant clear or pale cytoplasm and uniform nuclei with inconspicuous nucleoli [18]. Type 2 PRCC is composed of tumor cells with voluminous cytoplasm and pseudostratified high-grade nuclei with prominent nucleoli [18]. These subtypes also differ in their immunohistochemical phenotypes. CK7 is positive in 87% of type 1 and 20% of type 2 lesions [19]; EMA, Vimentin, and AMACR are typically positive in both types [4]. The tumor in our case was diagnosed as a type 2 PRCC due to its morphological features, lack of expression for CK7, and positivity for EMA, Vimentin, and AMACR. Due

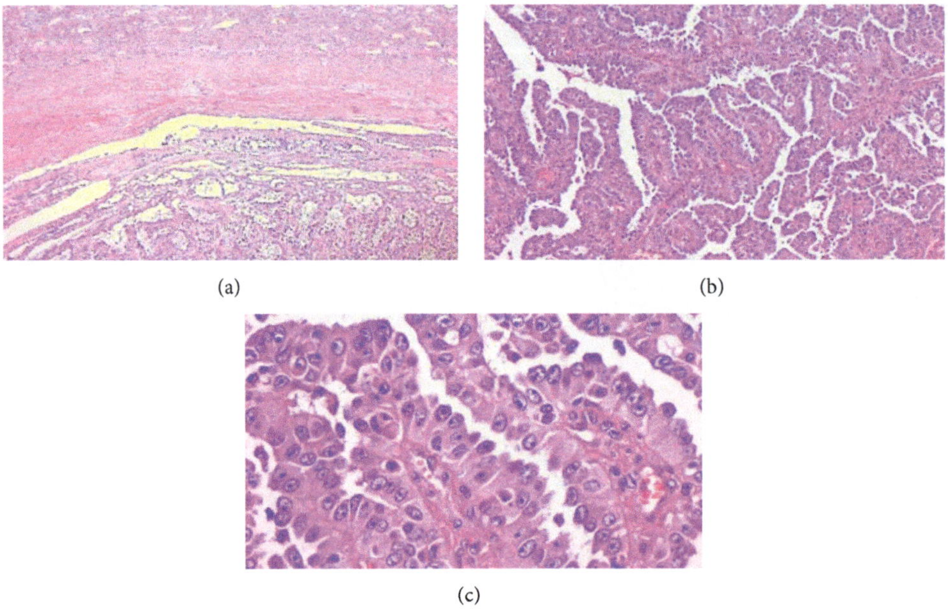

FIGURE 3: (a) Tumor pseudocapsule composed of fibrous tissue. H&E stain, ×50. (b) Papillae covered by large cells with abundant eosinophilic cytoplasm. H&E stain, ×100. (c) Pseudostratified high-grade nuclei with prominent nucleoli. H&E stain, ×400.

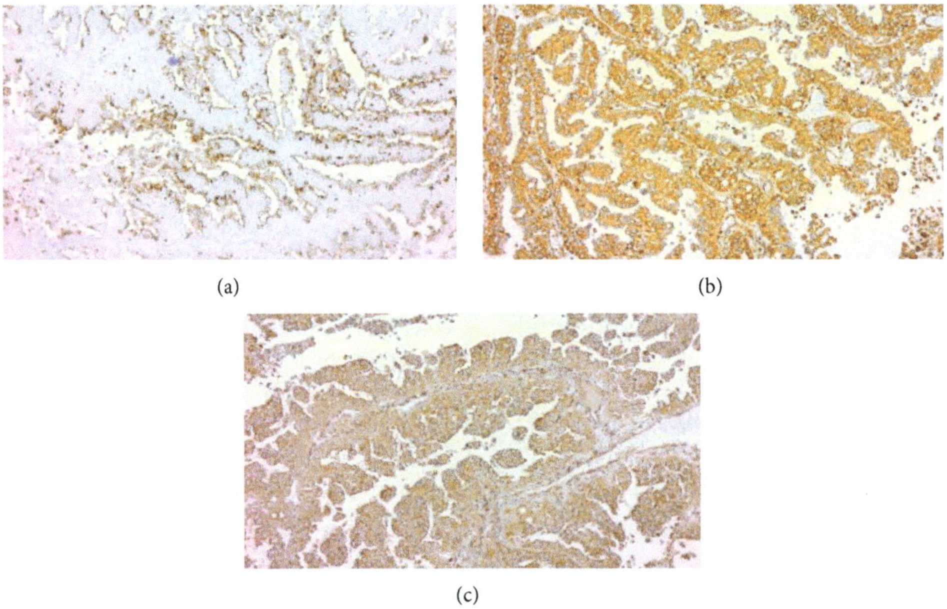

FIGURE 4: (a) Reactivity to EMA. Immunohistochemical stain with anti-EMA antibody, ×100. (b) Reactivity to Vimentin. Immunohistochemical stain with anti-Vimentin antibody, ×100. (c) Reactivity to AMACR. Immunohistochemical stain with anti-AMACR antibody, ×100.

to the age of our patient and the type of RCC he presented, it is important to mention an autosomal dominant syndrome known as hereditary leiomyomatosis and renal cell cancer, in which early age at onset and type 2 PRCCs are common [20]. In this syndrome patients also develop multiple cutaneous leiomyomas in almost all cases and definitive diagnosis is only made by the presence of a germline mutation in the fumarate hydratase gene [21]. Our patient, however, did not present any cutaneous nodules on physical examination nor did he have a family history of this syndrome.

Not much is known about treatment and outcome of the different subtypes of childhood RCC. It appears to have a similar stage-for-stage outcome to RCC in adults [22], but more data is needed to establish this. Neither chemotherapy nor radiation therapy have demonstrated significant activity in adult or pediatric patients with metastatic or residual RCC, regardless of the histologic type. For this reason, adjuvant therapy is not currently recommended for children with PRCC and no residual tumor [4]. Concerning the outcome of a patient with a tumor in a horseshoe kidney, presenting the anomaly does not seem to affect prognosis [10].

Consent

Written informed consent was obtained from the patient for publication of this case report and the accompanying images. A copy of the written consent is available upon request for review.

Conflict of Interests

The authors have no conflict of interests to declare.

References

[1] J. N. Eble, G. Sauter, J. I. Epstein, and I. A. Sesterhenn, *World Health Organization Classification of Tumours: Pathology and Genetics of Tumours of the Urinary System and Male Genital Organs*, IARC Press, Lyon, France, 2004.

[2] J. I. Geller and J. S. Dome, "Local lymph node involvement does not predict poor outcome in pediatric renal cell carcinoma," *Cancer*, vol. 101, no. 7, pp. 1575–1583, 2004.

[3] P. Indolfi, M. Terenziani, F. Casale et al., "Renal cell carcinoma in children: a clinicopathologic study," *Journal of Clinical Oncology*, vol. 21, no. 3, pp. 530–535, 2003.

[4] E. J. Perlman, "Pediatric renal cell carcinoma," *Surgical Pathology Clinics*, vol. 3, no. 3, pp. 641–651, 2010.

[5] M. D. Carcao, G. P. Taylor, M. L. Greenberg et al., "Renal-cell carcinoma in children: a different disorder from its adult counterpart," *Medical and Pediatric Oncology*, vol. 31, no. 3, pp. 153–158, 1998.

[6] L. R. Barros, S. Glina, and L. F. Mello, "Renal cell carcinoma in childhood," *Official Journal of the Brazilian Society of Urology*, vol. 30, no. 3, pp. 227–229, 2004.

[7] A. Z. Weizer, A. D. Silverstein, B. K. Auge et al., "Determining the incidence of horseshoe kidney from radiographic data at a single institution," *The Journal of Urology*, vol. 170, no. 5, pp. 1722–1726, 2003.

[8] A. Alamer, "Renal cell carcinoma in a horseshoe kidney: radiology and pathology correlation," *Journal of Clinical Imaging Science*, vol. 3, article 12, 2013.

[9] S. Ying-Long, X. Yue-Min, X. Hong, and X. Xiao-Lin, "Papillary renal cell carcinoma in the horseshoe kidney," *Southern Medical Journal*, vol. 103, no. 12, pp. 1272–1274, 2010.

[10] J. R. Briones, R. R. Pareja, F. S. Martin, G. C. Toniolo, J. H. Perez, and H. V. Mavrich, "Incidence of tumoural pathology in horseshoe kidneys," *European Urology*, vol. 33, no. 2, pp. 175–179, 1998.

[11] E. K. Yaber-Gomez, Y. Cortes-Arcos, F. G. Gonzalez-Ruiz et al., "Clear cell carcinoma in horseshoe kidney: a case report and literature review," *Revista Mexicana de Urología*, vol. 70, no. 2, pp. 111–115, 2010.

[12] P. Argani, J. Hicks, A. M. De Marzo et al., "Xp11 translocation renal cell carcinoma (RCC): extended immunohistochemical profile emphasizing novel RCC markers," *The American Journal of Surgical Pathology*, vol. 34, no. 9, pp. 1295–1303, 2010.

[13] P. Argani, M. Laé, B. Hutchinson et al., "Renal carcinomas with the t(6;11)(p21;q12): clinicopathologic features and demonstration of the specific alpha-TFEB gene fusion by immunohistochemistry, RT-PCR, and DNA PCR," *The American Journal of Surgical Pathology*, vol. 29, no. 2, pp. 230–240, 2005.

[14] P. Argani and M. Ladanyi, "Kideny: t(6; 11)(p21; q12) in renal cell carcinoma," *Atlas of Genetics and Cytogenetics in Oncology and Haematology*, vol. 9, no. 3, pp. 259–262, 2005.

[15] Q. Rao, B. Liu, L. Cheng et al., "Renal cell carcinomas with t(6;11)(p21;q12): a clinicopathologic study emphasizing unusual morphology, novel alpha-TFEB gene fusion point, immunobiomarkers, and ultrastructural features, as well as detection of the gene fusion by fluorescence in situ hybridization," *The American Journal of Surgical Pathology*, vol. 36, no. 9, pp. 1327–1338, 2012.

[16] L. Chen, F. N. M. Deng, J. Melamed, and M. Zhou, "Differential diagnosis of renal tumors with tubulopapillary architecture in children and young adults: a case report and review of literature," *American Journal of Clinical and Experimental Urology*, vol. 2, no. 3, pp. 266–272, 2014.

[17] W. R. Sukov, C. M. Lohse, B. C. Leibovich, R. H. Thompson, and J. C. Cheville, "Clinical and pathological features associated with prognosis in patients with papillary renal cell carcinoma," *The Journal of Urology*, vol. 187, no. 1, pp. 54–59, 2012.

[18] F. M. Deng, M. X. Kong, and M. Zhou, "Papillary or pseudopapillary tumors of the kidney," *Seminars in Diagnostic Pathology*, vol. 32, no. 2, pp. 124–139, 2015.

[19] B. Delahunt and J. N. Eble, "Papillary renal cell carcinoma: a clinicopathologic and immunohistochemical study of 105 tumors," *Modern Pathology*, vol. 10, no. 6, pp. 537–544, 1997.

[20] K. Y. Van Spaendonck-Zwarts, S. Badeloe, S. F. Oosting et al., "Hereditary leiomyomatosis and renal cell cancer presenting as metastatic kidney cancer at 18 years of age: implications for surveillance," *Familial Cancer*, vol. 11, no. 1, pp. 123–129, 2012.

[21] L. S. Schmidt and W. M. Linehan, "Hereditary leiomyomatosis and renal cell carcinoma," *International Journal of Nephrology and Renovascular Disease*, vol. 2014, article 7, pp. 253–260, 2014.

[22] D. C. Aronson, I. Medary, J. L. Finlay, H. W. Herr, P. R. Exelby, and M. P. La Quaglia, "Renal cell carcinoma in childhood and adolescence: a retrospective survey for prognostic factors in 22 cases," *Journal of Pediatric Surgery*, vol. 31, no. 1, pp. 183–186, 1996.

16

Occult Breast Lobular Carcinoma with Numerous Circulating Tumor Cells in Peripheral Blood

Kanako Ogura,[1] Maki Amano,[2] Toshiharu Matsumoto,[1] Asumi Sakaguchi,[1] Taijiro Kosaka,[3] Toshiaki Kitabatake,[3] and Kuniaki Kojima[3]

[1]*Department of Diagnostic Pathology, Juntendo University Nerima Hospital, Tokyo 177-8521, Japan*
[2]*Department of Radiology, Juntendo University Nerima Hospital, Tokyo 177-8521, Japan*
[3]*Department of Breast Surgery, Juntendo University Nerima Hospital, Tokyo 177-8521, Japan*

Correspondence should be addressed to Kanako Ogura; kanakogu@juntendo-nerima.jp

Academic Editor: Janina Kulka

We experienced a very rare case of occult breast lobular carcinoma with numerous circulating tumor cells in peripheral blood. The diagnosis was very difficult because there were no symptoms of breast cancer and the preceding chief complaints such as general fatigue and weight loss or abnormality of peripheral blood findings were suggestive of a hematological disease. We could make a correct diagnosis of this case by checking the findings of complete blood count and bone marrow biopsy at the same time using immunohistochemistry.

1. Introduction

Invasive lobular carcinoma (ILC) accounts for about 6% of breast cancer, which is the second most common type after invasive ductal carcinoma (IDC) [1, 2]. It is well known that the pattern of metastatic spread of ILC is different from that of IDC, so scrupulous attention to metastasis to unusual foci such as the gastrointestinal tract, uterus, ovary, and meninges is required [3].

There are some reports of breast cancers with bone marrow metastases. Kopp et al. analyzed 22 of such cases, in which 7 cases were ILC [4]. Seventeen cases were diagnosed by bone marrow histology and the other 5 cases were revealed because of leukoerythroblastic blood smear.

On the other hand, occult breast carcinoma accounts for 0.3 to 1% of breast cancer [5]. It is defined as breast carcinoma with an axillary lymph node metastasis as the first clinical manifestation of the disease. Recently, diagnostic imaging has dramatically improved, so it has been recommended for occult breast carcinoma to perform mammography repeatedly or magnetic resonance imaging (MRI). The prognosis of occult breast cancer seemed to be similar to that of usual and overt breast cancer with lymph node metastasis.

We experienced a unique case of occult invasive lobular carcinoma with identification of circulating tumor cells in peripheral blood count. There have been very few reports that tumor cells themselves were identified in peripheral blood count, even if secondary change such as leukoerythroblastosis in peripheral blood smear was shown.

2. Case Presentation

The patient was a 65-year-old woman, with chief complaints of general fatigue and weight loss. The findings of peripheral blood test are summarized in Table 1. The number of leukocytes was high (22,200/μL) and atypical unclassified cells were identified in her peripheral blood count. Those cells were counted as "other" at a level of 7.5%. The atypical cells were noncohesive and had round nuclei and cytoplasm with microvilli resembling lymphocytes or plasma cells in form (Figure 1). The serum calcium level was high (13.4 mg/dL). Such findings leaded her physician into the suspicion of hematological disease such as lymphoma or myeloma although the serum level of CEA was also high (621 ng/mL).

TABLE 1: The patient's peripheral blood data.

WBC	22200	/μL
Neutrophil	64.5	%
Lymphocyte	20	%
Monocyte	7.5	%
Eosinophil	0	%
Basophil	0	%
Other	7.5	%
Myelocyte	0.5	%
Hb	13.7	g/dL
Ht	42.4	%
Plt	315×10^4	/μL
TP	8.2	g/dL
Alb	3.4	g/dL
AST	57	IU/L
ALT	20	IU/L
LDH	373	IU/L
ALP	973	IU/L
BUN	29	mg/dL
Cre	1.2	mg/dL
Na	135	mEq/L
K	4.9	mEq/L
Cl	94	mEq/L
Ca	13.4	mg/dL
CEA	621	ng/mL

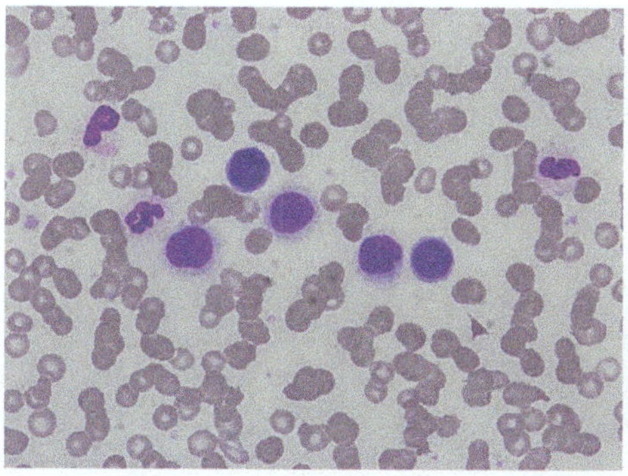

FIGURE 1: Tumor cells in peripheral blood smear. Noncohesive round tumor cells resembling lymphocytes were identified.

Her physician performed a bone marrow puncture. The bone marrow specimen showed so-called "packed bone marrow" and fibrosis was also shown, so aspiration failed (so-called "dry tap"). In the biopsy specimen, numerous small round cells that were the same as the cells in the peripheral blood had grown with proliferation of reticular fibers (Figures 2(a) and 2(b)). We continued histological investigation using immunohistochemistry. These tumor cells were negative for LCA but positive for AE1/AE3. Furthermore, tumor cells were also positive for GCDFP15, ER, and (Figure 2(c)) PgR but negative for E-cadherin. On the basis of the result of immunohistochemistry, we diagnosed the bone marrow lesion as metastatic lobular carcinoma of the breast.

TABLE 2: Immunohistochemical findings of this case.

	Bone marrow	Axial lymph node	Stomach
AE1/AE3	+	+	+
ER	+	+	+
PR	+	+	+
HER2	Score 1+	Score 1+	Score 1+
Mammaglobin	−	−	−
GCDFP15	+	+	+
CK7	+	+	+
CK20	−	−	−
CDX2	−	−	−

Subsequently, the patient underwent detailed examination concentrating on imaging study. However, no lesion in either breast was identified by mammography (Figure 3(a)), ultrasonography, and even contrast-enhanced CT or MRI (Figure 3(b)). Enhanced CT images showed swelling of left axillary, right internal mammary, and perigastric lymph nodes and diffuse thickening of gastric wall like "Bormann 4 tumor" (Figure 4). T1-weighted MRI revealed generalized bone marrow metastasis. Fatty bone marrow was diffusely occupied by low-intensity lesion (Figure 5). Furthermore, bone scintigraphy also revealed generalized osseous metastasis by so-called "beautiful bone sign." Biopsies from an enlarged left axillary lymph node and from gastric mucosa were performed, resulting in the finding of metastatic lobular carcinoma that we confirmed by immunohistochemistry including ER, PgR, and GCDFP15 (Figures 6 and 7). We summarized the immunohistochemical findings of bone marrow, axillary lymph node, and gastric biopsy specimens in Table 2. Carcinoma from accessory breast tissue in axilla was also ruled out.

Finally, this case was diagnosed as occult breast lobular carcinoma with multiple metastases to bone, bone marrow, left axillary lymph nodes, and stomach with many circulating tumor cells in peripheral blood.

After the diagnosis, combination chemotherapy with docetaxel, cyclophosphamide, and zoledronic acid hydrate was applied. During chemotherapy, diffuse thickening of upper dermis of the left breast appeared. Since the patient refused skin biopsy, the underlying cause of the skin swelling remains obscure. The symptoms such as swelling of axillary lymph nodes and thickening of dermis and gastric wall were improved by chemotherapy. Although enhanced CT has been repeatedly performed, there has been no lesion in either breast. At the time of writing the paper, the patient is still undergoing treatment.

3. Discussion

This case was difficult to diagnose because of an unusual clinical presentation, that is, identification of massive amount of nonhematological tumor cells in peripheral blood count and "occult" breast carcinoma.

Pentheroudakis et al. recommended performing mammography repeatedly or magnetic resonance imaging (MRI) for occult breast carcinoma [6]. They documented that

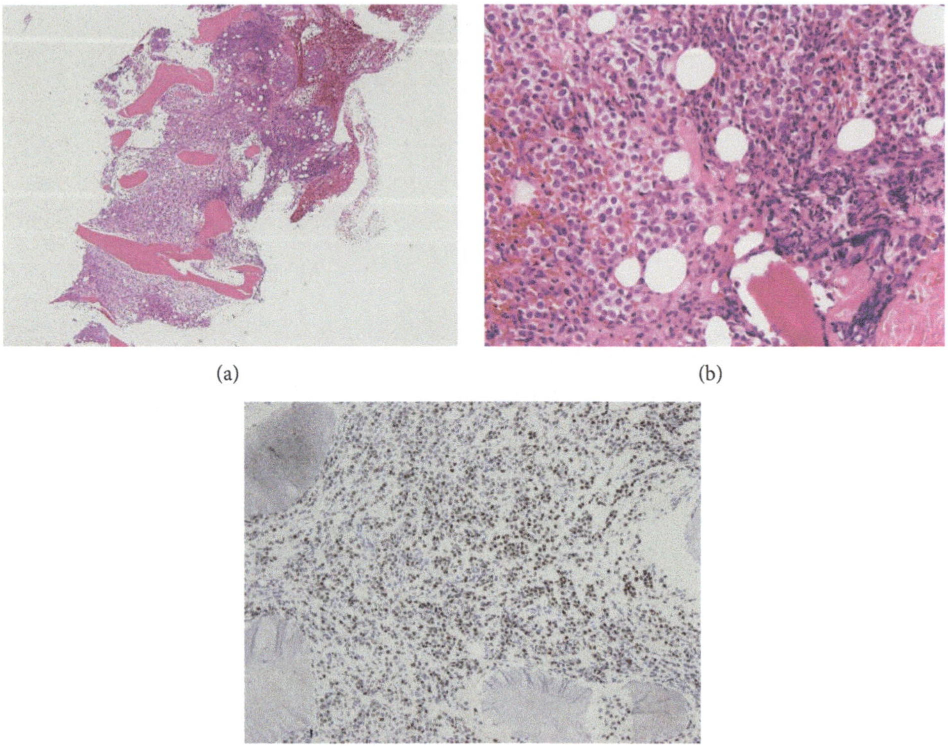

(a) (b)

(c)

FIGURE 2: Bone marrow biopsy specimen. (a) H-E stain. Hypercellular bone marrow. (b) H-E stain. Monotonous tumor cells invaded bone marrow space accompanied by fibrosis. (c) Immunohistochemical stain of estrogen receptor. Tumor cells were diffusely positive.

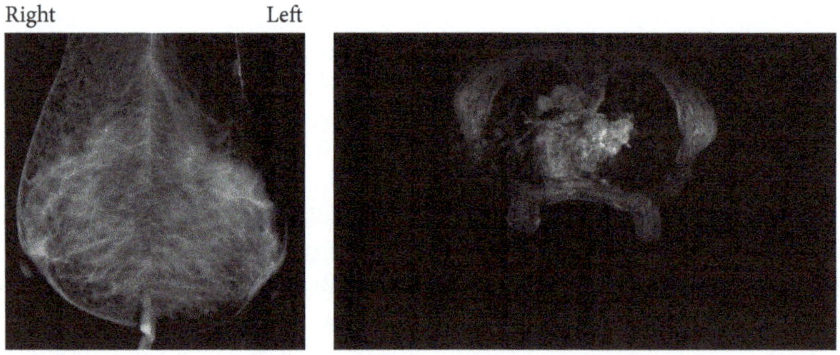

(a) (b)

FIGURE 3: (a) Mammography. There was no lesion in either breast. (b) Enhanced MRI. There was also no lesion in either breast.

primary small foci in both breasts were identified in 59% of cases of occult breast cancer that they reviewed by MRI imaging. They also revealed that a small breast primary focus was identified histologically in 72% of cases treated with mastectomy. However, primary foci were sometimes not identified. In our case, there was no lesion in either breast regardless of performing various modalities such as mammography, ultrasonography, CT, or MRI. Our case was thought of as true occult breast carcinoma. Neal et al. reported occult breast carcinoma (ILC) presenting as gastrointestinal metastases without lesions in the breasts [7]. Invasive lobular carcinoma has a tendency to metastasize to gastrointestinal tract. Metastatic breast lobular carcinoma can easily be mistaken for a primary gastrointestinal cancer. Metastatic "occult" lobular carcinoma is even more difficult to identify. They documented that immunohistochemistry could allow accurate diagnosis. In our case, tumor cells metastasized to stomach, axillary lymph node, and bone marrow. We could perform immunohistochemistry to all samples from stomach, lymph node, and bone marrow and compare the results. Immunohistochemistry was also powerful diagnostic tool in our case.

Such a situation when circulating tumor cells are visible in peripheral blood smear is extremely rare. In our case, hematological disease was suspected at the initial visit because of the many noncohesive tumor cells (7.5% of all

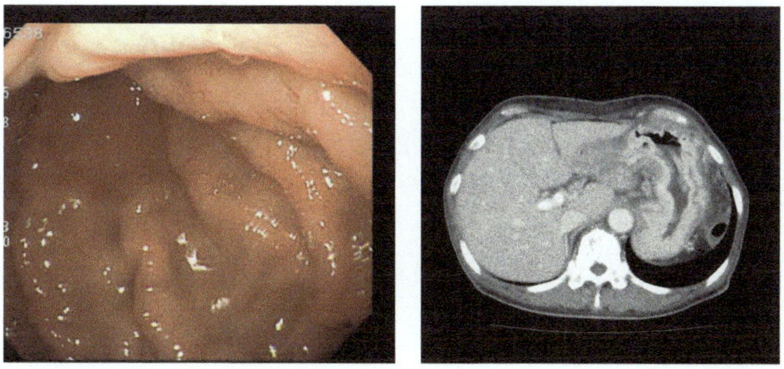

(a) (b)

FIGURE 4: (a) Upper endoscopy. Mucosal rugae were edematous and thickened. (b) Contrast-enhanced CT revealed diffuse thickening of gastric wall.

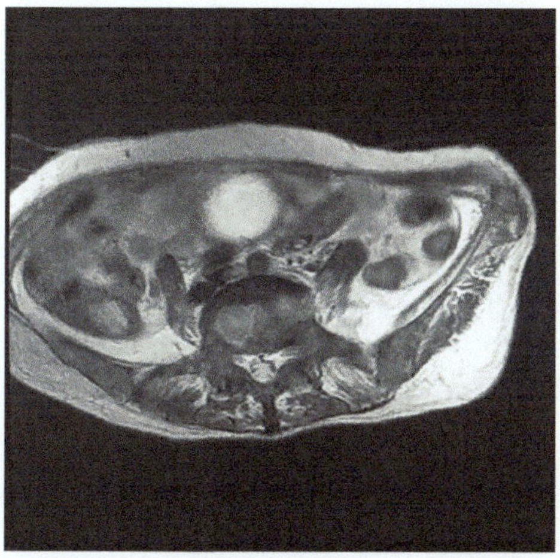

FIGURE 5: T1-weighted MRI revealed low-intensity lesion occupying lumbar spine and iliac bone diffusely.

blood cells) seen in the peripheral blood smear, suggesting hematological malignancy. There are reports of circulating tumor cells in primary breast cancer. However, the methods for the identification of circulating tumor cells are almost all molecular ones, such as RT-PCR. Fortunato et al. revealed that RT-PCR of the BM is an independent prognostic factor for disease-free survival of breast cancer patients [8]. This is the first case report of breast carcinoma with "countable" nonhematological tumor cells in a peripheral blood smear. In our case, bone marrow biopsy was also performed, so we could compare the circulating atypical cells in both peripheral blood smear and the biopsy sample with performing immunohistochemistry. It contributed to prompt and correct diagnosis of this difficult case.

Kopp et al. warned that bone marrow involvement has to be considered in breast cancer patients, in particular in those with bone metastases and otherwise unexplained cytopenia [4]. They also documented that full blood exam can serve as a simple diagnostic tool. Cotta et al. documented that lung, breast, and prostate cancers are prone to bone metastasis in adults [9]. If a carcinoma metastasises to bone marrow, leukoerythroblastic reaction can sometimes be found on full blood exam.

In our case, the patient was not suspected of having breast cancer at the first visit and bone marrow puncture proved to be the decisive tool in correct diagnosis. It may be necessary for breast cancer patients to perform not only complete blood count but also bone marrow puncture if some abnormalities on full blood exam are identified. Cotta et al. also documented that circulating tumor cells sometimes mimic the clinical appearance of acute leukemia. In cases of breast cancer, lobular carcinomas do metastasize to skeletal system in higher frequency. The tumor cells can be difficult to identify because they can be small and scant, with an appearance that is difficult to distinguish from that of lymphocytes or blast cells. Indeed, we also suspected lymphoma or plasmacytoma at first.

Lyda et al. documented that keratin immunohistochemistry (IHC) detected clinically significant metastases in bone marrow biopsy specimens in women with lobular breast carcinoma [10]. They divided the cases of ILC into three groups based on hematoxylin and eosin (H-E) staining and keratin IHC results. They showed that prognosis was worse in the order of H-E-negative/IHC-negative, H-E-negative/IHC-positive, and H-E-positive/IHC-positive. They concluded that routine morphologic examination without the aid of keratin IHC was unreliable in detecting clinically relevant metastatic lobular carcinoma in bone marrow biopsies. According to Lyda et al., our case was categorized into H-E positive/IHC positive case, so the patient's prognosis was to be expected as unfavorable. Immunohistochemistry in our case was not so much useful for prognostic prediction but helped in accurate diagnosis. We could reconsider the origin of the tumor cells by the immunohistochemical reactions: LCA was negative and ER, PR, and GCDFP15 were positive in the atypical cells in bone marrow, axillary lymph node, and gastric biopsy specimens. It was also important to check the findings of complete blood count and bone marrow biopsy specimen at the same time. Misdiagnosis or delay of diagnosis might have occurred if the diagnosis based on complete blood count preceded bone marrow biopsy.

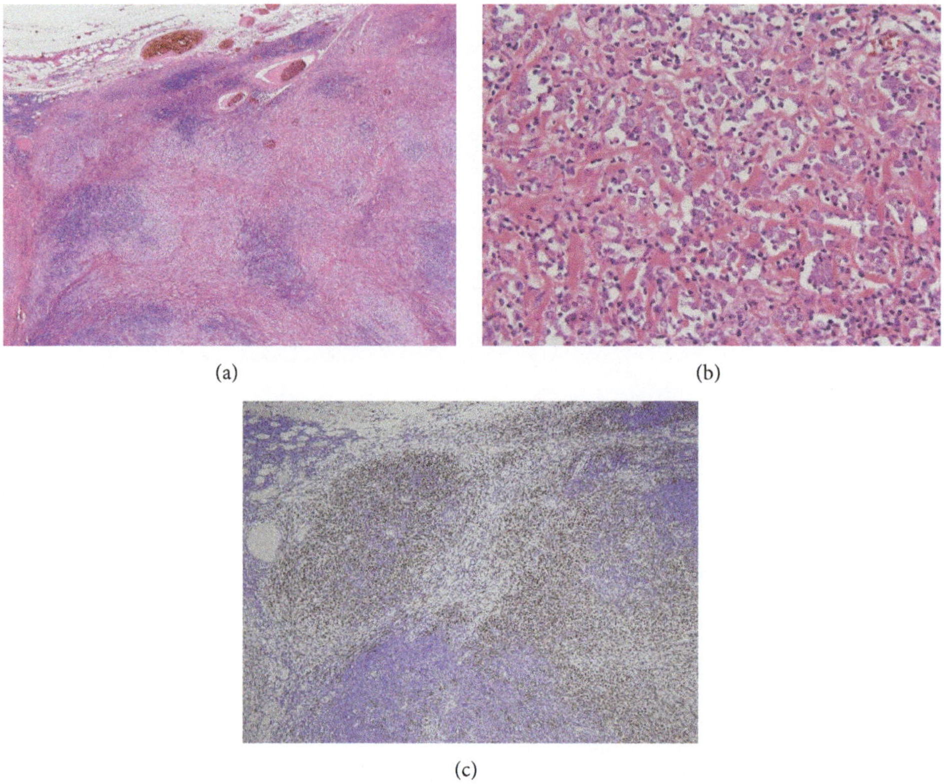

FIGURE 6: Axillary lymph node specimen. (a) H-E stain. Low power field. Tumor cells invaded lymph node parenchyma. (b) H-E stain. High power field. Monotonous tumor cells and fibrotic area. (c) Immunohistochemical stain of estrogen receptor. Tumor cells were diffusely positive.

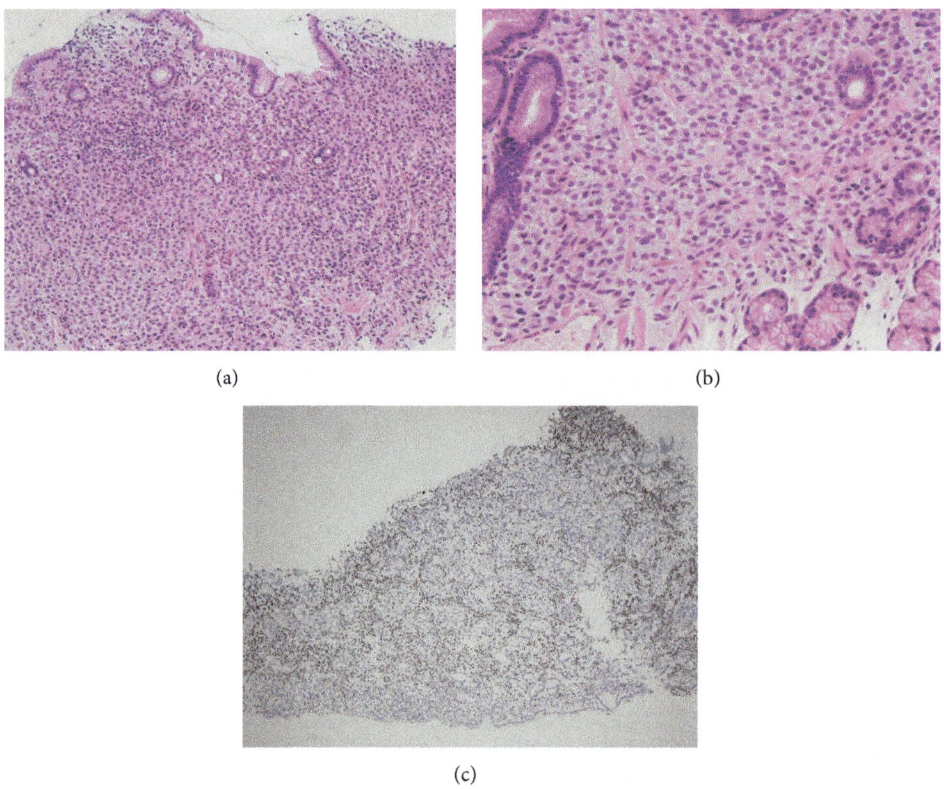

FIGURE 7: Gastric biopsy specimen. (a) H-E stain. Low power field. Tumor cells infiltrated the lamina propria. (b) H-E stain. High power field. Monotonous round tumor cells resembling the tumor cells seen in bone marrow and axillary lymph nodes. (c) Immunohistochemical stain of estrogen receptor. Tumor cells were diffusely positive.

In conclusion, we experienced a case of occult breast lobular carcinoma with numerous circulating tumor cells in peripheral blood count. Although the diagnosis was difficult because circulating tumor cells were abundant and mimicked lymphocytes or blast cells, immunohistochemistry was very useful for the correct diagnosis. We could also make a diagnosis quickly because we checked the patient's peripheral blood smear and bone marrow biopsy specimen at the same time.

Conflict of Interests

The authors declare that there is no conflict of interests regarding the publication of this paper.

Acknowledgment

The authors thank Mr. Daniel Mrozek (Medical English Service, Kyoto, Japan) for organizing the English revision of this paper.

References

[1] B. C. Pestalozzi, D. Zahrieh, E. Mallon et al., "Distinct clinical and prognostic features of infiltrating lobular carcinoma of the breast: combined results of 15 International Breast Cancer Study Group clinical trials," *Journal of Clinical Oncology*, vol. 26, no. 18, pp. 3006–3014, 2008.

[2] M. S. Moran, Q. Yang, and B. G. Haffty, "The yale university experience of early-stage invasive lobular carcinoma (ILC) and invasive ductal carcinoma (IDC) treated with breast conservation treatment (BCT): analysis of clinical-pathologic features, long-term outcomes, and molecular expression of COX-2, Bcl-2, and p53 as a function of histology," *The Breast Journal*, vol. 15, no. 6, pp. 571–578, 2009.

[3] S. R. Lakhani, E. Rakha, and P. T. Simpson, "Invasive lobular carcinoma," in *WHO Classification of Tumours of the Breast*, S. R. Lakhani, I. O. Ellis, S. J. Schnitt, P. H. Tan, and M. J. van de Vijver, Eds., pp. 40–42, IARC, 4th edition, 2012.

[4] H. G. Kopp, K. Krauss, T. Fehm et al., "Symptomatic bone marrow involvement in breast cancer—clinical presentation, treatment and prognosis: a single institution review of 22 cases," *Anticancer Research*, vol. 24, pp. 1593–1599, 2009.

[5] S. Lanitis, K. A. Behranwala, R. Al-Mufti, and D. Hadjiminas, "Axillary metastatic disease as presentation of occult or contralateral breast cancer," *Breast*, vol. 18, no. 4, pp. 225–227, 2009.

[6] G. Pentheroudakis, G. Lazaridis, and N. Pavlidis, "Axillary nodal metastases from carcinoma of unknown primary (CUPAx): a systematic review of published evidence," *Breast Cancer Research and Treatment*, vol. 119, no. 1, pp. 1–11, 2010.

[7] L. Neal, N. Sookhan, and C. Reynolds, "Occult breast carcinoma presenting as gastrointestinal metastases," *Case Reports in Medicine*, vol. 2009, Article ID 564756, 3 pages, 2009.

[8] L. Fortunato, A. Mascaro, A. Baldi et al., "Positive bone marrow biopsy is associated with a decreased disease-free survival in patients with operable breast cancer," *Annals of Surgical Oncology*, vol. 16, no. 11, pp. 3010–3019, 2009.

[9] C. V. Cotta, S. Konoplev, L. J. Medeiros, and C. E. Bueso-Ramos, "Metastatic tumors in bone marrow: histopathology and advances in the biology of the tumor cells and bone marrow environment," *Annals of Diagnostic Pathology*, vol. 10, no. 3, pp. 169–192, 2006.

[10] M. H. Lyda, M. Tetef, N. H. Carter, D. Ikle, L. M. Weiss, and D. A. Arber, "Keratin immunohistochemistry detects clinically significant metastases in bone marrow biopsy specimens in women with lobular breast carcinoma," *American Journal of Surgical Pathology*, vol. 24, no. 12, pp. 1593–1599, 2000.

17

A Dilemma in Staging of Esophageal Cancer: How Should We Stage ypT0 N2 M0 Esophageal Cancer after Neoadjuvant Therapy?

Sebahattin Celik,[1] Remzi Erten,[2] Abdulsamed Batur,[3] and Burak Suvak[4]

[1]*Department of General Surgery, Yüzüncü Yıl University, 65200 Van, Turkey*
[2]*Department of Pathology, Yüzüncü Yıl University, 65200 Van, Turkey*
[3]*Department of Radiology, Yüzüncü Yıl University, 65200 Van, Turkey*
[4]*Department of Gastroenterology, Yüzüncü Yıl University, 65200 Van, Turkey*

Correspondence should be addressed to Sebahattin Celik; drsebahattincelik@hotmail.com

Academic Editor: Yoji Nagashima

Background. Since neoadjuvant treatment in esophageal cancer began to become popular, a complete pathological response at the primary tumour site has been commonly reported. An issue of conflict is whether complete response in the esophageal lumen means that the esophagus is completely tumour-free. Another important issue is whether lymph nodes that are retrieved from pathologically complete response cases are also tumour-free or not. There is a gap in the esophageal cancer staging system for ypT0 N2 M0 tumours that have received neoadjuvant therapy. Here, we will discuss the problem about staging of esophageal cancer associated with neoadjuvant therapy. *Case.* A female aged 40 years complaining of dysphagia was diagnosed as having locally advanced thoracic esophageal cancer. Neoadjuvant therapy decision was taken by oncology committee. Six weeks after neoadjuvant therapy, with a curative intention, minimal invasive surgery was performed. The pathology report was as follows. "There were no neoplastic cells in the suspected area of the esophageal mucosa upon examination with all staining. There was no cancer at resection margins. Four metastatic lymph nodes were infiltrated with squamous cell cancer." *Conclusion.* Despite the growing use of neoadjuvant treatment in locally advanced esophageal cancer in world, we do not have a protocol for the evaluation of these patients' pathology reports. We believe that new studies and new ideas are needed to resolve this dilemma associated with neoadjuvant therapy.

1. Scientific Background

There is no question that the presence of lymph node (LN) metastasis in esophageal cancer is one of the most powerful prognostic indicators. Esophageal cancer staging is defined by the American Joint Committee on Cancer (AJCC) Staging System, which establishes tumor-node-metastasis (TNM) subclassifications based on the depth of invasion of the primary tumor (T), lymph node involvement (N), and extent of metastatic disease (M). The most recent 7th edition of the AJCC Cancer Staging Manual for esophageal and esophagogastric junction cancers was developed based on a database of 4627 esophagectomy patients who were not treated with induction or adjuvant therapy [1]. Because of the poor prognosis of surgery alone in esophageal cancer, multimodality treatments have become popular [2, 3]. There are conflicts about the adequacy of the AJCC Staging System in patients who received chemoradiotherapy (CRT) as neoadjuvant [4]. In the provocative study of Swisher et al., it was stated that pathological complete response to CRT before surgery was an independent prognostic factor for survival and they also proposed a revision of the 6th AJCC Staging System for esophageal cancer [4]. In that study, the authors reported 12 cases whose primary tumour sites were free from malignant cells, while lymph nodes (N1) were positive. The authors suggested "stage 2A" for such cases (ypT0, N1, M0, P0). But there has been no change in the 7th AJCC Staging System for esophageal cancer in that direction. In that case, what

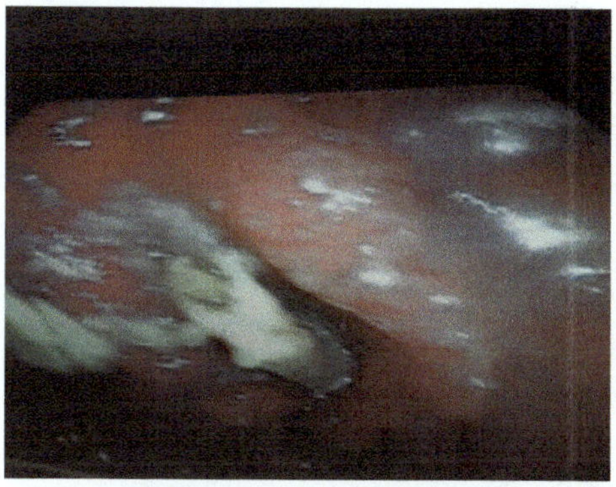

FIGURE 1: Upper endoscopy of patient showing an ulcerative lesion located between 25 and 38 cm of the esophagus.

should we do? With the case report below, we would like to complicate the situation to some degree by presenting an esophageal cancer CRT-treated patient whose pathologic report was ypT0, N2, M0.

2. Case

A 40-year-old female complaining of dysphagia came to our gastroenterology outpatient clinic. In her upper endoscopy, an ulcerative mass was found between 25 and 38 cm from the incisors (Figure 1). After initial work-up and also after the pathology report of an endoscopic biopsy (which was squamous cell cancer), the case was discussed in the oncologic committee. All blood tests (biochemistry, complete blood count) were in the normal range. Pretreatment computed tomography (CT) was as seen in Figure 2. Positron emission tomography (PET) was performed for occult distant metastases and there were no metastases. The patient's performance status was good and she had no comorbidities. Unfortunately, there is no endoscopic ultrasound unit (EUS) in our hospital so this modality was not performed.

After our case was discussed in the oncologic committee that gathered every week on Thursday, it was decided to characterize the clinical stage of the tumour as T3 or T4a, NX, M0 according to the 7th AJCC Staging System. As expected, for this advanced esophageal tumor, a neoadjuvant CRT decision was taken. In our oncology clinic, chemotherapy and simultaneous radiotherapy were given as follows: Paclitaxel (50 mg/m^2), Carboplatin (target AUC = 2 mg/Ml·min) plus radiotherapy (41.4 Gy in 23 fractions for 5 days per week). This chemotherapy protocol was given on the first day of radiotherapy and once a week until reaching 5 weeks. After the patient had completed the whole CRT protocol, a control CT was performed (Figure 3). According to the CT report, there was more than 50% response.

Six weeks after CRT, with a curative intention, minimal invasive surgery (MIS) was performed (thoracoscopic esophageal mobilization done first and then gastric mobilization and tube formation performed with laparotomy and cervical anastomosis). There was no tumour or any other lesion when the specimen was examined intraoperatively. No intraoperative complications occurred. However, on the 5th postoperative day, elevated temperature (38.7°C) and tachycardia (145 beats/min) developed. In radiological examination and with methylene blue test, we found a leak in the stapler line on the gastric wall that was formed while creating a gastric tube. Subsequently, despite all interventions and reoperation she was still in the intensive care unit and was intubated at the time of this writing.

The pathology report was as follows. "There were no neoplastic cells in the suspected area of the esophageal mucosa upon examination with HMWCK, P63, PAS, and dPAS staining. There were areas of ulceration and severe chronic inflammation and fibrosis in the esophageal lumen: perineural invasion (–), lymphovascular invasion (–). There was no cancer at resection margins. Four metastatic lymph nodes (Figures 4 and 5) were infiltrated with squamous cell cancer. The other 21 harvested lymph nodes were reactive." We then consulted with the pathologist and requested reevaluation of the specimen and of course the lymph nodes. Nevertheless, the pathological reevaluation was the same.

3. Discussion and Conclusion

Interesting proposals about the stage of this case were suggested when the case was discussed in the oncologic committee. One of the proposals was as follows. "It should be evaluated as "ypT4a or T3 and N2, M0" since before CRT the first stage was at this level and after CRT the tumour was present in four lymph nodes, so nothing changed." Another suggestion was as follows. "Although the pathologists have decided that the esophagus was free from tumour, I believe there are occult cancer foci that could not be examined, so it should be considered as ypTis, N2, M0."

If it would be decided to evaluate such cases in accordance with the National Comprehensive Cancer Network (NCCN) Guideline version 2.2012, which uses the AJCC Staging System, the part entitled "ESOPH-6" should be considered [5]. In that part, "Observe" is suggested for squamous cell cancer patients who received CRT and were node positive. The clinician would start to "observe" the patient with four metastatic lymph nodes.

If Swisher et al. were called for help, they would suggest that "...the group of patients treated with CRT who are found to have a complete pathologic response at the primary but involved nodes in the specimen (ypT0, N1, M0) should be classified a favourable stage 2 prognosis or a stage 2A..." [4]. Interestingly, all patients reported in the above-mentioned study had 1 or 2 positive (N1) lymph nodes, while in our case report there were 4 (N2) positive lymph nodes. If we think in this way, we must accept our own case as an advanced stage, for example, between stages 3A and stage 3C.

In the study conducted by Rizk et al., which analysed patients with esophageal adenocarcinoma who received CRT before esophagectomy, it was shown that involved lymph nodes and metastatic disease were the best predictors of survival and that depth of invasion and degree of treatment response were less predictive [6]. We think there is a similar tendency in the squamous cell cancer type of esophageal cancer as well. We also believe that although complete pathological response may be seen in post-CRT esophageal specimens,

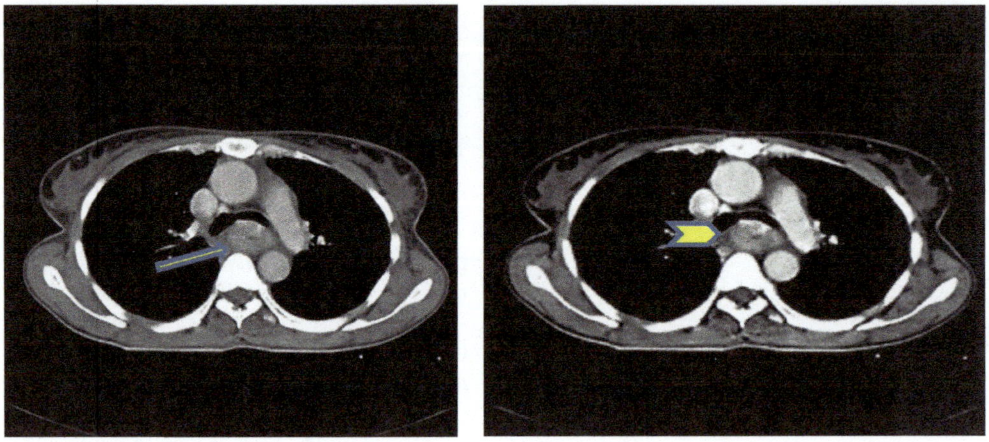

(a) (b)

FIGURE 2: Computed tomography of esophageal mass (arrows) before neoadjuvant therapy.

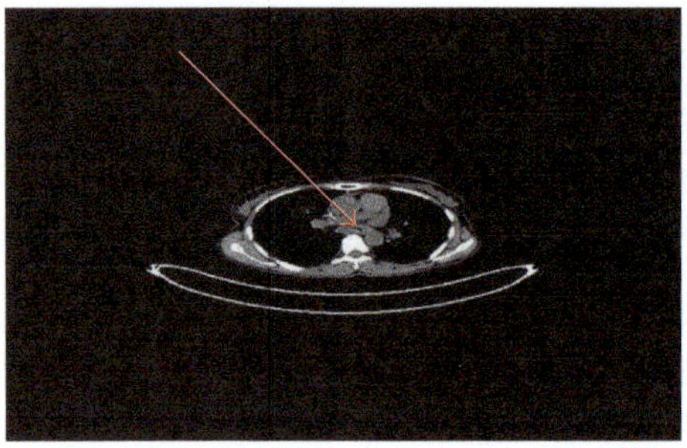

FIGURE 3: After neoadjuvant therapy, control CT of regressed mass (arrow).

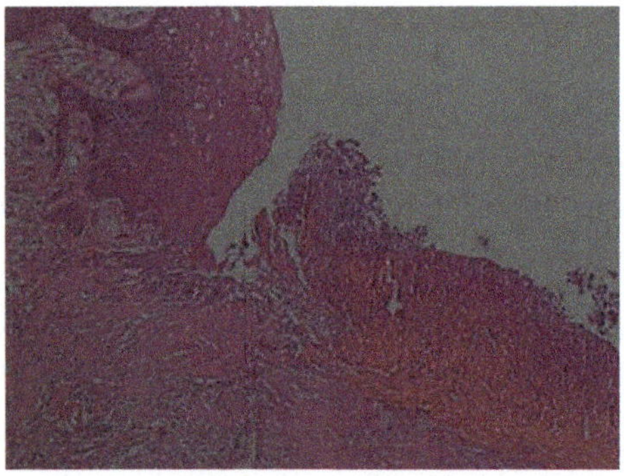

FIGURE 4: In the upper-left part, there is normal, well-preserved esophageal mucosa, while in the lower-right region there is an ulcer field disrupting the mucosa (H&E stain, ×100).

the number of retrieved lymph nodes and the number of metastatic lymph nodes are more important for later treatment and follow-up plans.

Someone can ask, although the exact advantages and disadvantages of CRT have not yet been demonstrated completely, how can we consider the response of tumour to CRT as a prognostic criterion? We think there is huge confusion about multimodality therapies and about the consequences of

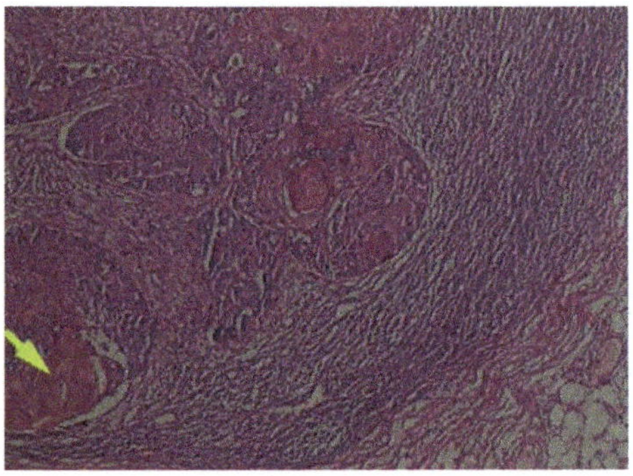

FIGURE 5: In the lower-right part, a well-preserved lymph node with its peripheral adipose tissue is seen but in the upper-left and lower-left (arrow shows central keratinization) parts of the same lymph node there are squamous cell cancer foci (neoplastic cells with large nuclei, wide eosinophilic cytoplasmic cells).

those therapies. As we have shown by this case report, there is still no consensus about prognosis and staging of patients who have received CRT.

Consequently, despite the growing use of neoadjuvant treatment in locally advanced esophageal cancer in our institute, we do not have a protocol for the evaluation of these patients' pathology reports. We believe that new studies and new ideas are needed to resolve this dilemma associated with CRT.

Consent

Written informed consent was obtained from the patient's husband (because she was intubated) for publication of this case report and any accompanying images. A copy of the written consent is available for review.

Conflict of Interests

All authors declare that they have no competing interests.

Authors' Contribution

Conception of work has been done by Dr. Sebahattin Celik, Dr. Remzi Erten, and Dr. Burak Suvak. Interpretation of data for the work has been done by Dr. Sebahattin Celik, Dr. Abdulsamed Batur, and Dr. Burak Suvak. Drafting the work has been done by Dr. Sebahattin Celik, Dr. Remzi Ertan, and Dr. Abdulsamed Batur.

References

[1] T. W. Rice, V. W. Rusch, H. Ishwaran, and E. H. Blackstone, "Cancer of the esophagus and esophagogastric junction: data-driven staging for the seventh edition of the American Joint Committee on Cancer/International Union Against Cancer Cancer Staging Manuals," *Cancer*, vol. 116, no. 16, pp. 3763–3773, 2010.

[2] Medical Research Council Oesophageal Cancer Working Party. Writing Committee, J. Bancewicz, P. I. Clark, D. B. Smith, and R. J. Donnelly, "Surgical resection with or without preoperative chemotherapy in oesophageal cancer: a randomised controlled trial," *The Lancet*, vol. 359, pp. 1727–1733, 2002.

[3] J. D. Urschel and H. Vasan, "A meta-analysis of randomized controlled trials that compared neoadjuvant chemoradiation and surgery to surgery alone for resectable esophageal cancer," *The American Journal of Surgery*, vol. 185, no. 6, pp. 538–543, 2003.

[4] S. G. Swisher, W. Hofstetter, T. T. Wu et al., "Proposed revision of the esophageal cancer staging system to accommodate pathologic response (pP) following preoperative chemoradiation (CRT)," *Annals of Surgery*, vol. 241, no. 5, pp. 810–820, 2005.

[5] http://www.nccn.org/professionals/physician_gls/pdf/esophageal.pdf.

[6] N. P. Rizk, E. Venkatraman, M. S. Bains et al., "American Joint Committee on Cancer staging system does not accurately predict survival in patients receiving multimodality therapy for esophageal adenocarcinoma," *Journal of Clinical Oncology*, vol. 25, no. 5, pp. 507–512, 2007.

18

Mature Cystic Teratoma in Douglas' Pouch

Kenji Ohshima,[1] Anna Umeda,[2] Ayako Hosoi,[2] Toshiya Yamamoto,[2] and Satoru Munakata[1]

[1]*Department of Pathology, Sakai City Hospital, 1-1-1 Minami-Yasui-Cho, Sakai-Ku, Sakai, Osaka 590-0064, Japan*
[2]*Department of Obstetrics and Gynecology, Sakai City Hospital, 1-1-1 Minami-Yasui-Cho, Sakai-Ku, Sakai, Osaka 590-0064, Japan*

Correspondence should be addressed to Kenji Ohshima; ohshima-path@umin.org

Academic Editor: Kyung-Un Choi

Mature cystic teratoma is one of the most common ovarian neoplasms, but extragonadal teratoma is rare. Teratoma in Douglas' pouch is extremely rare, and only 12 cases have been reported since the first case was described in 1978. We report a 20-year-old woman with a multicystic mass in Douglas' pouch that was treated via laparoscopic resection. The tumor consisted of cysts lined by stratified squamous epithelium with an accumulation of keratin debris and various mature tissues. No immature elements or malignancy was found in the tumor, confirming the pathologic diagnosis of a mature cystic teratoma. The teratoma contained no ovarian tissues and both of the ovaries were intact on laparoscopy. These findings suggest that the teratoma originated primarily in Douglas' pouch rather than being caused by autoamputation of a previously existing ovarian teratoma. This is the first case that simultaneously showed normal ovaries and a teratoma in Douglas' pouch on laparoscopy.

1. Introduction

Mature cystic teratoma is the most commonly encountered ovarian neoplasm. However, teratomas in Douglas' pouch are extremely rare. Only 12 cases have been reported since Lefkowitch et al. described the first case in 1978 [1–5]. In most of these cases, the causes of the teratomas were thought to be autoamputation resulting from torsion with subsequent reimplantation in Douglas' pouch, because, in these cases, one of the ovaries was small or absent, or the teratomas contained ovarian tissues [2–5]. Other hypotheses have been proposed, such as teratomas in Douglas' pouch that may originate from an ectopic ovary or from displaced primordial germ cells. In this report, we present a case of teratoma in Douglas' pouch and discuss the etiology of the teratoma.

2. Case Presentation

A 20-year-old woman without a medical history presented with lower abdominal pain that had persisted for two weeks. A general physical examination was unremarkable except for tenderness of the lower abdomen. Transvaginal ultrasonography showed swelling of both of the ovaries, with the right ovary measuring 8 cm and the left, which was solid and multicystic, measuring 6 cm. Right ovarian hemorrhage and a left ovarian tumor were suspected. Because her vital signs were stable and the pain was mild, she was followed as an outpatient. A follow-up ultrasonography examination revealed that while both of the ovaries had decreased in size, the left ovary still measured 4 cm. The patient underwent a more detailed examination and we performed magnetic resonance imaging (MRI). MRI revealed a multicystic mass in Douglas' pouch while both of the ovaries were normal in size. The levels of tumor markers (CA-125, CA-19-9, alpha-fetoprotein, and carcinoembryonic antigen) were all normal. Subsequent contrast enhanced computed tomography (CT) showed fatty and calcified components in the mass, and the diagnosis of a teratoma was mainly considered (Figures 1(a) and 1(b)). Both MRI and CT scans showed that both of the ovaries were normal. Laparoscopic resection was performed, revealing a multilobular tumor in Douglas' pouch, free from surrounding tissues with a vascular pedicle arising from the retroperitoneum. Both of the ovaries were normal considering the patient's age (Figure 2). The tumor was resected without rupture. Macroscopically, the tumor was whitish, multilobular, and solid. The size of the tumor was $7.0 \times 6.5 \times 2.5$ cm, and the tumor contained teeth, gingiva, and hair (Figure 3). On microscopic examination, the tumor showed remarkable

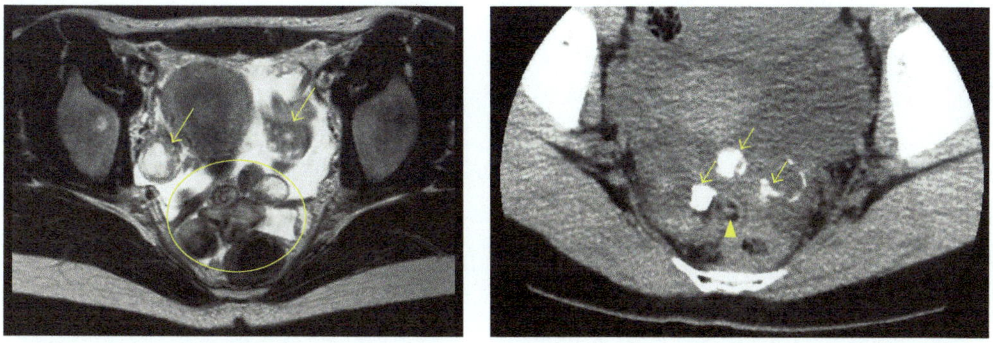

(a) (b)

FIGURE 1: (a) T2 weighted magnetic resonance imaging showing a multicystic mass (circle) and normal ovaries (arrows). (b) Computed tomography showing calcified (arrows) and fatty (arrow head) components in the mass.

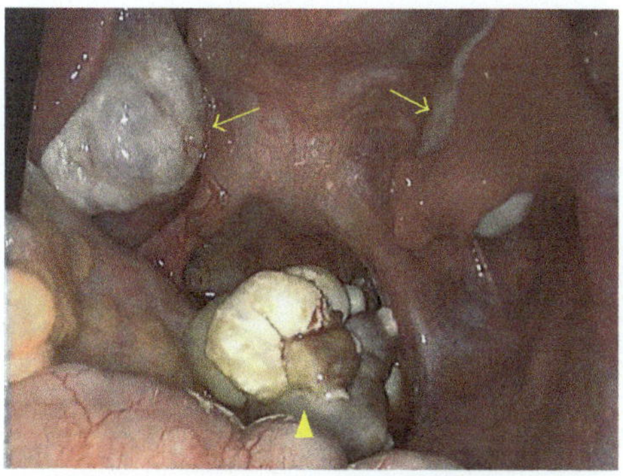

FIGURE 2: Laparoscopy showing normal ovaries (arrows) and a multilobular tumor in Douglas' pouch (arrow head).

hyalinization (Figure 4(a)). It consisted of cysts lined by stratified squamous epithelium with an accumulation of keratin debris and various mature tissues such as hair, teeth, cartilage, neural tissue, fat, foreign body granuloma, and granulation tissue (Figures 4(b)–4(d)). The tumor contained no ovarian tissues. No immature elements or malignancy was found in the tumor, confirming the final pathologic diagnosis of mature cystic teratoma. The patient had an uneventful postoperative course.

3. Discussion

Mature cystic teratoma is one of the most common ovarian neoplasms, accounting for approximately 20% of all adult ovarian neoplasms [6]. Teratomas may occur at extragonadal sites, usually along the midline of the body such as the mediastinum. However, extragonadal teratomas in the abdominal cavity are extremely rare, and the most commonly reported cases are in the omentum, 32 cases in total [7, 8]. Only 12 cases of teratomas in Douglas' pouch have been reported to date [1–5]. This is the first case that simultaneously showed normal ovaries and a teratoma in Douglas' pouch on laparoscopy.

The symptoms observed in this patient were abdominal pain with bilateral ovarian enlargement on transvaginal ultrasonography. The right ovary decreased in size but the left sustained a size up to 4 cm on ultrasonography. The patient was not receiving any medication and her menstrual cycle was regular, so the possibilities of ovarian hyperstimulation syndrome or polycystic ovary syndrome were excluded. We thought that right ovarian hemorrhage had caused the abdominal pain and that a left ovarian tumor had been found incidentally. However, MRI, CT, and laparoscopy revealed normal ovaries and a multicystic mass in Douglas' pouch. This most likely indicated that the left ovarian tumor we had first recognized on transvaginal ultrasonography was actually the tumor in Douglas' pouch.

Differential diagnoses of a cystic mass in Douglas' pouch include cystic mesothelioma, cystic lymphangioma, and endometriotic cyst. It is difficult to establish a diagnosis of teratoma in Douglas' pouch preoperatively. The preoperative diagnostic indication of teratoma is the presence of fat and calcification on CT images. Other differential diagnoses of a tumor with multifocal calcification and fat tissue components of Douglas' pouch are malignant peritoneal mesothelioma, liposarcoma, and metastasis of carcinoma. In our case, we observed the presence of fat and calcified components on the CT images. We considered the diagnosis of teratoma first, taking into account the patient's age, sex, and laboratory data. The tumor was successfully treated via laparoscopic resection, and pathological diagnosis of mature cystic teratoma was finally made. Pathological examination is important. Immature teratoma or teratoma with malignant transformation must be differentiated.

The etiology of extragonadal teratomas is poorly understood but is thought to arise from primordial germ cells or early embryonic cells or from totipotent cells [9]. Three main theories have been proposed to explain the etiology of extragonadal teratomas. The first theory is that extragonadal teratomas may be autoamputated into the abdominal cavity. When one of the ovaries is small or absent, or teratomas contain ovarian tissues, autoamputation has been thought to be a possible cause. This theory is widely accepted as the etiology of extragonadal teratomas in the abdominal cavity and 6 cases of teratomas in Douglas' pouch have been thought to be due to autoamputation [2–5]. However, in our case, the teratoma contained no ovarian tissues and both of the ovaries were

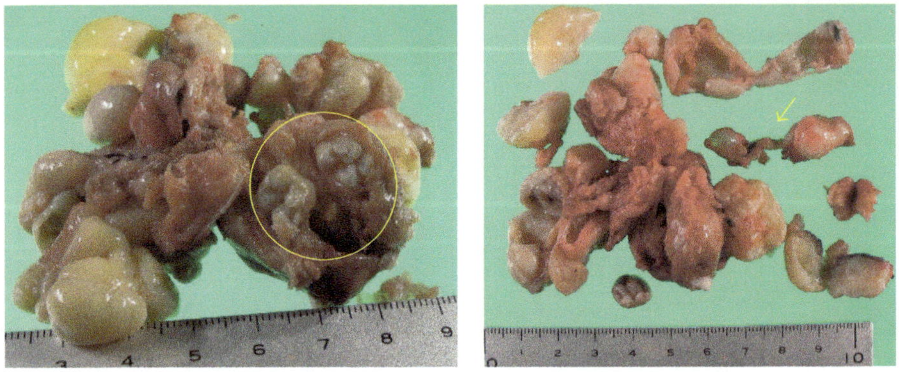

(a) (b)

FIGURE 3: (a) Resected tumor (7.0 × 6.5 × 2.5 cm) and (b) cut surfaces. The tumor was multilobular and contained teeth, gingiva (circle), and hair (arrow).

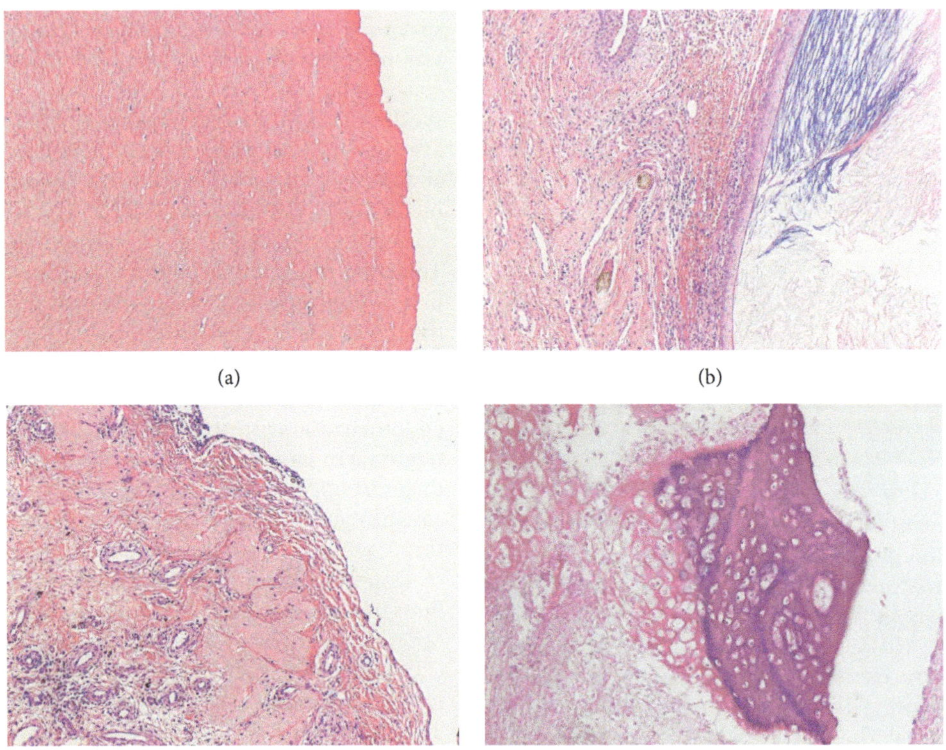

FIGURE 4: Microscopic findings of the tumor: (a) the tumor showed hyalinization. The main components of the tumor were (b) cysts and hair, (c) neural tissue, and (d) cartilage. (Hematoxylin and Eosin staining, original magnification ×4 (a, b, c), ×10 (d)).

intact on laparoscopy. Thus, autoamputation may not be a reasonable theory in our case. The second theory is that extragonadal teratomas may occur in an ectopic ovary [5]. An ectopic ovary is thought to arise congenitally or following a surgical procedure or inflammation within the pelvis. Our patient had no history of laparotomy, and the tumor contained no ovarian tissues. Therefore, this theory is not applicable. The third theory is that extragonadal teratomas may originate from displaced primordial germ cells. During fetal development, primordial germ cells migrate from the yolk sac along the hindgut, to the midline of the body, towards the genital ridge. Primordial germ cells may stop during migration and then may cause a teratoma later [9]. We think this theory is most applicable to our case, even though it is difficult to prove. During migration to the genital ridge, DNA methylation of primordial germ cells is erased and then reestablished during gametogenesis [10]. The results of genomic imprinting research have indicated that each group of germ cell tumors has a different imprinting status [11]. For example, teratoma/yolk sac tumors in infants and teratomas of the ovary in adults have a different status of imprinting. If we could have investigated the imprinting status of the teratoma in our case, it may have been helpful in understanding the origin of the tumor.

In conclusion, we report an extremely rare case of the teratoma in Douglas' pouch. Because the teratoma had no ovarian tissues and both of the ovaries were normal in size; the teratoma was considered to originate primarily in Douglas' pouch.

Conflict of Interests

The authors declare that there is no conflict of interests regarding the publication of this paper.

References

[1] J. H. Lefkowitch, C. M. Fenoglio, and R. M. Richart, "Benign cystic teratoma of the retrouterine pouch of Douglas," *The American Journal of Obstetrics and Gynecology*, vol. 131, no. 7, pp. 818–820, 1978.

[2] H. Matsushita, T. Kurabayashi, T. Yanase, and H. Hideki, "Autoamputation of an ovarian cyst: a case report," *The Journal of Reproductive Medicine*, vol. 54, no. 11-12, pp. 709–711, 2009.

[3] C. E. Bartlett, A. Khan, and N. Pisal, "Parasitic dermoid cyst managed laparoscopically in a 29-year-old woman: a case report," *Journal of Medical Case Reports*, vol. 3, article 63, 2009.

[4] A. Peitsidou, P. Peitsidis, N. Goumalatsos, R. Papaspyrou, G. Mitropoulou, and N. Georgoulias, "Diagnosis of an autoamputated ovary with dermoid cyst during a Cesarean section," *Fertility and Sterility*, vol. 91, no. 4, pp. 1294.e9–1294.e12, 2009.

[5] M. Kusaka and M. Mikuni, "Ectopic ovary: a case of autoamputated ovary with mature cystic teratoma into the cul-de-sac," *The Journal of Obstetrics and Gynaecology Research*, vol. 33, no. 3, pp. 368–370, 2007.

[6] A. Talerman and R. Vang, "Germ cell tumors of the ovary," in *Blaustein's Pathology of the Female Genital Tract*, R. J. Kurman, Ed., pp. 967–1033, Springer, New York, NY, USA, 5th edition, 2008.

[7] P. Hegde, "Extragonadal omental teratoma: a case report," *Journal of Obstetrics and Gynaecology Research*, vol. 40, no. 2, pp. 618–621, 2014.

[8] B. N. Wani, V. Rathod, P. Banode, and A. Bhole, "An omental teratoma in a young girl," *Clinics and Practice*, vol. 1, no. 4, article e129, 2011.

[9] J. W. Oosterhuis, H. Stoop, F. Honecker, and L. H. J. Looijenga, "Why human extragonadal germ cell tumours occur in the midline of the body: old concepts, new perspectives," *International Journal of Andrology*, vol. 30, no. 4, pp. 256–264, 2007.

[10] M. S. Bartolomei and A. C. Ferguson-Smith, "Mammalian Genomic Imprinting," *Cold Spring Harbor Perspectives in Biology*, vol. 3, no. 7, Article ID a002592, 2011.

[11] S. Sievers, K. Alemazkour, S. Zahn et al., "IGF2/H19 imprinting analysis of human germ cell tumors (GCTs) using the methylation-sensitive single-nucleotide primer extension method reflects the origin of GCTs in different stages of primordial germ cell development," *Genes Chromosomes and Cancer*, vol. 44, no. 3, pp. 256–264, 2005.

Adipocyte-Like Differentiation in a Posttreatment Embryonal Rhabdomyosarcoma

Dana Balitzer,[1] Timothy H. McCalmont,[2] and Andrew E. Horvai[3]

[1]*Department of Pathology, University of California, San Francisco, 505 Parnassus, M580, San Francisco, CA 94143, USA*
[2]*Departments of Pathology and Dermatology, University of California, San Francisco, 1701 Divisadero Street, Suite 280, San Francisco, CA 94115, USA*
[3]*Department of Pathology, University of California, San Francisco, 1825 4th Street, M2354, San Francisco, CA 94143, USA*

Correspondence should be addressed to Andrew E. Horvai; andrew.horvai@ucsf.edu

Academic Editor: Khin Thway

We describe a 16-year-old boy with rhabdomyosarcoma, consistent with embryonal subtype, of the lower extremity who received systemic neoadjuvant chemotherapy and subsequent excision. Microscopic sections of the postchemotherapy excision demonstrated diffuse, prominent, and immature adipocyte-like differentiation, in addition to skeletal muscle differentiation. Adipocyte-like differentiation was confirmed by a combination of positive Oil Red O and adipophilin immunohistochemical staining. To our knowledge, this represents the first report of an unusual phenomenon of differentiation of a soft tissue rhabdomyosarcoma into adipocyte-like cells after chemotherapy.

1. Introduction

Rhabdomyosarcoma is an aggressive mesenchymal neoplasm, most common in children, that frequently requires multimodality therapy consisting of surgery and chemotherapy [1]. So-called "cytodifferentiation" after neoadjuvant chemotherapy is a well-described phenomenon in rhabdomyosarcoma and consists of more prominent rhabdomyoblasts and decreased primitive, proliferating cells [2–4]. Rhabdomyosarcoma with adipocyte-like cells has been rarely observed in unusual ovarian carcinosarcomas [5]. However, to our knowledge, the present case represents the first example of a soft tissue rhabdomyosarcoma with adipocyte-like cells after chemotherapy.

2. Case Presentation

One year prior to presentation, a 16-year-old boy with no significant medical history noticed a lump, which progressively enlarged over the course of several months, at his posterior left knee. Magnetic resonance imaging demonstrated a 13-centimeter mass in the left posteroinferior thigh, centered in the region of the semitendinosus muscle and extending to the long head of the biceps femoris muscle.

A fine-needle aspiration of the tumor demonstrated a heterogeneous population of ovoid to tapered spindled cells with variable amounts of densely eosinophilic cytoplasm and occasional multinucleated cells (Figure 1(a)). No lipogenic differentiation was noted on any of the smears or cell block. Immunohistochemical stains for desmin (Figure 1(b)) and myogenin (Figure 1(c)) were positive, whereas staining for CD68, keratin, S-100, SOX-10, HMB-45, and Melan-A was negative (not shown). A diagnosis of rhabdomyosarcoma was made. Fluorescence in situ hybridization was negative for a *FOXO1* 13q14 rearrangement. Based on the cytomorphology and lack of *FOXO1* rearrangement, an embryonal subtype was favored. He received chemotherapy per intermediate risk protocol ARST0531 with vincristine/irinotecan for 10 weeks.

Following chemotherapy, the tumor was completely excised. Grossly, the mass was mixed, cystic and solid, and separated from the surrounding skeletal muscle by a thin white capsule (Figure 1(d)). Routine hematoxylin and eosin (H&E) sections demonstrated diffuse sheets of round tumor cells with variable amounts of dense, eosinophilic

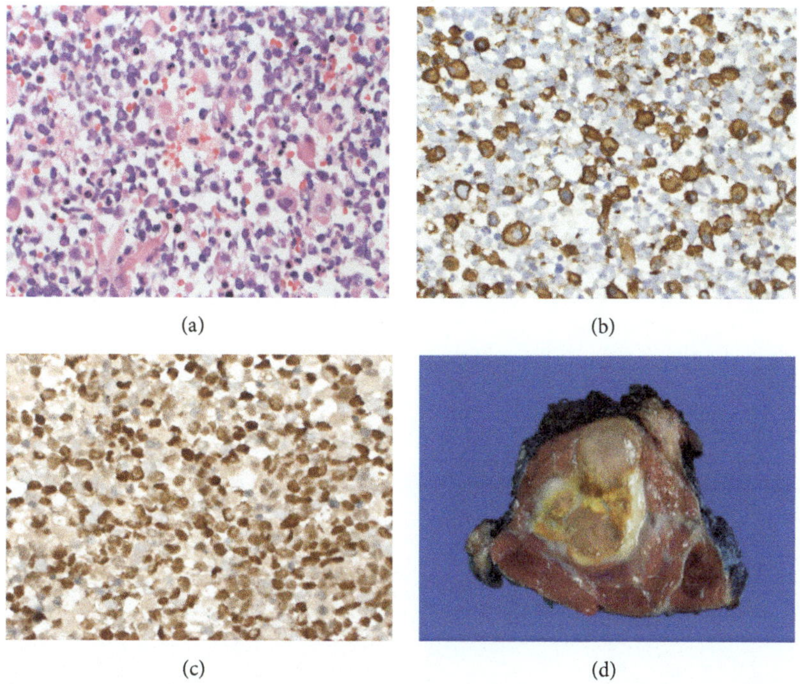

Figure 1: Gross and microscopic findings. (a) Hematoxylin and eosin (H&E) stain from fine-needle aspiration sample, prior to chemotherapy treatment, reveals a heterogeneous population of ovoid to slightly spindled cells (H&E, ×100 original magnification), (b) a subset of tumor cells are positive for desmin immunostain (×400 original magnification), and (c) most tumor cells are positive for myogenin (myogenin immunostain, ×400 original magnification). (d) Gross appearance of resected tumor after adjuvant chemotherapy treatment.

rhabdomyoblastic cytoplasm with large nuclei (Figure 2(a)). Diffusely throughout all sections of the tumor, a subset of cells showed a spectrum of vacuolation. The vacuolation ranged from small intracytoplasmic vacuoles to cells with multiple vacuoles indenting the nucleus thereby resembling adipocytes or lipoblasts (Figure 2(b)). The vacuolated cells were positive for adipophilin (Figure 2(c)), Oil Red O (Figure 2(d)), and S-100 protein (Figure 2(e)). Adipophilin is a ubiquitous component of lipid droplets and is a specific marker for lipid accumulation, which has been reported in cells of lactating mammary epithelium, adrenal cortex, male reproductive system (Sertoli and Leydig cells), steatotic hepatocytes in alcoholic cirrhosis, and liposarcomas [6]. The vacuoles in the adipocyte-like cells did not stain with periodic acid-Schiff, with or without diastase (not shown). An immunostain for desmin demonstrated staining within the cytoplasm of adipocyte-like cells (Figure 2(f)), while immunostaining for myogenin was negative within the nuclei of adipocyte-like cells (Figure 2(g)). Table 1 lists the antibody sources and dilutions used. Cystic change, scattered histiocytes, and extracellular hemosiderin consistent with treatment effect were also present. Mitotic activity was low (1 mf/10 hpf). No coagulative necrosis was identified.

Table 1: Antibody sources and dilutions.

Antibody	Source	Clone	Dilution
Adipophilin	Cell Marque, Rocklin, CA	Polyclonal	Undiluted
Desmin	Cell Marque	D33	1:5
Myogenin	Cell Marque	F5D	Undiluted
S-100 protein	DAKO, Carpinteria, CA	Polyclonal	1:2000

3. Discussion

Rhabdomyosarcoma is the most common soft tissue malignancy in children and adolescents and consists of a biologically and genetically diverse group of sarcoma [7]. Standard treatment regimens for rhabdomyosarcoma include local control with surgery or radiation therapy in conjunction with multiagent chemotherapy [1]. When the tumor is locally advanced, most protocols recommend a biopsy followed by neoadjuvant chemotherapy prior to excision [8].

Several studies have described the range of microscopic treatment related changes in rhabdomyosarcoma. Nonspecific treatment effect, such as necrosis, macrophage infiltrate, fibrosis, and skeletal muscle atrophy are commonly observed. A decrease in proliferative activity is also often present [9]. Rhabdomyosarcoma can also undergo histologic differentiation after treatment. Specifically, rhabdomyoblasts and strap cells become more prominent [2] while undifferentiated, primitive round cells become less conspicuous. Some authors have suggested that these apparently differentiated neoplastic cells may represent terminally differentiated elements withdrawn from the cell cycle after chemotherapy [10].

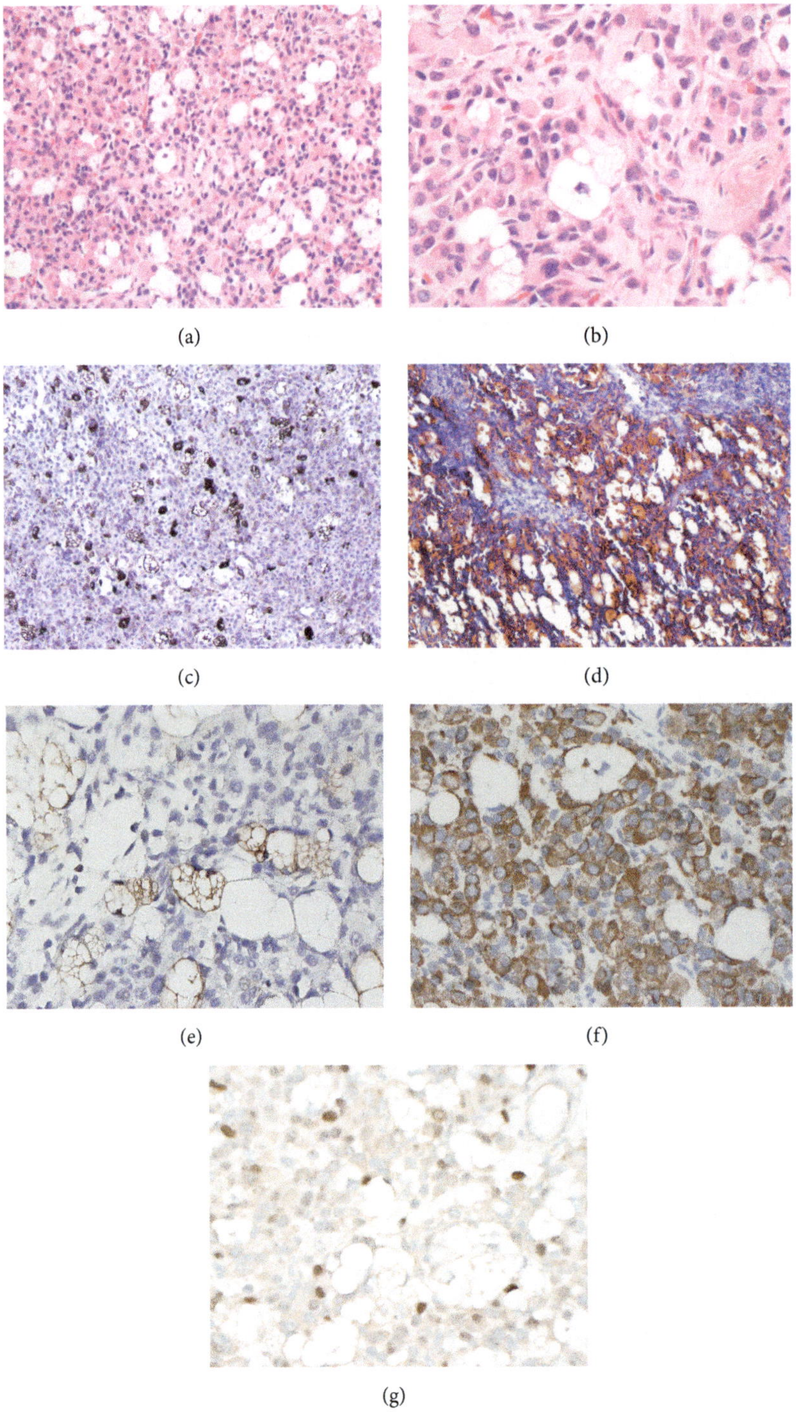

(a) (b) (c) (d) (e) (f) (g)

Figure 2: Histochemical and immunohistochemical studies in posttreatment rhabdomyosarcoma. (a) Microscopic appearance of resected tumor after adjuvant chemotherapy, demonstrating diffuse sheets of round tumor cells (H&E, ×200 original magnification) and (b) vacuolated adipocyte-like cells (H&E, ×400 original magnification). (c) Adipophilin demonstrates strong membrane staining within adipocyte-like cells (adipophilin immunostain, ×100 original magnification). (d) Oil Red O histochemical stain highlights intracytoplasmic lipid within the adipocyte-like cells (Oil Red O, ×200 original magnification). (e) The adipocyte-like cells stain with S-100 protein (S-100 protein immunostain, ×400 original magnification). (f) A subset of vacuolated adipcoyte-like cells show focal cytoplasmic desmin positivity (desmin immunostain, ×400 original magnification) but myogenin (g) is negative in vacuolated cells, staining only the nuclei of rhabdomyoblasts (myogenin immunostain, ×400 original magnification).

The presence of so-called postchemotherapy "cytodifferentiation" is thought to be more frequent in embryonal and botryoid rhabdomyosarcoma than other subtypes [3, 4].

In addition to the phenomenon of cytodifferentiation, vacuolated cells have been previously noted in cases of treated rhabdomyosarcoma. Coffin et al. described the presence of vacuolated cells in a rhabdomyosarcoma [9]. Likewise, a case report of an ovarian carcinosarcoma with pleomorphic rhabdomyosarcomatous differentiation noted the presence of "pseudolipoblasts" after neoadjuvant chemotherapy [5]. The presence of cells with morphology intermediate between rhabdomyoblasts and multivacuolated adipocyte-like cells suggested that the chemotherapy induced differentiation in the rhabdomyosarcomatous component of the carcinosarcoma, representative of a posttreatment phenomenon [5].

In our differential diagnosis, we also considered the possibility of clear cell rhabdomyosarcoma, or glycogen-rich rhabdomyosarcoma [11]. However, several lines of evidence argue against this possibility. First, clear cell rhabdomyosarcoma has not been reported as a treatment related change. Second, the histochemical and immunohistochemical features of the posttreatment excision support lipid accumulation rather than glycogen in the vacuolated cells. Rare examples of lipid-rich rhabdomyosarcomas have also been described, in untreated tumors but not as a morphologic change induced by chemotherapy [12, 13]. The presence of S-100 protein immunostaining, though not highly specific, is at least supportive of adipocytic differentiation. Furthermore, regenerating skeletal muscle can mimic rhabdomyosarcoma and sometimes demonstrate vacuolation. However, in the present case, the resection lacks other characteristic features of muscle regeneration such as sarcolemmal ghosts or necrotic myofibers [14]. We also considered the possibility that lipogenic differentiation was already present, but not sampled, in the FNA biopsy. Although it is impossible to completely exclude this possibility, the FNA yielded abundant cells using a "cone biopsy" technique that samples multiple regions of tumor [15, 16]. Yet, the biopsy contained no vacuolated cells whereas such cells were present diffusely in every section of the excision specimen. Finally, the decrease in density of myogenin positive cells after chemotherapy suggests a different expression pattern in the posttreated tumor compared to the pretreatment biopsy.

Rhabdomyoblastic differentiation is well described in a variety of mesenchymal tumors, including malignant mixed Mullerian tumors of the uterus and carcinosarcomas, as well as neuroectodermal neoplasms such as malignant Triton tumor or medulloblastomas. Intriguingly, rhabdomyoblastic differentiation has been reported in liposarcoma [17, 18], but the reverse (i.e., differentiation of rhabdomyoblasts into lipoblasts or adipocytes) appears extremely rare. Adipocyte-like cells have been previously reported in a primary ovarian rhabdomyosarcoma [19]. Recent cell culture studies suggest that rhabdomyosarcomas can arise from adipocyte progenitors via Smd activation, providing a model whereby embryonal rhabdomyosarcoma can arise in sites devoid of skeletal muscle [20]. Lineage tracing and clonal analysis studies have demonstrated that adult skeletal muscle stem cells are bipotential and can give rise to brown adipogenic and myogenic progenitors presumably under the correct genetic and epigenetic mechanisms [21].

To our knowledge, this is the first reported case of a soft tissue rhabdomyosarcoma with evidence to support adipocyte-like cells as a posttreatment phenomenon and expand the spectrum of cytodifferentiation that can be observed in treated rhabdomyosarcoma.

Conflict of Interests

The authors declare that there is no conflict of interests regarding the publication of this paper.

References

[1] D. S. Hawkins, A. A. Gupta, and E. R. Rudzinski, "What is new in the biology and treatment of pediatric rhabdomyosarcoma?" *Current Opinion in Pediatrics*, vol. 26, no. 1, pp. 50–56, 2014.

[2] W. M. Molenaar, J. W. Oosterhuis, and W. A. Kamps, "Cytologic 'differentiation' in childhood rhabdomyosarcomas following polychemotherapy," *Human Pathology*, vol. 15, no. 10, pp. 973–979, 1984.

[3] C. M. Coffin, J. Rulon, L. Smith, C. Bruggers, and F. V. White, "Pathologic features of rhabdomyosarcoma before and after treatment: a clinicopathologic and immunohistochemical analysis," *Modern Pathology*, vol. 10, no. 12, pp. 1175–1187, 1997.

[4] L. M. Smith, J. R. Anderson, and C. M. Coffin, "Cytodifferentiation and clinical outcome after chemotherapy and radiation therapy for rhabdomyosarcoma (RMS)," *Medical and Pediatric Oncology*, vol. 38, no. 6, pp. 398–404, 2002.

[5] K. Thway, S. Hazell, S. Banerjee, and C. Fisher, "Rhabdomyosarcoma with pseudolipoblasts arising in ovarian carcinosarcoma: a distinctive postchemotherapy morphologic variant mimicking pleomorphic liposarcoma," *Case Reports in Pathology*, vol. 2014, Article ID 238545, 5 pages, 2014.

[6] H. W. Heid, R. Moll, I. Schwetlick, H.-R. Rackwitz, and T. W. Keenan, "Adipophilin is a specific marker of lipid accumulation in diverse cell types and diseases," *Cell and Tissue Research*, vol. 294, no. 2, pp. 309–321, 1998.

[7] D. M. Parham, "Pathologic classification of rhabdomyosarcomas and correlations with molecular studies," *Modern Pathology*, vol. 14, no. 10, pp. 506–514, 2001.

[8] G. Cecchetto, G. Bisogno, F. De Corti et al., "Biopsy or debulking surgery as initial surgery for locally advanced rhabdomyosarcomas in children?: the experience of the Italian Cooperative Group studies," *Cancer*, vol. 110, no. 11, pp. 2561–2567, 2007.

[9] C. M. Coffin, A. Lowichik, and H. Zhou, "Treatment effects in pediatric soft tissue and bone tumors: practical considerations for the pathologist," *American Journal of Clinical Pathology*, vol. 123, no. 1, pp. 75–90, 2005.

[10] E. S. d'Amore, M. Tollot, V. Stracca-Pansa et al., "Therapy associated differentiation in rhabdomyosarcomas," *Modern Pathology*, vol. 7, no. 1, pp. 69–75, 1994.

[11] F. Boman, J. Champigneulle, C. Schmitt, P. Beurey, J. Floquet, and L. Boccon-Gibod, "Clear cell rhabdomyosarcoma," *Pediatric Pathology and Laboratory Medicine*, vol. 16, no. 6, pp. 951–959, 1996.

[12] C. Quincey, S. S. Baneriee, B. P. Eyden, and K. S. Vasudev, "Lipid rich rhabdomyosarcoma," *Journal of Clinical Pathology*, vol. 47, no. 3, pp. 280–282, 1994.

[13] C. W. Zuppan, G. W. Mierau, and D. A. Weeks, "Lipid-rich rhabdomyosarcoma—a potential source of diagnostic confusion," *Ultrastructural Pathology*, vol. 15, no. 4-5, pp. 353–359, 1991.

[14] L. Guillou, M. Coquet, P. Chaubert, and J. M. Coindre, "Skeletal muscle regeneration mimicking rhabdomyosarcoma: a potential diagnostic pitfall," *Histopathology*, vol. 33, no. 2, pp. 136–144, 1998.

[15] R. M. DeMay, *The Art and Science of Cytopathology*, ASCP Press, Chicago, Ill, USA, 1996.

[16] W. F. Symmans, M. Ayers, E. A. Clark et al., "Total RNA yield and microarray gene expression profiles from fine-needle aspiration biopsy and core-needle biopsy samples of breast carcinoma," *Cancer*, vol. 97, no. 12, pp. 2960–2971, 2003.

[17] D. Govender and P. Pillay, "Primary myxoid liposarcoma with rhabdomyoblastic differentiation," *Archives of Pathology and Laboratory Medicine*, vol. 122, no. 8, pp. 740–742, 1998.

[18] J. H. Shanks, S. S. Banerjee, and B. P. Eyden, "Focal rhabdomyosarcomatous differentiation in primary liposarcoma," *Journal of Clinical Pathology*, vol. 49, no. 9, pp. 770–772, 1996.

[19] D. S. Allende and B. Yang, "Primary ovarian rhabdomyosarcoma with heterologous elements: a case report," *International Journal of Gynecological Pathology*, vol. 27, no. 3, pp. 402–406, 2008.

[20] K. Kikuchi and C. Keller, "The not-so-skinny on muscle cancer," *Cancer Cell*, vol. 22, no. 4, pp. 421–422, 2012.

[21] H. Yin, A. Pasut, V. D. Soleimani et al., "MicroRNA-133 controls brown adipose determination in skeletal muscle satellite cells by targeting Prdm16," *Cell Metabolism*, vol. 17, no. 2, pp. 210–224, 2013.

20

Metastasis of Malignant Melanoma to Urinary Bladder: A Case Report and Review of the Literature

Rashna Meunier,[1] Gyan Pareek,[2] and Ali Amin[1]

[1] *Department of Pathology and Laboratory Medicine, Rhode Island Hospital, The Warren Alpert Medical School, Brown University, Providence, RI 02903, USA*
[2] *University Urological Associates, The Warren Alpert Medical School, Brown University, Providence, RI 02904, USA*

Correspondence should be addressed to Rashna Meunier; rashna55@gmail.com

Academic Editor: Piero Tosi

Aims. Metastatic malignant melanoma of the urinary bladder is a rare clinical entity, with only twenty-three published cases to date. We present a case of this rare entity, a thorough review of the literature, and differential diagnosis of melanoma in the bladder. *Methods and Results.* A 55-year-old woman with a history of malignant melanoma of the right thigh, excised eight years ago, presented with back pain, fatigue, and hematuria. She underwent computed tomography (CT) scan and was found to have metastases within the liver, spleen, lungs, and urinary bladder. She underwent cystoscopy and transurethral resection of three polypoid lesions. Histologic and immunohistochemical examination revealed metastatic malignant melanoma involving bladder mucosa. *Conclusions.* This case illustrates the importance of including malignant melanoma in the differential diagnosis of high grade neoplasms of bladder, especially in cases where the relevant clinical history is not available.

1. Introduction

Metastasis of malignant melanoma to the bladder is extremely rare in clinical practice. Although many recent review papers report less than ten cases in the past thirty years, our thorough review of the current literature reveals 23 confirmed cases published to date. This indicates that the incidence is likely higher than previously thought and may be due to the fact that many patients are asymptomatic and only found at autopsy. In 1964, Das Gupta and Brasfield performed an autopsy series of 125 patients with metastatic melanoma and found that 18% had metastases to the bladder [1]. Similarly in 2000, Bates and Baithun described five postmortem cases of melanoma metastasizing to the urinary bladder among 153 autopsy cases [2]. Symptomatic patients, on the other hand, usually present with painless gross hematuria [3]. The most common sites of metastasis include regional lymph nodes, lungs, liver, and brain. Malignant melanoma is extremely diverse in its histologic, cytological, and architectural appearances and is often known as the "great mimicker." This holds true for metastases to the urinary bladder. Our case highlights the importance of including malignant melanoma in the differential diagnosis of high grade urothelial lesions. Although a clinical history of melanoma is often the first clue to the diagnosis, this clinical information is not always readily available.

2. Materials and Methods

A 55-year-old woman presented with back pain, generalized fatigue, and hematuria. Her past medical history was significant for malignant melanoma of the right thigh, diagnosed eight years ago, for which she underwent wide local excision and sentinel lymph node biopsy. Biopsy revealed that the melanoma was 1.05 mm in thickness, Clark's level IV, and without ulceration. One sentinel lymph node was removed which was negative for metastatic disease. Reexcision revealed the presence of scar with no evidence of residual disease. She was followed up regularly and remained asymptomatic, until eight years later when she developed back pain and generalized fatigue. She was evaluated by her primary care physician and tested negative for Lyme disease.

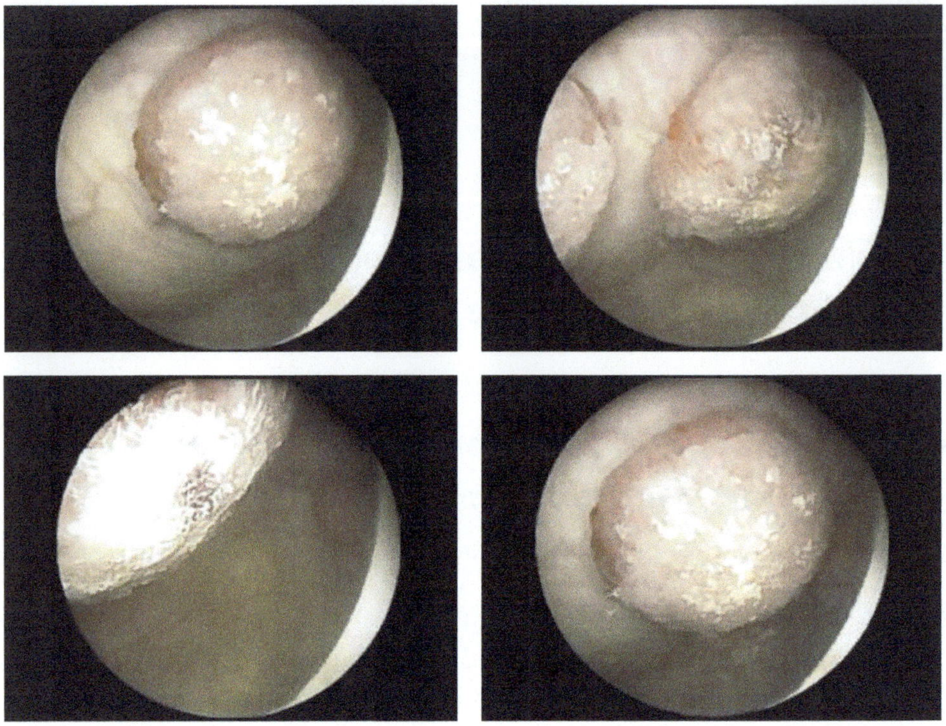

FIGURE 1: Cystoscopy revealed three polypoid masses, each protruding from a stalk.

Shortly afterwards, she developed hematuria and was referred to urology for further evaluation. Urinalysis ruled out infection and confirmed the presence of hematuria. She also had computed tomography (CT) scan of the chest, abdomen, and pelvis, which revealed multiple liver and splenic lesions, multiple subcentimeter bilateral pulmonary nodules suspicious for metastatic disease, and several masses within the bladder, measuring up to 1.9 cm in greatest dimension. Urine cytology identified atypical cells, but evaluation was limited by scant cellularity. She underwent cystoscopy, which revealed three polypoid, spherical lesions, each protruding from a stalk (Figure 1). Two of these lesions were located along the left anterior bladder dome and measured approximately 2 cm each. A third smaller lesion, located along the left lateral bladder wall, measured approximately 1 cm. There was no evidence of discoloration in the lesions or elsewhere in the bladder. Monopolar loop electrocautery was used to excise the tumors and the bases of the lesions were fulgurated.

3. Results

Histologic examination revealed diffuse hypercellular sheets and nests of basophilic medium to large tumor cells with high nuclear to cytoplasmic ratio, moderate nuclear pleomorphism, irregular nuclear contours, abundant intranuclear and cytoplasmic pseudoinclusions, vesicular chromatin, and occasional prominent nucleoli (Figure 2). Brisk mitotic activity was noted with atypical mitotic figures. Tumor cells were noted to engulf other tumor cells (tumor cannibalism). Numerous apoptotic bodies and karyorrhectic debris were present, along with patchy areas of geographic tumor necrosis

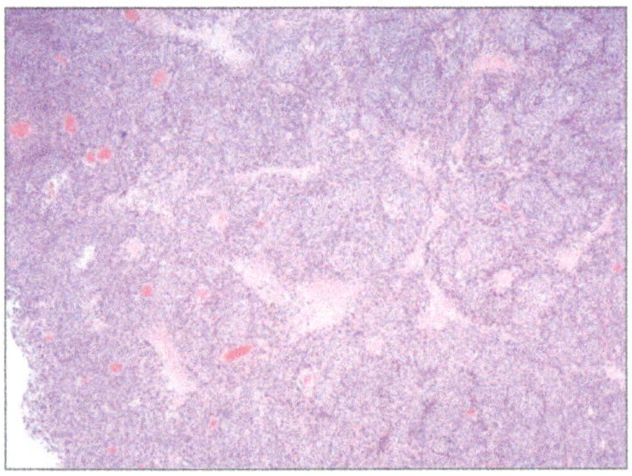

(a)

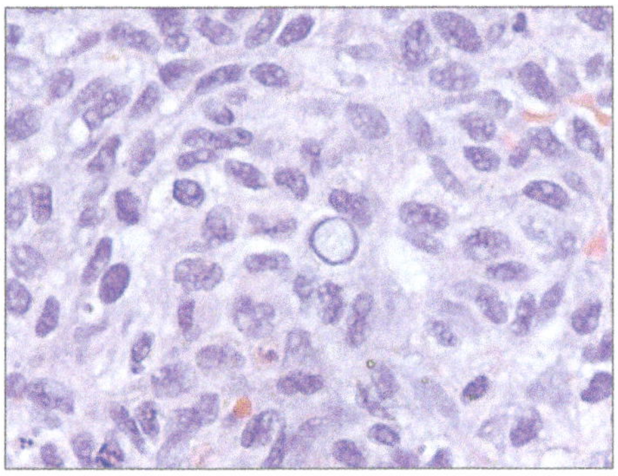

(b)

FIGURE 2: (a) Sheets and nests of tumor cells interspersed with patchy areas of necrosis (hematoxylin-eosin, 40x). (b) The tumor cells have a moderate degree of nuclear pleomorphism and occasionally demonstrate intranuclear and cytoplasmic pseudoinclusions (hematoxylin-eosin, 400x).

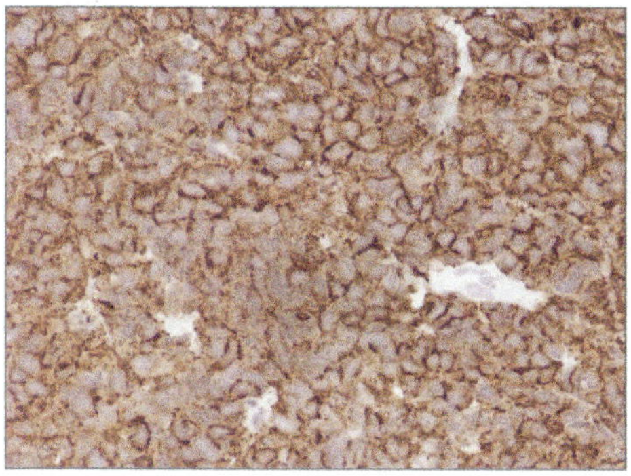

FIGURE 3: Tumor cells are strongly and diffusely positive for Melan-A.

with tumor cells palisading around necrotic foci. The sheets of tumor cells invaded into the muscularis propria of the bladder wall. There was no evidence of intracytoplasmic melanin pigmentation or pigment incontinence. Due to surface ulceration, no evidence of superficial urothelium was identified. Biopsy of the patient's previous skin lesion was not available for comparative review.

Immunohistochemistry (IHC) of the bladder lesion revealed diffuse positivity with Melan-A (Cell Marque, Rocklin, CA) and S100 protein (Dako, Carpinteria, CA) (Figure 3). Tumor cells did not stain with p63 (BioGenex Laboratories, San Ramon, CA) or cytokeratin 34BE12 (Enzo Life Sciences, New York, NY). A final histopathological diagnosis of metastatic malignant melanoma involving bladder mucosa was rendered.

4. Discussion

The presence of metastatic malignant melanoma within the urinary bladder is an exceedingly rare finding. A literature review by Efesoy and Cayan in 2011 states that there are less than ten cases reported in the last 30 years in the English literature [4]. Similarly, in 2014, Rishi et al. stated that there are "less than score of cases" [5]. This number is cited as slightly higher in a case report by Paterson et al. in which fourteen cases are listed [3]. We conducted a thorough PUBMED search and found that there are a total of twenty-three reported cases (Table 1). Patient age ranged from 28 to 84 years with a mean age of 56.5 years. Men were more commonly affected than women (M : F = 15 : 8). Not surprisingly, the most common primary site of disease was the skin. Sixteen cases had synchronous metastases of melanoma in other sites, five of which were considered "widespread." The most common presenting symptom in bladder metastasis was hematuria, present in sixteen cases.

While the most common imaging modality for bladder tumors is magnetic resonance imaging, cystoscopy is useful in its ability to visualize the bladder mucosa. However, there are cases in which the mucosa is uninvolved and the metastatic melanoma only involves the bladder wall [6]. Of all the cases published to date, synchronous metastases were present in all but four patients. Unfortunately, the long term followup for the patients without synchronous metastases was not available for comparison with those having synchronous disease.

In cases where the clinical history of primary melanoma is noted, the diagnosis of bladder metastases is often straightforward and can be confirmed by immunohistochemical stains. However, in the absence of a clinical history of melanoma, other lesions with an infiltrative growth pattern and similar cytomorphology may be considered. The possible list of differential diagnoses includes high grade urothelial carcinoma, prostatic carcinoma in male, Müllerian carcinomas in female, lung carcinoma, breast carcinoma, and rare entities like paraganglioma and sarcomatoid carcinoma.

When faced with this diagnostic challenge, there are certain morphological features that can be helpful in differentiating metastatic melanoma from high grade urothelial carcinoma. Malignant melanoma usually presents as a nodule devoid of mucosal excrescences and papillary fronds. The overlying urothelium is mostly unremarkable without any in situ components. In general, the absence of a superficial urothelial lesion overlying a poorly differentiated tumor is an important clue to secondary bladder neoplasia, including metastatic melanoma [5]. The presence of intramucosal atypical melanocytes has been reported in primary bladder melanomas and is considered a prerequisite finding for the diagnosis of primary bladder origin [7]; however, there is no report of such lesions in secondary bladder melanoma.

Tumor cells in melanoma are predominantly comprised of epithelioid cells with rare spindle cell morphology. They reveal macronuclei with marked variation in nuclear size and shape. Nuclei are hyperchromatic with prominent large eosinophilic nucleoli. A helpful feature is the conspicuous presence of intranuclear inclusions. The stroma surrounding melanoma is usually desmoplastic and inflamed, with melanophage aggregation. Intracytoplasmic pigments are useful when present. Atypical mitoses and lymphovascular invasion can also point to secondary bladder tumors including melanoma. It is noteworthy that none of the above-mentioned morphological findings are pathognomonic and a multimodal approach should be considered when confronting a suspicious secondary bladder tumor. The diagnosis can be confirmed using a panel of IHC (vide infra).

Urothelial carcinoma on the other hand is usually associated with a papillary or flat carcinoma in situ (CIS) component on the surface of the lesion that is continuous with the invasive component. Urothelial lesions commonly show glandular or squamous differentiation without cytoplasmic pigmentation or pigment incontinence around tumor nests. IHC staining for high molecular weight cytokeratin (34BE12 and CK5/6), p63, uroplakin, thrombomodulin, and GATA3 supports urothelial origin.

Prostate adenocarcinoma in males lacks cellular pleomorphism. Tumor cells are typically uniform and form glandular and cribriform arrangements. There is generally a high tendency for invasion into perineural spaces in the tumor. IHC staining for prostate-specific antigen (PSA), prostate-specific membrane antigen (PSMA), alpha methylacyl-CoA racemase (AMACR), and prostein (P501s) can be very helpful in differential diagnosis.

TABLE 1: Cases of malignant melanoma metastatic to urinary bladder previously reported in the English literature.

Author	Year	Age	Sex	Presenting symptom	Primary	Synchronous metastases	Treatment
Weston and Smith [10]	1964	69	M	Urinary retention	Right lower eyelid	Widespread	None
Bartone [18]	1964	70	F	Hematuria	Left thumb	Lymph nodes, brain	Partial cystectomy
Amar [19]	1964	33	M	Hematuria	Maxillary	Anterior neck	Partial cystectomy
Meyer [9]	1974	69	M	None	Unknown	Widespread	Chemotherapy
Meyer [9]	1974	60	F	Hematuria	Skin, left arm	Unknown	Surgery
Meyer [9]	1974	42	M	Incidental	Skin, right upper back	Widespread	TURBT
Silverstein et al. [20]	1974	56	M	Hematuria	Axillary lymph nodes	Absent	BCG
Tolley et al. [21]	1975	48	F	Hematuria	Vulva	Absent	Radical cystectomy
Stein and Kendall [22]	1984	50	M	Hematuria	Left arm	Absent	TURBT + chemotherapy
Irisawa et al. [23]	1987	77	M	Occult blood	Eye	Diffuse	TURBT
Arapantoni-Dadioti et al. [24]	1995	28	F	Dysuria	Axillary lymph node	Skin (abdomen, limbs), lung, and brain	TURBT
Demirkesen et al. [25]	2000	45	F	Frequency, hematuria	Right heel	Widespread	Chemotherapy
López et al. [26]	2002	75	M	Hematuria, lower urinary symptoms	Skin, scapula	Unknown	Cystectomy
Lee et al. [27]	2003	46	M	Hematuria	Skin, back	Lungs, liver, and mesenteric lymph nodes	Removed tumor and then IL-2 therapy
Fink et al. [28]	2003	38	M	Hematuria	Skin, left upper leg	Tonsils, cervical lymph nodes, esophagus, stomach, and skin	Embolization of nutrient vessels
Maeda et al. [29]	2008	65	M	Hematuria, urinary obstruction	Skin, foot	Unknown	TURBT
Nohara et al. [30]	2009	62	M	Hematuria	Skin, breast	Lymph nodes	Unknown
Efesoy and Cayan [4]	2011	60	F	Hematuria, weight loss	Skin, right middle finger	Brain, lung, and retroperitoneal and pelvic lymph nodes	TURBT
Nair et al. [6]	2011	54	M	Hematuria	Conjunctiva	Widespread	TURBT, chemo, and radiation for brain metastases
Charfi et al. [31]	2012	54	M	Unknown	Esophagus	Lumbar lymph nodes	Unknown
Paterson et al. [3]	2012	84	M	Rectal bleeding	Skin, upper back	Lungs	
Ikeda et al. [32]	2013	54	F	Hematuria	Skin, leg	Absent	TURBT
Rishi et al. [5]	2014	61	F	Dysuria, hematuria	Skin, mid-back	Brain, lung, and skin	Tumor resection, brain radiotherapy, and temozolomide
Meunier (current case)	2014	55	F	Hematuria	Skin, thigh	Liver, spleen, and lung	Ipilimumab + anti-PD-1 immunotherapy trial

Metastatic Müllerian tumors are diverse and, based on the subtype and organ of origin, can show variable morphologies. Some variants like high grade serous carcinoma can show marked cellular pleomorphism and extension beyond the organ of origin. Such tumors show micropapillary clusters with psammomatous calcifications. These tumors are usually cytokeratin positive and based on the site of origin can express PAX8, estrogen (ER), and progesterone (PR) receptors.

Breast carcinoma can be seen metastasizing into bladder and other pelvic organs. Arrangement of tumor cells in single file, discohesive tumor cells, and intracytoplasmic vacuoles can often be seen in metastasizing lobular breast carcinoma. However, some other carcinomas like lung may not show any specific morphological features to suggest a secondary tumor. In such situations, IHC is very helpful in the differential diagnosis. In the case of breast cancer, ER, PR, GATA3, and mammaglobin can be helpful, while TTF1 and napsin-A can point toward lung adenocarcinoma.

Paraganglioma of the bladder can also mimic melanoma. Occasionally these tumors cause prominent clinical symptoms. Morphologically, bladder paraganglioma is composed of a monomorphic cell population with or without cytoplasmic clearing and rare mitosis without atypical forms. IHC for chromogranin-A and synaptophysin is helpful in the diagnosis [8].

Rishi et al. suggest that metastatic melanoma often has nonrefractile green-brown pigment on gross examination [5]. In the available literature, only five case reports have noted the presence of grossly pigmented dark blue or black lesions on cystoscopy [3, 9–11]. The current case did not show any evidence of discoloration within the lesion. The histologic presence of pigment within lesional cells or surrounding histiocytes should prompt the pathologist to consider metastatic melanoma in the differential diagnosis.

Melanosis, both with and without atypia, has been reported in about a dozen cases in the literature [12]. Although melanosis usually occurs independently without any associated or adjacent lesions, it may be seen with other malignancies. One must keep in mind that the presence of melanosis within the bladder does not necessarily confer the diagnosis of melanoma. There are two reported cases of melanosis with subsequent development of urothelial carcinoma and one reported case of melanosis with subsequent development of multifocal malignant melanoma [13–15].

Sarcomatoid carcinoma may mimic metastatic melanoma with spindle cell morphology. The cells of sarcomatoid carcinoma are often large, spindled, and pleomorphic and may appear similar to the pleomorphic melanocytes of melanoma. However, the presence of heterologous elements such as cartilage or bone should point towards a diagnosis of sarcomatoid carcinoma. To confirm the diagnosis, areas of the tumor with epithelial differentiation should be cytokeratin positive, whereas melanoma will be negative.

To confirm the diagnosis of metastatic malignant melanoma, IHC is invaluable. S100 protein is a sensitive but not very specific marker and should be confirmed by more specific markers including Melan-A, HMB45, and MITF. One must be aware of the variable expression of melanoma markers in metastatic melanoma. The heterogeneity of melanoma associated antigens can even be seen within a single lesion. Therefore, we recommend the use of more than one melanoma marker. Cytokeratin expression, on the other hand, has been reported in up to 2% of melanomas [16]; therefore, this marker can be reliably used to rule out other carcinomas.

When confronting a malignant melanoma of the bladder in the absence of any clinical evidence of a primary lesion, one must keep primary malignant melanoma of the bladder within the differential diagnosis. Primary malignant melanoma of the genitourinary tract is very rare and most frequently involves the distal urethra [17], with less than thirty cases reported in the literature. In addition, one must be wary of collision tumors in which a melanoma metastasizes to a primary bladder tumor. Although uncommon, there is a single case report of a melanoma metastasizing to a preexisting urothelial carcinoma [11].

In summary, to date there are 24 known cases of malignant melanoma metastatic to the urinary bladder. As "the great mimicker," melanoma can take on various histologic appearances and it is important to keep this entity in the differential diagnosis of high grade infiltrative urothelial lesions without a papillary or in situ component. Immunohistochemical stains and a thorough clinical history and examination can provide further assurance in making the diagnosis.

Abbreviations

IHC: Immunohistochemistry
CIS: Carcinoma in situ
TURBT: Transurethral resection of bladder tumor.

Conflict of Interests

The authors declare that they have no conflict of interests.

Authors' Contribution

Dr. Gyan Pareek was the urologist of the patient, provided the tumor material, and provided clinical history. Dr. Ali Amin signed out the case and reviewed and edited the paper. Dr. Rashna Meunier wrote the paper and took the microscopic photographs.

References

[1] T. Das Gupta and R. Brasfield, "Metastatic melanoma. A clinicopathological study," *Cancer*, vol. 17, pp. 1323–1339, 1964.

[2] A. W. Bates and S. I. Baithun, "Secondary neoplasms of the bladder are histological mimics of nontransitional cell primary tumours: clinicopathological and histological features of 282 cases," *Histopathology*, vol. 36, no. 1, pp. 32–40, 2000.

[3] A. Paterson, M. Sut, A. Kaul et al., "Metastatic malignant melanoma of the urinary bladder: case report and literature review," *Central European Journal of Urology*, vol. 65, no. 4, pp. 232–234, 2012.

[4] O. Efesoy and S. Cayan, "Bladder metastasis of malignant melanoma: a case report and review of literature," *Medical Oncology*, vol. 28, supplement 1, pp. S667–S669, 2011.

[5] A. Rishi, T. A. Anderson, A. M. Kirschenbaum, and P. D. Unger, "Metastatic malignant melanoma to urinary bladder: a potential pitfall for high-grade urothelial carcinoma," *International Journal of Surgical Pathology*, vol. 22, no. 4, pp. 347–351, 2014.

[6] B. C. J. Nair, N. C. Williams, C. Cui et al., "Conjunctival melanoma: bladder and upper urinary tract metastases," *Journal of Clinical Oncology*, vol. 29, no. 9, pp. e216–e219, 2011.

[7] A. M. Ainsworth, W. H. Clark, M. Mastrangelo, and K. B. Conger, "Primary malignant melanoma of the urinary bladder," *Cancer*, vol. 37, no. 4, pp. 1928–1936, 1976.

[8] M. Zhou, J. I. Epstein, and R. H. Young, "Paraganglioma of the Urinary Bladder: A Lesion That May Be Misdiagnosed as Urothelial Carcinoma in Transurethral Resection Specimens," *American Journal of Surgical Pathology*, vol. 28, no. 1, pp. 94–100, 2004.

[9] J. E. Meyer, "Metastatic melanoma of the urinary bladder," *Cancer*, vol. 34, no. 5, pp. 1822–1824, 1974.

[10] P. A. Weston and B. J. Smith, "Metastatic melanoma in the bladder and urethra," *The British Journal of Surgery*, vol. 51, pp. 78–79, 1964.

[11] P. Arapantoni-Dadioti, J. Panayiotides, P. Kalkandi, C. Christodoulou, and G. S. Delides, "Metastasis of malignant melanoma to a transitional cell carcinoma of the urinary bladder," *European Journal of Surgical Oncology*, vol. 21, no. 1, pp. 92–93, 1995.

[12] C. B. Willys, D. C. Winkle, and K. M. Kerr, "Urinary bladder melanosis: case report of a rare mucosal lesion," *Pathology*, vol. 43, no. 2, pp. 164–166, 2011.

[13] S. L. Sanborn, G. MacLennan, M. M. Cooney, M. Zhou, and L. E. Ponsky, "High-grade transitional cell carcinoma and melanosis of urinary bladder: case report and review of the literature," *Urology*, vol. 73, no. 4, pp. 928.e13–928.e15, 2009.

[14] J. A. Harikrishnan, S. Chilka, and S. Jain, "Urinary tract transitional cell carcinoma and melanosis of the bladder: a case report and review of the literature," *Annals of the Royal College of Surgeons of England*, vol. 94, no. 4, pp. e152–e154, 2012.

[15] S. W. Kerley, M. L. Blute, and G. L. Keeney, "Multifocal malignant melanoma arising in vesicovaginal melanosis," *Archives of Pathology and Laboratory Medicine*, vol. 115, no. 9, pp. 950–952, 1991.

[16] R. King, K. Busam, and J. Rosai, "Metastatic malignant melanoma resembling malignant peripheral nerve sheath tumor: report of 16 cases," *American Journal of Surgical Pathology*, vol. 23, no. 12, pp. 1499–1505, 1999.

[17] A. K.-G. Venyo, "Melanoma of the urinary bladder: a review of the literature," *Surgery Research and Practice*, vol. 2014, Article ID 605802, 13 pages, 2014.

[18] F. F. Bartone, "Metastatic melanoma of the bladder," *Journal of Urology*, vol. 91, pp. 151–155, 1964.

[19] A. D. Amar, "Metastatic melanoma of the bladder," *The Journal of Urology*, vol. 92, pp. 198–200, 1964.

[20] M. J. Silverstein, J. DeKernion, and D. L. Morton, "Malignant melanoma metastatic to the bladder. Regression following intratumor injection of BCG vaccine," *Journal of the American Medical Association*, vol. 229, no. 6, p. 688, 1974.

[21] D. A. Tolley, J. E. Castro, and I. D. Anseli, "Malignant metastatic melanoma of the bladder," *British Journal of Clinical Practice*, vol. 29, no. 10, pp. 276–278, 1975.

[22] B. S. Stein and A. R. Kendall, "Malignant melanoma of the genitourinary tract," *The Journal of Urology*, vol. 132, no. 5, pp. 859–868, 1984.

[23] C. Irisawa, Y. Onmura, and S. Matsushita, "Metastatic malignant melanoma of the urinary bladder: a case report," *Hinyokika Kiyo*, vol. 33, no. 3, pp. 424–427, 1987.

[24] P. Arapantoni-Dadioti, J. Panayiotides, P. Kalkandi, C. Christodoulou, and G. S. Delides, "Metastasis of malignant melanoma to a transitional cell carcinoma of the urinary bladder," *European Journal of Surgical Oncology*, vol. 21, no. 1, pp. 92–93, 1995.

[25] O. Demirkesen, O. Yaycioglu, N. Uygun, G. Demir, and V. Yalcin, "A case of metastatic malignant melanoma presenting with hematuria," *Urologia Internationalis*, vol. 64, no. 2, pp. 118–120, 2000.

[26] V. M. López, R. A.-V. García, M. S. Arqués, and P. C. González, *Archivos Españoles de Urología*, vol. 55 of *1279*, 1277, 10 edition, 2002.

[27] C. S. Lee, I. K. Komenaka, K. S. Hurst-Wicker, G. Deraffele, J. Mitcham, and H. L. Kaufman, "Management of metastatic malignant melanoma of the bladder," *Urology*, vol. 62, no. 2, p. 351, 2003.

[28] W. Fink, A. Zimpfer, and S. Ugurel, "Mucosal metastases in malignant melanoma," *Onkologie*, vol. 26, no. 3, pp. 249–251, 2003.

[29] T. Maeda, Y. Uchida, T. Kouda et al., "Metastatic malignant melanoma of the urinary bladder presenting with hematuria: a case report," *Acta Urologica Japonica*, vol. 54, no. 12, pp. 787–790, 2008.

[30] T. Nohara, A. Sakai, H. Fuse, and Y. Imamura, "Metastatic malignant melanoma of the urinary bladder: a case report," *Nihon Hinyokika Gakkai Zasshi*, vol. 100, no. 7, pp. 707–711, 2009.

[31] S. Charfi, S. Ellouze, H. Mnif, A. Amouri, A. Khabir, and T. Sellami-Boudawara, "Plasmacytoid melanoma of the urinary bladder and lymph nodes with immunohistochemical expression of plasma cell markers revealing primary esophageal melanoma," *Case Reports in Pathology*, vol. 2012, Article ID 916256, 5 pages, 2012.

[32] A. Ikeda, T. Miyagawa, M. Kurobe et al., "Case of metastatic malignant melanoma of the urinary bladder," *Hinyokika Kiyo*, vol. 59, no. 9, pp. 579–582, 2013.

Malakoplakia of the Pancreas with Simultaneous Colon Involvement: Case Report and Review of the Literature

Surya Guha and Haiyan Liu

Geisinger Medical Center, 100 North Academy Avenue, Danville, PA 17821, USA

Correspondence should be addressed to Surya Guha; surya_iswar@yahoo.com

Academic Editor: Katsuyuki Aozasa

Although malakoplakia has been reported to occur at various body sites, pancreatic malakoplakia with simultaneous colonic involvement is very rare. Lesions of malakoplakia can masquerade as tumor masses leading to unwanted resections. Nevertheless, malakoplakia can occur in association with frank carcinomas, especially in the colon. By reporting a case of pancreatic malakoplakia diagnosed by fine needle aspiration cytology, this paper aims to describe cytologic features of malakoplakia and to further review findings from previous reported cases of pancreatic malakoplakia in the literature. With advances in minimally invasive, image-guided aspiration technologies, cytomorphological analyses can diagnose lesions of malakoplakia. This may help avoid surgeries that would have otherwise been carried out due to a misleading impression of tumor. However challenges remain as to the further management of patients diagnosed with this condition. More studies are necessary to determine the probability of malignancies arising in association with malakoplakia, in order to devise appropriate treatment protocols.

1. Introduction

A seemingly indolent disorder of immune function, malakoplakia, has been known to occur in various body sites, most commonly involving the urinary tract (in at least 70% of cases), with isolated reports of involvement of the colon, stomach, liver, pancreas, skin, and brain. On several occasions, malakoplakia presents as a "mass lesion" misleading clinicians toward a suspicion of a tumor. Conversely, malakoplakia has been shown to occur in organs otherwise harboring a malignancy (usually a carcinoma). In these instances, the malakoplakia occurs either as a response to the tumor or as an inciting agent. Other notable associations of malakoplakia include immune deficiency disorders, autoimmune conditions, organ transplantation (as a consequence of immunosuppression), and metabolic syndromes. Malakoplakias involving the pancreas are rare and may be diagnosed incidentally during elective cholecystectomy procedures [1]. Malakoplakias are infrequently diagnosed by cytological studies [2]. Diagnosis on cytology is further dependent upon the organ of involvement, which in turn determines the feasibility of performing fine needle aspirations. Reports of simultaneous or sequential organ involvement by malakoplakia are rare. We report a case of simultaneous involvement of the sigmoid colon and pancreas in a 59-year-old male with no known risk of immunodeficiency. Diagnosis of the sigmoid colon malakoplakia was performed on a surgical biopsy/polypectomy while the pancreatic involvement was diagnosed on fine needle aspiration. To our knowledge this is the first reported case of pancreatic malakoplakia to be diagnosed on cytology.

2. Case Presentation

A 59-year-old gentleman presented to our institution with anemia (hemoglobin: 9.4 g/dL) noted during preoperative evaluation for a cataract surgery. He was asymptomatic and had no history of immunodeficiency. His only previous history was a cholecystectomy performed 11 years prior to his current admission. He was noted to have a positive fecal occult blood test prompting colonoscopic evaluation revealing an 8 mm sessile polyp in the sigmoid colon which was resected. A second polyp, 3 mm in size, was identified within the ascending colon. No other large masses or mucosal ulcerations were identified. A few weeks later, the patient

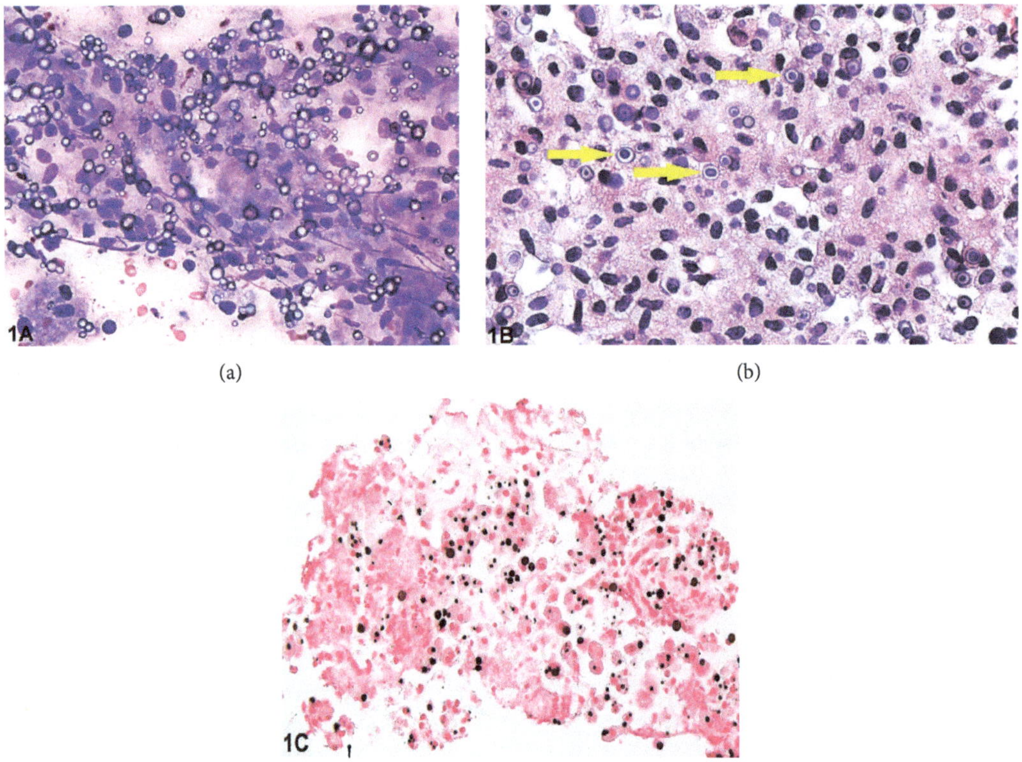

(a) (b) (c)

FIGURE 1: (a) Pancreatic fine needle aspirate showing many histiocytes with admixed lymphocytic tangles. Many refractile bodies with concentric laminations are identified (Diff-Quik, original magnification ×400). (b) Cellblock from pancreatic fine needle aspirate showing a granuloma containing many targetoid Michaelis-Gutmann bodies (arrows) (hematoxylin and eosin, original magnification ×400). (c) Von-Kossa stain highlighting the Michaelis-Gutmann bodies (original magnification ×400).

presented with abdominal pain and nausea, and a Computed Tomography (CT) scan of the abdomen was performed which revealed a vague mass like area within the pancreas. This was followed up with an endoscopic ultrasound which revealed a 33 × 32 mm mass with well-defined borders involving the pancreatic head. No cystic areas were present within the mass. No other abnormalities were detected in the remainder of the pancreas, bile duct, or liver. A fine needle aspiration of the pancreatic mass was performed.

During the next 3-4 weeks, the patient developed gradually worsening abdominal pain, fatigue, and weight loss. A repeat abdominopelvic imaging study revealed ascites and the pancreatic mass which had slightly enlarged. Cultures of the ascitic fluid grew *Escherichia coli* and hence antibiotic therapy was initiated. Impaired glucose tolerance was detected in the ensuing hospital stay. His general condition remained unimproved and he continued to experience reduction in weight and loss of appetite. Having counseled the patient on the possibility of a malignancy occurring in association with malakoplakias and in the absence of any other cause for his cachectic symptoms, the patient elected to undergo a pancreaticoduodenal resection (Whipple procedure). The patient reported improvement in his symptoms following surgery. Three months after surgery, he developed recurrent ascites with no additional imaging abnormalities detected.

3. Pathologic Findings

The fine needle aspirate obtained from the pancreatic head revealed abundant histiocytes and few admixed lymphocytes. Majority of the histiocytes were present in large sheets. On the Diff-Quik stained smears, the histiocytes were found to contain refractile bodies (Figure 1(a)). Occasional granulomas and focal aggregates of neutrophils along with scant necrotic debris were also present. The background contained few ductal and acinar cells. Fibrous stromal tissue was also identified. No dysplastic changes or overt features of malignancy were present. The cellblock revealed many granulomas containing distinctive targetoid bodies (Michaelis-Gutmann bodies) within the histiocytes (Figure 1(b)). A Von-Kossa stain performed on the cellblock material revealed dark-brown to black staining of the Michaelis-Gutmann bodies (Figure 1(c)). No organisms were identified by special stains (acid-fast stain, Grocott's methenamine silver stain). A CD68 immunoperoxidase stain highlighted the histiocytes.

The sigmoid colon polyp showed lymphohistiocytic infiltration of the lamina propria and submucosa (Figure 2(a)). Few scattered Michaelis-Gutmann bodies were identified (Figure 2(b)). Occasional neutrophils and eosinophils were present. The colonic mucosal epithelium was unremarkable. The polyp resected from the ascending colon showed a tubular adenoma.

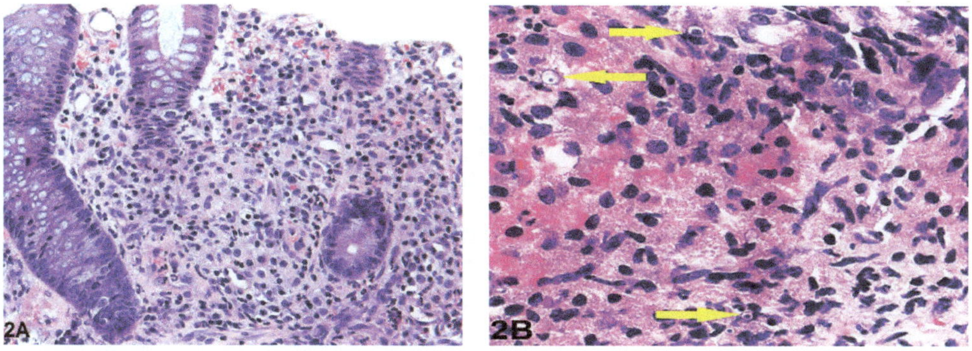

(a) (b)

FIGURE 2: (a) Sigmoid colon biopsy showing lymphohistiocytic infiltration of lamina propria (hematoxylin and eosin stain, original magnification ×200). (b) Higher power view of sigmoid colon biopsy showing Michaelis-Gutmann bodies (arrows) (hematoxylin and eosin, original magnification ×400).

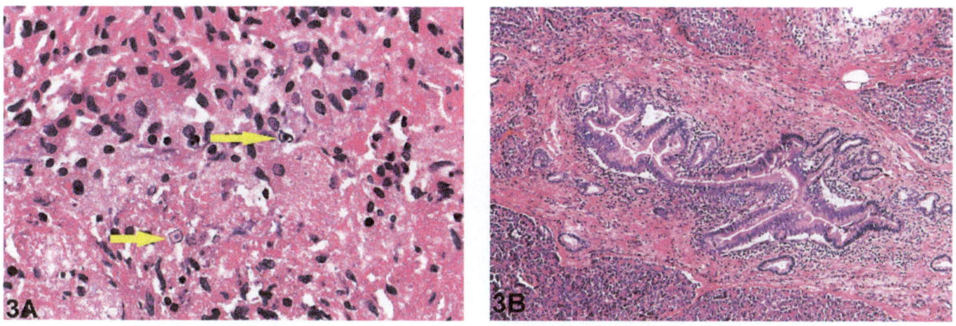

(a) (b)

FIGURE 3: (a) Section from pancreatic resection showing histiocytes with Michaelis-Gutmann bodies (arrows) (hematoxylin and eosin, original magnification ×400). (b) Focus of pancreatic intraepithelial neoplasia, PanIN-2 (hematoxylin and eosin, original magnification ×600).

On gross examination of the Whipple specimen, the pancreatic parenchyma was indurated and mildly congested. No discrete mass was present. No mucosal abnormalities were visible within the distal stomach, duodenum, or the common bile duct. On light microscopy, sections from the pancreatic head revealed established chronic pancreatitis with many areas of lymphocytic inflammation, acinar and ductal atrophy, and fibrosis. Few scattered plasma cells were present. Additional areas of malakoplakia adjacent to atrophied pancreatic acini were identified (Figure 3(a)). Interestingly, focal low-intermediate grade pancreatic intraepithelial neoplasia (PanIN-2) was observed (Figure 3(b)). No evidence of high grade dysplasia or adenocarcinoma was identified in the pancreas or ampullary region after thorough histopathological examination. The duodenal mucosa and bile duct epithelia were unremarkable. The surgical resection margins were benign. Fifteen peripancreatic lymph nodes were examined and were found to be benign.

4. Discussion

In recognition of the original discoverers of this condition, malakoplakia is ubiquitously characterized by the presence of targetoid mineralized bodies known as Michaelis-Gutmann bodies. In fact a diagnosis of malakoplakia may be missed in the setting of a paucity of these characteristic bodies [3]. These represent undigested products from phagocytosed bacteria which, owing to their mineralization by calcium and iron, stain positively with the Von-Kossa and Prussian blue stains. *Escherichia coli* infection has been identified in many cases of malakoplakia involving the urinary tract, although other bacteria, viruses, and even protozoa have been implicated [4]. Malakoplakias are commonly observed to occur in immunocompromised patients. Why the great majority of immune deficient patients do not present with the lesions of malakoplakia remains unclear; specific errors in mechanisms involving the cyclic guanosine monophosphate pathway that regulates lysosomal function appear to play a determining role. Our patient was noted to have frank diabetes soon after his diagnosis of pancreatic malakoplakia. It is uncertain whether the diabetes was the causative factor for, or end result of, the pancreatic malakoplakia. Occasional reports of malakoplakia affecting immunocompetent individuals also exist in the literature. Systemic involvement by malakoplakia has been rarely reported. Our case may be the fourth in a series of case reports detailing systemic involvement by

Table 1: Summary of features of pancreatic malakoplakia in the literature.

Reference article number	Age (in years) and gender of patient	Clinical presentation	Additional findings	Clinical progression
[1]	75, male	Pancreatic mass detected during elective cholecystectomy	No other organ involvement	No complications after excision of pancreatic mass
[3]	49, male	Weight loss and anemia	Retroperitoneal malakoplakia	Bone recurrence of malakoplakia
[5]	6 weeks, male	Immunodeficiency	Adrenal and colonic involvement by malakoplakia	Expired due to military tuberculosis
[6]	74, male	Fever and abdominal pain, pancreatic tail mass	Peripancreatic lymph nodes involved by malakoplakia	Well, 13 months after distal splenopancreatectomy
[7]	45, female	Recurrent abdominal pain	Moderately differentiated pancreatic ductal adenocarcinoma with metastasis	Expired 10 months after Whipple procedure

malakoplakia. Previous reports include a 49-year-old male who presented with retroperitoneal malakoplakia and subsequent bone involvement [3], a 6-week-old male with congenital immunodeficiency who presented with appendiceal and colonic malakoplakia, in addition to pancreatic involvement [5], and a 74-year-old male with pancreatic tail involvement by malakoplakia, along with spread to the peripancreatic lymph nodes [6].

The most common site of involvement of malakoplakia is the urinary tract. Malakoplakias involving the urinary bladder often present as white plaques noted on cystoscopic examination. The second most frequently involved site is the gastrointestinal tract, particularly the colon. Involvement of various other sites continues to be reported in the literature. As mentioned earlier, cases of malakoplakia involving the pancreas are relatively rare. A PubMed search revealed three publications reporting malakoplakia involving the pancreas. Zuk et al. [7] describe two additional cases of pancreatic malakoplakia in their review article. Relevant findings in these case reports are summarized in Table 1. Two patients [6, 7] presented with abdominal pain prompting further evaluation, while, in one patient, it was detected incidentally during elective cholecystectomy [1]. One of the patients described by Colby [3] was diagnosed with malakoplakia (secondary to *Corynebacterium equi* and *Klebsiella*) which presented as a retroperitoneal mass with additional involvement of the pancreatic tail and mesenteric root of the transverse colon. A year after antibiotic therapy he developed recurrent malakoplakia involving the right femur which also grew *Corynebacterium*, raising the possibility of immunodeficiency in the patient. Zuk et al. [7] described a patient with concurrent malakoplakia and moderately differentiated adenocarcinoma of the pancreas with widespread metastasis of the tumor and subsequent demise of the patient. Reports of malakoplakia involving lymph nodes have been described [6, 8] and it appears that diffuse lymph node involvement is usually more commonly seen in immunocompromised patients. The significance of lymph node involvement by malakoplakia is uncertain at present with some reports describing a poor prognostic implication [8], while in others [6] the patients have an uneventful postdiagnosis period.

Malakoplakia is notorious for mimicking a malignant neoplastic process. In fact, in a great majority of cases, the diagnosis first comes to light when a resection has been undertaken for the "malignant neoplasm." Conversely malakoplakias have been reported to occur in association with adenocarcinomas including those of the colon and prostate [9–12]. Malakoplakia can pose significant challenges in staging of tumors as overstaging due to an overestimation of the size of the tumor may occur. Interestingly, malakoplakia is reported to occur at sites of prior radiation treatment which can be falsely Positron Emission Tomography (PET) positive, leading to an impression of tumor metastasis or recurrence [13].

No specific treatment protocols have been established in the management of malakoplakia. Although primarily considered a disorder of immune function, malakoplakia by itself is not particularly debilitating and patients diagnosed with lesions of malakoplakia generally do well. Fluoroquinolones, among other classes of antibiotics, have been utilized in the management of malakoplakia, especially in immunocompromised patients or those with systemic involvement, due to their ability to achieve therapeutic concentrations within histiocytes [14, 15]. Malakoplakia occurring in patients rendered immunocompromised by posttransplant immunosuppressive therapy may experience an improvement in general well-being by a trial of reduction in immunosuppression.

Malakoplakias continue to be reported to occur at unusual sites, such as the spleen, nasal cavity, and oropharynx [16–18]. The exact frequency of the association of malakoplakia with malignancy is not known at present and whether all cases of malakoplakia are to be definitively managed with surgery due to this risk is open for deliberation. Perhaps the greatest significance of this condition lies in the fact that it can be frequently mistaken for malignancy. Hence minimally invasive techniques such as fine needle aspiration or biopsies wherever possible may be undertaken to examine the true nature of these mimickers of malignancy.

Disclosure

Surya Guha is the first author and Haiyan Liu is the coauthor.

Conflict of Interests

The authors declare that there is no conflict of interests regarding the publication of this paper.

References

[1] A. Kulatunga, A. P. Kyllönen, and K. Dammert, "Malakoplakia of the pancreas," *Acta Pathologica, Microbiologica et Immunologica Scandinavica: Section A*, vol. 95, pp. 127–129, 1987.

[2] M. Perez-Guillermo, J. Sola-Perez, and M. Rodriguez-Bermejo, "Malacoplakia and Rosai-Dorfman disease: two entities of histiocytic origin infrequently localized in the female breast—the cytologic aspect in aspirates obtained via fine-needle aspiration cytology," *Diagnostic Cytopathology*, vol. 9, no. 6, pp. 698–704, 1993.

[3] T. V. Colby, "Malakoplakia. Two unusual cases which presented diagnostic problems," *American Journal of Surgical Pathology*, vol. 2, no. 4, pp. 377–382, 1978.

[4] M. Jain, V. K. Arora, N. Singh, and A. Bhatia, "Malakoplakia of the appendix: an unusual association with eggs of Taenia species," *Archives of Pathology and Laboratory Medicine*, vol. 124, no. 12, pp. 1828–1829, 2000.

[5] C. S. Smith, L. B. Kahn, and S. Cywes, "Malakoplakia in childhood: case report with ultrastructural observations and review of literature," *Archives of Pathology & Laboratory Medicine*, vol. 99, no. 4, pp. 198–203, 1975.

[6] P. G. Nuciforo, L. Moneghini, P. Braidotti, L. Castoldi, P. De Rai, and S. Bosari, "Malakoplakia of the pancreas with diffuse lymph-node involvement," *Virchows Archiv*, vol. 442, no. 1, pp. 82–85, 2003.

[7] R. J. Zuk, J. W. Neal, and S. I. Baithun, "Malakoplakia of the pancreas," *Virchows Archiv A*, vol. 417, no. 2, pp. 181–184, 1990.

[8] P. A. Dervan, M. Teeling, J. Dempsey, I. M. Drury, E. O'Malley, and D. O'Connell, "Lymphadenopathy due to fatal histiocytic proliferative disorder containing Michaelis-Gutmann bodies," *Cancer*, vol. 57, no. 7, pp. 1337–1340, 1986.

[9] F. Karasavvidou, S. P. Potamianos, S. Barbanis et al., "Malakoplakia of the colon associated with colonic adenocarcinoma diagnosed in colonic biopsies," *World Journal of Gastroenterology*, vol. 13, no. 45, pp. 6109–6111, 2007.

[10] B. Asiyanbola, P. Camuto, and V. Mansourian, "Malakoplakia occurring in association with colon carcinoma," *Journal of Gastrointestinal Surgery*, vol. 10, no. 5, pp. 657–661, 2006.

[11] D. L. Répássy, A. Iványi, S. Csata, and G. Tamas, "Combined occurrence of prostate carcinoma and malacoplakia," *Pathology & Oncology Research*, vol. 8, no. 3, pp. 202–203, 2002.

[12] K. Pillay and R. Chetty, "Malakoplakia in association with colorectal carcinoma: a series of four cases," *Pathology*, vol. 34, no. 4, pp. 332–335, 2002.

[13] R. L. Kradin, T. A. Sheldon, P. Nielsen et al., "Malacoplakia of the tongue complicating the site of irradiation for squamous cell carcinoma with review of the literature," *Annals of Diagnostic Pathology*, vol. 16, no. 3, pp. 214–218, 2012.

[14] G. R. Dohle, J. Zwartendijk, and J. H. J. M. van Krieken, "Urogenital malacoplakia treated with fluoroquinolones," *Journal of Urology*, vol. 150, no. 5, part 1, pp. 1518–1520, 1993.

[15] R. van Furth, J. W. van't Wout, P. A. Wertheimer, and J. Zwartendijk, "Ciprofloxacin for treatment of malakoplakia," *The Lancet*, vol. 339, no. 8786, pp. 148–149, 1992.

[16] A. A. Mannan, M. C. Sharma, and S. Bahadur, "Malacoplakia of the vallecula masquerading as a malignancy," *Ear, Nose, & Throat Journal*, vol. 90, no. 3, pp. E17–E19, 2011.

[17] G. Akkuzu, E. Aydin, B. Bilezikçi, B. Akkuzu, and L. N. Ozluoglu, "Malakoplakia in nasal vestibule," *Otolaryngology—Head and Neck Surgery*, vol. 135, no. 4, pp. 636–637, 2006.

[18] W. O. Greaves and L. J. Wang, "Malakoplakia of the spleen: a case report," *International Journal of Surgical Pathology*, vol. 18, no. 6, pp. 584–587, 2010.

22

Hepatocellular Carcinoma with Both Fibrolamellar and Classical Components: An Unusual Morphological Pattern

Diana Castro-Villabón,[1] Luis E. Barrera-Herrera,[1] Paula A. Rodríguez-Urrego,[1,2] Rachel Hudacko,[3] Alonso Vera,[4] Johanna Álvarez,[1,2] Rafael Andrade,[1,2,5] and Rocío López[1,2]

[1]*Department of Pathology and Laboratories, Hospital Universitario Fundación Santa Fe de Bogotá, Calle 119 No. 7–75, Bogotá 110111, Colombia*
[2]*School of Medicine, University of Los Andes, Carrera 1 No. 18A-12, Bogotá 111711, Colombia*
[3]*Department of Pathology, Good Samaritan Regional Medical Center, 255 Lafayette Avenue, Suffern, NY 10901, USA*
[4]*Transplant and Hepatobiliary Surgical Service, Hospital Universitario Fundación Santa Fe de Bogotá, Calle 119 No. 7–75, Bogotá 110111, Colombia*
[5]*School of Medicine, National University of Colombia, Carrera 45 No. 26-85, Bogotá 111711, Colombia*

Correspondence should be addressed to Rocío López; rolopez@uniandes.edu.co

Academic Editor: Hiroko Kuwabara

Fibrolamellar carcinoma (FLC) is an uncommon form of primary liver malignancy with unique clinical, histological, and biological characteristics. It is usually seen in young adults without underlying liver disease. Histologically, it shows large cells with abundant eosinophilic cytoplasm, large vesicular nuclei, prominent nucleoli, and lamellar type fibrosis. In contrast, classical hepatocellular carcinoma (HCC) is typically present in elderly male patients with cirrhosis. It is the most common histological subtype, and it is characterized by its resemblance to the normal liver, both in its growth pattern and its cytology. The unusual case of a liver carcinoma that presented with histological features of both FLC and classical HCC is herein reported. This was the case of a 37-year-old female complaining of diffuse abdominal discomfort and epigastric pain for two months. She was referred to us for further management after she was diagnosed with HCC in a noncirrhotic liver. She underwent a left-sided hepatectomy. A yellow nodular mass with well-defined borders and a necrotic center was present in the resection specimen. The morphological features and immunohistochemical studies were consistent with a diagnosis of FLC mixed with classical HCC. The patient was followed up for five months, and no signs of recurrence were evident.

1. Introduction

Fibrolamellar carcinoma (FLC) is a rare variant of primary liver malignancy with unique clinical, histological, and biological characteristics. It was first reported as a separate entity by Hugh Edmondson in 1956, who described the typical gross and microscopic features of this neoplasm as "a liver cell carcinoma in which stroma is profuse and the similarity of the cancer cells to normal cells is striking" [1]. Since then, it has been further studied, and its diagnostic criteria have been clearly established, the tumor express characteristics of conventional hepatocellular carcinoma (HCC) including cytokeratin 7 a cholangiocellular marker; however studies suggest that no consistent mutation is known in FLC so far [2].

FLC accounts for up to 8% of all HCC, occurs predominantly in younger individuals, has no gender predilection, and develops in the absence of underlying liver disease [3–5]. It is considered to have a better prognosis, due to the fact that it is typically present in noncirrhotic patients with no other comorbid conditions [5]. In contrast to this distinct form of liver cancer, classical HCC represents the most common histologic subtype, occurring mainly in older men with underlying cirrhosis.

To our knowledge, only three cases of a liver carcinoma with elements of both classical HCC and FLC intimately mixed within one mass have been reported [6, 7]. Two other cases describe synchronous tumors [5, 8, 9]. Both the molecular background and the pathogenesis of FLC are obscure and limited, possibly owing to the relatively low number of cases studied by individual groups [10]. Herein, we present a new case of a mixed FLC and classical HCC.

2. Case Report

A 37-year-old female presented to our clinic with a two-month history of diffuse abdominal discomfort and epigastric pain. The abdominal ultrasound showed a 9.6 cm oval-shaped, well-demarcated, thin-walled, heterogeneous mass located in the left lateral segment of the liver (segments II and III). CT and MRI scans revealed a well-defined, encapsulated, nonenhancing mass with a central scar, surrounded by normal liver parenchyma. The radiologic diagnosis suggested a FLC in a noncirrhotic liver. Laboratory tests showed abnormally elevated transaminases. Serum tumor markers, including a-fetoprotein (AFP) and carcinoembryonic antigen (CEA), were within normal limits. Viral hepatitis and autoimmune markers were negative. A biopsy was performed at an outside institution before referral, and a diagnosis of classical HCC with a trabecular pattern in a noncirrhotic liver was rendered. The patient's past medical history was unremarkable, and she had no risk factors for chronic liver disease. Physical examination revealed a painful mass that comprised the upper abdomen.

The patient underwent an uneventful open left-lateral hepatectomy (Figure 1) and was discharged home two days after. Five months after surgery, the patient is alive with no clinical or radiological signs of recurrence.

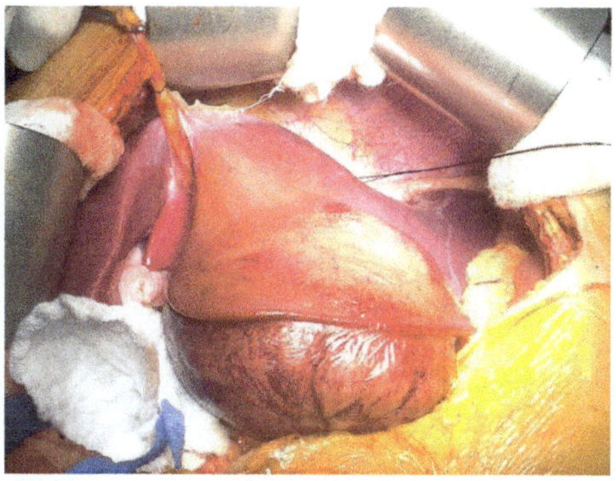

FIGURE 1: Surgical site showing tumor located in the left-lateral hepatic lobe next to grossly normal liver parechyma.

3. Materials and Methods

Macroscopic examination of the resected specimen revealed a multinodular, well-circumscribed, and partially encapsulated mass that measured 13 cm in greatest dimension. Cut surface showed a variegated appearance with some yellow discoloration and central necrosis. The surrounding liver parenchyma had a normal appearance and no evidence of fibrosis or nodularity was seen. The mass was located 3 cm from the surgical margin, and no other lesions were noted.

4. Microscopic Examination

Microscopically, the tumor had two different cell populations, one of which showed large, polygonal cells with eosinophilic cytoplasm, large nuclei, prominent nucleoli, and rare mitoses. In addition, there were scattered cytoplasmic inclusions with a ground-glass appearance, known as pale bodies. The tumor cells were surrounded by a fibrolamellar type stroma. These findings were consistent with FLC.

Adjacent to these areas, a second group of cells with marked cytologic atypia, nuclear pleomorphism, hyperchromatic nuclei, intracytoplasmic Mallory's hyaline and eosinophilic globules, and zones of necrosis was observed. Morphologically, these areas were consistent with classical HCC with a trabecular pattern. Vascular invasion and tumor thrombi were also present. The background liver showed no evidence of cirrhosis (Figure 2).

Immunohistochemical studies showed both components to be reactive for hepatocyte (Hepar-1) and to focally express AFP. Endothelial wrapping was highlighted with CD34, and a canalicular staining pattern was observed with polyclonal CEA. Both groups of neoplastic cells were positive for CK7 and negative for CK19. A diagnosis of a hepatocellular carcinoma with both FLC and classical HCC features was rendered.

5. Discussion

We present a case of a liver tumor with unusual morphology and features of both classical HCC and FLC in a patient with no predisposing factors. FLC is a malignant hepatocellular tumor with distinct clinical and pathologic characteristics that differ from classical HCC, predominantly in FLC there is no consistent mutation, and shows fewer chromosomal abnormalities compared with HCC [2].

To our knowledge, there are only five cases reporting the presence of classical HCC coexistent with FLC in the literature (Table 1). Two cases described two synchronous tumors of the liver. In the first case, one mass was located in the caudate lobe with FLC elements, and the other with classical HCC features located in the lateral segment [8]. The second case had two contiguous masses in the right lobe that were separated by a rim of fibrous tissue that surrounded the classical HCC component, which was the largest tumor. The smaller mass represented the FLC [9]. As in our case, there are only three previous reports that describe a single hepatic mass composed of the two mixed histologic subtypes [5–7].

FLCs have a predilection for the left lobe of the liver, and grossly, they tend to be yellow to pale tan and firm [3, 11, 12]. The average size ranges from 9 to 14 cm in greatest dimension, and a central scar may be found in up to 75% of cases [3]. Occasionally, these tumors can contain small foci of necrosis, hemorrhage, and calcifications [3, 13].

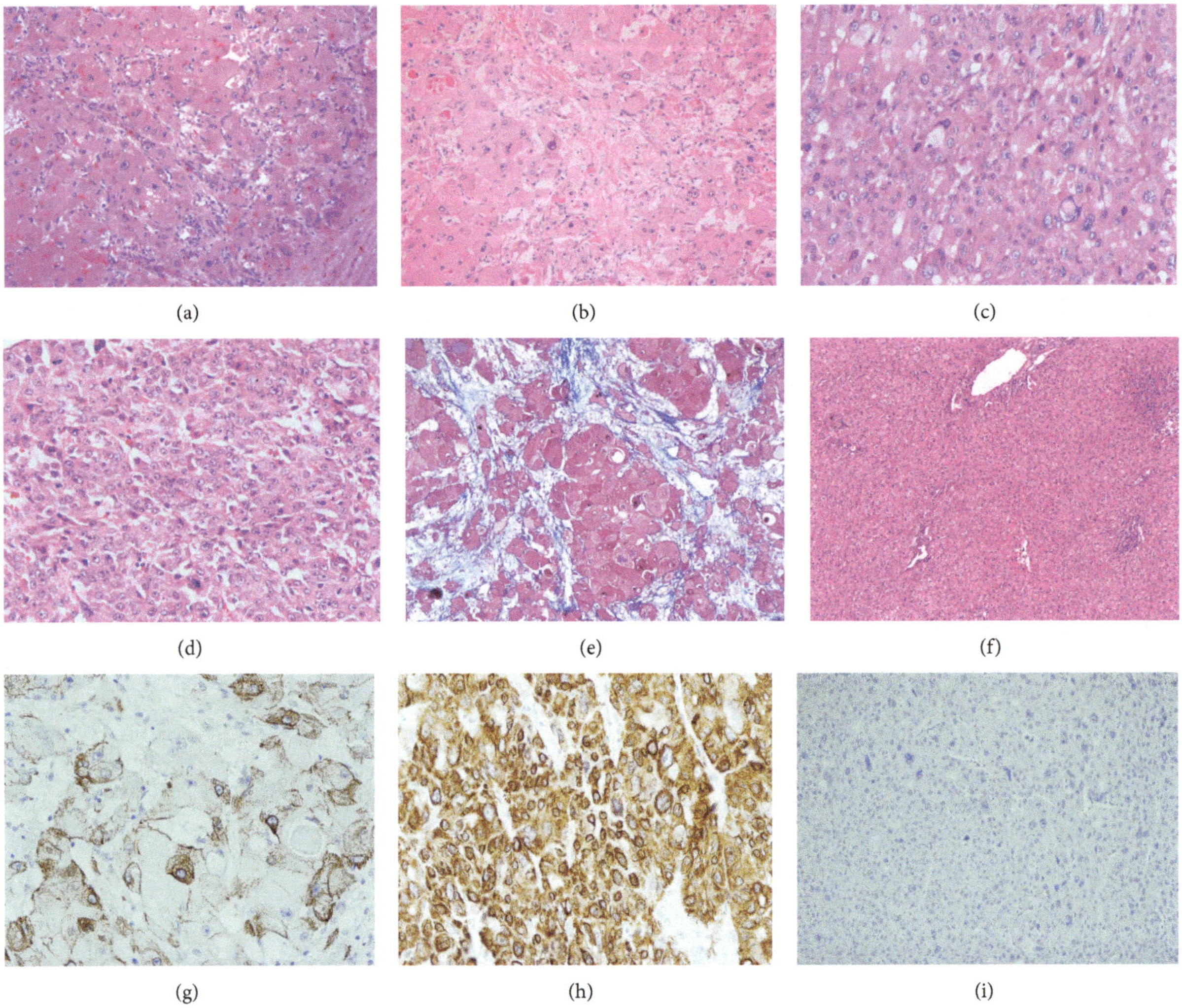

FIGURE 2: (a) (H and E stain, 200x) Mixed tumor composed of two different components, one with large, polygonal cells with eosinophilic cytoplasm, consistent with FLC (top left). Adjacent to it without transition (bottom right), the second component shows a neoplastic proliferation of hepatocytes with high N : C ratio and a trabecular pattern compatible with classical HCC. (b) (H and E stain, 200x) typical abundant lamellar connective tissue characterizing FLC. (c) (H and E stain, 400x) High power view of FLC component showing large neoplastic cells with abundant eosinophilic cytoplasm and pale bodies. (d) (H and E stain, 200x) Photograph of classical HCC showing nests of neoplastic hepatocytes with abnormal architecture showing thick liver plates and endothelial wraping. (e) (Masson's trichrome stain, 200x) Lamellar connective tissue in the FLC component. (f) (H and E stain, 100x) Low power view of adjacent liver parenchyma withouth fibrosis and few foci of nonspecific lymphocytic parenchymal inflammation with retained architecture. (g) (CK7-200x) Immunohistochemistry for CK7 showing positivity in FLC and (h) (CK7-400X) in the HCC. (i) (CK19-400X) Negative in HCC.

Microscopically, the defining features of FLCs are large polygonal cells with abundant eosinophilic (oncocytic) cytoplasm, large vesicular nuclei, large nucleoli, and lamellar type fibrosis [3, 11, 12]. Calcifications and round cytoplasmic inclusions (pale bodies) are seen in up to 50% of the cases [11]. Characteristically FLCs are strongly positive for CK7, and a recent study found that positivity for CD68 is highly sensitive [3, 14].

On the other hand, classical HCC is usually nodular with or without a fibrous capsule, and it is softer than the normal surrounding liver. It varies in color and can be yellow, green, brown, or heterogeneous [11].

Histologically, the main hallmark of classical HCC is its similarity to the normal liver both in its plate-like growth and its cytology [13]. It is characterized by plates of hepatocytes with eosinophilic or clear cytoplasm that are separated by sinusoid-like spaces lined by a single layer of endothelial cells that wrap around the plates of hepatocytes [11]. Architecturally, the cells are often arranged in trabecular, acinar/pseudoglandular, or solid/compact patterns [12]. Malignant hepatocytes are often pleomorphic, and cytoplasmic accumulations are commonly present, including Mallory's hyaline, bile, steatosis, iron, copper, and eosinophilic globules containing proteins such as a-1-antitrypsin [12].

Immunohistochemically, classical HCC is characterized by cytoplasmic positivity for Hepar-1 (approximately 90% of the cases), patchy AFP, fibrinogen, and cytokeratins 8 and 18. Polyclonal CEA and CD10 show canalicular patterns

TABLE 1: Summary of clinical findings of reported cases of coexistent FLC and classical HCC.

Author	Age (years)	Sex	Clinical presentation	Tumor size and lobe	Liver enzymes	AFP	CEA	HBV antigen titers	Non-neoplastic liver	Other findings	Type of tumor
Okada et al. [8]	56	M	Referral	1.9 cm left and 1.8 cm caudate	Elevated	Elevated	WNL	Negative	Cirrhosis	Leukopenia	Synchronous FLC and HCC
Singh and Ramakrishna [9]	14	M	Abdominal pain	10 cm right and 8 cm right	Elevated	WNL	WNL	Negative	None present	None	Synchronous FLC and HCC
Seitz et al. [5]	27	F	Epigastric pain	16 cm right	Elevated	WNL	NA	Negative	None present	None	Mixed FLC and HCC
Reuland et al. [6]	39	F	Incidental finding	NA	WNL	WNL	WNL	NA	None present	Leukocytosis and elevated ESR	Mixed FLC and HCC
Okano et al. [7]	52	M	Incidental finding	3.5 cm left	WNL	Elevated	WNL	Negative	None present	None	Mixed FLC and HCC
Castro-Villabón et al. (present case)	37	F	Abdominal distension and epigastric mass	13 cm left	Elevated	WNL	WNL	Negative	None present	None	Mixed FLC and HCC

AFP: a-fetoprotein; CEA: carcinoembryonic antigen; HBV: hepatitis B virus; ESR: erythrocyte sedimentation rate; WNL: within normal limits; NA: not available.

of positivity. Special stain for reticulin shows patchy or diffuse loss of the reticulin network [11]. CD34 highlights the endothelial wrapping. Immunostains for Glypican 3, heat shock protein, and glutamine synthetase are also positive in HCC. Usually, classical HCC is negative for CK7 (≥70% of cases).

In the present case, the patient had no evidence of underlying liver disease, she had no risk factors for HCC, AFP levels were within normal limits, HBV titers were negative, and imaging showed a mass in the left lobe of the liver, all of which are characteristic clinical features of FLC. In contrast, she presented with vague, nonspecific abdominal signs and symptoms, and with mild elevation of the liver function tests, which may be seen in both types of tumors. The age at presentation of the disease (37 years old) is not usual for either classical HCC or FLC.

Microscopically, the tumor showed distinct areas in which the morphological elements of classical HCC and FLC were mixed. However, the immunoreactivity for CK7, which was expected to be expressed solely by the FLC component, was positive in both groups of neoplastic cells. It should be noted that some (≤30%) classical HCCs may be reactive for CK7, in particular those in children and young adults [3, 15]. In this sense, the DNAJB1-PRKACA chimeric transcript that is missed in the domain that binds the regulatory subunits of PKA, may represent a diagnostic marker in FLC, nonetheless further research has to be done to define it as a therapeutic target [15].

Currently there are no molecular diagnostic tests for FLC; previous studies detected cAMP-dependent protein kinase A (PKA) in peripheral blood as a universal serum biomarker for cancers of various cell types [16]. The *DNAJB1-PRKACA* chimeric transcript that is missed in the domain that binds the regulatory subunits of PKA and may represent a diagnostic marker in FLC; nonetheless further research has to be done to define it as a therapeutic target [17].

We did not find any risk factors or environmental exposure in the patient's history that could explain the etiology of this neoplasm. As a matter of fact the surrounding liver parenchyma was normal and did not have any signs of cirrhosis or underlying liver disease.

In summary, we hope that our report will increase awareness of this combined entity in the liver and that further experience contributes in the establishment of prompt and accurate diagnoses involving not only proteins expression through immunohistochemistry but also genetic studies in future cases.

Conflict of Interests

The authors declare that there is no conflict of interests regarding the publication of this paper.

References

[1] H. A. Edmondson, "Differential diagnosis of tumors and tumor-like lesions of liver in infancy and childhood," *A.M.A. Journal of Diseases of Children*, vol. 91, no. 2, pp. 168–186, 1956.

[2] A. Patonai, B. Erdélyi-Belle, A. Korompay et al., "Molecular characteristics of fibrolamellar hepatocellular carcinoma," *Pathology & Oncology Research*, vol. 19, no. 1, pp. 63–70, 2013.

[3] M. Torbenson, "Fibrolamellar carcinoma: 2012 update," *Scientifica*, vol. 2012, Article ID 743790, 15 pages, 2012.

[4] J. R. Craig, R. L. Peters, H. A. Edmondson, and M. Omata, "Fibrolamellar carcinoma of the liver: a tumor of adolescents and young adults with distinctive clinico-pathologic features," *Cancer*, vol. 46, no. 2, pp. 372–379, 1980.

[5] G. Seitz, A. Zimmermann, H. Friess, and M. W. Bchler, "Adult-type hepatocellular carcinoma in the center of a fibrolamellar hepatocellular carcinoma," *Human Pathology*, vol. 33, no. 7, pp. 765–769, 2002.

[6] P. Reuland, K. P. Aicher, H.-J. Brambs et al., "Incidental finding of a hepatic lesion: differential diagnostic problems for fibrolamellar hepatic carcinoma," *Journal of Nuclear Medicine*, vol. 35, no. 8, pp. 1342–1346, 1994.

[7] A. Okano, K. Hajiro, H. Takakuwa, and Y. Kobashi, "Fibrolamellar carcinoma of the liver with a mixture of ordinary hepatocellular carcinoma: a case report," *The American Journal of Gastroenterology*, vol. 93, no. 7, pp. 1144–1145, 1998.

[8] K. Okada, Y. I. Kim, K. Nakashima et al., "Fibrolamellar hepatocellular carcinoma coexistent with a hepatocellular carcinoma of common type: report of a case," *Surgery Today*, vol. 23, no. 7, pp. 626–631, 1993.

[9] P. Singh and B. Ramakrishna, "Combined hepatocellular carcinoma and fibrolamellar carcinoma presenting as two adjacent separate lesions in a young boy: first case report from Asia," *Case Reports in Hepatology*, vol. 2013, Article ID 101862, 4 pages, 2013.

[10] A. Patonai, B. Erdélyi-Belle, A. Korompay et al., "Claudins and tricellulin in fibrolamellar hepatocellular carcinoma," *Virchows Archiv*, vol. 458, no. 6, pp. 679–688, 2011.

[11] N. D. Theise, "BFT. Pathology and Genetics of Tumours of the Digestive System," http://www.iarc.fr/en/publications/pdfs-online/pat-gen/bb2/.

[12] K. A. Mitchell, "Hepatocellular carcinoma: histologic considerations: pure, mixed, and motley," *Journal of Clinical Gastroenterology*, vol. 47, supplement, pp. S20–S26, 2013.

[13] V. Paradis, "Histopathology of hepatocellular carcinoma," in *Multidisciplinary Treatment of Hepatocellular Carcinoma*, vol. 190 of *Recent Results in Cancer Research*, pp. 21–32, Springer, Berlin, Germany, 2013.

[14] H. M. Ross, H. D. J. Daniel, P. Vivekanandan et al., "Fibrolamellar carcinomas are positive for CD68," *Modern Pathology*, vol. 24, no. 3, pp. 390–395, 2011.

[15] A. Durnez, C. Verslype, F. Nevens et al., "The clinicopathological and prognostic relevance of cytokeratin 7 and 19 expression in hepatocellular carcinoma. A possible progenitor cell origin," *Histopathology*, vol. 49, no. 2, pp. 138–151, 2006.

[16] J. N. Honeyman, E. P. Simon, N. Robine et al., "Detection of a recurrent *DNAJB1-PRKACA* chimeric transcript in fibrolamellar hepatocellular carcinoma," *Science*, vol. 343, no. 6174, pp. 1010–1014, 2014.

[17] M. V. Nesterova, N. Johnson, C. Cheadle et al., "Autoantibody cancer biomarker: extracellular protein kinase A," *Cancer Research*, vol. 66, no. 18, pp. 8971–8974, 2006.

23

Metachronous Bilateral Testicular Leydig-Like Tumors Leading to the Diagnosis of Congenital Adrenal Hyperplasia (Adrenogenital Syndrome)

Josip Vukina,[1] David D. Chism,[2,3] Julie L. Sharpless,[3,4] Mathew C. Raynor,[1] Matthew I. Milowsky,[2,3] and William K. Funkhouser[3,5]

[1]*Department of Urology, University of North Carolina, Chapel Hill, NC 27599, USA*
[2]*Division of Hematology and Oncology, Department of Medicine, University of North Carolina, Chapel Hill, NC 27599, USA*
[3]*Lineberger Comprehensive Cancer Center, Chapel Hill, NC 27599, USA*
[4]*Division of Endocrinology and Metabolism, Department of Medicine, University of North Carolina, Chapel Hill, NC 27599, USA*
[5]*Department of Pathology and Laboratory Medicine, University of North Carolina, Chapel Hill, NC 27599, USA*

Correspondence should be addressed to William K. Funkhouser; william.funkhouser@unchealth.unc.edu

Academic Editor: Zsuzsa Schaff

A 33-year-old male with a history of left testis Leydig cell tumor (LCT), 3-month status after left radical orchiectomy, presented with a rapidly enlarging (0.6 cm to 3.7 cm) right testicular mass. He underwent a right radical orchiectomy, sections interpreted as showing a similar Leydig cell-like oncocytic proliferation, with a differential diagnosis including metachronous bilateral LCT and metachronous bilateral testicular tumors associated with congenital adrenal hyperplasia (a.k.a. "testicular adrenal rest tumors" (TARTs) and "testicular tumors of the adrenogenital syndrome" (TTAGS)). Additional workup demonstrated a markedly elevated serum adrenocorticotropic hormone (ACTH) and elevated adrenal precursor steroid levels. He was diagnosed with congenital adrenal hyperplasia, 3β-hydroxysteroid dehydrogenase deficiency (3BHSD) type, and started on treatment. Metachronous bilateral testicular masses in adults should prompt consideration of adult presentation of CAH. Since all untreated CAH patients are expected to have elevated serum ACTH, formal exclusion of CAH prior to surgical resection of a testicular Leydig-like proliferation could be accomplished by screening for elevated serum ACTH.

1. Background

Testicular tumors in children and adults may be due to neoplasms or reactive hyperplasias. This paper considers the differential diagnosis of metachronous bilateral Leydig-like testicular tumors in an adult.

Primary testicular neoplasms are diverse, broadly categorized into germ cell tumors (seminoma, yolk sac tumor, embryonal carcinoma, choriocarcinoma, and teratoma) and sex cord/stromal tumors (Leydig cell tumors (LCT), Sertoli cell tumor, granulosa cell tumor, fibroma/thecoma, and undifferentiated tumors) [1]. Sex cord/stromal tumors are less common than germ cell tumors in children and adults [2]. LCTs represent 1–3% of all primary testicular tumors [3, 4] and up to 8% of pediatric primary testicular tumors [5]. LCTs in children and adults present as unilateral, unifocal testicular parenchymal masses in over 95% of cases [3]. Most are discrete solid tumors that displace adjacent parenchyma [3]. Microscopically, LCTs usually grow as sheets or septated lobules of minimally pleomorphic low N : C ratio cells with eosinophilic cytoplasm, cytologically bland nuclei, and prominent nucleoli [3–5]. Zona fasciculata-type vacuolated cells can be admixed or can predominate [3]. Spindle cell cytology, adipose metaplasia, and osseous metaplasia have been described [6]. Current immunohistochemical summary data predict that 85–95% of LCTs will show immunoreactivity for inhibin, Mart-1, and calretinin [7]. Two small series have

Table 1: Overlapping clinical presentations, morphologies, immunophenotypes, and associated endocrinopathies for LCTs and TARTs.

	Laterality	Gross appearance	Architecture	Cytology	Expected % cases with IHC reactivity	Expected serum ACTH	Expected serum testosterone
LCT	Unilateral	Intratesticular (parenchyma), solitary	Sheet-like or lobulated with fine fibrous bands	Leydig ± z. fascic. Reinke crystals in 30–40%	I 96% M 86% C 93% S < 10%	Normal	Increased
TART	Unilateral or Bilateral	Intratesticular (hilum), multifocal	Nodules with coarse fibrous bands	Leydig-like ± z. fascic. Reinke crystals absent	I (+) M (+) C (+) S > 88%	Increased	Increased/normal/low

z. fascic. = similar to adrenal zona fasciculata.
IHC = immunohistochemistry; I = inhibin; M = Mart-1; C = calretinin; S = synaptophysin.

shown that <10% of LCTs will show strong immunoreactivity for synaptophysin [8, 9].

Congenital adrenal hyperplasia (CAH) is a set of autosomal recessive genetic disorders characterized by loss-of-function defects in enzymes involved in the production of cortisol, aldosterone, and sex hormones [10, 11]. Roughly 90% of CAH cases are associated with loss-of-function mutations or translocations involving the *CYP21* gene that encodes the 21α-hydroxylase enzyme, and 5–8% are associated with loss-of-function mutations in the *CYP11B1* gene that encodes the 11β-hydroxylase enzyme [10, 12]. Less common yet are loss-of-function mutations in the *CYP17A1* gene that encodes the 17α-hydroxylase enzyme and loss-of-function mutations in the *HSD3β2* gene that encodes the 3β-hydroxysteroid dehydrogenase enzyme. Loss of function of these enzymes leads to decreased production of cortisol and other steroid hormones. Cortisol deficiency leads to increased hypothalamic secretion of corticotropin-releasing hormone (CRH) and increased anterior pituitary secretion of adrenocorticotropic hormone (ACTH).

Increased serum ACTH in undertreated CAH causes hyperplasia of normal adrenal cortex bilaterally [10], hyperplasia of ectopic adrenal rests [13], and hyperplasia of "steroid" cells occurring normally in the testicular hilum [4, 14]. ACTH-driven hyperplasia of the testicular hilar "steroid" cells usually presents as nodules of cytologically bland oncocytic cells similar to normal Leydig cells [4, 15] although subsets of cells with clear, vacuolated cytoplasm similar to z. fasciculata may be seen [15]. Like LCTs, these hyperplastic steroid cell nodules are expected to show immunoreactivity for inhibin, Mart-1, and calretinin; unlike LCTs, they are also expected to show immunoreactivity for synaptophysin [8, 9].

Testicular hilar steroid cell hyperplastic nodules occur in up to 94% of CAH patients [15, 16]. Treatment guidelines now recommend screening testicular ultrasounds because the growth of these tumors can lead to testicular failure that is reversible with medical treatment [17]. Traditionally, these testicular steroid cell hyperplastic nodules have been detected as synchronous bilateral testicular hilar tumors [15, 16]. However, current ultrasonographic screening approaches frequently detect these nodules as unilateral testicular tumors in preteens that can develop into metachronous bilateral disease over time [18].

Different terms have been used to describe these testicular steroid cell hyperplasias, including "testicular tumors of the adrenogenital syndrome (TTAGS)" [4, 5], "testicular adrenogenital tumors" [19], "testicular tumors in congenital adrenal hyperplasia" [19], "testicular adrenal rest tumors (TART)" [10], "bilateral nodular hyperplasia of testicular adrenal rests" [10], and "adrenogenital syndrome-associated tumors" [20]. There is a distinction made in the urologic pathology literature between adrenal rests and the testicular hilar steroid cell hyperplasias [4]. Because these testicular hilar steroid cell hyperplasias respond to ACTH similarly to adrenal cortex and extratesticular adrenal rests and because the term is commonly used in the endocrinology, radiology, and urology literatures, we elect to refer to these tumors hereafter as "testicular adrenal rest tumors (TARTs)."

Comparison and contrast of the clinical, gross, micro, IHC, and endocrine features of LCTs and TARTs are summarized in Table 1. LCTs and TARTs are expected to share a similar Leydig-like cytology and to share a core immunophenotype of immunoreactivity for inhibin, Mart-1, and calretinin. In contrast, LCTs and TARTs frequently differ in terms of tumor uni/bilaterality at presentation, tumor uni/multifocality, tumor location in the testis, Reinke crystal prevalence, lipofuscin prevalence, serum ACTH, serum testosterone, tumor responsiveness to ACTH, and synaptophysin immunoreactivity.

Because TARTs frequently mimic Leydig cells cytologically, a large unifocal unilateral TART that displaces testicular parenchyma could easily be confused with an LCT in an adult in whom CAH is unrecognized. This diagnostic puzzle is less likely in a child, because precocious puberty would usually prompt an endocrine workup that would distinguish LCT from TART. This paper describes a case in which an adult presented with metachronous bilateral Leydig cell-like testicular tumors, prompting a workup for congenital adrenal hyperplasia (CAH), and was ultimately found to have CAH due to 3β-hydroxysteroid dehydrogenase deficiency.

2. Case Presentation

A 33-year-old male presented with a 2-month history of left testicular pain and swelling. He reported a history of hypospadias repair and bilateral cryptorchidism status after orchiopexy as a child. A scrotal ultrasound (US) revealed a heterogeneous 2.5 cm left testis mass and an incidental markedly heterogeneous 0.6 cm right testis nodule. A computed tomography scan of the chest and abdomen revealed no significant lymphadenopathy. He underwent left radical orchiectomy at an outside hospital, demonstrating a unifocal 3.5 × 3.0 × 2.2 cm LCT, without extratesticular invasion or vascular invasion. Nuclear atypia was seen, but no mitotic activity, coagulative tumor cell necrosis, vascular invasion, or Reinke crystals were noted. The Leydig-like proliferation was interpreted as a Leydig cell tumor, likely benign, staged as pT1.

Two weeks after orchiectomy, he was referred to this institution for evaluation of a right testicular mass. He reported an unintentional 11-pound weight loss, night sweats, decreased libido, and erectile dysfunction. A repeat ultrasound of the right testis approximately 3.5 months after initial ultrasound revealed an increase in the size of the right testis nodule from 0.6 cm to 3.7 cm. No palpable mass was appreciated on initial or follow-up physical exams. The working clinical diagnosis at this juncture was a metachronous primary testicular malignancy. A metastatic workup was negative, and he underwent a right radical inguinal orchiectomy. Gross examination of the right testicular mass revealed a testicular hilar mass. Tissue sections showed nodules of oncocytic cells with low N : C ratios, prominent nucleoli, and focal lipofuscin, without Reinke crystals and without mitotic activity or coagulative necrosis (Figure 1). Immunostains showed reactivity for inhibin and synaptophysin. The pathologic diagnosis was "oncocytic proliferation, Leydig cell tumor versus testicular tumor of the adrenogenital syndrome," that is, metachronous bilateral LCT versus TARTs.

He was referred to endocrinology for concern for congenital adrenal hyperplasia, and additional history revealed facial hair as an adolescent, an early growth spurt, frequent asthma flairs that responded to steroid dosing, and salt craving without a history of hypertension. In retrospect, he suffered nausea and vomiting after both surgical procedures. The first episode was associated with fever and resolved after administration of antibiotics. The episode after the second surgery resolved after changing to a different pain medication. He also reported a grandfather with a similar early puberty. After his first orchiectomy, he attempted sperm banking but was azoospermic. More directed physical exam revealed tan skin (although he was of Hispanic descent), pale striae on the abdomen, mild acanthosis nigricans of the neck, and multiple hyperpigmented chicken pox scars. Further testing demonstrated normal sodium levels, although there were no postoperative measurements, cortisol of 0.3 mcg/dL (normal range 4.5–22.7 mcg/dL), ACTH of 3050 pg/mL (normal range 10–60 pg/mL), and DHEA-S of 145 mcg/dL (normal range 65–334 mcg/dL). He had an elevated 17-OH pregnenolone to 17-OH progesterone ratio, consistent with 3β-hydroxysteroid dehydrogenase deficiency (3BHSD). He also had elevated renin activity supporting the salt-wasting variant of 3BHSD. His spontaneous puberty and late presentation point to a mild 3BHSD deficiency. He was referred to genetic testing but unfortunately was lost to follow-up. The findings of metachronous bilateral Leydig-like tumors associated with depressed cortisol and elevated serum ACTH are most consistent with bilateral TARTs in a patient with unrecognized CAH.

3. Discussion

The first TART case was reported in 1940 in a 3-year-old boy with marked salt cravings, an enlarged penis and scrotum, and pubic hair who died in the hospital just days after admission [21]. Laboratory testing revealed serum sodium of 111 mEq/L. Autopsy revealed hyperplasia of the androgenic cells of the adrenal cortex and bilateral masses in the testicles consisting of aberrant adrenal tissue.

TART prevalence as high as 94% is reported in patients with CAH [16, 22–24] and TART is reported to be the most important cause of male infertility in CAH patients [25]. Although the condition is benign, it can lead to infertility via two separate mechanisms. The first mechanism is physical compression and obstruction of the seminiferous tubules by the hyperplastic nodules [26, 27]. The second mechanism is impaired secretion of gonadotropins due to overproduction of adrenal androgens, leading to hypogonadotropic hypogonadism [16].

Accurate distinction between TART and LCT in adults without known CAH can be problematic. This is particularly true if the TART is unilateral or bilateral with a metachronous presentation (as in the current case). Even with foreknowledge of CAH in a patient with bilateral testicular masses, morphologic features may not allow distinction between TART and LCT [28]. However, clinical distinction between these diseases is of paramount importance, because the treatment differs (cortisol and/or mineralocorticoid replacement therapy for CAH, versus partial or complete orchiectomy for LCT). The two challenging clinical scenarios are (1) milder forms of CAH in adults, in which the testicular lesion may be the first presentation of CAH, and (2) optimally treated CAH, in which the tumors do not regress, thereby elevating LCT in the differential diagnosis [28, 29].

Clinical and radiographic features can be used to distinguish TART from LCT. TART presentation varies with age. In boys, the lesions are often unilateral [22] and the incidence of bilaterality increases with age [30]. In contrast, LCTs are usually unilateral, independent of age. Therefore, bilaterality strongly favors TARTs over LCTs. Radiographically, TARTs are primary in the testicular hilum, never primary in the parenchyma. In contrast, LCTs are primary in the testicular parenchyma, never primary in the hilum. Scrotal imaging via US or MRI can demonstrate the hilar/paratesticular TART nodules in CAH patients [18]. Computer tomography done for LCT staging in patients with untreated CAH may show bilateral diffuse enlargement of the adrenal glands, but a mass-like appearance can also occur [31] and an enhancement pattern has not been well established [32].

Endocrine features can be used to distinguish TART from LCT. TARTs represent reactive hyperplasias that develop in response to supraphysiologic ACTH, whereas LCTs are not ACTH-responsive and are not associated with supraphysiologic ACTH. Thus, preoperative serum ACTH can be used to screen for background CAH in patients with uni- or bilateral testicular tumors. Both LCTs and TARTs can be

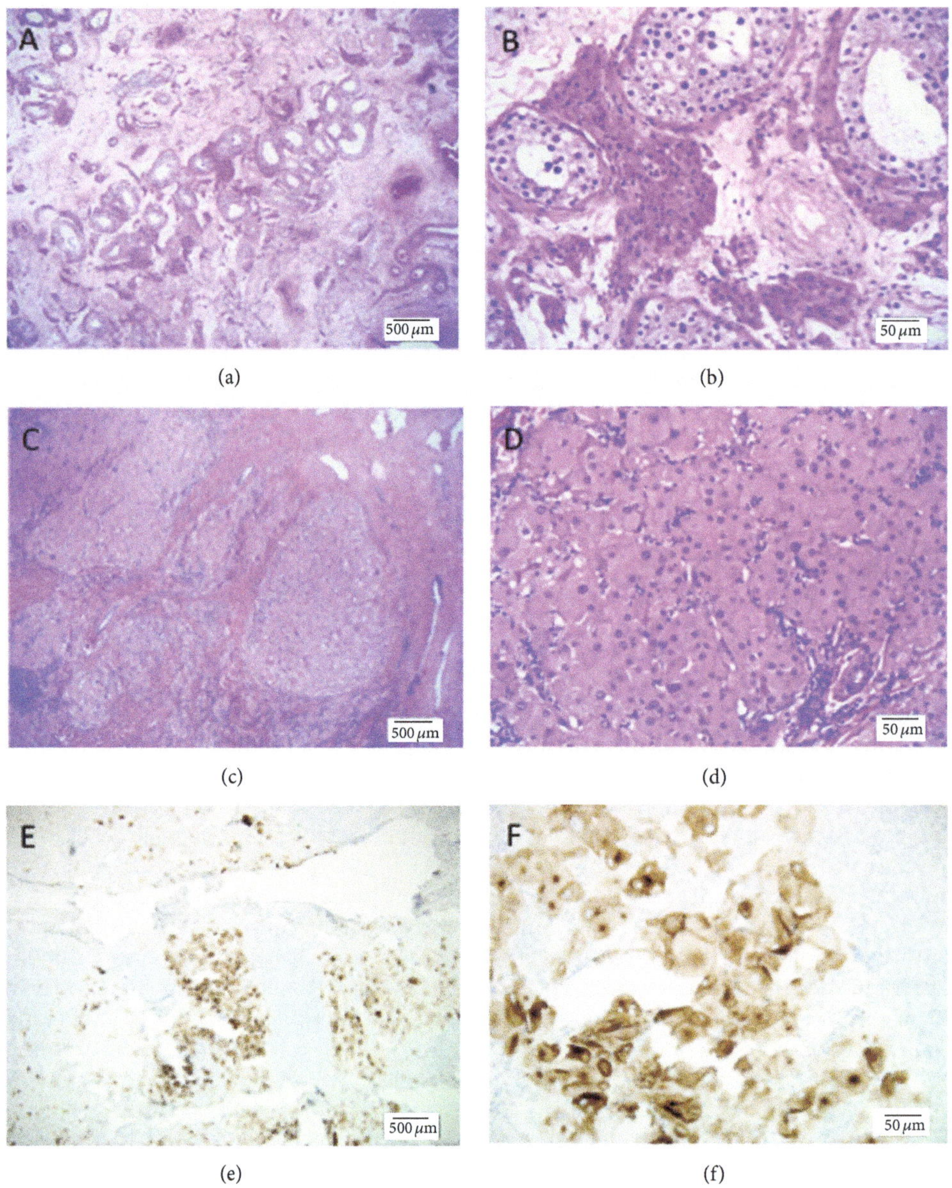

FIGURE 1: Morphology and IHC of the right testicular hilar tumor. (a) Uninvolved testis, H&E, 40x. (b) Uninvolved testis, H&E, 200x. (c) Testicular hilar tumor, H&E, 40x. (d) Testicular hilar tumor, H&E, 200x. (e) Testicular hilar tumor, synaptophysin, 40x. (f) Testicular hilar tumor, synaptophysin, 200x.

associated with alteration in serum testosterone. Most CAH is due to 21-hydroxylase deficiency, leading to high testosterone levels secreted by both the adrenals and the testes, until the TARTs get so big as to cause peritubular fibrosis leading to low testosterone. Thus, the serum testosterone in CAH is a function of the extent of testicular TART expansion [33, 34]. However, in our patient's rare form of CAH, 3BHSD type, his enzyme deficiency would limit production of testosterone. He had mildly elevated precursor steroids and slightly low testosterone level with elevated gonadotropins and azoospermia. This combination suggests two contributions to his gonadal dysfunction: first, partial enzyme deficiency as supported by his mild childhood course and late presentation and, secondly, testicular failure likely due to the TART. The elevated gonadotropins could also have further stimulated growth of the TART or differentiation toward LCT [35].

Gross and microscopic pathologic features can be used to distinguish TART from LCT. Bilaterality, multinodularity, dark brown color, hilar/paratesticular location, coarse fibrous stroma, and/or strong synaptophysin immunoreactivity favor TART over LCT [1, 8, 9]. Unifocality, yellow color, parenchymal location, scant/no fibrous stroma, and Reinke crystal formation favor LCT over TART. Leydig-like cytology, zona fasciculata-like cytology, adipose metaplasia, cytologic atypia, mitotic activity, lipofuscin pigment, and immunoreactivity for inhibin/Mart-1/calretinin are probably nonspecific findings [3, 4, 6, 8, 15]. Morphologic and immunophenotypic features of these Leydig-like proliferations overlap sufficiently that clinical and endocrinologic data become extremely valuable in achieving accurate pathologic diagnosis.

This patient's mild clinical symptoms of CAH likely contributed to the lack of clinical detection or treatment of his CAH, prolonging his exposure to high ACTH and further stimulating the ACTH-responsive steroid cells in the hilum of the residual testis. It has long been considered that growth of these lesions is due to chronic elevations of ACTH. TARTs have been shown to have ACTH receptors and to secrete steroids when stimulated with ACTH in vivo [36]. It can be speculated that the patient suffered worsening of his unrecognized adrenal insufficiency after his first surgery, which would have further raised his ACTH levels to the remarkably high levels documented when the diagnosis was finally considered. The rise in ACTH then stimulated growth of the second tumor after the first surgery. Workup leading to a CAH diagnosis will likely benefit this patient by assuring corticosteroid replacement during future stressful events such as surgical procedures. Interestingly, he was able to tolerate both anesthetics and procedures without issue, likely owing to their short duration and minimal morbidity. The postoperative nausea and vomiting could have been attributed to adrenal insufficiency; however other causes were plausible at the time.

4. Conclusions

We present a rare case in which pathology from a second orchiectomy led to a diagnosis of CAH due to (rare) 3β-HSD deficiency. This case highlights the challenges that urologists, radiologists, pathologists, and endocrinologists face when dealing with Leydig-like tumors in adults. We recommend a detailed history and physical examination as the first step in the evaluation of all patients with testicular masses, in addition to serum tumor markers and imaging. In this patient, the evolution of bilateral testicular masses over a short time interval could have prompted a more thorough discussion of past medical and family history, which would have revealed bilateral cryptorchidism, hypospadias, and a grandfather with early puberty. Taken together, this piece of information could have led to additional endocrine evaluation prior to surgical intervention. Because unilateral LCT and unilateral TART will share similar Leydig-like morphology and because both can involve the hilum and parenchyma, we recommend checking ACTH levels in all patients with a diagnosis of LCT with hilar involvement, as this may prompt formal preoperative workup for CAH.

Conflict of Interests

The authors declare that there is no conflict of interests regarding the publication of this paper.

References

[1] J. Eble, G. Sauter, J. Epstein et al., *World Health Organization Classification of Tumours. Pathology and Genetics of Tumours of the Urinary System and Male Genital Organs*, IARC Press, Paris, France, 2004.

[2] A. Wein, L. R. Kavoussi, A. C. Novick et al., "Neoplasm of the testis," in *Campbell-Walsh Urology*, chapter 31, 10th edition, 2010.

[3] I. Kim, R. H. Young, and R. E. Scully, "Leydig cell tumors of the testis. A clinicopathological analysis of 40 cases and review of the literature," *The American Journal of Surgical Pathology*, vol. 9, no. 3, pp. 177–192, 1985.

[4] T. M. Ulbright and R. H. Young, *Tumors of the Testis and Adjacent Structures*, AFIP Atlas of Tumor Pathology Series 4, Fascicle, American Registry of Pathology, 18th edition, 2013.

[5] H. Al-Ahmadie, "Testicular tumors," in *Pediatric Pathology*, Wolters Kluwer, Alphen aan den Rijn, The Netherlands, 2011.

[6] T. M. Ulbright, J. R. Srigley, D. K. Hatzianastassiou, and R. H. Young, "Leydig cell tumors of the testis with unusual features: adipose differentiation, calcification with ossification, and spindle-shaped tumor cells," *The American Journal of Surgical Pathology*, vol. 26, no. 11, pp. 1424–1433, 2002.

[7] Immunoquery, March 2015, http://www.immunoquery.com.

[8] R. A. Ashley, S. M. McGee, P. A. Isotaolo, S. A. Kramer, and J. C. Cheville, "Clinical and pathological features associated with the testicular tumor of the adrenogenital syndrome," *Journal of Urology*, vol. 177, no. 2, pp. 546–549, 2007.

[9] Z. Wang, S. Yang, H. Shi et al., "Histopathological and immunophenotypic features of testicular tumour of the adrenogenital syndrome," *Histopathology*, vol. 58, no. 7, pp. 1013–1018, 2011.

[10] R. Conran, E. Chung, L. Dehner et al., *Stocker and Dehner's Pediatric Pathology*, Edited by J. Stocker and L. Dehmer, Lipincott, 3rd edition, 2011.

[11] M. Wajnrajch and M. New, "Defects of adrenal steroidogenesis," in *Endocrinology*, J. Jameson and L. De Groot, Eds., Saunders, 6th edition, 1897–1920.

[12] P. C. White and P. W. Speiser, "Congenital adrenal hyperplasia due to 21-hydroxylase deficiency," *Endocrine Reviews*, vol. 21, no. 3, pp. 245–291, 2000.

[13] R. T. Kirkland, J. L. Kirkland, B. S. Keenan et al., "Bilateral testicular tumors in congenital adrenal hyperplasia," *Journal of Clinical Endocrinology and Metabolism*, vol. 44, no. 2, pp. 369–378, 1977.

[14] E. V. Dahl and R. C. Bahn, "Aberrant adrenal contical tissue near the testis in human infants," *The American Journal of Pathology*, vol. 40, pp. 587–598, 1962.

[15] J. L. Rutgers, R. H. Young, and R. E. Scully, "The testicular 'tumor' of the adrenogenital syndrome: a report of six cases and review of the literature on testicular masses in patients with adrenocortical disorders," *The American Journal of Surgical Pathology*, vol. 12, no. 7, pp. 503–513, 1988.

[16] N. M. M. L. Stikkelbroeck, B. J. Otten, A. Pasic et al., "High prevalence of testicular adrenal rest tumors, impaired spermatogenesis, and leydig cell failure in adolescent and adult males with congenital adrenal hyperplasia," *Journal of Clinical Endocrinology & Metabolism*, vol. 86, no. 12, pp. 5721–5728, 2001.

[17] P. W. Speiser, R. Azziz, L. S. Baskin et al., "Congenital adrenal hyperplasia due to steroid 21-hydroxylase deficiency: an endocrine society clinical practice guideline," *Journal of Clinical Endocrinology and Metabolism*, vol. 95, no. 9, pp. 4133–4160, 2010.

[18] N. M. M. L. Stikkelbroeck, H. M. Suliman, B. J. Otten, A. R. M. M. Hermus, J. G. Blickman, and G. J. Jager, "Testicular adrenal rest tumours in postpubertal males with congenital adrenal hyperplasia: sonographic and MR features," *European Radiology*, vol. 13, no. 7, pp. 1597–1603, 2003.

[19] E. Lack and E. Paal, "Neoplasm of the testis," in *Urologic Surgical Pathology*, D. G. Bostwick and L. Cheng, Eds., Elsevier Health Sciences, 3rd edition, 2014.

[20] N. Sabine, M. Malone, M. Ashworth et al., *Diagnostic Pediatric Surgical Pathology*, Elsevier, 2010.

[21] L. Wilkins, W. Fleischmann, and J. E. Howard, "Macrogenitosomia precox associated with hyperplasia of the androgenic tissue of the adrenal and death from corticoadrenal insufficiency. case report," *Endocrinology*, vol. 26, no. 3, pp. 385–395, 1940.

[22] H. L. Claahsen-van der Grinten, F. C. G. J. Sweep, J. G. Blickman, A. R. M. M. Hermus, and B. J. Otten, "Prevalence of testicular adrenal rest tumours in male children with congenital adrenal hyperplasia due to 21-hydroxylase deficiency," *European Journal of Endocrinology*, vol. 157, no. 3, pp. 339–344, 2007.

[23] A. Vanzulli, A. DelMaschio, P. Paesano et al., "Testicular masses in association with adrenogenital syndrome: US findings," *Radiology*, vol. 183, no. 2, pp. 425–429, 1992.

[24] M. D. Urban, P. A. Lee, and C. J. Migeon, "Adult height and fertility in men with congenital virilizing adrenal hyperplasia," *The New England Journal of Medicine*, vol. 299, no. 25, pp. 1392–1396, 1978.

[25] H. L. Claahsen-van der Grinten, B. J. Otten, A. R. M. M. Hermus, F. C. G. J. Sweep, and C. A. Hulsbergen-van de Kaa, "Testicular adrenal rest tumors in patients with congenital adrenal hyperplasia can cause severe testicular damage," *Fertility and Sterility*, vol. 89, no. 3, pp. 597–601, 2008.

[26] M. A. Rich and M. A. Keating, "Leydig cell tumors and tumors associated with congenital adrenal hyperplasia," *Urologic Clinics of North America*, vol. 27, no. 3, pp. 519–528, 2000.

[27] J. L. Knudsen, A. Savage, and G. E. Mobb, "The testicular 'tumour' of adrenogenital syndrome—a persistent diagnostic pitfall," *Histopathology*, vol. 19, no. 5, pp. 468–470, 1991.

[28] H. Ali, H. Arabi, and A. Samkari, "Testicular adrenal rest 'tumor' or Leydig cell tumor? A report of a challenging case with literature review," *Avicenna Journal of Medicine*, vol. 3, no. 1, p. 15, 2013.

[29] R. E. Emerson and T. M. Ulbright, "Morphological approach to tumours of the testis and paratestis," *Journal of Clinical Pathology*, vol. 60, no. 8, pp. 866–880, 2007.

[30] G. P. Finkielstain, M. S. Kim, N. Sinaii et al., "Clinical characteristics of a cohort of 244 patients with congenital adrenal hyperplasia," *Journal of Clinical Endocrinology and Metabolism*, vol. 97, no. 12, pp. 4429–4438, 2012.

[31] C. V. Harinarayana, G. Renu, A. C. Ammini et al., "Computed tomography in untreated congenital adrenal hyperplasia," *Pediatric Radiology*, vol. 21, no. 2, pp. 103–105, 1991.

[32] T. D. Barwick, A. Malhotra, J. A. W. Webb, M. O. Savage, and R. H. Reznek, "Embryology of the adrenal glands and its relevance to diagnostic imaging," *Clinical Radiology*, vol. 60, no. 9, pp. 953–959, 2005.

[33] H. L. C.-V. der Grinten, F. Dehzad, K. K.-V. Ulzen, and C. L. De Korte, "Increased prevalence of testicular adrenal rest tumours during adolescence in congenital adrenal hyperplasia," *Hormone Research in Paediatrics*, vol. 82, no. 4, pp. 238–244, 2014.

[34] N. Reisch, L. Flade, M. Scherr et al., "High prevalence of reduced fecundity in men with congenital adrenal hyperplasia," *Journal of Clinical Endocrinology and Metabolism*, vol. 94, no. 5, pp. 1665–1670, 2009.

[35] S. Benvenga, G. Smedile, F. Lo Giudice, and F. Trimarchi, "Testicular adrenal rests: Evidence for luteinizing hormone receptors and for distinct types of testicular nodules differing for their autonomization," *European Journal of Endocrinology*, vol. 141, no. 3, pp. 231–237, 1999.

[36] H. L. Claahsen-van der Grinten, B. J. Otten, F. C. G. J. Sweep et al., "Testicular tumors in patients with congenital adrenal hyperplasia due to 21-hydroxylase deficiency show functional features of adrenocortical tissue," *Journal of Clinical Endocrinology & Metabolism*, vol. 92, no. 9, pp. 3674–3680, 2007.

Anal Papilloma: An Exceptional Presentation of Fibrocystic Disease in Anogenital Mammary-Like Glands

Priya Subashchandrabose,[1] Muthuvel Esakkai,[1] Palani Venugopal,[2] Ilavarasan Kannaiyan,[2] Chitra Srinivasan,[1] Punuru Tejashwini Reddy,[1] and Evelyn Elizabeth Ebenezer[1]

[1]*Department of Pathology, Saveetha Medical College, Chennai 602105, India*
[2]*Department of Surgery, Saveetha Medical College, Chennai 602105, India*

Correspondence should be addressed to Priya Subashchandrabose; drspriya78@gmail.com

Academic Editor: Alp Usubutun

Previously ectopic breast tissue was thought to be derived from the caudal remnants of the primitive embryonic milk ridges; anogenital mammary-like glands are presently considered as normal constituents of the anogenital region. We report a case of young female, who presented with an anal papilloma. Histopathological examination revealed extensive fibrocystic changes in anogenital mammary-like glands. To date, a lot of benign changes and a wide range of benign and malignant neoplasms have been reported in these glands. However, extensive fibrocystic change of these glands in anal region is very rare. In addition, fibrocystic disease of anal mammary glands, masquerading clinically as an anal papilloma, has not been reported in literature. Hence, it is essential for clinicians and the pathologists to be aware of such a rare presentation. The features of fibrocystic disease in perianal region are also discussed.

1. Introduction

In anogenital region, mammary type glands constitute a normal component and are referred to as anogenital mammary-like glands (AGMLG) [1, 2]. These glands share several features in common with normal breast tissue like expression of estrogen and progesterone receptors [3]. Nonneoplastic lesions, benign, and malignant neoplasm arising in AGMLG are also similar to those arising in the breast. We report a case of young female, who presented with an anal papilloma on clinical examination, and the final histopathological evaluation revealed extensive fibrocystic changes (FCC) in the AGMLG.

2. Case Report

A 26-year-old female presented to the surgical outpatient department of our hospital with complaints of swelling in the anal region of one-year duration. Anal examination revealed a firm mobile mass at 3 o'clock position. Perrectal examination was normal and the clinical diagnosis was that of an anal papilloma. Excision biopsy of the papilloma was performed and the specimen was received in our pathology department in 10% neutral buffered formalin. Gross examination revealed a skin covered polypoidal mass measuring 3.5 × 2.5 cm. External surface was smooth (Figure 1(a)). Cut surface was gray white, firm, and lobulated with a focal tiny cyst measuring 0.5 cm in greatest dimension (Figure 1(b)). Routine histopathological examination of hematoxylin and eosin stained slides revealed skin with unremarkable epidermis and subepithelial tissue showing mammary-like glands composed of terminal duct lobular units (Figure 2(a)). The ducts were lined by bilayered epithelium, inner cuboidal epithelium, and outer myoepithelial cells (Figure 2(b)) with many of them exhibiting features of fibrocystic disease like adenosis (Figure 2(c)), cystic change (Figure 2(d)), apocrine metaplasia showing abundant eosinophilic cytoplasm with apical snouts (Figure 2(d), inset), and fibrosis in stroma.

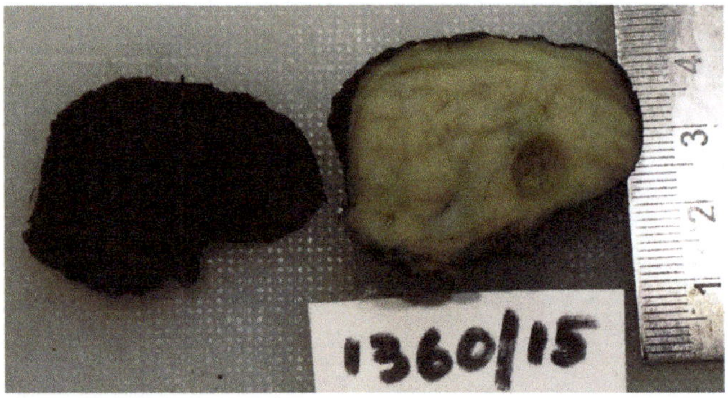

(a) (b)

Figure 1: Gross appearance. (a) Smooth external surface of the polyp. (b) Cut surface is gray white, firm, and lobulated with cystic spaces.

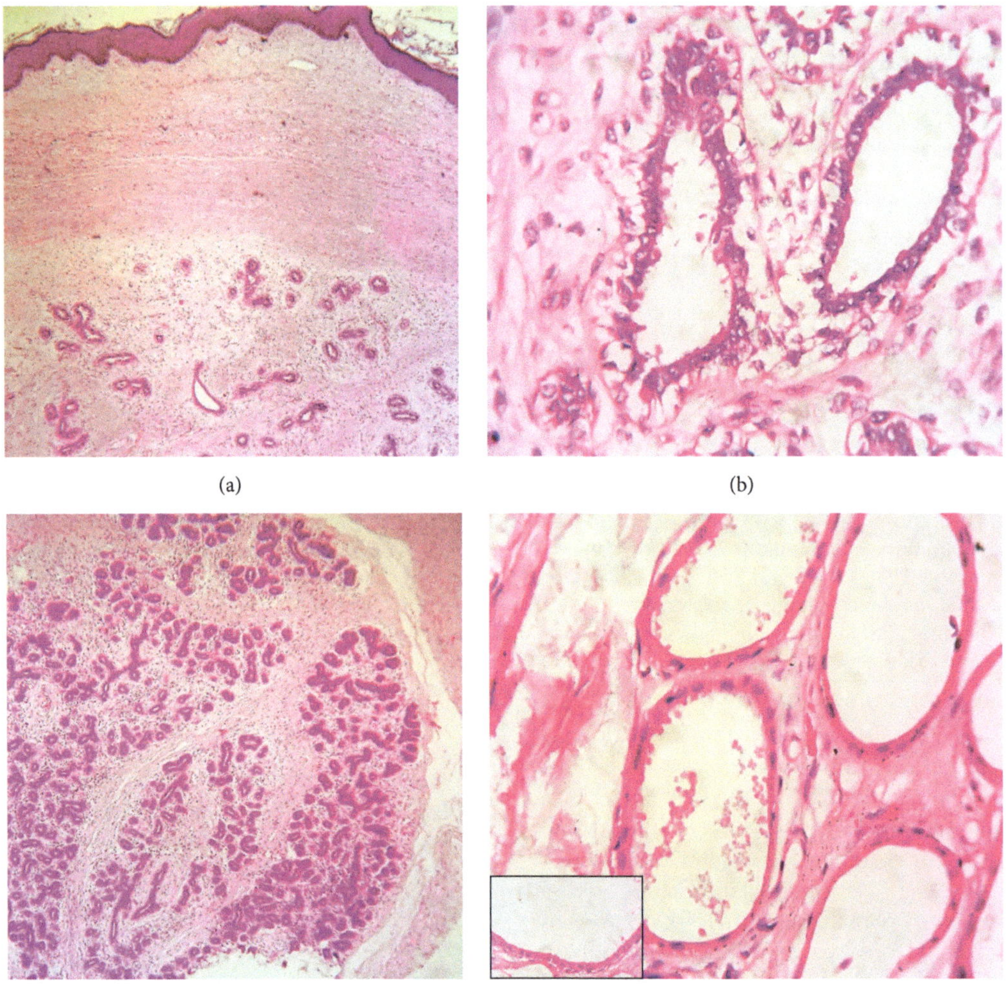

(a) (b) (c) (d)

Figure 2: Microscopic appearance. (a) Anal skin with subepithelial tissue showing terminal duct lobular units. H&E 40x. (b) Ducts lined by bilayered epithelium. H&E 100x. (c) Areas of adenosis. H&E 40x. (d) Areas of cystic change. H&E 100x. (Inset, apocrine change with apical snouts, H&E 400x).

3. Discussion

Ectopic breast tissue (EBT) may be present at any site along the primitive embryonic milk lines, extending from the axillary to the inguinal region [4]. Mammary type glands were reported in vulva by Hartung in 1872; these were for long considered as EBT representing the caudal remnants of the milk ridge [2]. But EBT can also be seen in anogenital regions or other unusual sites such as eyelid, nasal area, prostate gland, and gallbladder [5], which cannot be explained by the primitive milk line theory. Van der Putte proposed that, in the anogenital region, these mammary-like glands constitute a normal component [1, 2] and these glands are, at present, referred to as anogenital mammary-like glands (AGMLG).

The histology of these glands ranges from complex branching lobular units like those of normal breast to simple glandular structures surrounded by a loosely or densely fibrotic stroma [1]. Excretory system in these glands is also varied and the ducts have a luminal columnar cell lining exhibiting apocrine secretion and basal myoepithelial cell lining. Just before entering the epidermis, the ductal lining becomes stratified squamous epithelium and the myoepithelial cell layer is lost. Occasionally, small clear cells called Toker cells are present singly or in small nests surrounding the openings of these glands. These glands have mixed apocrine, eccrine, and mammary gland histology [2].

Nonneoplastic and neoplastic lesions occurring in AGMLG are similar to those arising in the breast [6]. A wide range of neoplasms can arise in these AGMLG including adenoma of lactating type, hidradenoma and syringocystadenoma papilliferum, fibroadenoma, phyllodes tumor, pseudoangiomatous stromal hyperplasia, extramammary Paget's disease, and other malignancies similar to those which arise in the breast [7]. These glands can also show nonspecific epithelial and stromal changes; a few of these are similar to the changes in the benign mammary diseases including lactation-like changes, columnar cell hyperplasia, columnar cell change, features like that of sclerosing adenosis, usual duct hyperplasia, atypical duct epithelial hyperplasia, flat epithelial atypia, satellitosis, fibrocystic change, epithelial-myoepithelial hyperplasia, lamprocyte-like changes, various metaplastic changes affecting epithelium like apocrine, oxyphilic, clear cell or squamous metaplasia, and stromal elastosis. Many of these changes do not have a clinical importance and however may lead to potential diagnostic pitfalls and hence clinicians and pathologists should be aware of such possibilities [7].

Fibrocystic change in the breast also referred to by many terms such as fibrocystic disease (FCD), fibrous or fibrocystic mastopathy, fibroadenosis cystic, and mammary dysplasia is a benign alteration in mammary tissue consisting of cystic change of the terminal duct lobular unit, with or without associated stromal fibrosis [8]. FCC is usually considered as an exaggerated physiologic response rather than a disease [9]. Microscopic features of FCC include cystically dilated round to oval spaces lined by a single or double layer of epithelial cells and attenuated myoepithelial cells: apocrine metaplasia in which the lining cells exhibit columnar morphology with abundant eosinophilic granular cytoplasm, uniform round to oval nuclei, and luminal cytoplasmic projections referred to as apical snouts: intralobular stroma showing prominent fibrosis and sclerotic changes: rupture of the cysts accompanied by secondary inflammatory reaction: microcalcifications which can be seen within the cyst lumen or in the surrounding connective tissue stroma; a mild degree of adenosis or microscopic expansion of the lobules by an increase in the number of acinar structures in the lobule that can be present [10, 11].

Anogenital mammary-like glands can undergo changes analogous to that of FCD of the breast including cystic change, periductal fibrosis, and apocrine metaplasia. FCD in AGMLG can have a wide range of microscopic features depending upon the predominant element of the disease [9]. However, the crucial histopathological alterations include cystic change, fibrosis, apocrine metaplasia, calcification, epithelial hyperplasia, and chronic inflammatory infiltrates. Similar to that of the mammary tissue, FCD-like changes can be seen focally in other lesions arising in the anogenital mammary-like glands [9].

4. Conclusion

To conclude, we report a case of fibrocystic change in anogenital mammary-like glands presenting as an anal papilloma. These clinically innocuous changes may however lead to potential diagnostic pitfalls and hence clinicians and pathologists should be aware of such possibilities.

Consent

The patient described in the case report has given her informed consent for the case report to be published.

Conflict of Interests

The authors declare that there is no conflict of interests regarding the publication of this paper.

References

[1] S. C. J. Van der Putte, "Anogenital 'sweat' glands: histology and pathology of a gland that may mimic mammary glands," *The American Journal of Dermatopathology*, vol. 13, no. 6, pp. 557–567, 1991.

[2] S. C. J. Van der Putte, "Mammary-like glands of the vulva and their disorders," *International Journal of Gynecological Pathology*, vol. 13, no. 2, pp. 150–160, 1994.

[3] S. Ahmed, R. M. Campbell, J. H. Li, L. J. Wang, and L. Robinson-Bostom, "Adenoma of anogenital mammary-like glands," *Journal of the American Academy of Dermatology*, vol. 57, no. 5, pp. 896–898, 2007.

[4] H. Ciralik, E. Bulbuloglu, O. Arican, and R. Citil, "Fibroadenoma of the ectopic breast of the axilla—a case report," *Polish Journal of Pathology*, vol. 57, no. 4, pp. 209–211, 2006.

[5] G. J. Solomon, S. J. Shin, and L. J. Romanzi, "A 65-year-old woman with a 'hemorrhoid'. Fibroadenoma of the anogenital region," *Archives of Pathology & Laboratory Medicine*, vol. 130, no. 2, pp. e30–e32, 2006.

[6] D. V. Kazakov, D. V. Spagnolo, C. J. Stewart et al., "Fibroadenoma and phyllodes tumors of anogenital mammary-like glands: a series of 13 neoplasms in 12 cases, including mammary-type juvenile fibroadenoma, fibroadenoma with lactation changes, and neurofibromatosis-associated pseudoangiomatous stromal hyperplasia with multinucleated giant cells," *The American Journal of Surgical Pathology*, vol. 34, no. 1, pp. 95–103, 2010.

[7] D. V. Kazakov, D. V. Spagnolo, D. Kacerovska, and M. Michal, "Lesions of anogenital mammary-like glands: an update," *Advances in Anatomic Pathology*, vol. 18, no. 1, pp. 1–28, 2011.

[8] J. V. Fiorica, "Fibrocystic changes," *Obstetrics and Gynecology Clinics of North America*, vol. 21, no. 3, pp. 445–452, 1994.

[9] S. M. Love, R. S. Gelman, and W. Silen, "Fibrocystic 'disease' of the breast—a nondisease?" *The New England Journal of Medicine*, vol. 307, no. 16, pp. 1010–1014, 1982.

[10] S. A. Bartow, W. C. Black, R. W. Waeckerlin, and F. A. Mettler, "Fibrocystic disease: a continuing enigma," *Pathology Annual*, vol. 17, pp. 93–111, 1982.

[11] H. Vorherr, "Fibrocystic breast disease: pathophysiology, pathomorphology, clinical picture, and management," *American Journal of Obstetrics & Gynecology*, vol. 154, no. 1, pp. 161–179, 1986.

Cytological Features of Mammary Analogue Secretory Carcinoma of the Parotid Gland in a 15-Year-Old Girl: A Case Report with Review of the Literature

Takako Inaba,[1] Yuki Fukumura,[2] Tsuyoshi Saito,[2] Junkichi Yokoyama,[3] Shinichi Ohba,[3] Atsushi Arakawa,[2] and Takashi Yao[2]

[1]*Division of Diagnostic Pathology, Juntendo University, 3-1-3 Hongo, Bunkyo-ku, Tokyo 113-0033, Japan*
[2]*Department of Human Pathology, Juntendo University School of Medicine, 1-1-19 Motomachi Bldg. 3F, Hongo, Bunkyo-ku, Tokyo 113-0033, Japan*
[3]*Department of Otorhinolaryngology, Juntendo University School of Medicine, 3-1-3 Hongo, Bunkyo-ku, Tokyo 113-0033, Japan*

Correspondence should be addressed to Yuki Fukumura; yfuku@juntendo.ac.jp

Academic Editor: Tibor Tot

Mammary analogue secretory carcinoma (MASC) is a recently recognized tumor of salivary glands characterized by the ETV6-NTRK3 fusion gene. This tumor is very rare in children and adolescents. We report a case of MASC in a 15-year-old girl, the fifth youngest case so far reported. The patient complained of a left infra-auricular mass that gradually enlarged for a year. Fine-needle aspiration cytology/imprint cytology showed individual tumor cells that had faintly eosinophilic granular cytoplasm with secretion granules sometimes seen adjacent to the tumor cells. These cytological features overlapped between those of zymogen granule-poor acinic cell carcinoma (AciCC) and MASC. In addition to the case report, we present a review of the related literature with a focus on the cytological features of MASC. The differential diagnostic clues are also discussed.

1. Introduction

Malignant tumors of the salivary gland are rare in the pediatric population. Of these, the most common histological types are mucoepidermoid carcinoma (MEC) and acinic cell carcinoma (AciCC) [1]. Mammary analogue secretory carcinoma (MASC) is a recently established salivary gland tumor, and it has been shown to affect both adult and child populations [2].

Herein, we report a case of parotid gland MASC in a 15-year-old girl along with a review of the literature on MASC in the young. Our case was cytologically diagnosed as "ACiCC, mostly composed of intercalated duct cell type." After surgical resection, it was successfully diagnosed as MASC of the parotid gland, by the detection of an *ETV6-NTRK3* fusion gene by RT-PCR. A retrospective review of the cytology indicated convincing features of MASC. We discuss here what could aid the diagnosis of MASC and the differentiation from acinic cell carcinoma (ACiCC), one of the most difficult salivary gland tumors to differentiate. As far as we know, only 7 cases of MASC have been reported with molecular confirmation below 19 years of age [3–8], and this is the 5th youngest case of it.

2. Case Presentation

A 15-year-old girl visited hospital for an otorhinolaryngology consultation because of a left infra-auricular mass, which had shown gradual enlargement for a year. Ultrasound-guided fine-needle aspiration (FNA) was performed and the diagnosis of possible ACiCC was rendered. The patient was introduced to our hospital in order to proceed onto surgery. The FNA materials obtained at the former hospital, consisting of 2 Papanicolaou-stained slides and 1 Giemsa-stained slide, were submitted to our hospital and ACiCC was again most strongly suspected by our cytological diagnosis. A CT scan showed a 2.8 cm sized mass in the left parotid gland (Figure 1). The patient underwent excision of her whole left parotid gland and imprint cytology was also obtained intraoperatively. This case had no metastasis in the regional lymph nodes of levels 1–4 and was staged as T1N0M0, Stage I. No adjuvant therapy was given, and the patient has no evidence of disease 40 months after surgery.

2.1. FNA and Imprint Cytology. The FNA specimen and imprint specimen showed similar cytological features; that is, the architecture of cells, individual cell appearance, and background were very similar between them. The cell clusters were mostly thin sheet-like, sometimes with slight accumulation, or were seen in an arborizing pattern with a vascular core (Figure 2(a)). Tubule formation was sometimes seen (Figure 2(b)). The cell adhesion between the tumor cells looked rather loose and they seemed easy to detach (Figure 2(c)). The cell border between the tumor cells was indistinct (Figure 2(d)). Individual tumor cells had slightly eosinophilic and granular cytoplasm (Figures 2(d) and 2(e)). Cytoplasmic vacuoles were not remarkable. Tumor cells were relatively uniform throughout, with little cellular pleomorphism. The nuclei of the tumor cells were round with no distortion and located mostly peripherally, containing small nucleoli. Although it was not recognized as such at the time of cytological diagnosis, retrospective review sometimes revealed a light-greenish material corresponding to material secreted by the tumor cells attached to the cell cluster (Figure 2(f)). Giemsa-stained specimen also showed that tumor cells had slightly eosinophilic and granular cytoplasm (Figure 2(g)). Pinkish material showing slight metachromacy was seen inside tubular structures/in the background (Figures 2(f) and 2(g)).

2.2. Surgical Specimen. Cut sections of the surgical specimen showed a 3.0 × 2.8 × 2.5-cm sized, uncircumscribed, whitish, elastic hard mass in both lobes of the left parotid gland (Figure 3(a)). Histopathologically, the tumor grew partially with a multinodular appearance but often showed invasive growth with fibrotic/hyalinized stroma (Figure 3(b)). In the tumor nodule, tumor cells formed small tubules or acini sometimes with secretory material inside (Figure 3(c)). Tumor cells were relatively uniform, similar to intercalated duct cells, and often had vacuolated cytoplasm (Figure 3(d)). A small portion of the tumor showed the aggregates of irregularly dilated glands with secretory material inside (Figure 3(e)). Only a few mitotic figures were observed. No lymphatic/vascular or perineural invasion was evident.

Periodic acid Schiff (PAS) stain showed positivity for the eosinophilic material inside the dilated tubule and the luminal site of the tumor tubules, but negativity for the cytoplasm, suggesting a lack of zymogen granules. Immunohistochemically, tumor cells were intensely positive for S-100 (Figure 3(f)), GCDFP-15, and mammaglobin (Figure 3(g)), while ER, PgR, HER2, and p63 were negative. The Ki-67 index of the tumor was 22%.

2.3. Molecular Pathology. A formalin-fixed, paraffin-embedded section obtained from the surgical specimen was submitted for RT-PCR studies. RNA was extracted and converted into cDNA. RT-PCR was performed using previously described primer pairs [9]. This analysis revealed the presence of an *ETV6-NTRK3* fusion transcript in this tumor (Figures 4(a) and 4(b)). The final diagnosis was MASC.

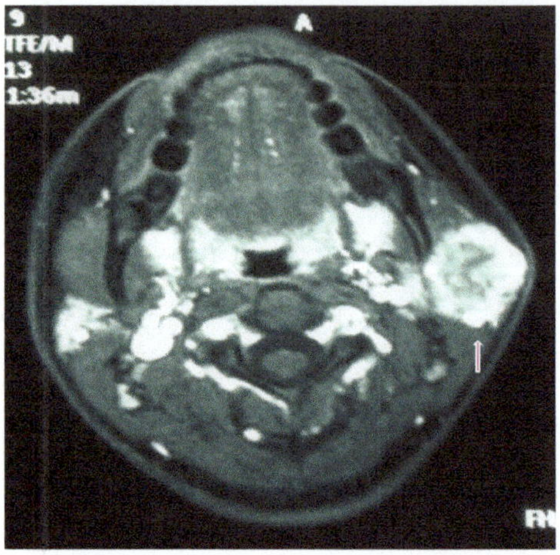

Figure 1: Contrast-enhanced computed tomography images of the tumor. A 2.8 cm sized tumor was present at the left parotid gland. The tumor was relatively circumscribed and contained a low-density area inside.

3. Discussion

MASC was first described by Skálová et al. in 2010 [9] and more than 90 cases have been reported in the last 2 years [2]. Unlike secretory breast carcinoma, which is usually seen in young patients, MASC occurs in both children and adults (13 to 72 years), with an average age of 44.2 years, and shows slight male predominance. The present case was a 15-year-old female with the complaint of an infra-auricular mass/swelling for one year and is the fifth youngest case of MASC so far reported with molecular conformation (Table 1). Although relatively rare, we need to keep this entity in mind for the differential diagnosis of salivary gland tumors in pediatric patients. In pediatrics, the majority of MASC occur in the parotid gland, but they can occur in other locations, such as lips, and are most often diagnosed as AciCC before molecular study [3–8].

The cytological distinction between zymogen granule-poor ACiCC and MASC without molecular study or immunohistochemical study is very difficult, since the cytology of MASC has many overlapping features with AciCC. However, there seem to be several cytological features suggestive of MASC, such as papillary structure, extracellular and intracellular mucinous material, vacuolated cytoplasm, tumor cells with low-grade nuclear atypia, and abundant vascularity [3–8, 10–12]. Retrospectively, three out of five of the above-mentioned features, mucinous material (extracellular, in this case), low-grade nuclear atypia, and abundant vascularity, were seen in the present case, which might have led to the diagnosis of MASC. According to Griffith et al.,

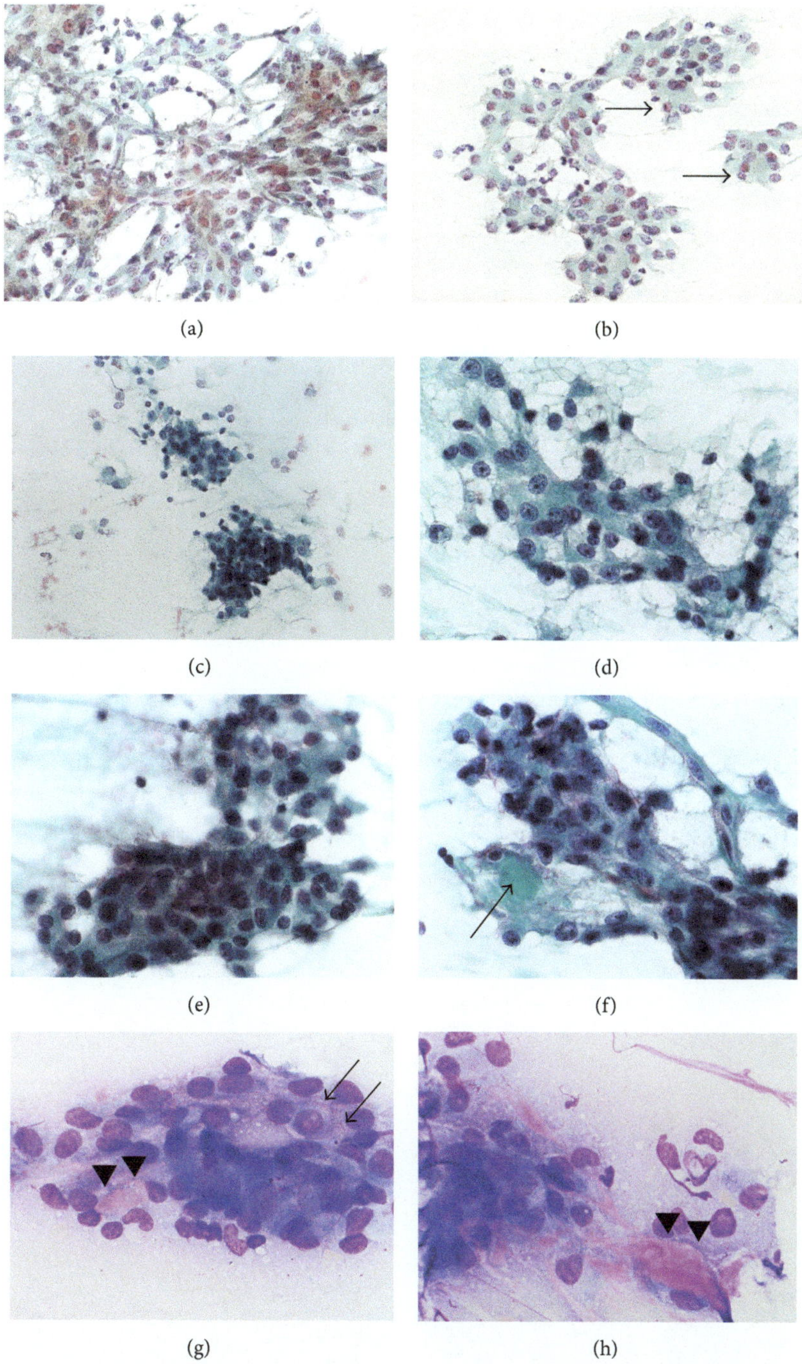

FIGURE 2: Cytomorphology of mammary analogue secretory carcinoma. Tumor cells were seen in a relatively flat sheet with abundant vascular supply (a). Tubules or rosette-like structures were sometimes seen (arrows, (b)). Tumor cells sometimes piled up with scattered detached cells peripherally (c). The cytoplasm of the tumor cells was slightly eosinophilic and the cell border between the tumor cells was indistinct ((d), (e)). Light-greenish material was sometimes observed at the periphery of the tumor cell cluster (arrow), which is now considered to correspond to material secreted by the tumor cells (f). With Giemsa stain, tumor cells showed slightly eosinophilic cytoplasm and intracytoplasmic granules (arrows) were rarely seen (g). Eosinophilic substance (arrowheads) showing slight metachromacy was seen inside tumor tubules/in the background ((g), (h)). (a) to (f) Papanicolaou stain; (a) and (b) FNA material; (c) to (f) imprint material; (g) and (h) Giemsa stain.

the subtle clues for discriminating MASC from ACiCC are prominent extracellular and intracellular mucin, greater size variability of cytoplasmic vacuoles, and clinical information such as the tumor's anatomic site and the sex of the patient [7]. The absence of basophilic cytoplasmic granules seen in ACiCC is also important.

In MASC, it is described that perineural invasion is uncommon and that lymphovascular invasion has not been

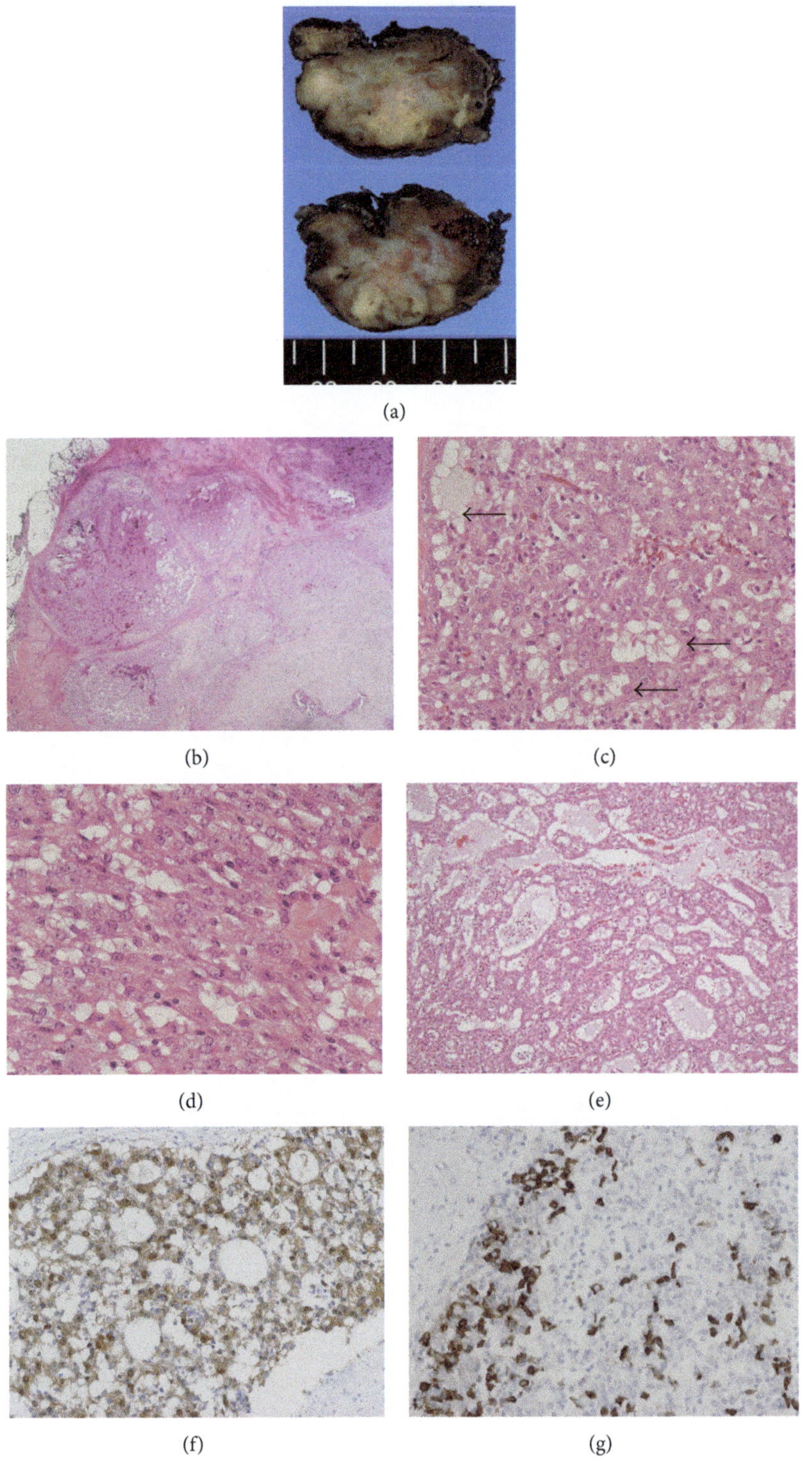

Figure 3: Macroscopic and histological morphology of mammary analogue secretory carcinoma. The cut section of the tumor was uncircumscribed and whitish, invading into the connective tissue surrounding the parotid gland (a). Microscopically, the tumor grew in a nodular fashion with abundant fibrous septa (b). The tumor formed small ducts or microcysts and often had vacuolated cytoplasm (arrows) (c). Tumor cells were relatively uniform and showed morphology similar to intercalated duct (d). Pinkish/mucin-like substances were sometimes seen inside the tumor tubules (e). Immunohistochemically, tumor cells were diffusely and intensely positive for S-100 (f) and partially/intensely positive for mammaglobin (g). (b) to (e) HE stain; (f) immunohistochemistry for S100; (g) immunohistochemistry for mammaglobin.

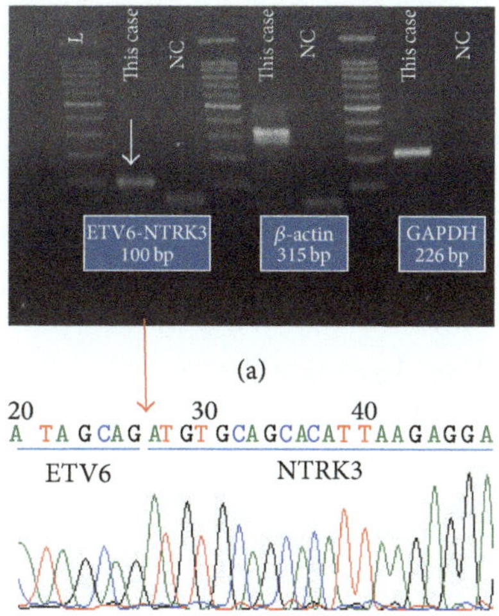

(a)

(b)

FIGURE 4: The analysis of *ETV6-NTRK3* fusion transcript. The results of the electrophoresis (a) and direct sequencing (b) revealed the presence of an *ETV6-NTRK3* fusion gene. In (a), the arrow indicates the PCR product of the *ETV6-NTRK3* transcript. PCR for *β-actin* and *GAPDH* was performed as a quality check of the extracted RNA. NC: negative control. L: ladder (molecular marker). In (b), the arrow indicates the fusion point of the *ETV6-NTRK3* transcript.

TABLE 1: Mammary analogue secretory carcinoma cases under 19 years old: summary of the reported cases (with molecular confirmation).

Age	Sex	Site[a]	Size[b]	Duration[c]	Outcome/FU[d]	Original Dx./procedure[e]	Others[f]	Reference
13	M	P	2.1	3 yr	No rec/8 mo	AciCC/His		[3]
14	M	P	2.0	1 yr	NA	Sal Neopl/His	Post-rad	[4]
14	F	P	2.8	NA	NA	AciCC/His		[5]
14	F	P	3.0	4 mo	No rec/1 yr	AciCC/His		[6]
15	F	P	3.0	1 yr	No rec	AciCC/FNA & His		This case
15	M	Lip, sp.	1.0	NA	NA	Neopl.NOS/NA		[7]
17	F	P	1.0	NA	Rec[g]	MEC/FNA		[8]
17	M	P	1.5	NA	No rec/NA	Pleo/FNA		[8]

[a] P: parotid gland; Lip, sp.: upper lip.
[b] Size in cm.
[c] Duration: duration before surgery; NA: duration before surgery was not available.
[d] rec: recurrence; No rec/NA: no recurrence/follow-up period is not available.
[e] AciCC: acinic cell carcinoma; Sal Neopl: salivary neoplasm with no further classification; Neopl NOS: neoplasm NOS; MEC: mucoepidermoid carcinoma; Pleo: pleomorphic adenoma; NA: not written in the literature; for procedure; His: by histology; FNA: by fine-needle aspiration cytology.
[f] Post-rad: postradiation therapy.
[g] Recurred 6 times during the 15 years after first surgery according to [8].

reported; therefore, MASC is currently regarded as a low-grade carcinoma, and its prognosis appears to be favorable [9]. The present case is alive and well with no evidence of disease 40 months after surgery. Skálová et al. recently showed that MASC can transform into a high-grade tumor [13]. Therefore, it should be considered by cytologists that tumor cells with high-grade nuclear atypia might appear in the cytological specimen of MASC.

In conclusion, the cytological features of MASC of the salivary gland of a 15-year-old girl were reported. Since preoperative FNA is increasingly and widely used for tumors of the salivary gland owing to its simplicity and safety, it is necessary for cytologists and pathologists to be aware of the cytology of recently established tumors such as MASC.

To the best of our knowledge, this is the fifth youngest case of MASC reported in the literature.

Conflict of Interests

The authors have no conflict of interests to declare.

Acknowledgments

The authors thank Dr. T. Nagao, Department of Human Pathology, Tokyo Medical University, for consultation on the histopathological diagnosis of this case. This work was supported in part by a Grant-in-Aid for General Scientific

Research from the Ministry of Education, Science, Sports and Culture (no. 26670286 to Tsuyoshi Saito), Tokyo, Japan.

References

[1] N. L. Shapiro and N. Bhattacharyya, "Clinical characteristics and survival for major salivary gland malignancies in children," *Otolaryngology—Head and Neck Surgery*, vol. 134, no. 4, pp. 631–634, 2006.

[2] R. Sethi, E. Kozin, A. Remenschneider et al., "Mammary analogue secretory carcinoma: update on a new diagnosis of salivary gland malignancy," *Laryngoscope*, vol. 124, no. 1, pp. 188–195, 2014.

[3] M. J. Hwang, P. R. Wu, C.-M. Chen, C.-Y. Chen, and C.-J. Chen, "A rare malignancy of the parotid gland in a 13-year-old Taiwanese boy: case report of a mammary analogue secretory carcinoma of the salivary gland with molecular study," *Medical Molecular Morphology*, vol. 47, no. 1, pp. 57–61, 2014.

[4] J. Woo, R. R. Seethala, and S. J. Sirintrapun, "Mammary analogue secretory carcinoma of the parotid gland as a secondary malignancy in a childhood survivor of atypical teratoid rhabdoid tumor," *Head and Neck Pathology*, vol. 8, no. 2, pp. 194–197, 2014.

[5] M. Urano, T. Nagao, S. Miyabe, K. Ishibashi, K. Higuchi, and M. Kuroda, "Characterization of mammary analogue secretory carcinoma of the salivary gland: discrimination from its mimics by the presence of the *ETV6-NTRK3* translocation and novel surrogate markers," *Human Pathology*, vol. 46, no. 1, pp. 94–103, 2015.

[6] J. C. Rastatter, K. R. Jatana, L. J. Jennings, and H. Melin-Aldana, "Mammary analogue secretory carcinoma of the parotid gland in a pediatric patient," *Otolaryngology—Head and Neck Surgery*, vol. 146, no. 3, pp. 514–515, 2012.

[7] C. C. Griffith, E. B. Stelow, A. Saqi et al., "The cytological features of mammary analogue secretory carcinoma: a series of 6 molecularly confirmed cases," *Cancer Cytopathology*, vol. 121, no. 5, pp. 234–241, 2013.

[8] M. J. Jung, S. Y. Kim, S. Y. Nam et al., "Aspiration cytology of mammary analogue secretory carcinoma of the salivary gland," *Diagnostic Cytopathology*, 2014.

[9] A. Skálová, T. Vanecek, R. Sima et al., "Mammary analogue secretory carcinoma of salivary glands, containing the etv6-ntrk3 fusion gene: a hitherto undescribed salivary gland tumor entity," *The American Journal of Surgical Pathology*, vol. 34, no. 5, pp. 599–608, 2010.

[10] J. A. Bishop, "Unmasking MASC: bringing to light the unique morphologic, immunohistochemical and genetic features of the newly recognized mammaryanaloguesecretorycarcinoma of salivary glands," *Head and Neck Pathology*, vol. 7, no. 1, pp. 35–39, 2013.

[11] R. Sethi, E. Kozin, A. Remenschneider et al., "Mammary analogue secretory carcinoma: update on a new diagnosis of salivary gland malignancy," *Laryngoscope*, vol. 124, no. 1, pp. 188–195, 2014.

[12] T. D. Samulski, V. A. LiVolsi, and Z. Baloch, "The cytopathologic features of mammary analog secretory carcinoma and its mimics," *CytoJournal*, vol. 11, no. 1, article 24, 2014.

[13] A. Skálová, T. Vanecek, H. Majewska et al., "Mammary analogue secretory carcinoma of salivary glands with high-grade transformation: report of 3 cases with the ETV6-NTRK3 gene fusion and analysis of TP53, β-catenin, EGFR, and CCND1 genes," *American Journal of Surgical Pathology*, vol. 38, no. 1, pp. 23–33, 2014.

26

Multiple Epithelioid Hemangiomas with Orbital Involvement

Branislava Miličić,[1] Tomaž Velnar,[2] Rado Pregelj,[3] and Clara Limbaeck-Stokin[1]

[1]*Faculty of Medicine, Institute of Pathology, University of Ljubljana, 1000 Ljubljana, Slovenia*
[2]*Department of Neurosurgery, University Medical Center Maribor, 2000 Maribor, Slovenia*
[3]*International Institute for Neurosurgery and Neurosciences, 1000 Ljubljana, Slovenia*

Correspondence should be addressed to Branislava Miličić; bibamilicic@gmail.com

Academic Editor: Imtiaz A. Chaudhry

Epithelioid hemangioma, also known as angiolymphoid hyperplasia with eosinophilia, is a cutaneous angioproliferative lesion that follows a benign clinical course. It is most frequently localized in the skin of the head and neck region; although it may sometimes arise deeper in soft tissues, orbital involvement is rare. Here we describe a patient who developed multiple epithelioid hemangiomas, including an intraorbital lesion. The histopathological parallels with other reactive and neoplastic lesions as well as therapeutic options are discussed.

1. Introduction

Epithelioid hemangioma (EH) is an uncommon vasoproliferative process of the skin and less frequently soft tissues that usually affects middle-aged adults [1]. EH typically presents as painless, erythematous nodules or plaques of the head and neck region, involving the dermis and subcutaneous tissue. The process tends to recur and roughly 50% of affected patients develop multiple lesions [1, 2]. Despite these worrisome features the clinical course of EH is benign; pathogenesis though remains unclear and its nature, whether it is a reactive process or a neoplasm, is still a matter of discussion.

A definitive diagnosis requires histological evaluation: EH has distinctive morphological features consisting of proliferation of blood vessels lined by abnormal endothelial cells, accompanied by lymphocytic and eosinophilic inflammatory infiltrate [2, 3]. Importantly, the endothelial cells are plump but do not show signs of atypia or increased mitotic activity [4]. Orbital involvement is very rare and appears to have a later onset. So far only few cases have been reported in the literature [5, 6].

2. Case Report

A 71-year-old woman with a history of sarcoidosis and non-Hodgkin lymphoma of the gastrointestinal tract was admitted to the neurosurgery department for crushing pain in the right eye, headaches, and double vision. A year before, a tumour of the right orbit was partially excised. Histopathological examination at that time showed fibrous tissue with vascular proliferation (Figure 1). The nature of the proliferation, reactive or neoplastic, was not definitively established at that time. Nevertheless the lesion was considered benign because histological parameters typical for malignant neoplasm—high mitotic activity, cellular atypia, necrosis, and infiltrative growth pattern—were not observed; therefore further treatment was not recommended. Symptoms, however, recurred after a few months and were progressively worsening.

At the time of admission to the hospital, exophthalmos of the right eye was evident with paresis of the third and fourth cranial nerves. Visual acuity was 0.8 and had not changed since previous hospitalization. The patient complained of double vision, which was exaggerated in the gaze directions of the affected orbital muscles. No other cranial nerve abnormalities were noted.

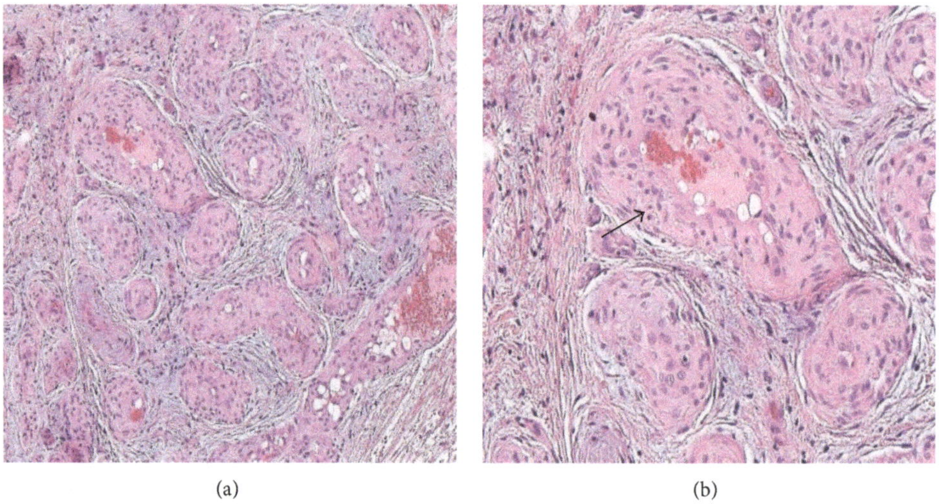

FIGURE 1: Representative histological images of the first biopsy: (a) HE: low magnification, showing numerous blood vessels. (b) HE: higher magnification, showing thick vessel walls with proliferated endothelium (arrow) and some inflammatory infiltrate.

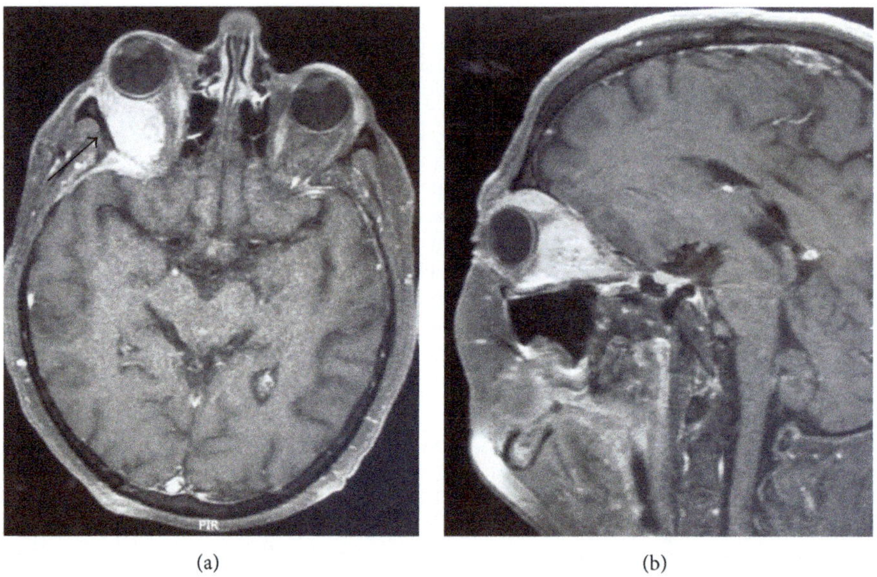

FIGURE 2: MRI: (a) T2-weighted MRI image of the head showing intraorbital mass and scar tissue (arrow) from previous operation. (b) On contrast T1-weighted image, the intraorbital mass may be clearly seen, as well as exophthalmos.

MRI of the head revealed a mass of the right orbit, about two centimetres in diameter (Figure 2). Some contrast staining was present in the operative field, indicating scar tissue from previous surgery. A CT scan showed a defect of the orbital roof bone, removed at the time of the first operation (Figure 3(a)). Surgical resection was indicated.

Surgery was performed through right pterional approach with retrepanation of the cranial bone and complete orbitotomy. A fibrous tumour was found in the periorbital adipose tissue, embedded in scar tissue and extending to the fibrous coverings of the globe, partially adherent to the extraocular muscles. The tumour was completely resected.

After surgery, exophthalmos and ocular pain slowly subsided, as did paresis of the third and fourth cranial nerves, although some minor deficit of ocular motion persisted (Figure 3(b)). Histopathological evaluation revealed a lesion composed of numerous blood vessels and fibrous tissue, accompanied by a dense, mixed inflammatory infiltrate including eosinophils, lymphocytes, and plasma cells. Focal lymphocyte aggregates were also present, while granulomas were not observed. The vascular walls were thick, lined by mildly polymorphic, plump endothelial cells with abundant eosinophilic cytoplasm and vesicular nuclei. Necrosis and mitoses were not seen (Figure 4). In comparison with

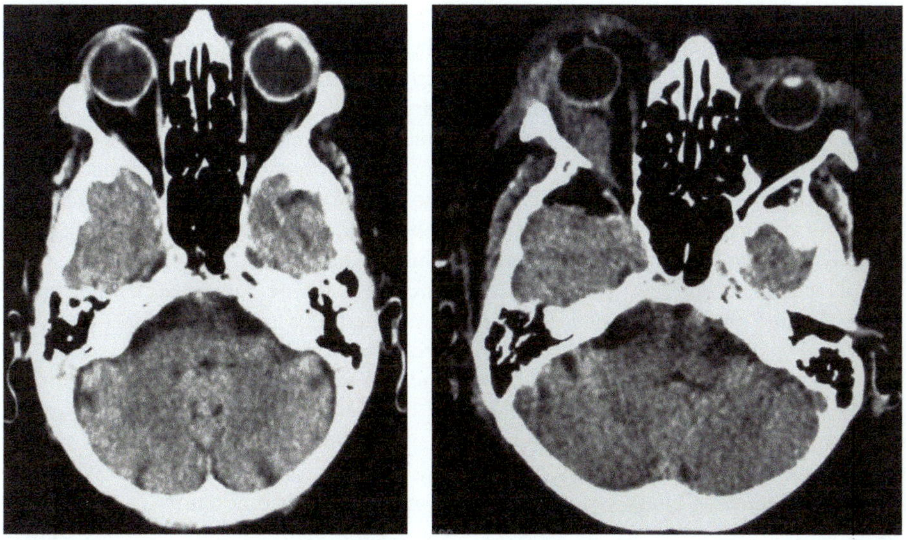

(a) (b)

Figure 3: CT, pre- and postoperative: (a) Preoperative CT: intraorbital mass (thick arrow) and partially removed bone of the orbital roof (thin arrow) are seen. (b) Postoperative CT: the intraorbital mass has been removed and the exophthalmos is less clearly evident in comparison to preoperative images.

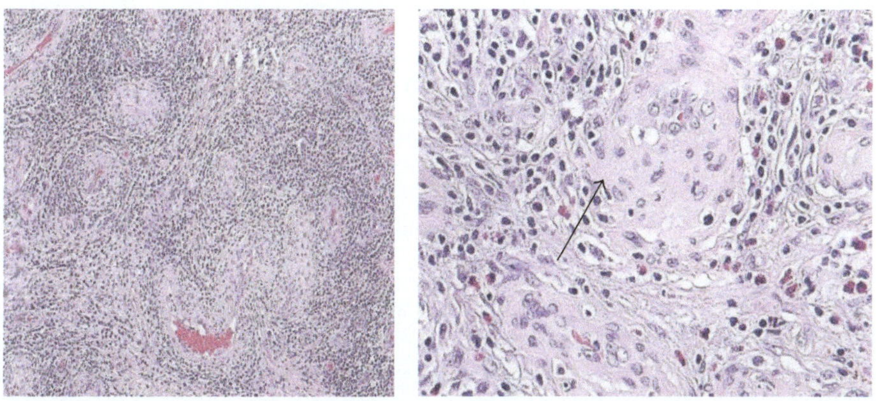

(a) (b)

Figure 4: Histological images of the second biopsy: (a) HE: lower magnification, compared to the first biopsy blood vessels are surrounded by a denser inflammatory infiltrate. (b) HE: higher magnification, showing marked endothelial proliferation. Endothelial cells are plump (arrow). Many eosinophils are seen.

the first biopsy (Figure 1), there was more inflammatory infiltrate, probably secondary to surgery, blood vessels displayed thicker walls and the epithelioid appearance of the endothelium was more pronounced. Based on these histopathological findings, a diagnosis of EH was made.

In addition, we retrieved two older biopsies of the same patient from our archives. Both were performed two years earlier; the first one was a skin biopsy of the scalp and the second was a biopsy of the right orbital adipose tissue and lacrimal gland. The lesion of the scalp also displayed histopathological features of EH, while interestingly in the lacrimal gland granulomatous inflammation turned out to be consistent with sarcoidosis.

Also, a new tumour localized on the eyelid has developed a few months after surgery. This lesion has not been histologically verified yet, but according to its clinical features, it could represent another EH.

3. Discussion

EH was first described in 1969 as angiolymphoid hyperplasia with eosinophilia [7, 8] and, although uncommon, it is now a well-recognised entity both at superficial and deep soft tissue sites, as well as in bones. Orbital involvement is rare, but when present symptoms such as exophthalmos, ocular pain, tearing, pruritus around the eye, blurred vision, and double vision have been described [5, 6]. These last two symptoms were observed in our patient and clearly reflect involvement of ocular cranial nerves.

The orbital tumour exhibited convincing histopathological elements of EH, evident in particular in the second biopsy and closely resembling the lesion previously excised from the scalp. Nevertheless, a differential diagnosis in particular with diseases that more commonly affect the orbit had to be considered. This included reactive processes, lymphoproliferative disorders, and some vascular neoplasms.

Several reactive processes had to be ruled out. In this category, the main differential diagnosis was with Kimura's disease (KD), since EH shares with KD some clinical and histologic features. Both KD and EH usually manifest as nodules or plaques in the head and neck region. KD probably represents an allergic or autoimmune response and, unlike EH, it often develops systemic features such as blood eosinophilia and nephrotic syndrome, asthma, tuberculosis, or Loeffler syndrome [9–11]. KD differs from EH also histologically, as in KD proliferate blood vessels do not display abnormal epithelioid endothelial cells [4].

Based on tumour location, the second major reactive process to be excluded was idiopathic orbital inflammation (IOI). IOI is characterized histologically by a mixed inflammatory infiltrate and in later stages fibrosis, but again abnormal endothelial proliferation is not seen [12].

Since the cellular infiltrate was rich in lymphoid cells, the second group of diseases to enter into the differential diagnosis was lymphoproliferative disorders. This diagnosis was excluded considering the reactive appearance of the infiltrate, which was composed of a mixed population of well-differentiated lymphatic cells.

Vascular tumours represent the third family of lesions that had to be considered. Among benign vascular tumours, especially arteriovenous hemangioma (cirsoid aneurism) had to be taken into account. Cirsoid aneurisms also present as a nodule or papule in the head and neck region of middle-aged or elderly adults. Histologically, they are characterised by a combination of thin and thick-walled blood vessels with no epithelioid endothelium. Malignant vascular neoplasms, in particular epithelioid hemangioendothelioma and angiosarcoma, also had to be excluded [1]; according to the benign histological features of the blood vessels observed in the biopsy (well-formed vessels, no cellular atypia of endothelial cells), this diagnosis was easily ruled out in our case.

The aetiology of EH remains unknown. It is either a benign neoplastic proliferation of blood vessels or a reactive hyperplasia of vascular structures, which develops in response to trauma, and possibly other triggers such as hyperestrogenic states (pregnancy or oral contraceptives) or infection [13–15]. It is interesting in our case that the patient had sarcoidosis with histologically confirmed involvement of the right lacrimal gland. We have not found any association between sarcoidosis and EH in the literature, but we cannot exclude a connection among the two processes considering that EH developed after granulomatous dacryoadenitis.

There are many treatment options for EH depending on the extent, location, and size of the lesions [6]. The most effective therapy is complete removal and follow-up [16]. Possible nonsurgical possible treatments include intralesional injections of isotretinoin, steroids, interferon alpha-2a, cytotoxic agents and irradiation therapy, carbon dioxide and argon laser, and electrodessication [13, 15–17]. Orbital lesions have also been treated successfully with surgical excision, as in our patient. Great care must be taken to avoid damage to orbital muscles, vessels, ocular nerves, and in particular the optic nerve, as the lesion in itself is benign and can be fully removed [16]. Prognosis after surgery is usually good. In our case, the ocular movements improved and double vision subsided as a result of orbital decompression and pressure release on the extraocular muscles. Additional steroids may accelerate recovery and are recommended in lower doses [2, 16].

In conclusion EH, although rare at this site, enters into the differential diagnosis of orbital masses. Histopathological examination is mandatory in order to exclude other tumours and tumour-like lesions. Despite being a benign process, its disrupting growth may cause severe symptoms, spontaneous regression is uncommon, and lesions often recur, so complete removal is the therapy of choice.

Conflict of Interests

The authors declare that there is no conflict of interests regarding the publication of this paper.

References

[1] S. D. Bilings and J. R. Goldblum, "Soft tissue tumors and the tumor like reactions," in *Dermatopathology*, K. J. Busam, Ed., pp. 546–558, Elsevier Saunders, 1st edition, 2010.

[2] V. V. Panicker, A. D. Dhramaratnam, and J. Kuruvilla, "Angiolymphoid hyperplasia with eosinophilia," *Indian Dermatology Online Journal*, vol. 3, no. 1, article 80, 2012.

[3] L. Shevchenko, T. Aaberg Jr., and H. E. Grossniklaus, "Conjunctival angiolymphoid hyperplasia with eosinophilia in a child," *Journal of Pediatric Ophthalmology and Strabismus*, vol. 49, pp. e66–e69, 2012.

[4] C. D. M. Fletcher, "Vascular tumors," in *Diagnostic Histopathology of Tumors*, pp. 54–55, Elsevier Saunders, Philadelphia, Pa, USA, 4th edition, 2013.

[5] B. F. Fernandes, A. Al-Mujaini, T. Petrogiannis-Haliotis, A. Al-Kandari, B. Arthurs, and M. N. Burnier Jr., "Epithelioid hemangioma (angiolymphoid hyperplasia with eosinophilia) of the orbit: a case report," *Journal of Medical Case Reports*, vol. 25, no. 1, article 30, 2007.

[6] T. M. McEachren, S. Brownstein, D. R. Jordan, V. A. Montpetit, and R. L. Font, "Epithelioid hemangioma of the orbit," *Ophthalmology*, vol. 107, no. 4, pp. 806–810, 2000.

[7] G. C. Wells and I. W. Whimster, "Subcutaneous angiolymphoid hyperplasia with eosinophilia," *British Journal of Dermatology*, vol. 81, no. 1, pp. 1–15, 1969.

[8] Y. Kurihara, H. Inoue, H. Kiryu, and M. Furue, "Epithelioid hemangioma (Angiolymphoid hyperplasia with eosinophilia) in zosteriform distribution," *Indian Journal of Dermatology*, vol. 57, no. 5, pp. 401–403, 2012.

[9] G. Cunniffe, T. Alonso, C. Dinares, F. J. Medina, and R. Medel, "Angiolymphoid hyperplasia with eosinophilia of the eyelid and

orbit: the Western cousin of Kimura's disease?" *International Ophthalmology*, vol. 34, no. 1, pp. 107–110, 2014.

[10] W.-S. Chong, A. Thomas, and C.-L. Goh, "Kimura's disease and angiolymphoid hyperplasia with eosinophilia: two disease entities in the same patient. Case report and review of the literature," *International Journal of Dermatology*, vol. 45, no. 2, pp. 139–145, 2006.

[11] D. L. Smith, M. C. Kincaid, and E. Nicolitz, "Angiolymphoid hyperplasia with eosinophilia (Kimura's Disease) of the orbit," *Archives of Ophthalmology*, vol. 106, no. 6, pp. 793–795, 1988.

[12] J. D. Hsuan, D. Selva, A. A. McNab, T. J. Sullivan, P. Saeed, and B. A. O'Donnell, "Idiopathic sclerosing orbital inflammation," *Archives of Ophthalmology*, vol. 124, no. 9, pp. 1244–1250, 2006.

[13] F. El Sayed, R. Dhaybi, A. Ammoury, and M. Chababi, "Angiolymphoid hyperplasia with eosinophilia: efficacy of isotretinoin?" *Head & Face Medicine*, vol. 4, no. 2, article 32, 2006.

[14] C. J. Miller, M. D. Ioffreda, and C. T. Ammirati, "Mohs micrographic surgery for angiolymphoid hyperplasia with eosinophilia," *Dermatologic Surgery*, vol. 30, no. 8, pp. 1169–1173, 2004.

[15] T. Kaur, K. Sandhu, S. Gupta, A. J. Kanwar, and B. Kumar, "Treatment of angiolymphoid hyperplasia with eosinophilia with the carbon dioxide laser," *Journal of Dermatological Treatment*, vol. 15, no. 5, pp. 328–330, 2004.

[16] G. Tchernev, T. Taneva, J. Ananiev et al., "Angiolymphoid hyperplasia with eosinophilia-an incidental fnding after surgical excision," *Wiener Medizinische Wochenschrift*, vol. 162, no. 19-20, pp. 448–451, 2012.

[17] M. S. Baker, R. B. Avery, C. R. Johnson, and R. C. Allen, "Methotrexate as an alternative treatment for orbital angiolymphoid hyperplasia with eosinophilia," *Orbit*, vol. 31, no. 5, pp. 324–326, 2012.

27

Isolated Ocular Manifestation of Relapsed Chronic Myelogenous Leukemia Presenting as Myeloid Blast Crisis in a Patient on Imatinib Therapy: A Case Report and Review of the Literature

Rohit Gulati, Yaser Alkhatib, Vijayalakshmi Donthireddy, Michelle Madden Felicella, Madhu P. Menon, and Kedar V. Inamdar

Henry Ford Hospital, 2799 W. Grand Boulevard, Detroit, MI 48202, USA

Correspondence should be addressed to Kedar V. Inamdar; kinamda1@hfhs.org

Academic Editor: Achille Pich

Blast phase in chronic myelogenous leukemia (CML) has rarely been reported to involve extramedullary sites like skin, lymph nodes, and central nervous system. Clinical history, characteristic hematologic findings (elevated leukocyte counts, myelocytic predominance, and basophilia), and Philadelphia chromosome are of high diagnostic significance especially in isolated extramedullary presentations. We describe a unique case of CML relapse with blast phase involving the eye. A 66-year-old man with a known diagnosis of CML on imatinib and in molecular remission for 3 years presented with a painful blind eye. Histologic examination revealed diffuse involvement of choroid, iris, vitreous humor, and the optic nerve by blast cells. The blasts expressed CD34, aberrant TdT, and a myeloid phenotype (CD13, CD33, and CD117). Fluorescence in situ hybridization (FISH) of vitreous fluid detected *BCR-ABL1* gene rearrangement. Additionally, trisomy 8 and gains of 9 and 22 were seen which were not present in the initial diagnostic marrow study 3 years ago. At relapse, the bone marrow, peripheral blood, and the cerebrospinal fluid were not involved by CML. Patient received induction chemotherapy and single dose prophylactic intrathecal methotrexate and was maintained on antityrosine kinase therapy and eventually underwent allogenic stem cell transplantation.

1. Introduction

Blast crisis in CML is defined by the presence of ≥20% blasts in the bone marrow or peripheral blood, large clusters of blasts in the bone marrow biopsy, or any extramedullary blast proliferation [1]. Extramedullary disease occurs in a small percent of CML cases and is found to manifest in its chronic, accelerated, or blast phase [2, 3]. It can occur at various sites including bone, lymph node, skin, soft tissue, and central nervous system (CNS) [3–6]. We describe an unusual case of relapsed chronic myelogenous leukemia (CML) in blast crisis presenting with isolated ocular involvement in a patient undergoing imatinib therapy and hematologically in morphologic, cytogenetic, and molecular remission at the time of relapse.

2. Case Presentation

Our patient is a 66-year-old male who was first diagnosed with CML after presenting to the emergency room with acute onset knee pain. During the investigation, he was found to have an elevated white blood cell count (64.4×10^9/L). The differential count revealed neutrophilia with left shift and basophilia. A subsequent bone marrow biopsy showed morphologic features consistent with chronic phase of CML. Conventional karyotyping and fluorescence in situ hybridization (FISH) on the bone marrow aspirate (Figure 9) showed evidence of t(9;22) *BCR-ABL1* rearrangement and real time quantitative PCR was positive for *M-BCR/ABL* t(9;22), p210 fusion transcript. The patient was started on imatinib 400 mg once a day. He achieved major molecular

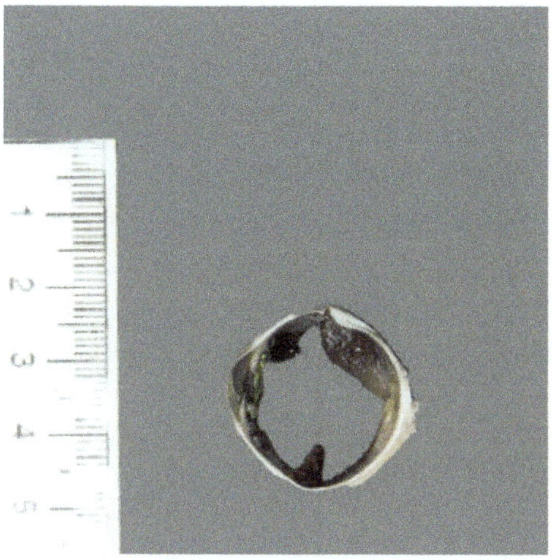

FIGURE 1: Gross photomicrograph depicting pupil-optic nerve (PO) section of enucleated eye which reveals diffuse thickening of the iris and part of the choroid layer.

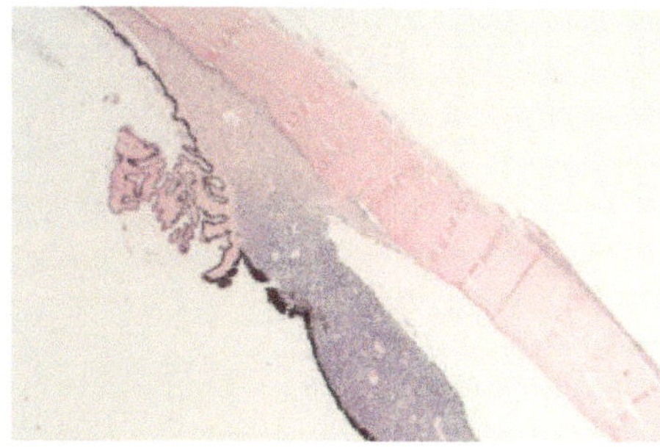

FIGURE 2: Blasts cells infiltrating the iris (H&E, magnification ×20).

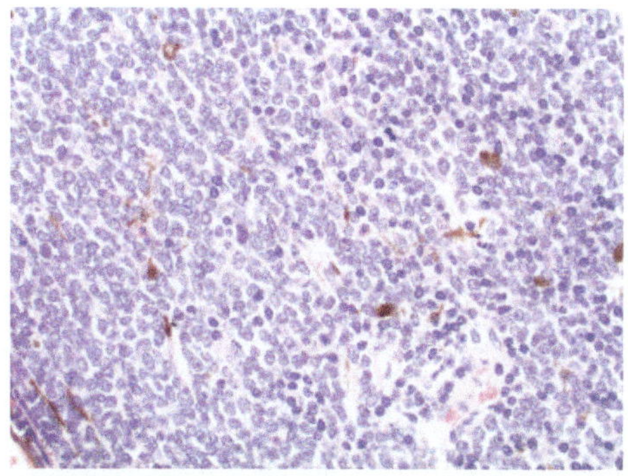

FIGURE 3: Sheets of monotonous mononuclear blast cells (H&E, magnification ×400).

response after 3 months of therapy and was followed up every 3-4 months thereafter with *M-BCR/ABL* [t(9;22), p210] fusion gene transcript levels in peripheral blood by real time quantitative PCR.

He remained in remission for three years after initial diagnosis, when he presented with sudden onset pain and loss of vision in the right eye. Magnetic resonance imaging (MRI) scan showed significant intraorbital and optic nerve enhancement. An infratemporal intraconal fat and intraorbital fat biopsy was negative for malignancy. The patient's symptoms improved with conservative management by posterior chamber decompression and steroid therapy but his vision never returned to baseline following this episode. A follow-up MRI 2 months later showed no residual signs of enhancement. Eight months following this episode, he presented with recurrent pain in the right eye, which did not resolve with conservative management. As a result, the patient underwent enucleation of his right eye.

On gross examination, a cross section of the eye showed diffuse circumferential thickening of the choroid (Figure 1). Microscopic examination revealed dense infiltration of the choroid and iris and optic nerve margin by a monotonous mononuclear cell infiltrate morphologically resembling blasts (Figures 2 and 3). By flow cytometry (Figure 4), the blasts were positive for CD34 and demonstrated myeloid immunophenotype expressing CD13, CD33, and CD11c. Blasts were negative for specific lymphoid markers including CD19, CD20, CD79a, CD2, cytoplasmic CD3, CD5, and CD10. However, CD7 was aberrantly coexpressed by the blasts. Interestingly, the blasts did not show cytoplasmic myeloperoxidase (MPO) and terminal deoxynucleotidyl transferase (TdT) expression by flow cytometry. By immunohistochemical staining (Figures 5–7), the blasts were positive for CD34 (Figure 5) with focal expression of variable intensity for CD117 (Figure 6) and strong and diffuse expression of TdT (Figure 7) but were negative for B- or T-lineage lymphoid antigen markers (CD20, CD3, and CD79a) (not shown). MPO expression was focal and weak (not shown). FISH cytogenetic analysis on vitreous fluid (Figure 8) demonstrated presence of *BCR/ABL1* [t(9;22)] gene rearrangement identical to the abnormalities detected in the original bone marrow (Figure 9) in which the diagnosis of CML was rendered. In addition to Philadelphia chromosome (Ph), a complex karyotype including trisomy 8 and gain of chromosomes 9 and 22 was also detected in this analysis. In view of the patient's history, a diagnosis of CML in blast phase was rendered. A subsequent bone marrow exam showed no morphologic, cytogenetic, or molecular evidence of CML or acute leukemia. Cytological evaluation and flow cytometry of cerebrospinal fluid were also negative for disease involvement. The patient underwent induction therapy with idarubicin and cytarabine and a single dose of intrathecal methotrexate. He was maintained on dasatinib 150 mg daily but was switched back to imatinib due to intolerance to dasatinib. He subsequently underwent allogenic stem cell transplantation after 5 months.

3. Discussion

Extramedullary blast crisis in CML is a rare occurrence. In a study of 235 CML patients by Specchia et al. [2], 16% developed extramedullary blast crisis. While both myeloid and lymphoid blast transformations are described, 80% of transformations are of myeloid origin, whereas lymphoblastic transformations account for approximately 20%. Among the latter, B-lymphoblastic transformations are more common than T-lymphoblastic crisis [4, 7]. A recent study looking

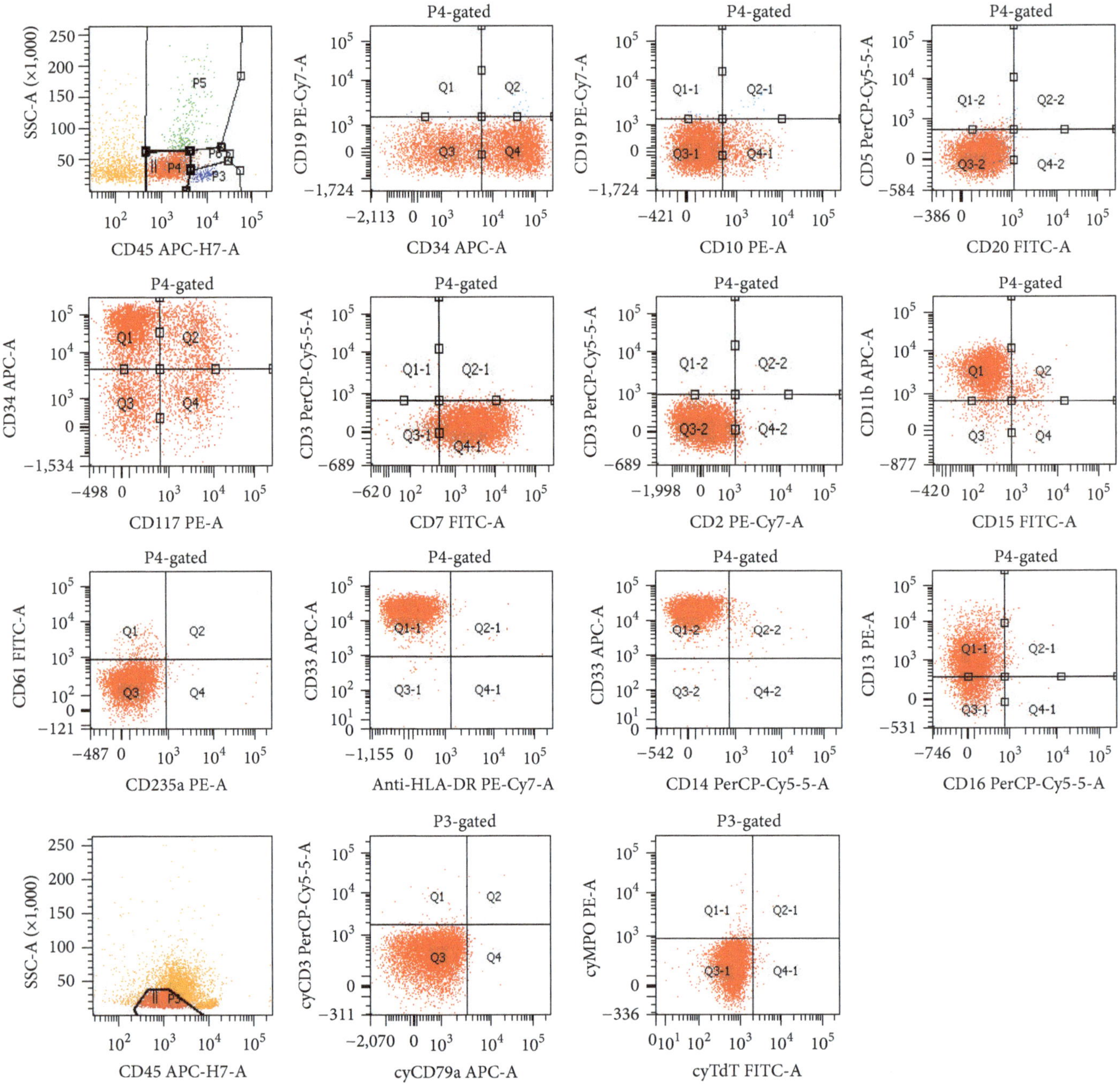

FIGURE 4: Flow cytometric immunophenotypic analysis of vitreous fluid: blast gate (P4 gate in the top line) represents the dim CD45+ cells with low side light scatter (SSC). Blast gate (P3 gate in the bottom line) represents the same population of blasts analyzed for cytoplasmic markers in a separate tube. The distinct cluster of blasts (red color population) exhibit the following immunophenotypic characteristics: *positive for* CD34, CD117, CD7, CD11b, CD13 (dim), and CD33; *negative for* CD19, CD10, CD20, CD3, CD5, CD15, CD16, CD61, CD235a, HLA-DR, CD14, cytoplasmic CD3, cytoplasmic CD79a, cytoplasmic MPO, and cytoplasmic TdT.

at outcomes found no significant difference in overall survival of CML in myeloid versus lymphoid blast crisis [7]. Ocular manifestations as presenting feature of CML have been previously described. The first case report of ocular involvement by CML in blast phase was published by Alegre et al. [8] but the patient had evidence of disease at other sites. Isolated ocular blast crisis was first described by Lipton et al. [9], who reported a case of relapsed CML presenting as lymphoid blast crisis. In their patient, lymphoid blast crisis was also the initial presentation of the disease at the time of diagnosis. Conversely, our patient initially presented in chronic phase of CML and relapsed with myeloid blast crisis in the eye. Immunophenotypically by flow cytometry, the blasts expressed CD34, CD13, and CD33 with a subset expressing CD117 whereas they were negative for cytoplasmic MPO, TdT, and B- (CD19, CD22, CD79a, and CD10) as well as

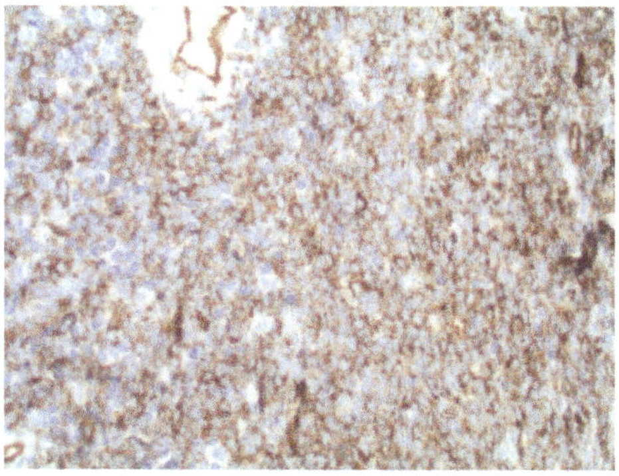

FIGURE 5: CD34 immunohistochemistry: sheets of monotonous CD34 positive blast cells (magnification ×400).

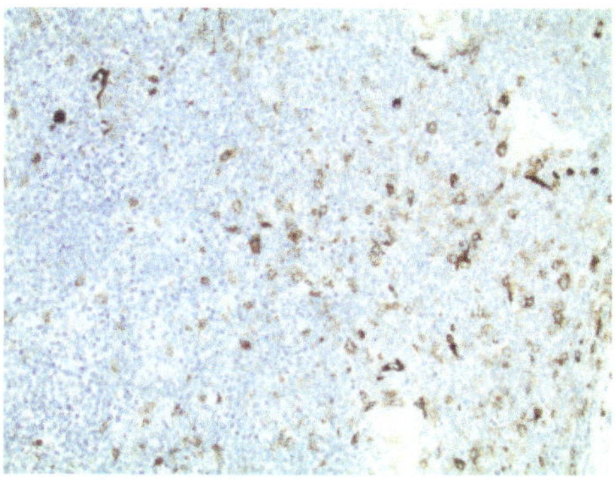

FIGURE 6: CD117 immunohistochemistry: focal and variable intensity of CD117 expression is seen in the blasts (magnification ×400).

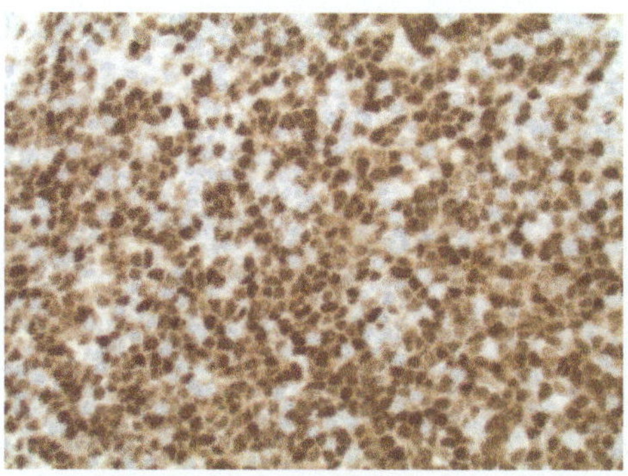

FIGURE 7: TdT immunohistochemistry: sheets of blasts showing nuclear expression of TdT (magnification ×400).

T-lymphoid antigen markers (cytoplasmic CD3). In contrast to flow cytometry, the blasts were strongly and uniformly positive for TdT by immunohistochemistry. The reason for this discrepancy is not entirely clear but we speculate that the lack of TdT expression by flow cytometry may be attributed to failure of permeabilization step in the protocol for assessment of cytoplasmic markers. The lack of expression of lymphoid markers and positivity for CD13, CD33, and CD117 was consistent with myeloid immunophenotype for the blasts.

In our case, the patient was treated with cytarabine/doxorubicin and intrathecal methotrexate. Imatinib mesylate is considered first-line therapy for treatment of CML in chronic

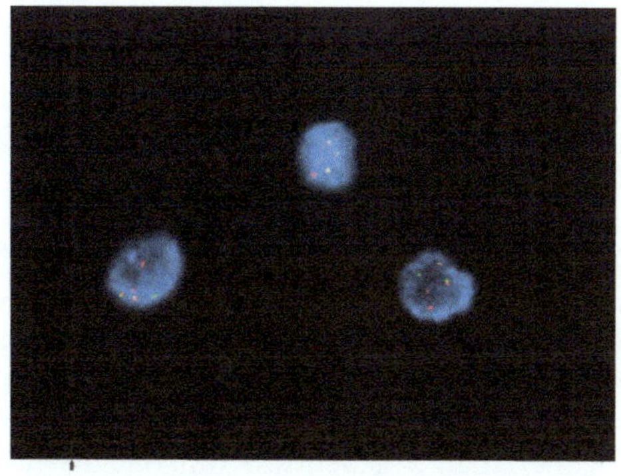

FIGURE 8: Fluorescence in situ hybridization assay on vitreous humor smear shows two BCR-ABL1 fusion signals, one BCR probe signal, and two ABL1 probe signals; thus a t(9;22) BCR-ABL1 gene rearrangement with gains of 9 and 22 [orange = 9q34 ABL1 probe; green = 22q11.2 BCR probe].

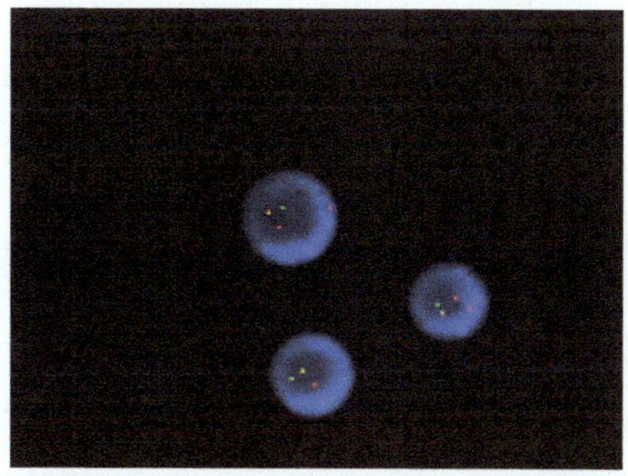

FIGURE 9: Fluorescent in situ hybridization on original diagnostic bone marrow aspirate shows one BCR-ABL1 fusion signal, two BCR probe signals, and three ABL1 probe signals in 90.5% of interphase cells.

phase with majority of patients achieving complete cytogenetic and major molecular response. Sudden evolution of disease into blast phase can rarely occur while the patient is on imatinib therapy [10]. Isolated CNS involvement by CML in blast phase has been reported in patients receiving imatinib mesylate treatment [11, 12]. It usually presents as a relapse following an initial complete remission on imatinib or after bone marrow transplant. In some patients, there may be no signs of disease involvement in the blood and bone marrow at time of CNS manifestation [12]. The central nervous system is relatively prone to disease involvement while on imatinib therapy and this is attributed mainly to poor permeability of imatinib through the blood brain barrier [11, 13]. The most common sites of CNS involvement are the lateral ventricular walls [14], meninges [15], and the optic nerve [16], causing symptoms such as headache, cognitive changes, raised intracranial pressure, and visual disturbances. Intraocular optic nerve involvement has been associated with poor prognosis and impermeability to intrathecal chemotherapeutic agents [17]. Increasing reports of CNS involvement by CML in different phases have necessitated broader disease monitoring, including BCR-ABL gene quantification in CSF [14]. Second-generation tyrosine kinase inhibitors (TKI) such as dasatinib are more effective in treating CNS disease [18] due to better penetration of the blood brain barrier [19]. For these reasons, dasatinib and nilotinib are now FDA-approved as first-line therapy in CML [20].

In our patient, the chromosome study was positive for t(9;22)(q34;q11) translocation, FISH showed *BCR/ABL* fusion gene, and RT-PCR assay was positive for major *BCR-ABL* mRNA expression. His previously documented diagnosis of chronic phase CML was helpful in diagnosing his ocular blast proliferation/myeloid sarcoma as a blast phase of CML rather than a genetically different de novo acute myeloid leukemia [4, 21, 22]. While blast proliferation in an extramedullary setting would be most consistent with a diagnosis of myeloid sarcoma, since our patient had a documented history of CML, we preferred to use the term blast phase of CML to guide therapeutic decisions. While t(9;22)(q34;q11) translocation is most commonly associated with CML or precursor B-ALL, its presence can be rarely seen in acute myeloid leukemia with a reported incidence of 1-2% of all AML cases. In the absence of a prior chronic or accelerated phase of CML, distinction between blast phase of CML and Philadelphia chromosome-positive (Ph+) AML can be difficult, as they exhibit a major overlap in their clinical presentation and genetic features [23]. Nevertheless, presence of splenomegaly, basophilia, and chromosomal abnormalities in addition to Philadelphia chromosome and a previous history of chronic or accelerated phase CML have all been attributed to blast phase of CML over Ph+ AML [24, 25].

At the time of relapse, in addition to t(9;22)(q34;q11) reciprocal translocation (Ph+), our patient demonstrated other chromosomal aberrancies including trisomy 8 and gains of chromosomes 9 and 22. Trisomy 8 has been frequently associated with clonal evolution in CML patients on imatinib who are otherwise in complete cytogenetic remission [26]. At the genetic level, trisomy 8 has been linked to alterations of *MYC* located at 8q24 [26]. Interestingly, no *MYC* alterations were detected in our patient. Gains of chromosomes 9 and 22 appear to be nonrandom chromosomal aberrations and perhaps contribute to overall genomic instability; however, the mechanisms of clonal evolution in CML are not well understood.

Using whole genome sequencing, Calabretta and Perrotti [26] found mutations in 9 genes, including GATA2, MAX, ENO1, and ANO5, which were linked to progression of CML to blast phase. Gain-of-function mutations in GATA2 were described in a previous study which reported myeloid blast transformation in CML [27]. *MAX* gene, through its complex interactions with *MYC* [28] and *CEBPA* [29], has been linked to tumor progression [30]. *ENO1* acts as a transcriptional repressor of *MYC* [31]. Recently it has been shown that transcription regulators, including Hes1 and Evi1, are involved in disease progression and even confer resistance to tyrosine kinase inhibitors [32, 33]. Many recent studies have identified potential markers as a means of better monitoring of disease progression. *SYK* gene activation is one such potential marker of disease progression and dasatinib resistance [34, 35].

4. Conclusions

While extramedullary manifestation of CML is rare, a high degree of suspicion is warranted in patients with CML on imatinib therapy who manifest CNS or ocular symptoms, even in the absence of any hematologic, cytogenetic, or molecular evidence of disease. Despite advances in molecular disease detection, more sensitive and effective methods of monitoring disease progression are still needed.

Abbreviations

CML: Chronic myelogenous leukemia
FISH: Fluorescent in situ hybridization
CNS: Central nervous system
PCR: Polymerase chain reaction
MRI: Magnetic resonance imaging
FDA: Food and Drug Administration.

Ethical Approval

The above study was approved by the Institutional Review Board at Henry Ford Hospital, Detroit, Michigan, USA.

Consent

Written informed consent was obtained from the patient for publication of the case report and any accompanying images.

Conflict of Interests

The authors declare that they have no competing interests.

Authors' Contribution

Rohit Gulati did the data collection, grossing of the surgical specimen in patient care, drafted the paper, and reviewed literature. Yaser Alkhatib helped in data collection from clinical aspects and helped in formulation of the paper. Michelle Madden Felicella conducted the grossing of the specimen supervising Rohit Gulati, helped in paper completion, and took images of the surgical specimen. Vijayalakshmi Donthireddy is the oncologist of the patient and helped collect pertinent points of patient clinical history and completing the paper. Madhu P. Menon played a significant role in paper completion and critically analyzing the review of the literature. Kedar V. Inamdar is the primary hematopathologist for the case and played a significant role in data collection, selecting microscopic images, critically analyzing the data, and reviewing literature and paper preparation.

References

[1] J. W. Vardiman, N. L. Harris, and R. D. Brunning, "The World Health Organization (WHO) classification of the myeloid neoplasms," *Blood*, vol. 100, no. 7, pp. 2292–2302, 2002.

[2] G. Specchia, G. Palumbo, D. Pastore, D. Mininni, A. Mestice, and V. Liso, "Extramedullary blast crisis in chronic myeloid

leukemia," *Leukemia Research*, vol. 20, no. 11-12, pp. 905–908, 1996.

[3] D. Inverardi, M. Lazzarino, E. Morra et al., "Extramedullary disease in PH'-positive chronic myelogenous leukemia: frequency, clinical features and prognostic significance," *Haematologica*, vol. 75, no. 2, pp. 146–148, 1990.

[4] G.-N. Jin, P. Zou, W.-X. Chen, Z.-Y. Ding, and H. Zhou, "Fluorescent in situ hybridization diagnosis of extramedullary nodal blast crisis," *Diagnostic Cytopathology*, vol. 41, no. 3, pp. 253–256, 2013.

[5] P. J. Van Dijken, M. Niazi, and R. H. Al-Asiri, "Extramedullary blastic transformation in a child with adult chronic myelocytic leukemia," *Cancer Genetics and Cytogenetics*, vol. 76, no. 2, pp. 151–153, 1994.

[6] S. Tsukamoto, S. Ota, C. Ohwada et al., "Extramedullary blast crisis of chronic myelogenous leukemia as an initial presentation," *Leukemia Research Reports*, vol. 2, no. 2, pp. 67–69, 2013.

[7] Y.-L. Liu, X. N. Wang, and H. S. Liu, "Differential analysis of BM cell morphology, immunophenotypic, cytogenetic characters and prognosis between myeloblastic and lymphoblastic crisis of CML," *Zhongguo Shi Yan Xue Ye Xue Za Zhi*, vol. 22, no. 3, pp. 629–633, 2014.

[8] A. Alegre, E. Ojeda, R. Mataix, and T. Molero, "Ocular infiltration as a presenting form of extramedullary blast crisis in CML," *Sangre*, vol. 35, no. 3, pp. 236–237, 1990.

[9] J. H. Lipton, H. D. Mcgowan, and D. G. Payne, "Ocular masquerade syndrome in lymphoid blast crisis of chronic myeloid leukemia," *Leukemia and Lymphoma*, vol. 20, no. 1-2, pp. 161–163, 1995.

[10] I. Voican, A. M. Vlădăreanu, H. Bumbea, and M. Begu, "Sudden blast crisis in a chronic myeloid leukemia patient during imatinib therapy," *Romanian Journal of Internal Medicine*, vol. 50, no. 3, pp. 241–244, 2012.

[11] Y. Isobe, K. Sugimoto, A. Masuda, Y. Hamano, and K. Oshimi, "Central nervous system is a sanctuary site for chronic myelogenous leukaemia treated with imatinib mesylate," *Internal Medicine Journal*, vol. 39, no. 6, pp. 408–411, 2009.

[12] S. Bujassoum, J. Rifkind, and J. H. Lipton, "Isolated central nervous system relapse in lymphoid blast crisis chronic myeloid leukemia and acute lymphoblastic leukemia in patients on imatinib therapy," *Leukemia and Lymphoma*, vol. 45, no. 2, pp. 401–403, 2004.

[13] J. F. Leis, D. E. Stepan, P. T. Curtin et al., "Central nervous system failure in patients with chronic myelogenous leukemia lymphoid blast crisis and Philadelphia chromosome positive acute lymphoblastic leukemia treated with imatinib (STI-571)," *Leukemia and Lymphoma*, vol. 45, no. 4, pp. 695–698, 2004.

[14] M. Fuchs, M. Reinhöfer, A. Ragoschke-Schumm et al., "Isolated central nervous system relapse of chronic myeloid leukemia after allogeneic hematopoietic stem cell transplantation," *BMC Blood Disorders*, vol. 12, article 9, 2012.

[15] T. K. Saikia, B. Dhabhar, R. S. Iyer et al., "High incidence of meningeal leukemia in lymphoid blast crisis of chronic myelogenous leukemia," *American Journal of Hematology*, vol. 43, no. 1, pp. 10–13, 1993.

[16] A. Thomas, C. K. Stein, T. C. Gentile, and C. M. Shah, "Isolated CNS relapse of CML after bone marrow transplantation," *Leukemia Research*, vol. 34, no. 4, pp. e113–e114, 2010.

[17] T. Sharma, J. Grewal, S. Gupta, and P. I. Murray, "Ophthalmic manifestations of acute leukaemias: the ophthalmologist's role," *Eye*, vol. 18, no. 7, pp. 663–672, 2004.

[18] M. J. Taylor and P. A. Schuffham, "Pharmacoeconomic benefits of dasatinib in the treatment of imatinib-resistant patients with chronic myelogenous leukemia," *Expert Review of Pharmacoeconomics and Outcomes Research*, vol. 9, no. 2, pp. 117–121, 2009.

[19] K. Porkka, P. Koskenvesa, T. Lundán et al., "Dasatinib crosses the blood-brain barrier and is an efficient therapy for central nervous system Philadelphia chromosome-positive leukemia," *Blood*, vol. 112, no. 4, pp. 1005–1012, 2008.

[20] C. Fava, G. Rege-Cambrin, and G. Saglio, "The choice of first-line chronic myelogenous leukemia treatment," *Annals of Hematology*, vol. 94, supplement 2, pp. S123–S131, 2015.

[21] S. H. Swerdlow, E. Campo, N. Harris et al., Eds., *WHO Classification of Tumours of Haematopoietic and Lymphoid Tissues*, IARC, Lyon, France, 2008.

[22] J. Wei, M. Huang, Y. Wang, and J. Zhou, "Sudden extramedullary blast crisis of chronic myeloid leukemia manifesting as T-Cell lymphoblastic lymphoma," *Onkologie*, vol. 36, no. 3, pp. 119–122, 2013.

[23] C. P. Soupir, J.-A. Vergilio, P. Dal Cin et al., "Philadelphia chromosome-positive acute myeloid leukemia: a rare aggressive leukemia with clinicopathologic features distinct from chronic myeloid leukemia in myeloid blast crisis," *American Journal of Clinical Pathology*, vol. 127, no. 4, pp. 642–650, 2007.

[24] R. Berger, "Differences between blastic chronic myeloid leukemia and ph-positive acute leukemia," *Leukemia and Lymphoma*, vol. 11, supplement 1, pp. 235–237, 1993.

[25] A. Cuneo, A. Ferrant, J.-L. Michaux et al., "Philadelphia chromosome-positive acute myeloid leukemia: cytoimmunologic and cytogenetic features," *Haematologica*, vol. 81, no. 5, pp. 423–427, 1996.

[26] B. Calabretta and D. Perrotti, "The biology of CML blast crisis," *Blood*, vol. 103, no. 11, pp. 4010–4022, 2004.

[27] S.-J. Zhang, L.-Y. Ma, Q.-H. Huang et al., "Gain-of-function mutation of GATA-2 in acute myeloid transformation of chronic myeloid leukemia," *Proceedings of the National Academy of Sciences of the United States of America*, vol. 105, no. 6, pp. 2076–2081, 2008.

[28] C. V. Dang, "MYC on the path to cancer," *Cell*, vol. 149, no. 1, pp. 22–35, 2012.

[29] A. A. Zada, J. A. Pulikkan, D. Bararia et al., "Proteomic discovery of Max as a novel interacting partner of C/EBPα: a Myc/Max/Mad link," *Leukemia*, vol. 20, no. 12, pp. 2137–2146, 2006.

[30] Y. Huang, J. Zheng, J. D. Hu et al., "Discovery of somatic mutations in the progression of chronic myeloid leukemia by whole-exome sequencing," *Genetics and Molecular Research*, vol. 13, no. 1, pp. 945–953, 2014.

[31] S. Feo, D. Arcuri, E. Piddini, R. Passantino, and A. Giallongo, "ENO1 gene product binds to the c-myc promoter and acts as a transcriptional repressor: relationship with Myc promoter-binding protein 1 (MBP-1)," *FEBS Letters*, vol. 473, no. 1, pp. 47–52, 2000.

[32] T. Sato, "Evi1 defines leukemia-initiating capacity and tyrosine kinase inhibitor resistance in chronic myeloid leukemia," *Oncogene*, vol. 33, no. 42, pp. 5028–5038, 2014.

[33] F. Nakahara, J. Kitaura, T. Uchida et al., "Hes1 promotes blast crisis in chronic myelogenous leukemia through MMP-9 upregulation in leukemic cells," *Blood*, vol. 123, no. 25, pp. 3932–3942, 2014.

[34] C. Bourgne, A. Janel, J. Berger et al., "Phosphorylation of spleen tyrosine kinase at tyrosine 348 (pSyk^{348}) may be a marker of advanced phase of Chronic Myeloid Leukemia (CML)," *Leukemia Research*, vol. 39, no. 3, pp. 329–334, 2015.

[35] F. El Rassi, J. D. Bergsagel, M. Arellano et al., "Predicting early blast transformation in chronic-phase chronic myeloid leukemia: is immunophenotyping the missing link?" *Cancer*, vol. 121, no. 6, pp. 872–875, 2015.

28

Microsatellite Genotyping to Distinguish Somatic β-HCG Secreting Carcinoma from Epithelioid Trophoblastic Tumor

Mary Anne Brett, Monalisa Sur, Dean Daya, Jefferson Terry, and Alice Lytwyn

Department of Pathology and Molecular Medicine, McMaster University, 1280 Main Street West, Room No. HSC-1N16, Hamilton, ON, Canada L8S 4L8

Correspondence should be addressed to Mary Anne Brett; mary.brett@medportal.ca

Academic Editor: Mojgan Devouassoux

Objective. Morphologically, β-HCG secreting somatic carcinoma can be difficult to distinguish from epithelioid trophoblastic tumors (ETT). However, their distinction is critical due to their potentially differing prognoses and choice of chemotherapy. Presence of biparental alleles in ETT can be identified with molecular testing. We describe a patient who presented with metastatic carcinoma and elevated serum β-HCG and contrast this to an ETT in another patient. *Data and Results.* A 32-year-old female with recent possible miscarriage presented with pulmonary emboli and was found to have an increased serum β-HCG, a retroduodenal mass, and multiple nodules in her lungs, liver, and para-aortic lymph nodes. Biopsy showed a β-HCG and p63 positive epithelioid neoplasm with otherwise noncontributory immunohistochemistry. Molecular testing for biparental alleles in repeated length polymorphisms was negative, consistent with somatic origin. The second patient was a 35-year-old pregnant female with increased serum β-HCG and a uterine epithelioid tumor positive for β-HCG. Clinical and pathologic findings were characteristic of ETT and molecular testing was not required. These 2 cases illustrate that β-HCG secreting tumors of different etiologies may have similar appearances, and when clinical and/or IHC findings are inconclusive, molecular testing may be useful.

1. Introduction

Epithelioid trophoblastic tumor (ETT) is a malignant gestational neoplasm first described as a distinct entity in 1998 by Shih and Kurman [1]. It is an exceedingly rare tumor with fewer than 100 cases reported in the literature [2]. Women diagnosed with ETT often present with unexplained vaginal bleeding, amenorrhea, and a uterine mass [2], even up to 30 years after their initial pregnancy [3]. After the placenta is delivered, placental nodules can remain embedded in the myometrium and are usually reabsorbed over time. Sometimes they can persist, develop atypical cytological features, and transform into ETT [4].

ETT can pose many diagnostic challenges due to its rarity, the young age of those affected, late presentation after pregnancy, and histological mimickers. Somatic carcinoma, both β-HCG secreting and nonsecreting, can be morphologically difficult to distinguish from ETT. Their distinction is critical due to differing treatment options. ETT can be surgically and medically managed with hysterectomy and chemotherapy (etoposide, methotrexate, dactinomycin, cyclophosphamide, and vincristine) [5], although those with metastatic disease tend to be less responsive to conventional chemotherapy options [6].

To correctly identify ETT, genetic testing modalities may be useful in order to determine the presence of biparental alleles. Microsatellite genotyping using repeat length polymorphisms (RLP) is a genetic test that can be used to determine similarity of tissues. RLP testing can distinguish maternal from fetal tissues by identifying paternal RLPs. This testing is valuable when the differential diagnosis includes both somatic (self) and trophoblastic (nonself) neoplasms. We describe 2 cases of β-HCG secreting malignancy in young women that exemplify the potential value of RLP analysis as an adjunctive test in separating somatic carcinoma from gestational trophoblastic tumor.

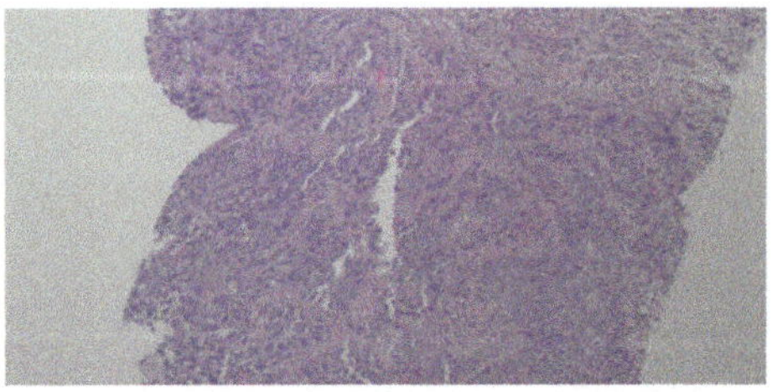

FIGURE 1: H & E. Liver core biopsy with nests of malignant epithelioid cells with eosinophilic cytoplasm.

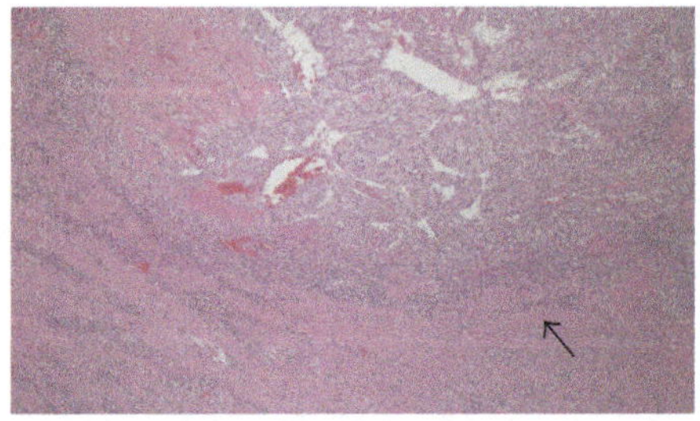

FIGURE 2: H & E. Mononucleate epithelioid tumor cells, rimmed by a lymphocytic infiltrate (arrow).

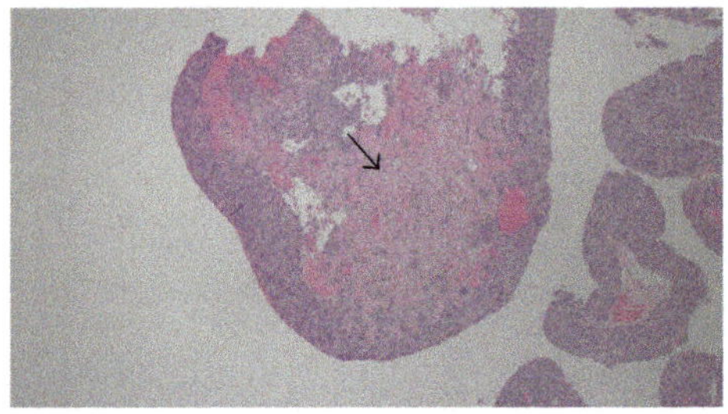

FIGURE 3: Tumor cells surrounded by eosinophilic hyaline-like material (arrow).

2. Material and Methods: Case Presentations

Case 1 (β-HCG secreting carcinoma). A 32-year-old female, with a history of an unconfirmed miscarriage, presented to the hospital with acute onset shortness of breath. A CT scan revealed bilateral pulmonary emboli and small pulmonary nodules (1 to 4 mm). An incidental elevated serum β-HCG (32 mIU/mL) was discovered during admission and continued to rise abnormally to a peak level of 169 mIU/mL. Subsequently, an ultrasound of the pelvis and liver showed a nongravid uterus and multiple small liver lesions. MRI confirmed the presence of metastatic hepatic nodules, as well as mesenteric masses and para-aortic nodal disease.

Biopsy of the liver lesions showed nests of malignant epithelioid cells with oval to round nuclei, abundant eosinophilic cytoplasm, and extensive necrosis (Figure 1). The malignant cells showed immunohistochemical (IHC) staining that was diffusely positive for β-HCG and p63. It was also positive for CD10, EMA, CK7, AE1/AE3, CK5/6, p16, CA-125, and p53 (patchy). Negative stains included inhibin, PLAP, AFP, CD30, CK20, CDX2, mucin, HepPar, BRST2, ER, Napsin, TTF1, WT1, S100, HMB45, CD117, and CD34.

To determine if the malignancy was of gestational origin, a maternal blood sample and the paraffin embedded liver core biopsy containing the tumor were PCR amplified using QIAamp DNA kit (QIAGEN). Nine polymorphic microsatellite loci from 9 chromosomes, including the locus for XY determination, were amplified and analyzed. No nonmaternal (nonself) alleles were discovered in the tumor. Genetic testing supported the diagnosis of poorly differentiated carcinoma with trophoblastic differentiation.

The patient was initially started on chemotherapy with etoposide, methotrexate, and daptomycin for presumed ETT. Once the diagnosis of somatic carcinoma was made, she was switched to oxaliplatin, leucovorin, and 5-fluorouracil (FOLFOX). A repeat CT scan showed extensive worsening of disease and a new splenic lesion (1.2 cm). The patient was discharged home with palliative measures and died 3 months after her initial presentation.

Case 2 (epithelioid trophoblastic tumor). A 35-year-old female (gravida 1) presented to her family physician with a positive pregnancy test. Her β-HCG was aberrantly elevated when compared to the expected gestational age of the fetus. Ultrasound of the pelvis showed a nonviable pregnancy, so she underwent a dilation and curettage (D&C). Despite the procedure, the patient's serum β-HCG level rose to 6541 mIU/mL and follow-up ultrasound showed a 1.9 cm echogenic vascular mass in the uterus. She then underwent a hysterectomy, bilateral salpingectomy, and pelvic lymph node dissection. Her serum β-HCG levels continually declined after the surgical management.

Pathology from the D&C and hysterectomy specimens were consistent with an epithelioid trophoblastic tumor and did not require further genetic testing. The tumor was composed of cells which showed a relatively monotonous, large, mononucleate epithelioid morphology with abundant cytoplasm within the endometrium and extending into the myometrium. The tumor had a circumscribed boarder with surrounding lymphocytic infiltrate (Figure 2). The tumor cells were surrounded by eosinophilic hyaline-like material (Figure 3) and there were areas of geographic necrosis. Tumor cells were diffusely positive for β-HCG, focally positive for p63, and negative for CD10, inhibin, and PLAP and had a high Ki-67 labelling index (>70%).

3. Results and Discussion

Gestational trophoblastic diseases are a spectrum of neoplasms that include (1) benign tumors (placental site nodule and exaggerated placental site reaction), (2) partial, complete, and invasive hydatidiform moles, and (3) malignant tumors (choriocarcinoma, epithelioid trophoblastic tumor, and placental site trophoblastic tumor).

With regard to ETT, most patients present with abnormal vaginal bleeding and are found to have a uterine or cervical primary tumor [7]. These tumors tend to respond poorly to chemotherapy and can present late, with metastases to the lungs and vagina being the most common [8]. Rare metastases have been reported in the lymph nodes, brain, liver, and skin [8]. In the literature, there are 10 cases of primary ETT presenting as an isolated lung mass without evidence of gynecological disease [7]. These lung tumors pose diagnostic challenges due to their morphological similarity to carcinoma and are easily misdiagnosed as primary nonsmall cell carcinoma (including squamous cell and pleomorphic carcinoma) or primary or metastatic germ cell tumors with trophoblastic differentiation [7]. Another issue that may hinder correct identification is that 40% of lung carcinomas aberrantly secrete β-HCG in the serum and stain positive on immunohistochemical analysis [3]. Histological clues to aid in diagnosing ETT within a lung biopsy are mononuclear tumor cells infiltrating alveolar spaces with preserved alveolar septa and no cytoplasmic eosinophilia or intracellular bridges [9].

There are sparse case reports and limited research to explain why ETT can present as a primary lung mass without gynecological involvement. The 2 classical etiologies include de novo transformation of trophoblastic cells that travel to the lungs during pregnancy and spontaneous regression of uterine ETT after spreading to the lungs [7]. However, the delayed presentation of lung ETT (reported up to 30 years after pregnancy) suggests that placental cells circulate through the maternal bloodstream and transform into a malignancy only after they have reached the lungs and not in the uterus after spontaneous trophoblastic tumor resolution [3].

Microsatellite genotyping is an effective test to differentiate gestational from nongestational tumors by the presence or absence of biparental alleles. This distinction is important when examining other more common trophoblastic diseases, such as gestational and nongestational choriocarcinoma. Most choriocarcinomas are derived from pregnancies, with very few arising independently from gestation (primary/nongestational choriocarcinoma) [10]. It is imperative to correctly distinguish between these tumors due to differing sensitivity to chemotherapy and overall prognosis [10]. Using microsatellite genotyping, choriocarcinoma can display 3 genetic patterns: (1) nongestational choriocarcinoma where all tumor alleles match those of the patient, (2) gestational choriocarcinoma, originating from androgenesis, where all tumor alleles belong to the partner and none are derived from the patient, and (3) gestational choriocarcinoma, originating from a diploid embryo, where the tumor alleles are of biparental origin [10]. Genetic testing in this situation would impact patient care because gestational choriocarcinomas, containing both patient and paternal genetic material, tend to be more chemosensitive and have a better prognosis than those of uniparental origin [10].

We report 2 patients who presented with elevated β-HCG as a result of differing neoplastic processes and how microsatellite genotyping, as an adjunct test, was helpful in reaching the final diagnosis. Epithelioid trophoblastic tumor is a very rare malignancy and therefore poses diagnostic pitfalls which must be addressed.

Several factors made our first case an especially challenging diagnosis. (1) The patient's possible history of miscarriage and young age were more in keeping with GTD as opposed to a somatic neoplasm, which would be less likely in this age group. (2) The mild incidental increase in β-HCG could have been due to ectopic pregnancy, GTD, or an extrauterine malignancy with trophoblastic differentiation. (3) Her presentation of nodules in the lungs, liver, mesentery, para-aortic lymph nodes, and eventually spleen, without evidence of disease in the uterus, remained unusual for GTD. Nonetheless, there are several case reports of ETT presenting in unusual locations including the lungs [5, 11], with unremarkable reproductive organs. (4) On light microscopy, the malignant cells resembled those seen in ETT, having large epithelioid cells with abundant eosinophilic cytoplasm and large areas of necrosis. (5) Multiple IHC panels were overall inconclusive therefore molecular genotyping was necessary and valuable.

In our second case, the clinical presentation, morphology of the neoplastic cells, IHC profile, and site of primary tumor were all consistent with ETT. Molecular testing with repeat length polymorphisms was not required for diagnosis.

In young female patients with elevated β-HCG, somatic metastatic carcinoma is unusual, so it is important to consider other diagnoses including gestational trophoblastic tumor. When the primary tumor site is unknown, histology and immunohistochemistry fail to delineate the origin, and epithelioid trophoblastic tumor remains in the differential diagnosis, then microsatellite genotyping is recommended.

Conflict of Interests

The authors declare that there is no conflict of interests regarding the publication of this paper.

References

[1] I. M. Shih and R. J. Kurman, "Epithelioid trophoblastic tumor: a neoplasm distinct from choriocarcinoma and placental site trophoblastic tumor simulating carcinoma," *The American Journal of Surgical Pathology*, vol. 22, no. 11, pp. 1393–1403, 1998.

[2] F. Y. Fang, C. R. Lai, M. J. Yang et al., "Diagnostic challenges in cornual epithelioid trophoblastic tumor," *Taiwanese Journal of Obstetrics and Gynecology*, vol. 53, no. 2, pp. 235–238, 2014.

[3] P. Fénichel, C. Rouzier, C. Butori et al., "Extragestational βHCG secretion due to an isolated lung epithelioid trophoblastic tumor: microsatellite genotyping of tumoral cells confirmed their placental origin and oriented specific chemotherapy," *The Journal of Clinical Endocrinology & Metabolism*, vol. 99, no. 10, pp. 3515–3520, 2014.

[4] F. E. Froeling and M. J. Seckl, "Gestational trophoblastic tumours: an update for 2014," *Current Oncology Reports*, vol. 16, no. 11, article 408, 2014.

[5] B. Madhu, R. Gerbi, and R. Nabila, "Epithelioid trophoblastic tumor and its diagnostic dilemmas: a rare case report," *Gynecologic Oncology Case Reports*, vol. 2, no. 2, pp. 42–43, 2012.

[6] I. M. Shih, "Gestational trophoblastic neoplasia-pathogenesis and potential therapeutic targets," *The Lancet Oncology*, vol. 8, no. 7, pp. 642–650, 2007.

[7] S. N. Lewin, C. Aghajanian, A. L. Moreira, and R. A. Soslow, "Extrauterine epithelioid trophoblastic tumors presenting as primary lung carcinomas: Morphologic and immunohistochemical features to resolve a diagnostic dilemma," *American Journal of Surgical Pathology*, vol. 33, no. 12, pp. 1809–1814, 2009.

[8] M. E. Cole, R. Broaddus, P. Thaker, C. Landen, and R. S. Freedman, "Placental-site trophoblastic tumors: a case of resistant pulmonary metastasis," *Nature Clinical Practice Cardiovascular Medicine*, vol. 5, no. 3, pp. 171–175, 2008.

[9] S. Hamazaki, S. Nakamoto, T. Okino et al., "Epithelioid trophoblastic tumor: morphological and immunohistochemical study of three lung lesions," *Human Pathology*, vol. 30, no. 11, pp. 1321–1327, 1999.

[10] J. Zhao, Y. Xiang, X. R. Wan, F. Z. Feng, Q. C. Cui, and X. Y. Yang, "Molecular genetic analyses of choriocarcinoma," *Placenta*, vol. 30, no. 9, pp. 816–820, 2009.

[11] I. C. Okereke and S. Chen, "Primary epithelioid trophoblastic tumor of the lung," *Annals of Thoracic Surgery*, vol. 97, no. 4, pp. 1420–1421, 2014.

Unexpected Malignant Diagnosis in Colonic Biopsies: Malignant Transformation of Ovarian Mature Teratomas—Two Case Reports and Review of the Literature

Claudia P. Rojas, Parvin Ganjei-Azar, and Monica T. Garcia-Buitrago

Department of Pathology, University of Miami Miller School of Medicine, Jackson Memorial Hospital, 1611 NW 12th Avenue, Holtz 2042C, Miami, FL 33136, USA

Correspondence should be addressed to Claudia P. Rojas; crojas@med.miami.edu

Academic Editor: Tibor Tot

Colorectal adenocarcinoma is the second cause of cancer-related deaths in the United States. The occurrence of squamous cell carcinoma in the colorectum is extremely unusual. Malignant transformation from mature cystic teratoma of the ovary is a rare event. The most common transformation is squamous cell carcinoma, followed by adenocarcinoma. It occurs more often in elderly patients, who usually present with advance disease. We report two unusual cases of postmenopausal women diagnosed with squamous cell carcinoma in colon biopsies. After surgical resections, the carcinoma was proven to be the result of malignant transformation of ovarian mature cystic teratomas. Since squamous cell carcinoma of the colorectum is extremely rare, the presence of squamous cell carcinoma in a colonic biopsy in a female patient should alert the clinicians to other possible primary sites, as seen in these cases.

1. Introduction

Colon cancer is the third most commonly diagnosed cancer and the second leading cause of cancer death in men and women in the United States. The American Cancer Society estimated that about 136,830 people were diagnosed with colorectal cancer in the United States, and about 50,310 people were predicted to die of the disease in 2014. Adenocarcinomas are by far the most common histologic type of colorectal cancer. Squamous cell carcinoma (SCC) of the colon is a rare entity, representing only a small fraction of colorectal malignancies [1].

We report two unusual cases of postmenopausal women diagnosed with squamous cell carcinoma in colon biopsies that, in follow-up, were proven to be the result of a malignant transformation of ovarian mature cystic teratomas.

2. Case Presentation

2.1. Case 1. A 71-year-old Hispanic woman with history of diabetes mellitus and hypertension presented with slowly progressive constipation for 6 months, mild, dull, nonradiating, lower abdominal pain, increased abdominal girth, and 50-pound weight loss. A computed tomography scan of the abdomen and pelvis demonstrated a large 18.9 × 12.8 × 12.5 cm heterogeneous mass originating either from the right adnexa or the intestine (Figure 1(a)). The serum tumor markers were CA19.9: 119 U/mL and CEA: 7.2 ng/mL.

A colonoscopy revealed a necrotic mass located at 25 cm from the anal verge. The colonic biopsy showed minute detached fragments of dysplastic squamous epithelium, highly suspicious for squamous cell carcinoma (Figure 1(b)). She underwent a hysterectomy with bilateral salpingoophorectomy and partial colectomy.

Gross examination of the specimen revealed an 18 cm cystic mass, attached to a 14 cm segment of the colon. The cyst was filled with tan sebaceous material and black hair and was attached to the colonic wall, where a firm white 11 cm solid mass was noted (Figure 1(c)). Microscopic examination revealed an invasive moderately differentiated keratinizing squamous cell carcinoma invading up to the submucosa of the colon (Figure 1(d)). The cystic component shows a mature

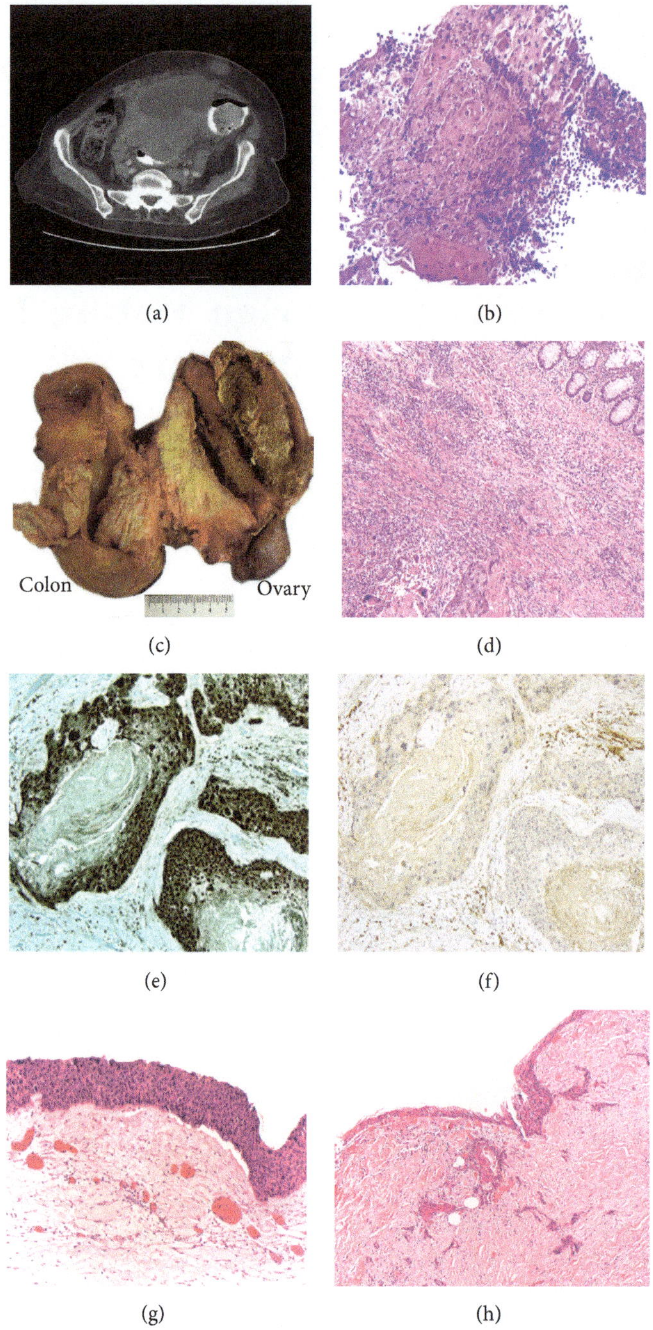

Figure 1: (a) Abdomen and pelvis CT showing a heterogenous mass with cystic and solid component. (b) Colon biopsy (H&E, 40x) showing a dysplastic squamous cell epithelium with keratin material, suspicious for squamous cell carcinoma. (c) Gross picture showing a cystic teratoma with sebaceous material and hair (right), the colon (left), and a firm white tan mass in between. (d) Squamous cell carcinoma (inferior left) invading into the colonic wall up to the submucosa (H&E, 20x). (e) P63 immunostain highlighting the tumor (20x). (f) Negative p16 immunostain (20x). (g) In situ squamous cell carcinoma (H&E 20x). (h) In situ squamous cell carcinoma with invasive component (H&E, 10x).

teratoma with in situ carcinoma in a squamous-lined cyst (Figures 1(d), 1(g), and 1(h)). The tumor cells were positive for p63 (Figure 1(e)) and negative for p16 (Figure 1(f)) by immunohistochemistry. The patient was deemed to be stage IIB and underwent 6 cycles of adjuvant chemotherapy with carboplatin and Taxotere. The tumor markers were still elevated one month after surgery; CA19-9 was 106.7 U/mL and CEA was 4.62 ng/mL. Two months later, an abdominal and pelvic CT scan revealed a new bilobed 5.5 cm mesenteric mass in the right hemipelvis, which was not separable from the adjacent bowel loops, an enlarged soft tissue mass in the left iliac fossa, and a subhepatic mesenteric mass. The patient

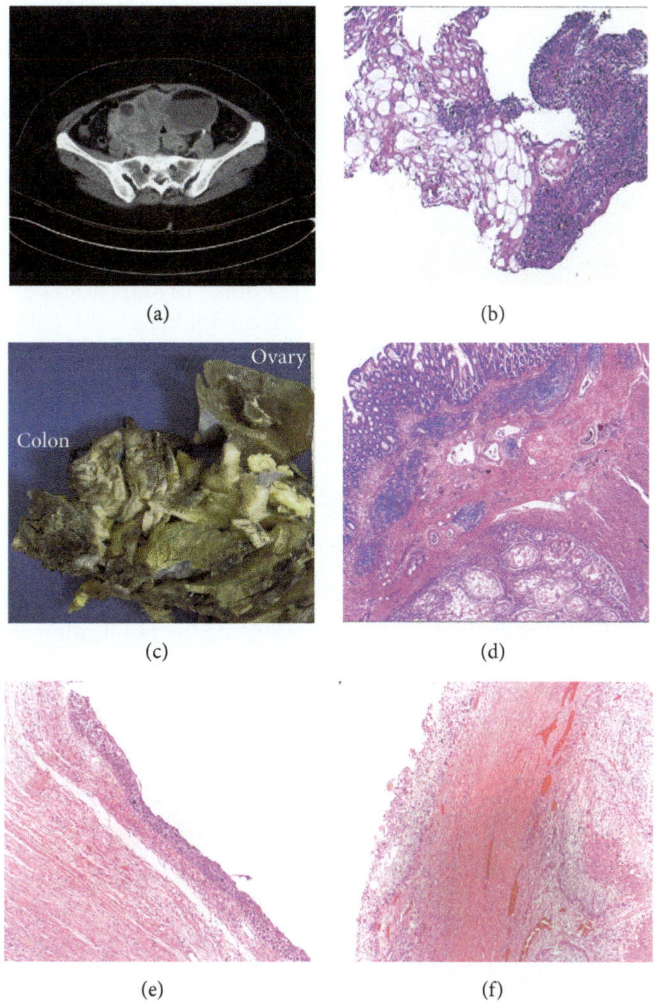

FIGURE 2: (a) Pelvis CT showing a mass with a cystic and solid component and internal septations. (b) Colon biopsy revealing an atypical squamous epithelium, suspicious for well-differentiated squamous cell carcinoma (H&E, 40x). (c) Gross picture showing a cystic ovarian mass (right) and (d) squamous cell carcinoma invading colonic wall (H&E, 20x). (e) In situ squamous cell carcinoma (H&E, 10x). (f) In situ squamous cell carcinoma and invasive component (H&E, 10x).

declined any type of additional chemotherapy, moved to a different city, and was lost in follow-up.

2.2. Case 2. A 55-year-old Hispanic female complained of pelvic pain, loss of appetite, weakness, and 40-pound weight loss in the last 5 months. She was also noted to have a small amount of bright blood per rectum.

A computed tomography scan of the abdomen showed a 17 × 14 × 11 cm pelvic mass with cystic and solid components and internal septations, which appeared to encase the sigmoid colon (Figure 2(a)).

A colonoscopy was performed to reveal a friable and hyperemic colonic mucosa at about 20 cm from the anus. A colonic biopsy showed fragments of a highly atypical squamous epithelium, suggestive of squamous cell carcinoma. No colonic mucosa was present (Figure 2(b)). The tumor markers were CA19.9: 50.1 U/mL and CEA: 3.7 ng/mL.

The patient underwent a hysterectomy with bilateral salpingoophorectomy and rectosigmoid resection with end-to-end anastomosis.

Gross examination of the specimen revealed a 16 cm multiloculated solid and cystic adnexal mass attached to a 12 cm segment of rectosigmoid colon. The heterogeneous cystic mass was filled with adipose tissue, hair, and sebaceous material. Upon opening, the segment of colon showed a large fistulous tract that measures 2 cm in diameter (Figure 2(c)).

Microscopic examination revealed a moderately differentiated squamous cell carcinoma invading up to submucosa of the colon (Figure 2(d)) and an in situ squamous cell carcinoma component in the lining of the ovarian cyst (Figures 2(e) and 2(f)). The patient was deemed to be stage IIIB and received six cycles of chemotherapy with cisplatin and taxol. She completed the chemotherapy and, after 8 months, there was no evidence of recurrence. After that, she was lost in follow-up.

3. Discussion

Primary colorectal squamous cell carcinoma is an exceedingly rare malignancy representing 0.25–1 per 1000 colorectal carcinomas [2]. To date, about 120 cases of SCC have been reported in the world literature [3]. Before the diagnosis of primary SCC of colorectum is made, certain criteria must be fulfilled as established by Williams et al. in 1979 [4]. These criteria include (A) absence of squamous cell carcinoma in any other part of the body, excluding potential metastasis to the colorectal site; (B) exclusion of any proximal extension of anal squamous cell carcinoma; (C) absence of fistulous tract lined by squamous cells; and (D) confirmation of SCC by histological analysis [1, 3].

Ovarian germ cell tumors account for about 20–25% of the ovarian neoplasms. Mature cystic teratoma (MCT) is the most common ovarian germ cell tumor, representing 10–20% of all ovarian tumors. Malignant transformation (MT) occurs in less than 2% of ovarian cystic teratomas, with squamous cell carcinoma being the most common type [5]. Most MCTs are detected 15 to 20 years before they undergo a secondary malignant transformation [6]. Thus, SCC in MCT is more common in postmenopausal patients. Historically, the carcinomas are diagnosed postoperatively because there is no particular sign or symptom characteristic of a malignancy arising in mature cystic teratomas. Presenting symptoms may include abdominal pain and distension secondary to a pelvic mass. The patient with advance disease may also present with bowel or bladder symptoms.

Studies performed by Kikkawa et al. and Dos Santos et al. concluded that a tumor diameter of 10 cm or greater or a tumor demonstrating rapid growth should be a cause for concern [7, 8]. Risk factors for MT of an MCT include patient's age, tumor size, imaging characteristics, and serum tumor markers [9]. Tumor stage is the most important prognostic factor, as most of the survivors presented with early-stage disease [7]. In a review of 188 patients, Ruey-Jien et al. reported a 5-year survival rate of 75,5%; 33,3%; 20,6%, and 0% for patients with stages I, II, III, and IV, respectively [10]. The prognosis of patients with advance squamous cell carcinoma of the ovary is poor regardless of the treatment received [11]. Due to the rare incidence of malignant transformation of mature cystic teratomas, adjuvant treatment has not been standardized; however, in a review paper, Sakuma et al. recommended the use of platinum/taxane chemotherapy [12]. It has been shown that the prognosis of MT is significantly worse than that of epithelial ovarian cancer, regardless of the use of adjuvant chemotherapy or radiotherapy [8]. Ovarian carcinomas composed entirely of squamous cells arise most often in dermoid cysts but have also been reported in association with endometriosis and in a pure de novo form [13]. In order to establish the diagnosis of pure primary ovarian squamous cell carcinoma, it is necessary to exclude extragenital and genital squamous cell carcinoma as well as endometriosis [14]. These tumors are usually diagnosed after resection with extensive histologic evaluation.

Few manuscripts have reported the use of imaging modalities to diagnose MT of MCT. Kido et al. reported the MRI findings for six MCT with MT. They described solid portions present in five out of six tumors; two of them were enhanced by gadolinium to varying degrees [15]. The presence of solid, friable, or variegated components, extensive transmural extension, and direct invasion of neighboring pelvic organs suggests the possibility of MT [16–18]. In our cases, the squamous cell carcinoma infiltrated the adjacent colon, precluding the identification of the origin of the tumor at the preoperative initial biopsy.

We conclude that, in postmenopausal patients with colorectal SCC, other sources should be considered including metastasis or tumor extension of cervical or vaginal carcinoma and malignant transformation of mature cystic teratoma. In our cases, the unusual finding of squamous cell carcinoma in the colonic biopsies creates a diagnostic dilemma and the pathologist should raise the possibility of secondary involvement. Malignant transformation of a MCT must be included in the differential diagnosis when squamous cell carcinoma is found above the anal verge, especially if present in conjunction with a large pelvic mass.

Conflict of Interests

The authors declare that there is no conflict of interests regarding the publication of this paper.

References

[1] T. Dyson and P. V. Draganov, "Squamous cell cancer of the rectum," *World Journal of Gastroenterology*, vol. 15, no. 35, pp. 4380–4386, 2009.

[2] C. S. R. Nahas, J. Shia, R. Joseph et al., "Squamous-cell carcinoma of the rectum: a rare but curable tumor," *Diseases of the Colon and Rectum*, vol. 50, no. 9, pp. 1393–1400, 2007.

[3] A. S. Sameer, N. Syeed, N. A. Chowdri, F. Q. Parray, and M. A. Siddiqi, "Squamous cell carcinoma of rectum presenting in a man: a case report," *Journal of Medical Case Reports*, vol. 4, article 392, 2010.

[4] G. T. Williams, A. J. Blackshaw, and B. C. Morson, "Squamous carcinoma of the colorectum and its genesis," *The Journal of Pathology*, vol. 129, no. 3, pp. 139–147, 1979.

[5] J. Rosai, *Rosai and Ackerman's Surgical Pathology*, vol. 2, Mosby, 9th edition, 2004.

[6] P. Russel and A. Farnsworth, "Teratomas with secondary malignant transformation," in *Surgical Pathology of the Ovaries*, pp. 545–551, Churchill Livingstone, New York, NY, USA, 2nd edition, 1997.

[7] F. Kikkawa, A. Nawa, K. Tamakoshi et al., "Diagnosis of squamous cell carcinoma arising from mature cystic teratoma of the ovary," *Cancer*, vol. 82, no. 11, pp. 2249–2255, 1998.

[8] L. Dos Santos, E. Mok, A. Iasonos et al., "Squamous cell carcinoma arising in mature cystic teratoma of the ovary: a case series and review of the literature," *Gynecologic Oncology*, vol. 105, no. 2, pp. 321–324, 2007.

[9] A.-J. Chiang, V. La, J. Peng, K.-J. Yu, and N. N. H. Teng, "Squamous cell carcinoma arising from mature cystic teratoma of the ovary," *International Journal of Gynecological Cancer*, vol. 21, no. 3, pp. 466–474, 2011.

[10] R.-J. Chen, K.-Y. Chen, T.-C. Chang, B.-C. Sheu, S.-N. Chow, and S.-C. Huang, "Prognosis and treatment of squamous cell carcinoma from a mature cystic teratoma of the ovary," *Journal of the Formosan Medical Association*, vol. 107, no. 11, pp. 857–868, 2008.

[11] M. Gainford, A. Tinker, J. Carter et al., "Malignant transformation within ovarian dermoid cysts: an audit of treatment received and patient outcomes. an Australia New Zealand gynaecological oncology group (ANZGOG) and gynaecologic cancer intergroup (GCIG) study," *International Journal of Gynecological Cancer*, vol. 20, no. 1, pp. 75–81, 2010.

[12] M. Sakuma, T. Otsuki, K. Yoshinaga et al., "Malignant transformation arising from mature cystic teratoma of the ovary: a retrospective study of 20 cases," *International Journal of Gynecological Cancer*, vol. 20, no. 5, pp. 766–771, 2010.

[13] G. Ben-Baruch, Y. Menashe, E. Herczeg, and J. Menczer, "Pure primary ovarian squamous cell carcinoma," *Gynecologic Oncology*, vol. 29, no. 2, pp. 257–262, 1988.

[14] M. R. Pins, R. H. Young, W. J. Daly, and R. E. Scully, "Primary squamous cell carcinoma of the ovary: report of 37 cases," *American Journal of Surgical Pathology*, vol. 20, no. 7, pp. 823–833, 1996.

[15] A. Kido, K. Togashi, I. Konishi et al., "Dermoid cysts of the ovary with malignant transformation: MR appearance," *American Journal of Roentgenology*, vol. 172, no. 2, pp. 445–449, 1999.

[16] K. B. Badmos, O. K. Ibrahim, A. P. Aboyeji, and J. A. Omotayo, "Squamous cell carcinoma arising in a mature cystic ovarian teratoma with bladder invasion: a case report," *African Health Sciences*, vol. 11, no. 2, pp. 285–287, 2011.

[17] W. Song and M. Conner, "Squamous cell carcinoma arising within a mature cystic teratoma with invasion into the adjacent small intestine: a case report," *International Journal of Gynecological Pathology*, vol. 31, no. 3, pp. 272–275, 2012.

[18] Y.-C. Lee, O. Abulafia, N. Montalto, K. Holcomb, R. Matthews, and R. W. Golub, "Malignant transformation of an ovarian mature cystic teratoma presenting as a rectal mass," *Gynecologic Oncology*, vol. 75, no. 3, pp. 499–503, 1999.

Beta-Human Chorionic Gonadotropin Producing Osteosarcoma of the Sacrum in a 26-Year-Old Woman: A Case Report and Review of the Literature

Ryan Glass, Jaya Ruth Asirvatham, Leonard Kahn, and Mohamed Aziz

Department of Pathology, North Shore Long Island Jewish, New Hyde Park, NY 11040, USA

Correspondence should be addressed to Ryan Glass; rglass01@gmail.com

Academic Editor: Katsuyuki Aozasa

Ectopic secretion of beta-human chorionic gonadotropin is considered a poor prognostic marker in epithelial tumors. However, very few cases have been reported in sarcomas. We present the case of a 26-year-old female who presented with a metastatic osteosarcoma. She underwent usual testing prior to starting treatment and was found to have elevated levels of beta-human chorionic gonadotropin. As the patient was not pregnant, another source of beta-human chorionic gonadotropin secretion had to be considered. The tumor cells demonstrated positive staining for beta-human chorionic gonadotropin by immunohistochemistry, and serum levels of beta-human chorionic gonadotropin were used to monitor tumor progression and response to chemotherapy. We review the literature and discuss a potential role of beta-human chorionic gonadotropin in the treatment of such patients.

1. Introduction

Beta-human chorionic gonadotropin (β-hCG) is normally produced by syncytiotrophoblasts of the placenta and may also be secreted by germ cell neoplasms. Ectopic secretion of β-hCG by epithelial tumors, including bladder, lung, and colorectal cancers, is a recognized phenomenon associated with a poorer prognosis [1]. However, ectopic β-hCG expression has been less frequently reported in sarcomas, with very few known in osteosarcomas. We present a case of a female patient with an osteosarcoma who was incidentally discovered to have elevated serum β-hCG levels. Immunohistochemical staining identified the tumor as the source of the hormone and serum levels were used to monitor the tumor's response to treatment and progression.

2. Case Report

A 26-year-old female presented to an outside institution with pelvic pain over the previous several months. A CT scan revealed a large lytic lesion in the pelvis, multiple paraspinal soft tissue masses, parasacral soft tissue masses, and a lytic lesion in the L4 vertebral body (Figures 1(a) and 1(b)), with a chest X-ray showing multiple lung lesions. Biopsies of the paraspinal masses revealed a high-grade sarcoma. She was seen at our institution approximately one month later. Biopsies taken from the pelvic mass showed identical features to those of the paraspinal masses. During the initial workup, the patient was found to have serum β-hCG levels of 693 mIU/mL and pregnancy was suspected. However, pregnancy was ruled out as her menstrual bleeding was 3 weeks earlier and she had never been sexually active. The possibility of a β-hCG secreting tumor was considered, and the tumor cells stained strongly positive for β-hCG. The final diagnosis was that of a β-hCG secreting osteogenic sarcoma. As metastases were present at the time of diagnosis, the patient was not a surgical candidate. Chemotherapy with methotrexate and ifosfamide was initiated. Serum β-hCG levels, which were monitored throughout the patient's course, transiently fell after each treatment. This drop correlated with radiologic response to treatment. However, as this was an aggressive tumor, it tended to regrow in spite of treatment. These periods of growth were accompanied by rising β-hCG levels.

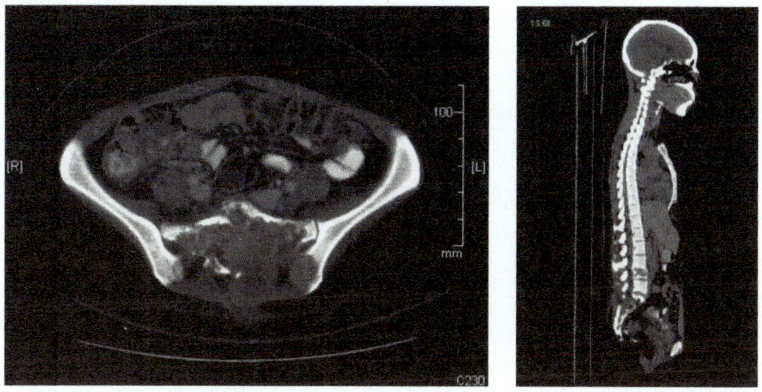

(a) (b)

FIGURE 1: CT Scan showing tumor invasion of sacrum: left and right surrounding parasacral soft tissue (a), and L4 vertebral body (b).

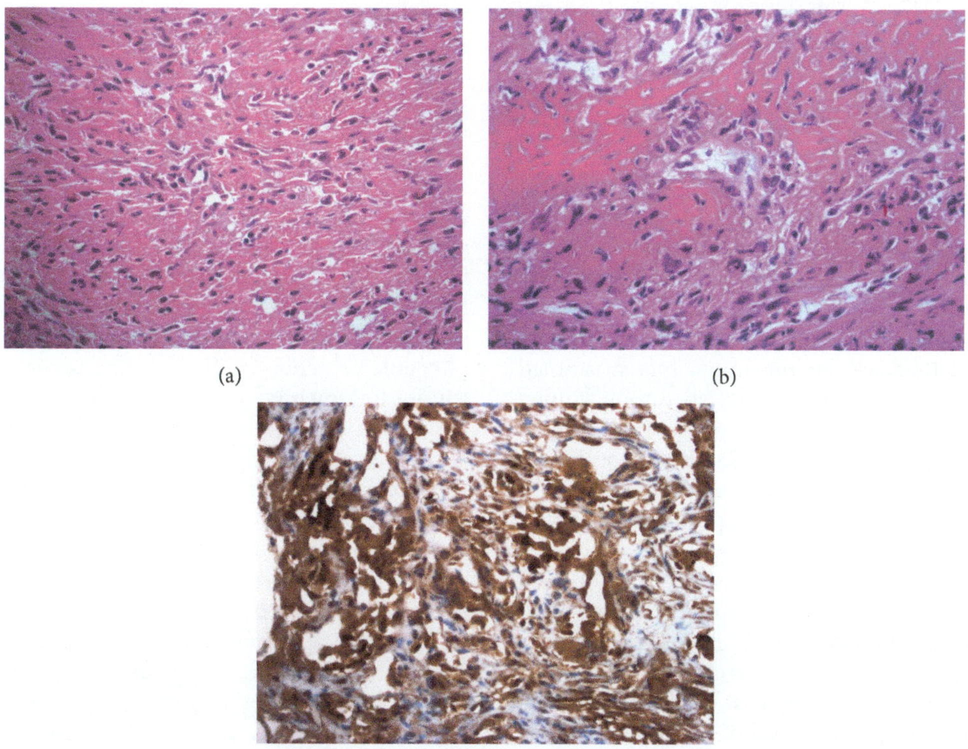

(a) (b) (c)

FIGURE 2: Osteosarcoma of pelvis demonstrating hyperchromatic spindle-shaped tumor cells associated with matrix production (a) and osteoid formation (b). Tumor stains positive for β-hCG (c) (Hematoxylin-eosin [a, b], original magnifications ×4 [c], ×20 [a-b]).

3. Microscopic Description

Microscopic examination of the biopsy specimens revealed a mass composed primarily of malignant spindle cells, infiltrating bone and soft tissue with no recognizable architectural pattern. The tumor cells appeared cytologically atypical with focal areas of pleomorphism and mitoses up to 4 per 10 high-power fields. Multiple areas of osteoid formation and scattered benign appearing giant cells were noted within the tumor (Figures 2(a) and 2(b)). Initial studies were positive for vimentin, focally positive for CD68, and negative for cytokeratin, CK7, CD34, and S100.

Additional studies were requested after the patient was found to have high levels of β-hCG (Figure 2(c)). These revealed the tumor to be positive for β-hCG and negative for placental alkaline phosphatase, epithelial membrane antigen, smooth muscle antigen, desmin, myogenin, and CD31.

4. Discussion

To the best of our knowledge, very few cases of β-hCG secreting osteosarcomas exist in the literature (Table 1). The mean age of these patients was 22 years (range: 5–57 years) with

Table 1: Previously reported cases of β-hCG producing osteosarcoma.

Author	Age	Sex	Chemotherapy	Status
Kalra et al. [2]	21	F	Vinblastine, bleomycin, and cisplatin	Died during treatment
Tuy et al. [3]	37	F	None	Died from disease progression
Boss et al. [4]	57	F	Doxorubicin and cisplatin; ifosfamide and etoposide; Cyclophosphamide and imatinib; E7080	Initial success with E7080, followed by disease progression
Masrouha et al. [5]	17	F	Regimen unknown	Lung metastases
	14	M	Regimen unknown	Died during treatment
	17	F	Regimen unknown	No recurrence
	17	M	Regimen unknown	Lung metastases
	5	M	Regimen unknown	Died during treatment
Leidinger et al. [6]	18	F	COSS-96; COSS-96 with carboplatin, etoposide, and RT	Lost to follow-up
Oshrine et al. [7]	14	F	Doxorubicin and ifosfamide, cisplatin regimen	Disease free after 6 months
Ordonez et al. [8]	26	F	Unknown	Unknown
Our case	26	F	Methotrexate and ifosfamide	Died from progressive disease

nine females and three males. In cases where serum β-hCG testing was performed, levels as high as 5000 mIU/mL have been reported although the significance of this is unclear [2]. Of the ten patients with available follow-up, eight have died or experienced lung metastases. One of Masrouha et al.'s patients, however, experienced a complete response although it should be noted that cells of the initial biopsy stained weakly positive and those from the excised tumor stained negative [5]. Leidinger et al.'s patient also remained disease free, although follow-up was only available for six months [6]. As the majority of these tumors demonstrated an unfavorable rapidly progressing course, this paraneoplastic feature may portend poor prognosis in osteosarcomas.

It is difficult to ascertain the true incidence of β-hCG producing osteosarcomas. As most cases in the literature (as well as ours) were discovered incidentally by urine pregnancy screening, it is likely that many others are missed, especially in male patients. To determine the rate of β-hCG positivity, Ordonez et al. retrospectively stained 11 osteosarcoma specimens for β-hCG, finding that only two (18.2%) stained positive [8]. In a more recent study, by Masrouha et al., 5 of 32 (15.6%) retrospectively stained specimens showed β-hCG positivity, 3 of which were from male patients [5].

The significance of β-hCG-staining in tumor cells as well is unclear. While it has been shown that staining intensity in carcinomas correlates with tumor grade [1], it is unknown if this relationship holds in osteosarcomas as very few studies have examined this. Leidinger et al. reported positive staining in dedifferentiated metastases of negatively staining primary tumors [6], and Masrouha et al. reported that four of the five cases stained positively in histologically high-grade tumors [5]. However, Oshrine et al. reported no morphological differences between β-hCG-positive and β-hCG-negative cells within the same tumor [7]. In our case, the tumor appeared of low-grade and, similar to Orhrine's findings, no noticeable differences were seen between β-hCG-positive and β-hCG-negative areas.

X-ray crystallography of β-hCG revealed a quaternary structure containing a "cysteine knot," making it structurally similar to other members of the "cysteine knot growth factors" (CKGF) super family such as transforming growth factor beta (TGFβ), platelet derived growth factor (PDGF), vascular endothelial growth factor (VEGF), and bone morphogenic proteins [1]. This finding is consistent with observations linking high serum hCG levels with tumor neovascularization [9], as well as studies showing that addition of hCG may reverse the proapoptotic effects of TGFβ [10]. hCG may therefore stimulate growth of these tumors through agonistic and antagonistic interactions with receptors of other CKGFs.

Currently, the role of beta-hCG in osteosarcoma management is not well established. However, several prior studies demonstrated that β-hCG expressing tumors respond poorly to chemotherapy, and changes in serum levels correlate with relapse and response to treatment [3, 5, 6]. In Boss et al.'s patient, it was found that initial drops followed by increases in β-hCG levels corresponded with radiologic response to E7080, an investigational tyrosine kinase inhibitor that targets VEGFR-2 and VEGFR-3 with secondary activity against PDGFR-β, FGFR-1, and C-KIT. Taking these observations together, they hypothesized that β-hCG could mediate resistance to VEGF inhibition [3], consistent with prior reports of β-hCG interactions with CKGF superfamily receptors.

Conflict of Interests

The authors declare that there is no conflict of interests.

References

[1] R. K. Iles, P. J. Delves, and S. A. Butler, "Does hCG or hCGβ play a role in cancer cell biology?" *Molecular and Cellular Endocrinology*, vol. 329, no. 1-2, pp. 62–70, 2010.

[2] J. K. Kalra, R. Mir, L. B. Kahn, Z. Wessely, and A. B. Shah, "Osteogenic sarcoma producing human chorionic

gonadotrophin. Case report with immunohistochemical studies," *Cancer*, vol. 53, no. 10, pp. 2125–2128, 1984.

[3] B. E. Tuy, A. A. Obafemi, K. S. Beebe, and F. R. Patterson, "Case report: elevated serum beta human chorionic gonadotropin in a woman with osteosarcoma," *Clinical Orthopaedics and Related Research*, vol. 466, no. 4, pp. 997–1001, 2008.

[4] D. S. Boss, H. Glen, J. H. Beijnen et al., "Serum β-HCG and CA-125 as tumor markers in a patient with osteosarcoma: case report," *Tumori*, vol. 97, no. 1, pp. 109–114, 2011.

[5] K. Z. Masrouha, R. Khattab, A. Tawil et al., "A preliminary investigation of beta-hCG expression in patients with osteosarcoma," *Journal of Bone and Joint Surgery—Series B*, vol. 94, no. 3, pp. 419–424, 2012.

[6] B. Leidinger, S. Bielack, G. Koehler, V. Vieth, W. Winkelmann, and G. Gosheger, "High level of beta-hCG simulating pregnancy in recurrent osteosarcoma: case report and review of literature," *Journal of Cancer Research and Clinical Oncology*, vol. 130, no. 6, pp. 357–361, 2004.

[7] B. R. Oshrine, L. M. Sullivan, and N. J. Balamuth, "Ectopic production of β-hCG by osteosarcoma: a case report and review of the literature," *Journal of Pediatric Hematology/Oncology*, vol. 36, no. 3, pp. e202–e206, 2014.

[8] N. G. Ordonez, A. G. Ayala, A. K. Raymond, C. Plager, R. S. Benjamin, and N. A. Samaan, "Ectopic production of the β-subunit of human chorionic gonadotropin in osteosarcoma," *Archives of Pathology & Laboratory Medicine*, vol. 113, no. 4, pp. 416–419, 1989.

[9] O. Arrieta, R. M. Michel Ortega, J. Ángeles-Snchez et al., "Serum human chorionic gonadotropin is associated with angiogenesis in germ cell testicular tumors," *Journal of Experimental and Clinical Cancer Research*, vol. 28, no. 1, article 120, 2009.

[10] S. A. Butler, M. S. Ikram, S. Mathieu, and R. K. Iles, "The increase in bladder carcinoma cell population induced by the free beta subunit of human chorionic gonadotrophin is a result of an anti-apoptosis effect and not cell proliferation," *British Journal of Cancer*, vol. 82, no. 9, pp. 1553–1556, 2000.

31

A Rare Case of Erdheim-Chester Disease and Langerhans Cell Histiocytosis Overlap Syndrome

Shahzaib Nabi,[1] Adeel Arshad,[2] Tarun Jain,[1] Fawad Virk,[1] Rohit Gulati,[3] and Rana Awdish[4]

[1]*Department of Internal Medicine, Henry Ford Health System, 2799 W. Grand Boulevard, Detroit, MI 48202, USA*
[2]*Department of Internal Medicine, Hamad Medical Corporation, Weill Cornell University, Doha, Qatar*
[3]*Department of Pathology, Henry Ford Health System, 2799 W. Grand Boulevard, Detroit, MI 48202, USA*
[4]*Department of Pulmonary and Critical Care Medicine, Henry Ford Health System, 2799 W. Grand Boulevard, Detroit, MI 48202, USA*

Correspondence should be addressed to Shahzaib Nabi; snabi1@hfhs.org

Academic Editor: Hiroko Kuwabara

A 48-year-old woman with a past medical history of seizures and end-stage renal disease secondary to obstructive uropathy from retroperitoneal fibrosis presented to the emergency department with seizures and altered mental status. A Glasgow Coma Scale of 4 prompted intubation, and she was subsequently admitted to the intensive care unit. Magnetic resonance imaging of the brain performed to elucidate the aetiology of her seizure showed a dural-based mass within the left temporoparietal lobe as well as mass lesions within the orbits. Further imaging showed extensive retroperitoneal fibrosis extending to the mediastinum with involvement of aorta and posterior pleural space. Imaging of the long bones showed bilateral sclerosis and cortical thickening of the diaphyses. Imaging of the maxillofacial structures showed osseous destructive lesions involving the mandible. These clinical and radiological features were consistent with a diagnosis of Erdheim-Chester disease; however, the patient's skin biopsy was consistent with Langerhans cell histiocytosis.

1. Introduction

Both Erdheim-Chester disease (ECD) and Langerhans cell histiocytosis (LCH) are histiocytic disorders and are extremely rare. Review of the literature shows cases of overlap between ECD and LCH. The purpose of writing this case report is to strengthen the limited knowledge of such an overlap syndrome. Moreover, such case reports suggest that these 2 disorders might not be completely separate entities and, hence, can lead to a better understanding of the pathophysiology of these disorders.

More importantly, such case reports aid clinicians in making an accurate diagnosis when faced with this rare group of disorders. Early diagnosis and prompt treatment can confer improved outcomes, both clinically and in terms of patient satisfaction.

2. Case Presentation

Our patient is a 48-year-old female with a past medical history of end-stage renal disease secondary to obstructive uropathy from retroperitoneal fibrosis (with bilateral ureteral stents). She also had a past medical history of intermittent seizures. She presented to the hospital with altered mental status that had been waxing and waning for the past 2 weeks.

On physical examination in the emergency department, she was found to have a temperature of 39.2°Celsius, pulse of 110 beats/minute, respiratory rate of 22 breaths/minute, and blood pressure of 83/42 mmHg. On neurological examination, the patient was found to be alert to person, but not to time or place. She was moving all 4 extremities without any apparent focal neurological deficit. Reflexes were normal in both upper and lower extremities. The rest of the neurological

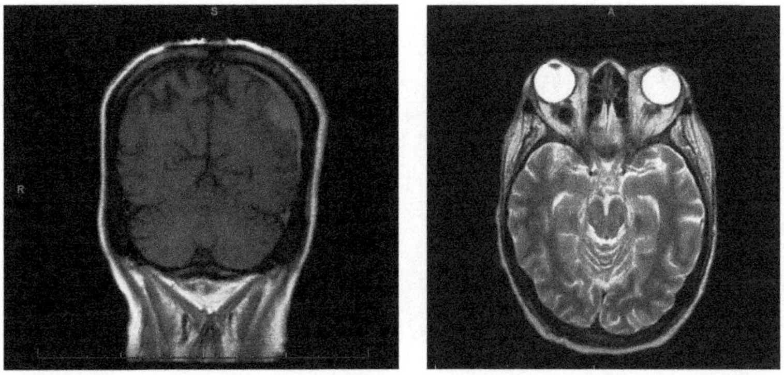

(a) (b)

FIGURE 1: MRI brain coronal section (a) and transverse section (b) showing dural-based mass in the left temporoparietal region as well as mass lesions within the orbits.

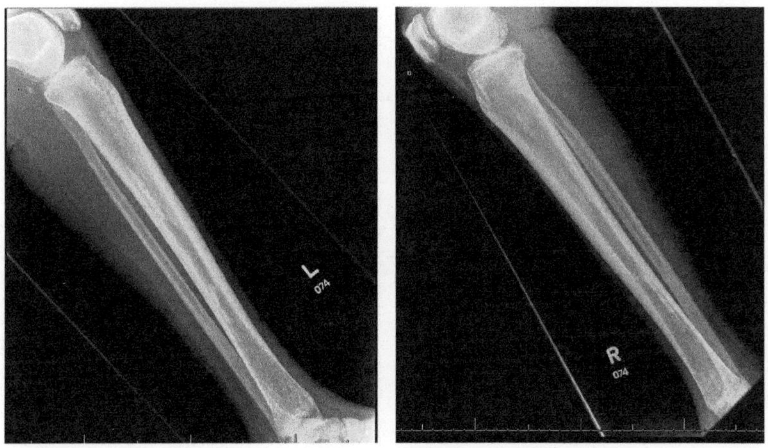

FIGURE 2: X-ray of both legs showing regions of sclerotic cortical thickening identified in the posterior distal metadiaphysis and anterior metadiaphysis of the tibia with additional sclerosis of the metadiaphyseal regions of the fibula.

examination was limited as the patient was unable to follow commands. Cardiovascular examination showed normal S1 and S2 with no added sounds. Respiratory and abdominal examinations were unremarkable. Skin examination showed chronic ulcers on the lower extremities in different stages of healing. She was also found to have scaly erythematous papules in her right axillary skin fold.

Her family history was unremarkable. She was a lifelong nonsmoker and nonalcoholic and never used any illicit drugs. She was on levetiracetam for seizures, which she was taking as prescribed (according to the family).

Patient was found to be in septic shock secondary to infected ureteral stents. She was admitted to the intensive care unit and her ureteral stents were removed. She received broad spectrum intravenous antibiotics and aggressive fluid resuscitation with resolution of her septic shock and normalization of her hemodynamics. However, her mental status did not improve with resolution of the sepsis. Imaging studies showed a dural-based mass in the left temporoparietal region as well as mass lesions within the orbits. Further work-up showed lytic lesions involving the mandible and axilla. Bilateral cortical thickening and sclerosis of the long bones of the extremities was also noted. Her retroperitoneal fibrosis was found to be extending into her mediastinum with encasement of the vessels and pleural involvement. These findings were consistent with a diagnosis of ECD; however, the patient's skin biopsy was consistent with a diagnosis of LCH.

3. Investigations

3.1. Pertinent Imaging Investigations. Magnetic resonance imaging of the brain showed a dural-based mass within the left temporoparietal lobe. Evidence of mass lesions within the orbits with tram track appearance was found on fluid-attenuated inversion recovery imaging (Figure 1). X-rays of the long bones of the extremities displayed evidence of sclerosis and cortical thickening involving the bilateral radial and ulnar diaphyses. Regions of metadiaphyseal sclerosis and cortical thickening were identified in the bilateral tibias and fibulas (Figure 2).

Radiographic imaging of the skull showed large lytic lesions involving the alveolar regions of bilateral maxillae, as well as symphysis, body, and alveolar ridge of the mandible

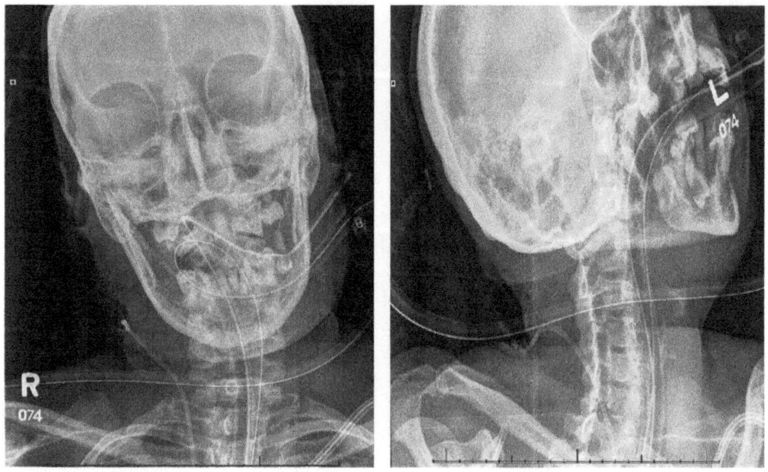

FIGURE 3: X-ray of the skull, showing lytic lesions in the mandible and bilateral maxillae.

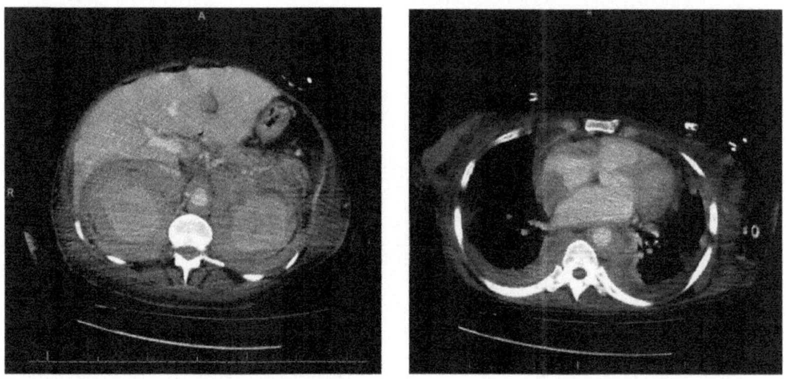

(a) (b)

FIGURE 4: CT of the abdomen (a) showing extensive retroperitoneal soft tissue (fibrosis) surrounding the kidney and vessels. The soft tissue is seen extending into the mediastinum with involvement of the pleura, heart, and vessels (b).

bilaterally (Figure 3). Extensive soft tissue surrounding both of the kidneys, the aorta, and the retroperitoneum, extending along the great peritoneal vessels, was found on computed tomography of the abdomen and pelvis. Computed tomography of the chest further showed that the soft tissue from the retroperitoneal region extended into the mediastinum and was surrounding the heart, the aorta, and pulmonary arteries and extending along the paraspinal region (Figure 4).

3.2. Pertinent Laboratory Investigations. Complete blood count (on presentation) showed a white blood cell count of 28,000/mm^3 and haemoglobin of 7.7 gm/dL (anemia secondary to end-stage renal disease). Basic metabolic panel is as follows: normal electrolytes and creatinine of 4.4 mg/dL (due to end-stage renal disease). IgG 4 level was found to be 37 mg/dL. Triglycerides and fibrinogen level was within normal limits.

Retroperitoneal/perirenal soft tissue biopsy showed evidence of fibrosis with abundance of foamy macrophages (Figure 5). CD68 immunostain was positive. Immunostains were negative for S100, CDla, and cytokeratins (Figure 6). We were unable to assess the BRAF status as the biopsy specimen was insufficient to test for BRAF status.

Axillary skin punch biopsy showed numerous Langerhans' cells in the epidermis and superficial dermis (Figure 7). Immunostains were positive for CD68, S100, and CDla (Figure 8). These findings were consistent with a diagnosis of LCH.

4. Treatment

The patient was started on broad spectrum antibiotics and aggressive intravenous fluid resuscitation. Her vital signs stabilized after completing the course of antibiotics and adequate fluid resuscitation; however, her mental status did not improve. She was ultimately intubated for airway protection as well as volume overload from aggressive fluid hydration. She ultimately required a tracheostomy as well as a percutaneous endoscopic gastrostomy tube placement.

The oncology team was consulted for consideration of therapy for ECD-LCH. However, given the patient's poor performance status, she was deemed a poor candidate for interferons/chemotherapy. The benefits and risks of therapy were

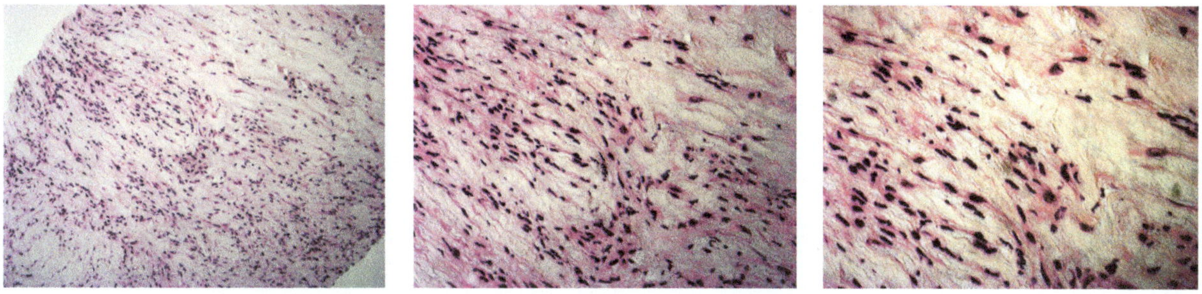

(a) (b) (c)

FIGURE 5: Retroperitoneal biopsy, H&E stain, ×200 (a), ×400 (b), and ×600 (c) showing fibrotic tissue and abundance of foamy macrophages.

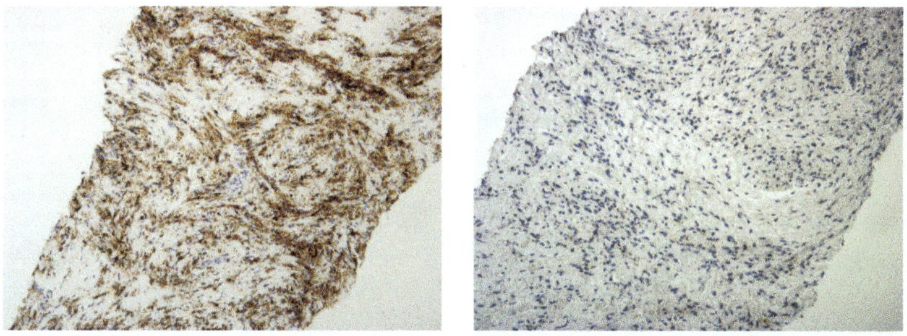

(a) (b)

FIGURE 6: Retroperitoneal biopsy: immunohistochemical stain showing positivity for CD68 (a) and negativity for S100 (b).

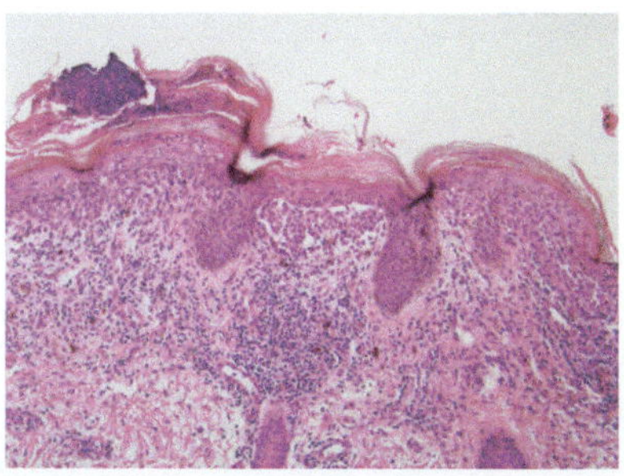

FIGURE 7: Skin biopsy, H&E stain (×200): dense deposit of Langerhans cells with eosinophilic cytoplasm and indented nuclei in the superficial dermis and epidermis highlights epidermotropism.

discussed with the family and their decision was to continue with conservative measures. The patient's acute issues subsequently resolved. She was ultimately transferred to a long term acute care facility due to her poor performance status. Follow-up visits with her primary care physician have shown clinical stability without any acute issues. She is being managed conservatively (without any aggressive therapies) based on her family's wishes.

5. Discussion

Histiocytic disorders are exceedingly rare entities which arise from either Langerhans' dendritic cells (antigen-presenting cells) or the monocyte-phagocytic cells (antigen-processing cells) [1]. Such disorders, based on their genesis, are divided into LCH or non-LCH (ECD being the prototype) [2].

Erdheim-Chester disease, first described in 1930 by Jakob Erdheim and William Chester as "lipid granulomatosis," is a multisystem histiocytosis (non-Langerhans cell type) with a myriad of clinical presentations, distinct radiological findings, and unique immunohistological features [3]. It is a rare variant of non-LCH [3]. The limited reports would suggest it primarily affects individuals between their fifth and seventh decades of life (average 54 years), with a slight predilection towards males [3]. It carries a high mortality (around 60%) in 5 years, which is worse than that found in LCH [3].

ECD is characterized by the symmetrical multifocal osteosclerotic lesions in the diametaphyseal regions of the long bones (especially of the lower extremities), which is virtually pathognomonic for it [4]. More than 650 cases have been described in the literature worldwide [5]. In contrast, the osseous involvement of LCH is typically lytic lesions which can involve any bone of the body [6, 7]. The skeletal or extraskeletal lesions in ECD are the result of infiltration of foamy macrophages (which do not bear the characteristic markers of Langerhans' cells) into these structures. Our patient had evidence of bilateral osteosclerotic lesions of the long bones in her upper and lower extremities. Her maxillae and mandible had evidence of large lytic lesions, which can be seen in both ECD and LCH [8, 9].

The etiology of ECD is not clear, but a multihit hypothesis is favoured. It is hypothesized that either infection or other inciting factors in a genetically predisposed individual can lead to aberration in the regulation of the immune system,

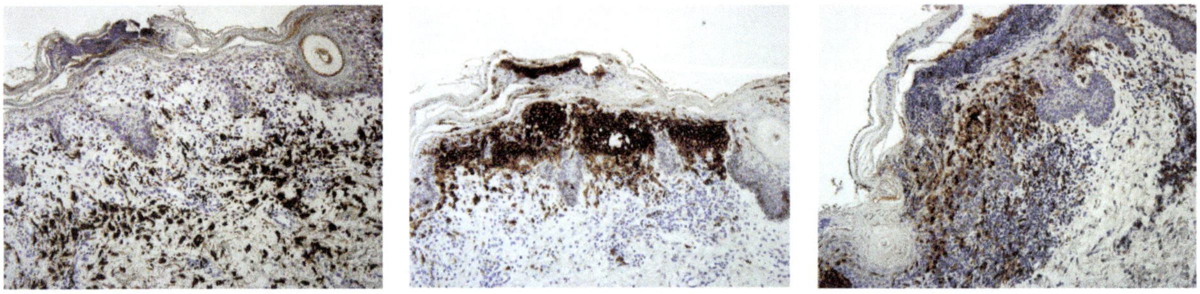

(a) (b) (c)

Figure 8: Skin biopsy: immunohistochemical stain showing positivity for CD68 (a), CD1a (b), and S100 (c).

which results in initiation and propagation of chemokine induced histiocytic invasion of different sites of the body. Chester proposed histiocyte infiltration to be responsible for multisystem sclerosis and fibrosis, a concept which if manipulated can affect the management and prognosis.

Skeletal involvement is the hallmark of ECD (96%). Pain in bones and/or joints is the most common presenting complaint (around 50%). Almost all of the patients also have extraskeletal involvement (maxillary sinus, heart and great vessels, retroperitoneum, kidneys, lungs, and central nervous system including pituitary and orbit) which determines the supplemental clinical features which the patient exhibits as well as the prognosis of the disease with cardiovascular and/or central nervous system affliction carrying the worst outcomes [10].

ECD is diagnosed on the basis of radiological and immunohistochemical features interpreted in the background of clinical context. One retrospective case series showed that ECD can involve (in order of decreasing frequency) the long bones (95%); maxilla, large vessels, and retroperitoneum (59%); heart (57%); lungs (46%); central nervous system (41%); skin (27%); and orbit (22%) [11, 12].

The bony lesions of ECD can be readily picked up by radiographs and Technetium-99m bone scintigraphs [13]. Immunohistochemical analysis of the bone lesions demonstrates the presence of mononuclear foamy histiocytes, from monocyte-macrophage lineage, which are CD68 positive but negative for CD1a, S100 protein, and Birbeck granules, in contradistinction to the Langerhans' cells [4, 14].

Even rarer in ECD is the coexistence of Langerhans' cells along with the CD1a negative foamy macrophages, on either the same site or different ones [15]. One possible explanation of this additional infiltration of Langerhans' cells in ECD is the chemokines (CCL19, CCL21, and more) released by the foamy macrophages. "Mixed histiocytosis," a term vaguely used to highlight the presence of features of both LCH and ECD in a single patient, is being increasingly recognized recently. There is evidence to suggest that misguided differentiation of myeloid precursors plays a role in development of ECD and LCH leading to the term "inflammatory myeloid neoplasms" [5, 16]. Fewer than 10 cases had been reported before the work of Hervier et al., who later presented a series of 23 biopsy proven "mixed histiocytosis" cases and also emphasized the importance of BRAF mutations [15, 17–22].

Table 1: Pertinent differences between the two varieties of histiocytic disorders.

Clinical and immunohistochemical features	Histiocytosis: Langerhans' cell	Histiocytosis: Non-Langerhans' cell
Incidence	Higher	Lower
Mortality	Lower (10%)	Higher (57%)
Culprit cells	Langerhans' cells	Foamy macrophages
Culprit lineage	Langerhans-dendritic cell lineage	Monocyte-macrophage lineage
CD 68	+	+
CD 1a	+	–
S100	+	–
Central nuclear groves	+	–
Birbeck granules	+	–
Age of onset	Children or young adults	The elderly (50s–70s)
Skin involvement	More	Less
Skeletal involvement	Asymmetric osteolytic lesion of skull and flat bones	Symmetric osteosclerotic lesions of long bones
Proliferative index	2–60%	<3%

A few striking features noted in mixed histiocytosis which are dissimilar to both ECD and LCH are age, skeletal involvement, and the underlying culprit cells (Table 1).

Age: patients reported in case reports describing mixed histiocytosis are found to have an age between 27 and 43 years. In contrast, ECD is a disease of the elderly with the majority of patients being in the fifth to seventh decades of their life (average 53 years). On the other hand, LCH most commonly afflicts children or younger adults. Skeletal involvement: ECD is characterized by symmetrical osteosclerotic lesions in the diametaphyseal regions of the long bones, especially the femur, tibia, and fibula, whereas asymmetrical osteolytic lesions of the flat bones and the skull are characteristic of LCH. Patients with "mixed histiocytosis" show a combination of osteosclerotic and osteolytic lesions in the bones, at either the same site or a different site.

Underlying culprit cell: in LCH, the causal cell is derived from the Langerhans dendritic cell lineage whereas the monocyte-macrophage system (i.e., foamy macrophages) is the culprit in the pathogenesis of ECD. Patients showing features of both LCH and ECD are thought to have an abnormality in CD 34+ cells, which are progenitors for both cell types described and can be steered in either pathway when cultured in vitro. BRAF (V600E) mutations have been shown to play an important role in the development of these disorders [23].

Most recognized "overlap" cases describe the presence of both disease states simultaneously in the patient, but existence of both of them spaced apart in time has been reported which could represent evolution of LCH into ECD, reflecting the old concept of ECD being "late-stage healing" of Langerhans as was proposed by Pineles et al. [18, 21, 22].

Treatment of ECD is not well established. Interferon alpha, either conventional or pegylated, is the preferred treatment for symptomatic patients, especially those with extraosseous system involvement. In patients with BRAF V600E mutations, vemurafenib (a BRAF inhibitor) has shown promising results [24, 25]. Other options, though controversial, include systemic chemotherapy, glucocorticoids, and radiation therapy [23, 26, 27].

In conclusion, ECD with overlapping features of LCH might represent different spectra of the same disorder. Increasing recognition and reporting of such cases can help clinicians to have a better understanding of the pathophysiology involved, which ultimately can be translated into better management of the therapeutic options. Diagnosis of either of these rare syndromes requires a high index of suspicion, and when suspected these should be evaluated by radiological and immunohistopathological analysis.

Conflict of Interests

The authors declare that there is no conflict of interests regarding the publication of this paper.

References

[1] P. S. Furmanczyk, J. D. Bruckner, T. Gillespy III, and B. P. Rubin, "An unusual case of Erdheim-Chester disease with features of Langerhans cell histiocytosis," *Skeletal Radiology*, vol. 36, no. 9, pp. 885–889, 2007.

[2] H. D. Dorfman and B. Czerniak, "Bone cancers," *Cancer*, vol. 75, supplement 1, pp. 203–210, 1995.

[3] R. D. Mazor, M. Manevich-Mazor, and Y. Shoenfeld, "Erdheim-Chester Disease: a comprehensive review of the literature," *Orphanet Journal of Rare Diseases*, vol. 8, article 137, 2013.

[4] M. Cives, V. Simone, F. M. Rizzo et al., "Erdheim-Chester disease: a systematic review," *Critical Reviews in Oncology/Hematology*, vol. 95, no. 1, pp. 1–11, 2015.

[5] J. Haroche, F. Cohen-Aubart, F. Charlotte et al., "The histiocytosis Erdheim-Chester disease is an inflammatory myeloid neoplasm," *Expert Review of Clinical Immunology*, vol. 11, no. 9, pp. 1033–1042, 2015.

[6] I. Baumgartner, A. von Hochstetter, B. Baumert, U. Luetolf, and F. Follath, "Langerhans'-cell histiocytosis in adults," *Medical and Pediatric Oncology*, vol. 28, no. 1, pp. 9–14, 1997.

[7] S. Toro Galván, A. Planas Vilaseca, T. Michalopoulou Alevras, A. Torres Díaz, J. Suárez Balaguer, and C. Villabona Artero, "Endocrine changes in histiocytosis of the hypothalamic-pituitary axis," *Endocrinologia y Nutricion*, vol. 62, no. 2, pp. 72–79, 2015.

[8] Y.-A. Cho, H.-J. Yoon, S.-D. Hong, J.-I. Lee, and S.-P. Hong, "Hypothetical pathogenesis of eosinophilic infiltration in Langerhans cell histiocytosis of the jaw," *Oral Surgery, Oral Medicine, Oral Pathology and Oral Radiology*, vol. 116, no. 6, pp. 734–742, 2013.

[9] M. Kambouchner, T. V. Colby, C. Domenge, J. P. Battesti, P. Soler, and A. Tazi, "Erdheim-Chester disease with prominent pulmonary involvement associated with eosinophilic granuloma of mandibular bone," *Histopathology*, vol. 30, no. 4, pp. 353–358, 1997.

[10] L. Arnaud, B. Hervier, A. Néel et al., "CNS involvement and treatment with interferon-α are independent prognostic factors in Erdheim-Chester disease: a multicenter survival analysis of 53 patients," *Blood*, vol. 117, no. 10, pp. 2778–2782, 2011.

[11] L. Arnaud, G. Gorochov, F. Charlotte et al., "Systemic perturbation of cytokine and chemokine networks in Erdheim-Chester disease: a single-center series of 37 patients," *Blood*, vol. 117, no. 10, pp. 2783–2790, 2011.

[12] C. Veyssier-Belot, P. Cacoub, D. Caparros-Lefebvre et al., "Erdheim-Chester disease. Clinical and radiologic characteristics of 59 cases," *Medicine*, vol. 75, no. 3, pp. 157–169, 1996.

[13] O. Adib, E. Baroth, L. Perard et al., "Imaging features of osseous and extra-osseous involvement in Erdheim-Chester disease," *Journal de Radiologie*, vol. 92, no. 7-8, pp. 671–680, 2011.

[14] A. J. M. Egan, L. A. Boardman, H. D. Tazelaar et al., "Erdheim-Chester disease: clinical, radiologic, and histopathologic findings in five patients with interstitial lung disease," *The American Journal of Surgical Pathology*, vol. 23, no. 1, pp. 17–26, 1999.

[15] H. Naruse, H. Shoda, A. Okamoto, T. Oka, and K. Yamamoto, "A case of osteoarthropathy due to Erdheim-Chester disease with overlapping Langerhans' cell infiltration," *Internal Medicine*, vol. 49, no. 12, pp. 1225–1228, 2010.

[16] M. L. Berres, M. Merad, and C. E. Allen, "Progress in understanding the pathogenesis of Langerhans cell histiocytosis: back to Histiocytosis X?" *British Journal of Haematology*, vol. 169, no. 1, pp. 3–13, 2015.

[17] V. P. Andrade, C. C. V. Nemer, A. N. L. Prezotti, and W. S. L. Goulart, "Erdheim-Chester disease of the breast associated with Langerhans-cell histiocytosis of the hard palate," *Virchows Archiv*, vol. 445, no. 4, pp. 405–409, 2004.

[18] S. L. Pineles, G. T. Liu, X. Acebes et al., "Presence of Erdheim-Chester disease and Langerhans cell histiocytosis in the same patient: a report of 2 cases," *Journal of Neuro-Ophthalmology*, vol. 31, no. 3, pp. 217–223, 2011.

[19] J.-W. Tsai, J.-H. Tsou, L.-Y. Hung, H.-B. Wu, and K.-C. Chang, "Combined Erdheim-Chester disease and Langerhans cell histiocytosis of skin are both monoclonal: a rare case with human androgen-receptor gene analysis," *Journal of the American Academy of Dermatology*, vol. 63, no. 2, pp. 284–291, 2010.

[20] C. Vital, P. Bioulac-Sage, F. Tison et al., "Brain stem infiltration by mixed langerhans cell histiocytosis and Chester-Erdheim disease: more than just an isolated case?" *Journal of Clinical & Experimental Pathology*, vol. 47, no. 2, pp. 71–76, 1999.

[21] R. J. Waite, P. W. Doherty, M. Liepman, and B. Woda, "Langerhans cell histiocytosis with the radiographic findings of Erdheim-Chester disease," *American Journal of Roentgenology*, vol. 150, no. 4, pp. 869–871, 1988.

[22] B. Hervier, J. Haroche, L. Arnaud et al., "Association of both Langerhans cell histiocytosis and Erdheim-Chester disease linked to the BRAFV600E mutation," *Blood*, vol. 124, no. 7, pp. 1119–1126, 2014.

[23] J. Haroche, F. Charlotte, L. Arnaud et al., "High prevalence of BRAF V600E mutations in Erdheim-Chester disease but not in other non-Langerhans cell histiocytoses," *Blood*, vol. 120, no. 13, pp. 2700–2703, 2012.

[24] P. Euskirchen, J. Haroche, J. F. Emile, R. Buchert, S. Vandersee, and A. Meisel, "Complete remission of critical neurohistiocytosis by vemurafenib," *Neurology: Neuroimmunology & Neuroinflammation*, vol. 2, no. 2, article e78, 2015.

[25] J. Haroche, F. Cohen-Aubart, J.-F. Emile et al., "Reproducible and sustained efficacy of targeted therapy with vemurafenib in patients with $BRAF^{V600E}$-mutated Erdheim-Chester disease," *Journal of Clinical Oncology*, vol. 33, no. 5, pp. 411–418, 2015.

[26] I.-S. Jeon, S. S. Lee, and M. K. Lee, "Chemotherapy and interferon-α treatment of Erdheim-chester disease," *Pediatric Blood and Cancer*, vol. 55, no. 4, pp. 745–747, 2010.

[27] L. Monti, J. Haroche, A. Sciarra et al., "Interferon-alpha in cardiac Erdheim-Chester disease," *Journal of the American College of Cardiology*, vol. 58, no. 25, p. 2695, 2011.

32

Retained Placenta Accreta Mimicking Choriocarcinoma

Maureen P. Kohi,[1] Gabrielle A. Rizzuto,[2] Nicholas Fidelman,[1] Jennifer Lucero,[3] and Mari-Paule Thiet[4]

[1] *Department of Radiology and Biomedical Imaging, University of California, San Francisco, San Francisco, CA 94143, USA*
[2] *Department of Pathology and Laboratory Medicine, University of California, San Francisco, San Francisco, CA 94143, USA*
[3] *Department of Anesthesia and Perioperative Care, University of California, San Francisco, San Francisco, CA 94143, USA*
[4] *Department of Obstetrics, Gynecology and Reproductive Sciences, University of California, San Francisco, San Francisco, CA 94143, USA*

Correspondence should be addressed to Maureen P. Kohi; maureen.kohi@ucsf.edu

Academic Editor: George Adonakis

This case demonstrates a rare event of retained invasive placenta masquerading as choriocarcinoma. The patient presented with heavy vaginal bleeding following vaginal delivery complicated by retained products of conception. Ultrasound and computed tomography demonstrated a vascular endometrial mass, invading the uterine wall and raising suspicion for choriocarcinoma. Hysterectomy revealed retained invasive placenta.

1. Introduction

Abnormally invasive placenta is a life-threatening condition that occurs when chorionic villi adhere to the uterine myometrium without normal intervening decidua basalis [1]. The most common complication of invasive placenta is postpartum hemorrhage (PPH), which often requires hysterectomy [2].

Retained products of conception (RPOC) or placental fragments are a common cause of PPH with an incidence of 3%–5% after routine vaginal delivery [3]. Ultrasound (US) is the primary modality during the antepartum period and the modality of choice to evaluate for PPH [4]. Combined gray-scale and color Doppler US allow real-time assessment of the uterine cavity and blood flow, which aid in the diagnosis of RPOC. Early diagnosis is critical for directing clinical management and for preventing associated immediate complications, such as infection, as well as future obstetric complications [5].

Herein, we present a case of retained invasive placenta, which was undetected in the antepartum and mimicked choriocarcinoma in the postpartum period, ultimately resulting in hysterectomy.

2. Case Report

A 39-year-old gravida 3 nulliparous female with a dichorionic diamniotic twin pregnancy at 36 weeks and 4 days was admitted to our institution for induction of labor secondary to intrauterine growth restriction (IUGR) of both infants. Her obstetrical history was significant for two prior dilatation and curettage (D&C) procedures. Her antenatal ultrasounds demonstrated two normal placentas without evidence of previa or placental invasion.

She progressed to spontaneous rupture of membranes 18 hours following administration of oxytocin and placement of a transcervical Foley balloon. Once US confirmed vertex lie of both infants, the patient was moved to the operating room (OR) where labor progressed normally with delivery of two female infants weighting 2085 g (Apgar scores of 8 and 8 at 1 and 5 minutes) and 1945 g (Apgar scores of 4 and 8 at 1 and 5 minutes), respectively.

The third stage of labor was complicated by retained placenta, which was extracted manually and with banjo curettage under ultrasound guidance. At the end of the procedure, a thin endometrium was confirmed by US.

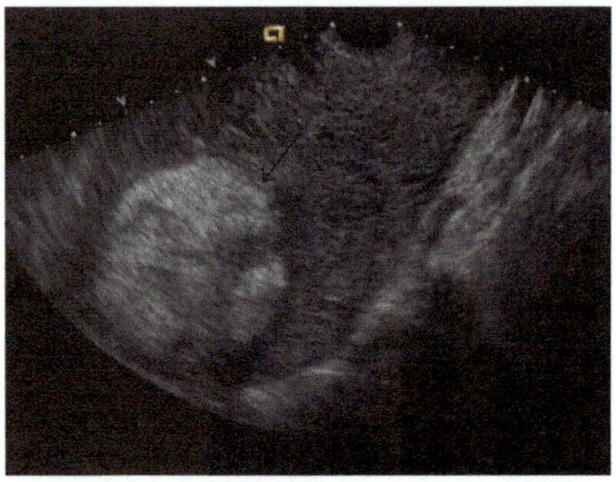

Figure 1: Gray-scale US demonstrates an echogenic mass in the endometrial cavity (black arrow).

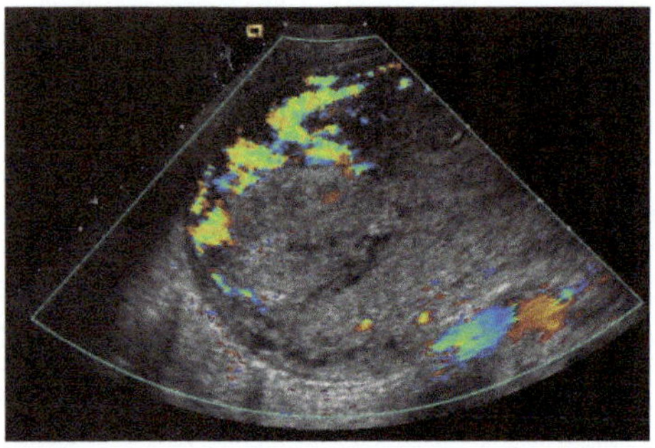

Figure 2: Color Doppler US image demonstrates vascularity in the echogenic mass with extensive vascularity surrounding the mass.

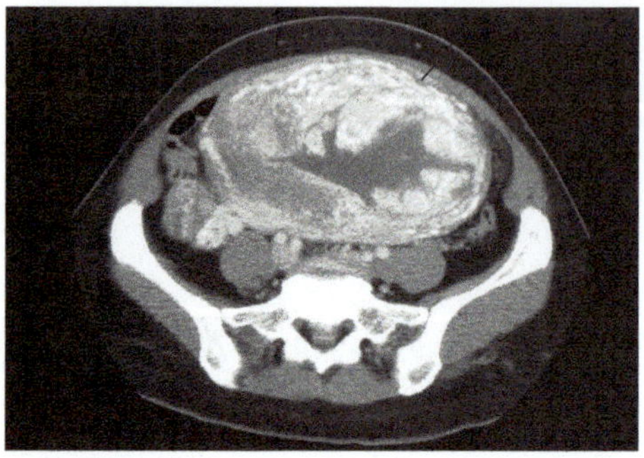

Figure 3: Contrast-enhanced CT image demonstrates hypervascular uterine mass. Note loss of plane between the mass and the uterine wall (white arrow).

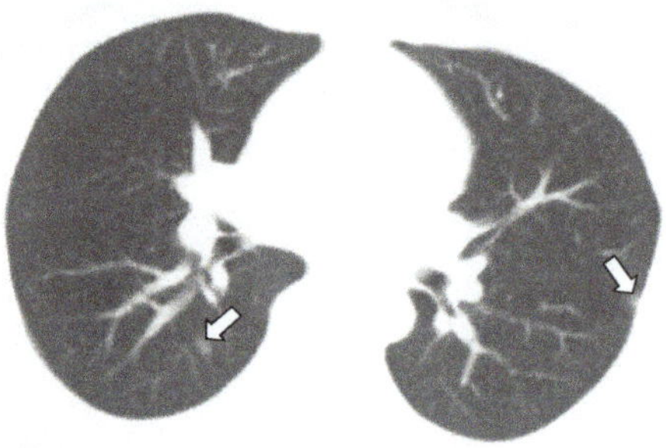

Figure 4: CT image of the chest demonstrates ground glass opacities in the lungs (open arrows).

Initially, the postpartum course was uncomplicated, and the patient was discharged on postpartum day two in stable condition. However, on postpartum day five, while visiting her infants in the hospital, the patient passed an orange-sized blood clot. A repeat US demonstrated a thin endometrial stripe. For the next several weeks, light bleeding continued.

At the routine 6-week postpartum visit, the patient again passed a large blood clot and her uterus was palpable 2 cm below the umbilicus. At that time, serum quantitative human chorionic gonadotropin (hCG) level was 203 IU/L, and hematocrit was 33%.

Transvaginal US showed a large echogenic mass within the endometrial cavity, measuring 9.4 × 8.5 × 6.7 cm (Figure 1). Color Doppler US demonstrated vascularity, predominately in the periphery of the mass (Figure 2). Computed tomography (CT) demonstrated a large hypervascular and heterogeneously enhancing uterine mass measuring 10.4 × 15 × 16.8 cm with diffuse myometrial invasion (Figure 3) and CT chest demonstrated bilateral ground glass nodules (Figure 4). Differential diagnoses included gestational trophoblastic disease versus RPOC, but choriocarcinoma was favored given the hypervascularity noted on CT, the degree of uterine invasion, and the presence of pulmonary nodules, which is worrisome for metastases. RPOC was considered less likely in light of manual and instrumental placental extractions and thin stripe noted US performed in the OR.

Management options included transcervical biopsy for diagnosis (D&C) with frozen section with subsequent hysterectomy in case of malignancy or outright hysterectomy. The patient and her husband did not desire future fertility and preferred hysterectomy.

The patient underwent total abdominal hysterectomy, and pathology demonstrated placenta accreta (Figures 5(a) and 5(b)). The postoperative course was uncomplicated, and the patient was discharged on postoperative day four.

3. Discussion

Invasive placenta is a condition caused by placental invasion into the uterine wall. Three distinct types of invasive placenta exist, based on the degree of placental villi invasion into the myometrium: placenta accreta (superficial invasion of the basalis layer), placenta increta (deeper invasion of the myometrium), and placenta percreta (deeper invasion involving the serosa and other surrounding organs such as the bladder) [6]. Risk factors for invasive placentation include placenta previa, previous history of cesarean delivery, advanced maternal age, previous uterine surgery, and multiparity [7]. The incidence of invasive placentation has increased fivefold over the past few decades from 1 in 2510 in the 1980s to currently about 1 in 533 pregnancies [7]. The major contributing factor to this is likely the increase in the rate of cesarean delivery and uterine instrumentation [8].

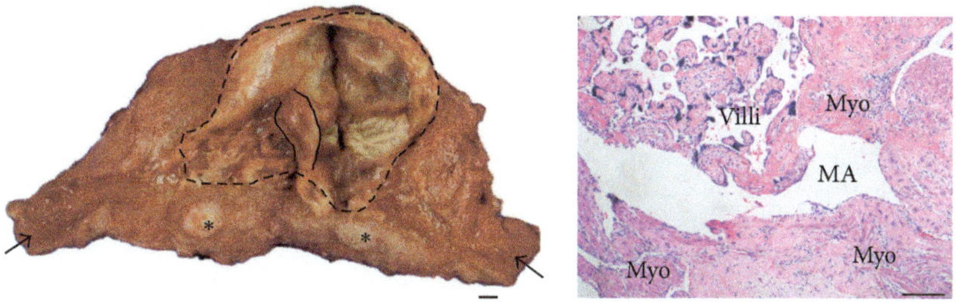

(a) (b)

FIGURE 5: Grossly retained placenta with microscopic evidence of placenta accreta. (a) Gross photograph of hysterectomy specimen bisected in coronal plane shows ~12 × 11 × 3 cm fundal placenta (outlined in dashed lines) with ~3.5 cm umbilical cord (outlined in solid lines) (arrows at cervical os, * = leiomyoma). (b) Hematoxylin and eosin stained microscopic section demonstrates degenerating placental villous parenchyma [villi] adjacent to large bands of myometrial smooth muscle [myo] without intervening decidua [MA = maternal myometrial artery]. Scale bars: (a) 1 cm and (b) 100 microns. Note: due to extensive tissue degeneration at the placenta/myometrial interface, the depth of accreta could not be accurately determined on pathologic examination.

Antenatal diagnosis of invasive placentation is critical and has been shown to decrease maternal morbidity [9]. US is the primary imaging modality for the diagnosis of invasive placenta in the antepartum period [10] with sensitivity of 91% and specificity of 97% [11]. Findings suggestive of invasive placentation on US include intraplacental lacunar spaces, lack of normal retroplacental clear zone, irregularity and attenuation of the uterine-bladder interface, retroplacental myometrial thickness, and bridging vessels between the placenta and bladder wall when using color Doppler [12].

RPOC refers to intrauterine tissue that persists after delivery or termination of pregnancy and is often of placental trophoblastic origin and a common cause of PPH [5]. US is the primary modality for the diagnosis of RPOC. On gray-scale US, the presence of a thickened endometrial echo complex (EEC) of at least 10 mm has a diagnostic sensitivity of 80% [13] and presence of an endometrial or intrauterine mass has a diagnostic sensitivity of 79% [14]. Additionally, color Doppler US can further enhance the diagnosis of RPOC as any vascularity detected in a thickened EEC or mass increases the likelihood of RPOC [5].

CT or magnetic resonance imaging (MRI) can serve as diagnostic adjuncts in complicated cases. However, there is variability of postcontrast enhancement on CT imaging and of T1- and T2-weighted signal intensity depending on the degree of hemorrhage and tissue necrosis [14, 15].

Gestational trophoblastic disease is a rare complication of pregnancy encompassing a group of interrelated diseases ranging from premalignant partial and complete hydatidiform mole to malignant diseases of an invasive mole, choriocarcinoma, and rare placental-site trophoblastic tumor and epithelioid trophoblastic tumor [16]. The serum and urine hCG levels are elevated in this disease process. Choriocarcinoma is a rare trophoblastic tumor characterized by myometrial and vascular invasion with high incidence of pulmonary metastasis in the form of nodules with surrounding ground glass opacities [17].

In the present case, the vascularity of the uterine mass in addition to the myometrial invasion suggested a malignant process as opposed to invasive placenta. In addition, the small ground glass pulmonary nodules in the setting of the invasive uterine mass suggested the diagnosis of choriocarcinoma.

Prior reports have described that retained invasive placenta may mimic acquired arteriovenous malformation [18], leiomyomata [19], and endometrial cancer [20]. Therefore, it is important to consider the diagnosis of retained invasive placenta in patients presenting with PPH who have risk factors for invasive placentation. This is particularly critical prior to performing a D&C for presumed RPOC, which in cases of retained invasive placenta may result in massive bleeding, necessitating an emergent hysterectomy.

Conflict of Interests

None of the authors have any relevant conflict of interests to disclose.

References

[1] T. Angstmann, G. Gard, T. Harrington, E. Ward, A. Thomson, and W. Giles, "Surgical management of placenta accreta: a cohort series and suggested approach," *American Journal of Obstetrics and Gynecology*, vol. 202, no. 1, pp. 38.e1–38.e9, 2010.

[2] Y. Oyelese and J. C. Smulian, "Placenta previa, placenta accreta, and vasa previa," *Obstetrics and Gynecology*, vol. 107, no. 4, pp. 927–941, 2006.

[3] T. D. Epperly, J. P. Fogarty, and S. G. Hodges, "Efficacy of routine postpartum uterine exploration and manual sponge curettage," *The Journal of Family Practice*, vol. 28, no. 2, pp. 172–176, 1989.

[4] J. S. Abramowicz and E. Sheiner, "In utero imaging of the placenta: importance for diseases of pregnancy," *Placenta*, vol. 28, pp. S14–S22, 2007.

[5] M. A. Sellmyer, T. S. Desser, K. E. Maturen, R. B. Jeffrey Jr., and A. Kamaya, "Physiologic, histologic, and imaging features of retained products of conception," *Radiographics*, vol. 33, no. 3, pp. 781–796, 2013.

[6] L. Sentilhes, F. Goffinet, and G. Kayem, "Management of placenta accreta," *Acta Obstetricia et Gynecologica Scandinavica*, vol. 92, no. 10, pp. 1125–1134, 2013.

[7] E. Adler, R. Madankumar, M. Rosner, and S. E. Reznik, "Increased placental trophoblast inclusions in placenta accreta," *Placenta*, vol. 35, no. 12, pp. 1075–1078, 2014.

[8] R. M. Silver, K. A. Fox, J. R. Barton et al., "Center of excellence for placenta accreta," *American Journal of Obstetrics & Gynecology*, vol. 212, no. 5, pp. 561–568, 2015.

[9] M. Tikkanen, J. Paavonen, M. Loukovaara, and V. Stefanovic, "Antenatal diagnosis of placenta accreta leads to reduced blood loss," *Acta Obstetricia et Gynecologica Scandinavica*, vol. 90, no. 10, pp. 1140–1146, 2011.

[10] G. Calì, L. Giambanco, G. Puccio, and F. Forlani, "Morbidly adherent placenta: evaluation of ultrasound diagnostic criteria and differentiation of placenta accreta from percreta," *Ultrasound in Obstetrics and Gynecology*, vol. 41, no. 4, pp. 406–412, 2013.

[11] F. D'Antonio, C. Iacovella, and A. Bhide, "Prenatal identification of invasive placentation using ultrasound: systematic review and meta-analysis," *Ultrasound in Obstetrics and Gynecology*, vol. 42, no. 5, pp. 509–517, 2013.

[12] M. W. F. Rac, J. S. Dashe, C. E. Wells, E. Moschos, D. D. McIntire, and D. M. Twickler, "Ultrasound predictors of placental invasion: the Placenta Accreta Index," *American Journal of Obstetrics & Gynecology*, vol. 212, no. 3, pp. 343.e1–343.e7, 2015.

[13] E. Ustunyurt, O. Kaymak, C. Iskender, O. B. Ustunyurt, C. Celik, and N. Danisman, "Role of transvaginal sonography in the diagnosis of retained products of conception," *Archives of Gynecology and Obstetrics*, vol. 277, no. 2, pp. 151–154, 2008.

[14] K. M. Elsayes, A. T. Trout, A. M. Friedkin et al., "Imaging of the placenta: a multimodality pictorial review," *RadioGraphics*, vol. 29, no. 5, pp. 1371–1391, 2009.

[15] H. Fleming, A. G. Ostör, H. Pickel, and D. W. Fortune, "Arteriovenous malformations of the uterus," *Obstetrics and Gynecology*, vol. 73, no. 2, pp. 209–214, 1989.

[16] F. E. M. Froeling and M. J. Seckl, "Gestational trophoblastic tumours: an update for 2014," *Current Oncology Reports*, vol. 16, article 408, 2014.

[17] S. Martínez-Jiménez, M. L. Rosado-de-Christenson, C. M. Walker et al., "Imaging features of thoracic metastases from gynecologic neoplasms," *RadioGraphics*, vol. 34, no. 6, pp. 1742–1754, 2014.

[18] A. Kido, K. Togashi, T. Koyama et al., "Retained products of conception masquerading as acquired arteriovenous malformation," *Journal of Computer Assisted Tomography*, vol. 27, no. 1, pp. 88–92, 2003.

[19] A. Ekiz, I. Polat, S. Mumusoglu, B. Aydiner, C. Ozdemir, and H. S. Arslan, "A case of placenta increta mimicking submucous leiomyoma," *Case Reports in Obstetrics and Gynecology*, vol. 2014, Article ID 429406, 3 pages, 2014.

[20] S. Lim, S. Ha, K. Lee, and J. Lee, "Retained placenta accreta after a first-trimester abortion manifesting as an uterine mass," *Obstetrics & Gynecology Science*, vol. 56, no. 3, pp. 205–207, 2013.

33

High Grade (Large Cell) Neuroendocrine Carcinoma of the Nasopharynx: Novel Case Report with Touch Preparation Cytology and Positive EBV Encoded Early RNA

Charles D. Sturgis,[1] Brian B. Burkey,[2] Suhael Momin,[2] and Aaron P. Hoschar[1]

[1]*Cleveland Clinic, Tomsich Pathology Institute, 9500 Euclid Avenue L25, Cleveland, OH 44195, USA*
[2]*Cleveland Clinic, Head and Neck Institute, 9500 Euclid Avenue A71, Cleveland, OH 44195, USA*

Correspondence should be addressed to Charles D. Sturgis; sturgic@ccf.org

Academic Editor: Paolo Perrini

Fewer than five case reports of primary large cell neuroendocrine carcinoma of the nasopharynx are known to the authors. No previous reports have included examples of cytomorphology or have proven association with Epstein-Barr virus. We herein illustrate MRI findings, histopathologic features, immunohistochemical characterization, cytologic details, and in situ hybridization studies from a unique case of primary large cell neuroendocrine carcinoma of the nasopharynx in a 38-year-old Caucasian male patient. Recognition of rare tumor types of the nasopharynx allows for refinements in disease management and prognostication.

1. Introduction

The current World Health Organization (WHO) classification of tumors of the head and neck lists three categories of primary malignant epithelial neoplasms in the nasopharynx. These categories are nasopharyngeal carcinomas (NPC), nasopharyngeal papillary adenocarcinomas, and salivary gland-type carcinomas [1]. The first category of nasopharyngeal carcinoma is subdivided into "nonkeratinizing" carcinoma, keratinizing squamous carcinoma, and basaloid squamous carcinoma. The "nonkeratinizing" group is generally further divided into differentiated and undifferentiated (more common) subtypes [1]. In examples of older literature, nasopharyngeal carcinomas are sometimes referred to as lymphoepithelial carcinomas or undifferentiated carcinomas with lymphoid stroma. Common symptoms and physical signs of NPC include neck masses (enlarged lymph nodes), nasal obstruction with bleeding, and sometimes aural changes. A near constant association exists between NPC and Epstein-Barr virus (EBV) infection with strong evidence to support a carcinogenic role of the virus. The presence of host incorporated EBV can be of diagnostic importance and also has therapeutic implications [1, 2]. While they do exist, neuroendocrine carcinomas of the nasopharynx are not included in the WHO classification. Such tumors are known to exist but are seen rarely and can mimic other blue cell tumors such as lymphomas, neuroblastomas, mucosal melanomas, and primitive neuroectodermal tumors [3]. In the lungs (where neuroendocrine tumors are more common), these neoplasms can be divided into carcinoid tumor, atypical carcinoid tumor, large cell neuroendocrine carcinoma, and small cell carcinoma. Case reports of nasopharyngeal primary tumors ranging the morphologic spectrum of these neuroendocrine lung tumors have been reported [4–7]. To our knowledge, only three cases of primary large cell (non-small cell) neuroendocrine carcinoma of the nasopharynx have been reported in the literature, and the reports of these have not included examples of cytomorphology (as opposed to histomorphology) or substantiated associations with EBV [8, 9]. We herein report an EBV positive case of primary large cell neuroendocrine carcinoma of the nasopharynx in a 38-year-old man in which touch preparation cytology studies were integral to establishing a definitive diagnosis.

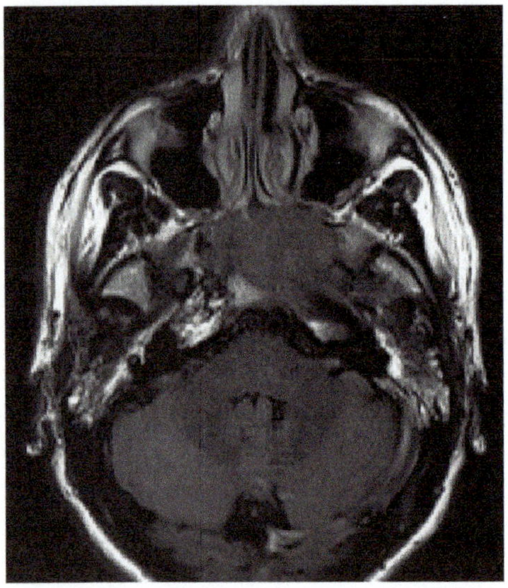

Figure 1: Magnetic resonance imaging of the head and neck revealed a nasopharyngeal mass with extension into the left pterygopalatine fossa. Bony involvement of the greater wings of the sphenoid and clivus was described.

2. Case Presentation

The patient is a 38-year-old, single, Caucasian male who presents with a 2-month history of painless bilateral neck swelling and "muffled" hearing. He reports being recently previously treated with a course of oral antibiotics without resolution of symptoms. He is a current, every-day cigarette smoker with a 15-pack-year history of tobacco use. The patient denies weight loss, fever, night sweats, fatigue, head ache, and visual disturbances. Firm submandibular masses (5 to 8 cm, bilaterally) are reported on physical examination. Imaging studies of the head and neck demonstrate bulky homogenous soft tissue mass-like lymphadenopathy in the bilateral neck as well as a nasopharyngeal mass with erosive changes of the left pterygopalatine fossa and left skull base. Imaging studies are interpreted as "concerning for lymphoma" (Figure 1). Endoscopic nasopharyngeal biopsies are performed.

3. Discussion

Multiple biopsies were obtained from a nasopharyngeal mass in this case. The tissue sample measured 2.0 × 1.0 × 0.4 cm in aggregate. The specimen was sent fresh to the frozen section area for intraoperative consultation, and both touch preparations and frozen sections were performed on portions of the sample, confirming the presence of lesional material. The neoplastic proliferation was felt to be nonlymphoid at the time of intraoperative assessment, and the entire sample was then submitted for routine histologic processing. Hematoxylin and eosin stained tissue sections from the permanent tissue block revealed marked crush artifact with more than 80% of tumor nests being significantly distorted. In focal areas, well-preserved sheets of lesional cells were seen set within a fibrous/desmoplastic stroma that contained mixed

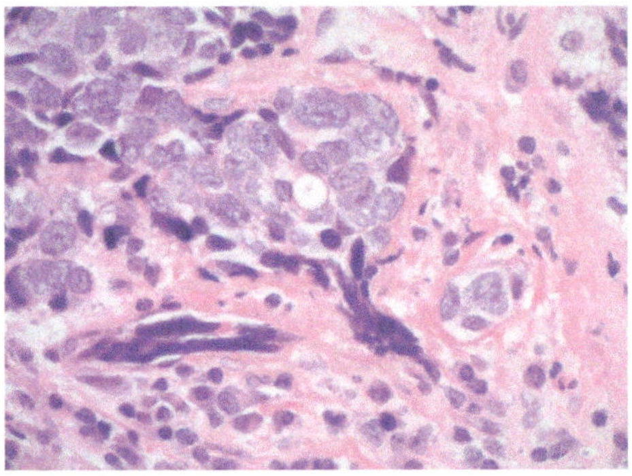

Figure 2: Tissue section from the nasopharyngeal biopsy showed a nested histoarchitecture with crush artifact and a well-preserved region of lesional cells set in a fibrous stroma with accompanying lymphocytes and plasmacytoid cells. Tumor cell sizes were intermediate to large with minimal to moderate amounts of amphophilic cytoplasm, large nuclei with finely granular chromatin, and eosinophilic nucleoli (hematoxylin and eosin stain, 600x).

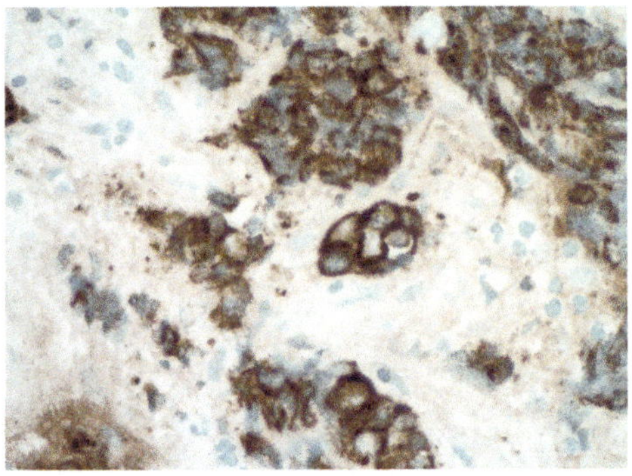

Figure 3: Ancillary testing revealed strong and diffuse tumor cell immunoreactivity for cytokeratin (CAM5.2 immunohistochemistry, 600x).

lymphoid cells. The lesional cells were intermediate to large in size and showed a variably solid to nested histoarchitecture with foci of necrosis. Rare vaguely acinar structures were noted. The lesional cells were noted to have fine, uniform chromatin which when coupled with the appearance of the crush artifact suggested a possible neuroendocrine phenotype (Figure 2). Mitotic counts were somewhat difficult because of crush artifact. Results of counts confirmed eight mitoses on average per 10 high power (40x objective) microscopic fields. Ancillary immunohistochemical (IHC) studies were performed, including cytokeratin AE1/AE3, cytokeratin CAM 5.2, cytokeratin 5/6, CD34, CD99, CD45, CD56, neuron specific enolase, synaptophysin, chromogranin, p63, S-100, desmin, and myogenin. The lesional cells (in both the well-preserved and crushed regions) showed diffuse and strong immunoreactivity for cytokeratin CAM5.2, supporting an epithelial phenotype (Figure 3). Cytokeratin AE1/AE3 was also positive. In addition, the lesional cells were shown to be immunoreactive with the pan-neuroendocrine markers neuron specific enolase, synaptophysin, and CD56 (Figures 4 and 5). All other IHC marker studies were nonreactive. Ki-67

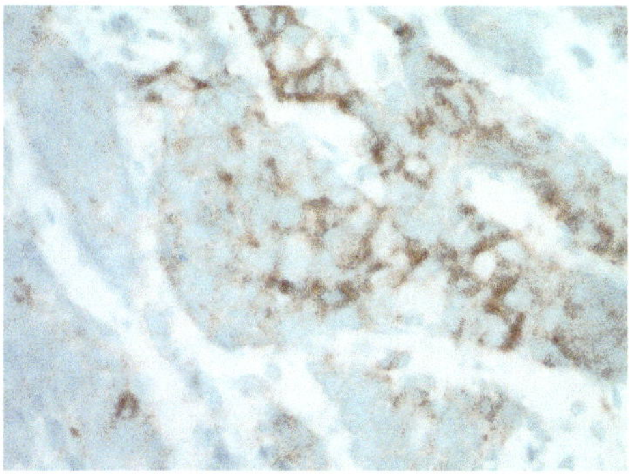

FIGURE 4: Ancillary testing confirmed immunoreactivity with synaptophysin (synaptophysin immunohistochemistry, 600x).

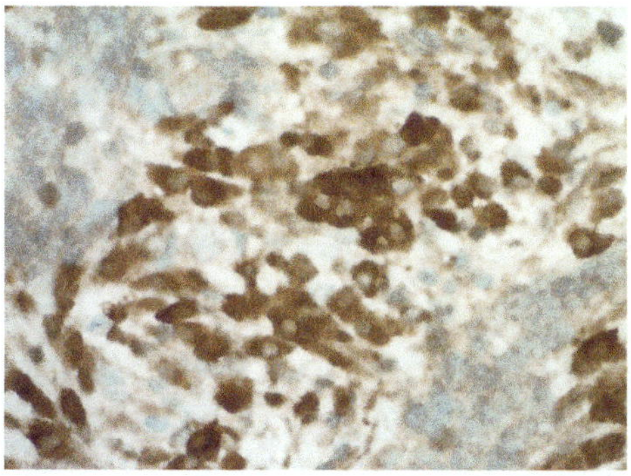

FIGURE 5: Ancillary testing demonstrated strong immunoreactivity with neuron specific enolase (NSE immunohistochemistry, 600x).

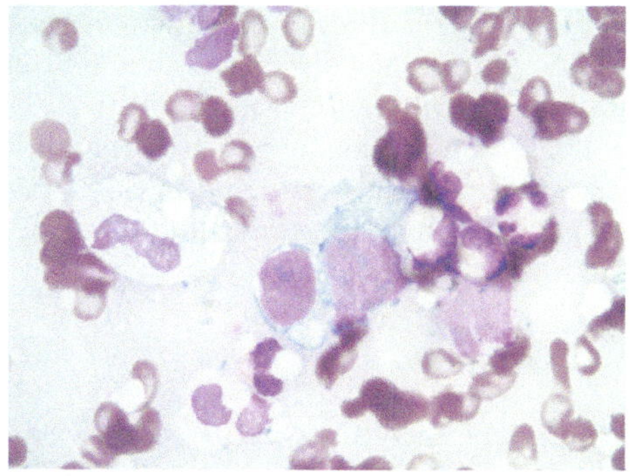

FIGURE 6: Large cell neuroendocrine carcinoma cytomorphology with moderately abundant pale blue to amphophilic cytoplasm, intermediate to large nuclei, and readily identified nucleoli (Modified Giemsa Stain, Touch Preparation, 1000x).

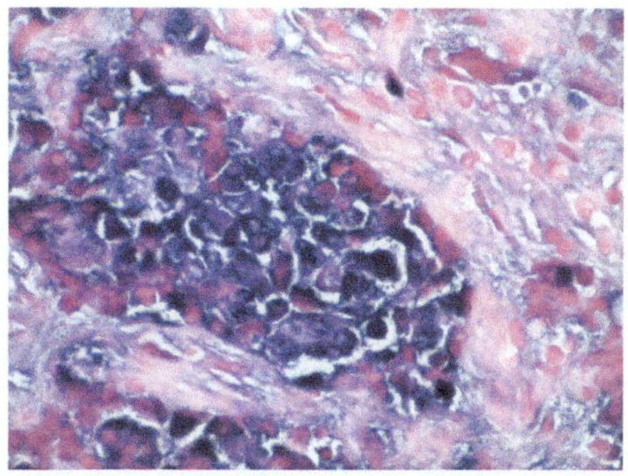

FIGURE 7: Positive chromogenic in situ hybridization for Epstein-Barr virus encoded early RNAs (slide based EBER CISH study, 600x).

studies were not pursued. The combined histomorphology and pattern of immunoreactivity were consistent with a high grade neuroendocrine carcinoma. With the limitations caused by crush artifact and the morphology of the cellular process, the two chief differential diagnostic considerations were small cell carcinoma and large cell neuroendocrine carcinoma.

The WHO classification of tumors of the lungs indicates that large cell neuroendocrine carcinomas show histologic features such as organoid nesting, trabecular growth, and palisaded patterns with the tumor cells generally being large in size and having moderate to abundant cytoplasm with nucleoli being present [10]. Characteristic cellular features of large cell neuroendocrine carcinoma of the lungs have also been described in needle aspiration and imprint cytology studies with emphases placed on nuclear size, nuclear/cytoplasmic ratios, and perceptibility of nucleoli in tumor cells [11–13]. Touch preparations were made during the time of the intraoperative consultation in this case. In some instances, touch preparations are used to establish the presence of lesional material and do not later influence diagnostic algorithms. In this case, the touch preparations were an important diagnostic adjunct, and preserved cells in the touch preparations were judged to be of larger size and greater cytoplasmic volume that would be seen in classical small cell carcinoma as well. In addition, lesional cells were noted to contain readily perceived nucleoli. These findings were even more evident on the cytology preparations than in the traditional histologic biopsies. To our knowledge, this report is the first in the literature specifically depicting the cytologic characteristics of cells from a primary nasopharyngeal large cell neuroendocrine carcinoma (Figure 6). In addition to cytologic, histologic, and immunohistochemical characterizations, the tumor in the case was also characterized as being EBV associated by confirming the presence of EBV encoded early RNAs (EBERs) (Figure 7). To our knowledge, this report is the first in the literature confirming an EBV related primary large cell neuroendocrine carcinoma of the nasopharynx.

While most commonly encountered in the lungs, primary high grade neuroendocrine carcinomas can occur at other body sites, including the salivary glands and other sites in the head and neck [14, 15]. High grade neuroendocrine tumors of the head and neck include small cell carcinomas and large cell neuroendocrine carcinomas. Some investigators have reported that, stage for stage, patients with large cell neuroendocrine cancers of the lung survive longer than patients with small cell cancers [16]. Separating high grade neuroendocrine tumors into small cell and non-small cell categories may have diagnostic and prognostic importance. Accurate diagnosis of these rare lesions requires careful clinicopathologic correlations as well as incorporation of pertinent radiographic and historic data. Metastases from a neuroendocrine primary at a distant site should be excluded. Light microscopic interpretations can be effectively enhanced by cytohistologic comparison of touch preparation slides, and ancillary studies including immunohistochemistry and chromogenic in situ hybridization studies for EBER are important in tumor typing.

Conflict of Interests

The authors declare that there is no conflict of interests regarding the publication of this paper.

References

[1] L. Barnes, J. W. Eveson, P. Reichert, and D. Sidransky, *WHO Classification of Tumors of the Head and Neck*, Internation Agency for Research on Cancer, Lyon, France, 2005.

[2] S. H. Hutajulu, J. Kurnianda, I. B. Tan, and J. M. Middeldorp, "Therapeutic implications of Epstein–Barr virus infection for the treatment of nasopharyngeal carcinoma," *Therapeutics and Clinical Risk Management*, vol. 10, pp. 721–736, 2014.

[3] O. Casiraghi and M. Lefèvre, "Undifferentiated malignant round cell tumors of the sinonasal tract and nasopharynx," *Annales de Pathologie*, vol. 29, no. 4, pp. 296–312, 2009.

[4] V. Vandist, F. Deridder, W. Waelput, P. M. Parizel, P. Van De Heyning, and C. Van Laer, "A neuroendocrine tumour of the sphenoid sinus and nasopharynx: a case report," *B-ENT*, vol. 6, no. 2, pp. 147–151, 2010.

[5] I.-H. Lin, C.-F. Hwang, H.-Y. Huang, and C.-Y. Chien, "Small cell carcinoma of the nasopharynx," *Acta Oto-Laryngologica*, vol. 127, no. 2, pp. 206–208, 2007.

[6] S. Deviprasad, A. Rajeshwari, M. Tahir, T. V. Adarsha, and S. Gangadhara, "Small-cell neuroendocrine carcinoma originating from the lateral nasopharyngeal wall," *Ear, Nose & Throat Journal*, vol. 87, no. 11, pp. E1–E3, 2008.

[7] L.-Y. Lee, K.-P. Chang, C.-L. Hsu, T.-C. Chen, and T.-T. Kuo, "Small-cell neuroendocrine carcinoma of the nasopharynx: report of a rare case lacking association with Epstein-Barr virus," *International Journal of Surgical Pathology*, vol. 19, no. 2, pp. 199–202, 2011.

[8] F. Elloumi, N. Fourati, W. Siala et al., "Large cell neuroendocrine carcinoma of the nasopharynx: a case report," *Cancer/Radiotherapie*, vol. 18, no. 3, pp. 208–210, 2014.

[9] I. Weinreb and B. Perez-Ordoñez, "Non-small cell neuroendocrine carcinoma of the sinonasal tract and nasopharynx: report of 2 cases and review of the literature," *Head and Neck Pathology*, vol. 1, no. 1, pp. 21–26, 2007.

[10] W. D. Travis, E. Brambilla, H. K. Muller-Hermelink, and C. C. Harris, *WHO Classification of Tumors of the Lung, Pleura, Thymus and Heart*, International Agency for Research on Cancer, Lyon, France, 2004.

[11] Y. J. Yang, C. T. Steele, X. L. Ou, K. P. Snyder, and L. J. Kohman, "Diagnosis of high-grade pulmonary neuroendocrine carcinoma by fine-needle aspiration biopsy: nonsmall-cell or small-cell type?" *Diagnostic Cytopathology*, vol. 25, no. 5, pp. 292–300, 2001.

[12] J. A. Jimenez-Heffernan, P. Lopez-Ferrer, B. Vicandi et al., "Fine-needle aspiration cytology of large cell neuroendocrine carcinoma of the lung: a cytohistologic correlation study of 11 cases," *Cancer*, vol. 114, no. 3, pp. 180–186, 2008.

[13] A. Iyoda, M. Baba, K. Hiroshima et al., "Imprint cytologic features of pulmonary large cell neuroendocrine carcinoma: comparison with classic large cell carcinoma," *Oncology Reports*, vol. 11, no. 2, pp. 285–288, 2004.

[14] T. Nagao, I. Sugano, Y. Ishida et al., "Primary large-cell neuroendocrine carcinoma of the parotid gland: immunohistochemical and molecular analysis of two cases," *Modern Pathology*, vol. 13, no. 5, pp. 554–561, 2000.

[15] N. Yamamoto, S. Minami, M. Kidoguchi, A. Shindo, Y. Tokumaru, and M. Fujii, "Large cell neuroendocrine carcinoma of the submandibular gland: case report and literature review," *Auris Nasus Larynx*, vol. 41, no. 1, pp. 105–108, 2014.

[16] L. Sun, S. Sakurai, T. Sano, M. Hironaka, O. Kawashima, and T. Nakajima, "High-grade neuroendocrine carcinoma of the lung: comparative clinicopathological study of large cell neuroendocrine carcinoma and small cell lung carcinoma," *Pathology International*, vol. 59, no. 8, pp. 522–529, 2009.

Synchronous Fibrolamellar Hepatocellular Carcinoma and Auricular Myxoma

Yessica M. González-Cantú,[1] Cristina Rodriguez-Padilla,[1] Martha Lilia Tena-Suck,[2] Alberto García de la Fuente,[1] Rosa María Mejía-Bañuelos,[3] Raymundo Díaz Mendoza,[1] Samuel Quintanilla-Garza,[4] and Yolaester Batisda-Acuña[5]

[1]*Laboratorio de Inmunología y Virología, Facultad de Ciencias Biológicas, Universidad Autónoma de Nuevo León, Avenida Manuel L. Barragán S/N, Ciudad Universitaria, 66451 San Nicolás de los Garza, NL, Mexico*
[2]*Departamento de Neuropatología, Instituto Nacional de Neurología y Neurocirugía, Manuel Velasco Suárez, Avenida Insurgentes Sur 3877, Colonia La Fama, 14269 Delegación Tlalpan, DF, Mexico*
[3]*Hospital General de Zona 17, Instituto Mexicano del Seguro Social, Fortunato Lozano y Roble Colonia Benito Juárez, 64420 Monterrey, NL, Mexico*
[4]*Unidad de Medicina Familiar No. 73, Instituto Mexicano del Seguro Social, Pablo de Mejía No. 526, Colonia Zona Centro, 25000 Saltillo, COAH, Mexico*
[5]*Hospital General Regional No. 1, Instituto Mexicano del Seguro Social, Bosques de los Olivos 101, 61301 Morelia, MICH, Mexico*

Correspondence should be addressed to Yessica M. González-Cantú; ymgc1301@gmail.com

Academic Editor: Tibor Tot

Synchronic occurrence of benign and malignant tumors is extremely rare. Fibrolamellar hepatocellular carcinoma represents 1% to 2% of all hepatocarcinomas, while myxomas represent about half of all the cases of primary tumors of the heart. We present the case of a 53-year-old woman with a left atrial myxoma that was surgically removed. Several weeks later, the patient returned to the hospital with abdominal pain. CT scan showed a mass in the left lobe of the liver that was resected and diagnosed as fibrolamellar hepatocellular carcinoma. As of this writing, the patient is healthy.

1. Introduction

Hepatocellular carcinoma (HCC) represents 80% to 90% of all liver cancers [1]. According to the International Classification of Disease for Oncology, HCC is categorized as HCC-not otherwise specified (HCC-NOS), scirrhous HCC, spindle cell variant HCC, clear cell HCC, pleomorphic HCC, and fibrolamellar HCC (FLHCC) [2]. FLHCC is a relatively rare form of HCC that affects mostly young people and is not associated with any diseases of the liver such as cirrhosis or hepatitis virus infection [3]. FLHCC is less aggressive than HCC [4].

Primary cardiac tumors are rare, representing 0.0017% to 0.19% of autopsy cases [5]. Myxomas represent about 50% of all cardiac tumors [6] and are located mostly in the left atrium (left-right ratio = 4 : 1) [5]. Most cardiac myxomas are sporadic, although a small percentage of them are familial and sometimes attributable to Carney syndrome.

Here we describe the case of a 53-year-old woman who was diagnosed with fibrolamellar hepatocellular carcinoma synchronous with left atrial myxoma.

2. Case Presentation

A 53-year-old female with no known medical conditions reported the start of symptoms 4 months before consultation. The patient reported palpitations that exacerbated by cardiovascular exercise and attenuated with rest. The cardiologist requested an ECG and diagnosed sinus tachycardia. Subsequently, a transthoracic echocardiography was performed, and a mass dependent on the left atrium compatible with

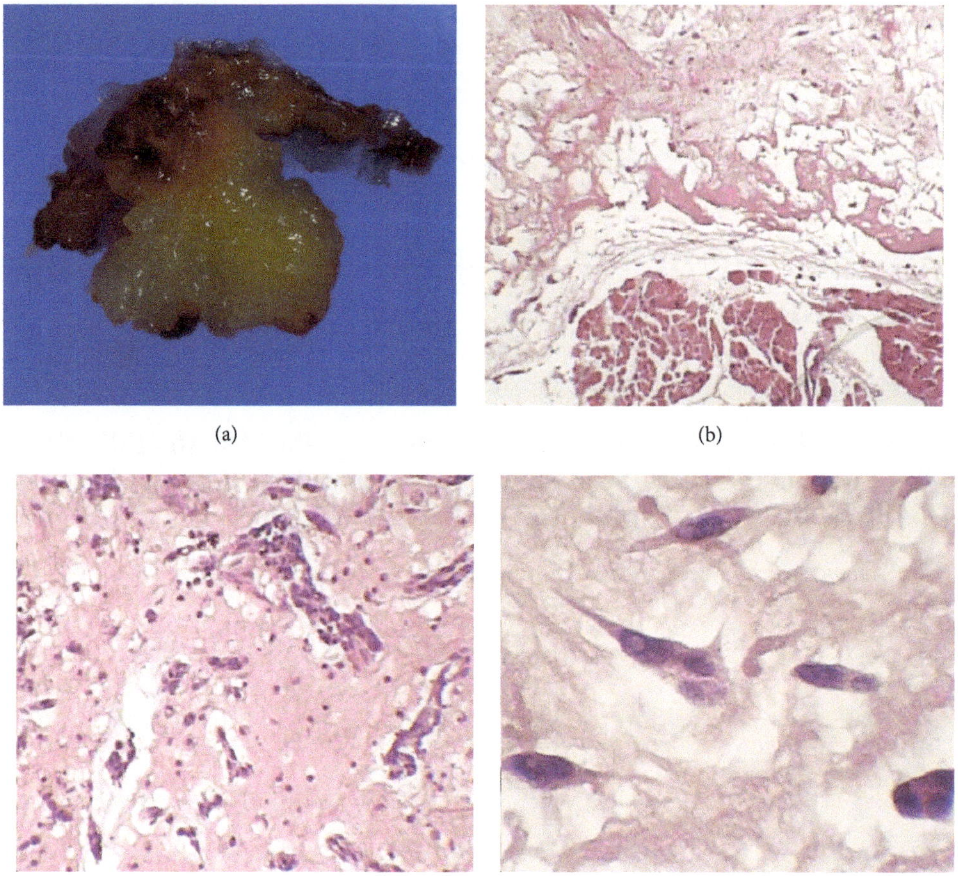

FIGURE 1: (a) Macroscopic image of the left auricular myxoma. (b) shows fusiform hyperchromatic cells immersed in a myxoid matrix and the cardiac muscle (H and E stain, 50x). (c) Groups of fusiform cells immersed in a myxoid matrix surrounded by abundant inflammatory cells (H and E stain, 100x). (d) Fusiform cells under higher magnification (H and E stain, 400x).

auricular myxoma was detected. The patient was scheduled for surgery, a median sternotomy for a transseptal approach to the right atrium was performed, and the patient began treatment with IMMUNEPOTENT CRP (bovine dialyzable leukocyte extract) which was administered orally to promote postsurgical recovery.

The patient underwent surgery without complications and was discharged from the hospital. The mass was diagnosed by pathology as left atrial myxoma with mural thrombus (Figure 1). Three months after discharge from the hospital, the patient presented epigastric abdominal pain of moderate intensity that irradiated to the mesogastrium and right upper quadrant, which was accompanied by postprandial pain, nausea, and constipation. The patient was admitted to the hospital to evaluate her abdominal pain. Her heart rate was 100 bpm and her blood pressure was 130/80 mmHg; all laboratory tests were normal.

A CT scan of the abdomen was performed, which showed $8 \times 8 \times 7.3$ cm mass in the left lobe of the liver (Figure 2(a)). The lesion was hypervascular and had central calcification and a tendency toward necrosis (Figures 2(b) and 2(c)). The patient underwent surgery for tumor resection.

After postoperative analysis from pathology, the diagnosis was of a 9 cm, Grade III moderately differentiated fibrolamellar hepatocellular carcinoma with clean resection borders (AJCC, T2, N0, Mx) (Figures 3(a)–3(d)). The patient is currently asymptomatic and receives annual check-ups.

3. Discussion

Multiple primary malignant neoplasms (MPMN) are defined as a diagnosis of two or more independent primary malignancies of different histologies/origins in an individual [7]. They are classified as MPMN according to the following criteria: tumors must be malignant, they must be located in different organs or tissues, and the possibility of metastasis must be ruled out completely. The incidence rate of MPNM varies from 0.7% to 11.7% [8]. The association of benign and malignant tumors, in absence of underlying genetic diseases, is extremely rare [9].

Fibrolamellar hepatocellular carcinoma and cardiac myxoma are a rare presentation of synchronous tumors. Ochoa et al. (2011) described one case of hepatocarcinoma synchronous with atrial myxoma [9]. There at least two cases

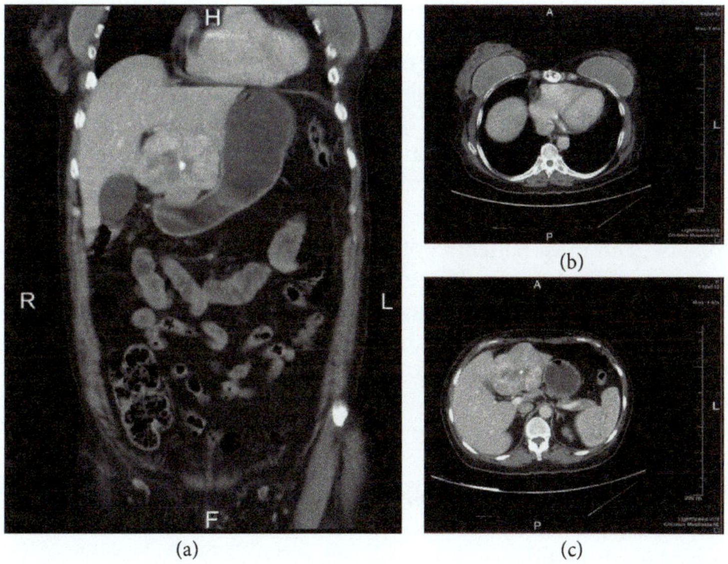

FIGURE 2: Images from the abdominal CT. (a) and (b) show the 8 × 8 × 7.3 cm tumor located in segment IV of the left lobe of the liver that laterally displaces the gallbladder. The lesion has defined lobular borders that show a heterogeneous peripheral areas and a hypodense center with calcification. (c) shows changes in the sternum with presence of surgical material.

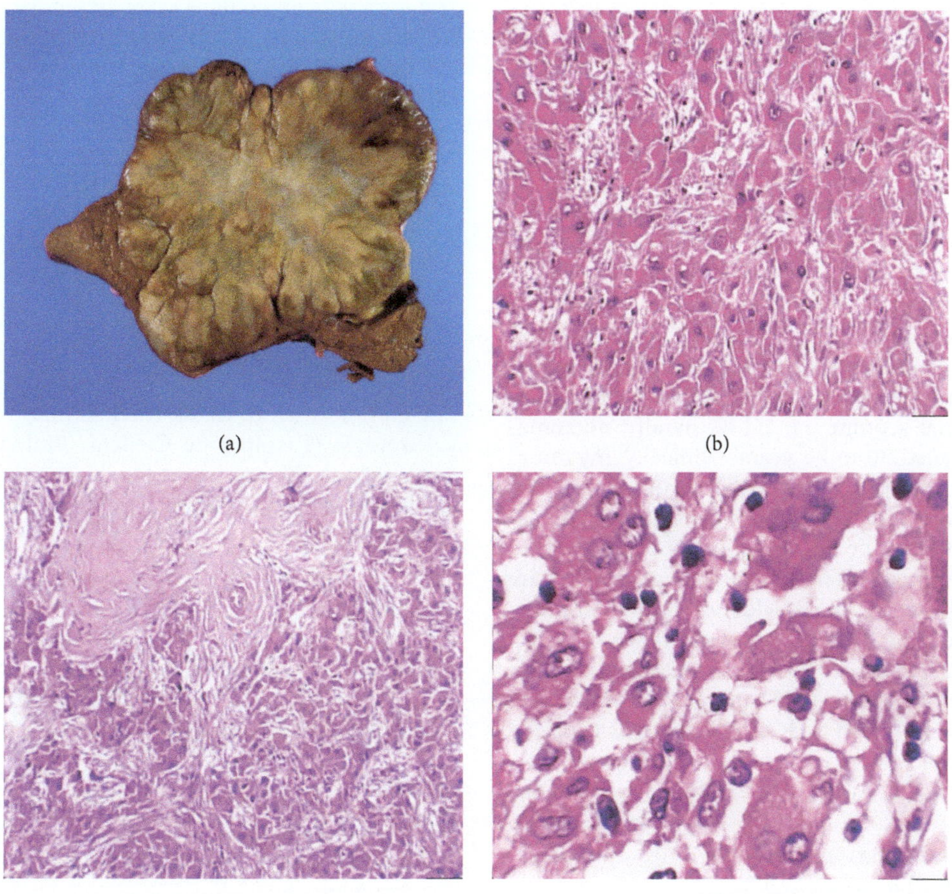

FIGURE 3: (a) Macroscopic image of the liver that shows a 9 × 7 cm, central yellowish lesion with diffuse, infiltrating borders with a whitish central lesion. (b) shows neoplastic cells separated into nodules by connective tissue (H and E stain, 50x). (c) Neoplastic cells with loss of the nucleus-cytoplasm relationship (H and E stain, 100x). (d) Image that shows the cellular and nuclear pleomorphism in greater detail (H and E stain, 400x).

of metastasis mimicking atrial myxoma in hepatocellular carcinoma [1, 10]. Fibrolamellar hepatocellular carcinoma (FLHCC) usually appears in younger patients (median age of 25 years) [11], although recent studies show two distinct peaks of incidence, the first at 10 to 30 years of age and the second at 70 to 79 years of age [2, 4]. At the moment of diagnosis, our patient was 53 years old, which is inconsistent with the data reported in the literature.

FLHCC is usually asymptomatic, and most patients visit a doctor when they note the presence of an abdominal mass. Those patients with symptomatology report vague symptoms such as weight loss and abdominal pain or discomfort [3]. Imaging studies, such as ultrasound, MRI, and CT scans, are an integral part of FLHCC diagnosis [4]. Our patient was diagnosed with FLHCC during a CT scan performed a few weeks after surgery to remove myxoma.

Liver function tests for patients with FLHCC are usually normal, although sometimes alpha-fetoprotein and aminotransferases show slightly increased levels [3, 12].

FHLCC prefers the left lobe of the liver, and, grossly, it is usually yellow to pale tan and firm, with an average size of 6–19 cm at its longest diameter. About 75% of tumors present a central scar; some tumors present foci of necrosis, hemorrhage, and calcification [3, 11].

Histopathologically, the tumor is composed of large polygonal cells with large vesicular nuclei containing marginalized chromatin and prominent nucleoli with eosinophilic (oncocytic) cytoplasm surrounded by distinctly lamellar stroma. Calcifications and pale bodies are seen in more than 50% of cases [11, 13]. Stainable copper is found in 75% of all FLHCC cases [12]. Immunohistochemical markers for FHLCC are CK7, EMA, mCEA, CA19-9, EpCAM, and CD68 [11, 13]. Whenever possible, complete surgical resection is the preferred treatment for FLHCC [4].

Myxomas represent 50% of the very rare cases of primary cardiac tumors. The most frequent location for myxomas is the left atrium, and they usually originate from the endocardium of the atrial septum [14, 15]. Generally, myxomas appear in women aged 30 to 70 years. Clinically, myxomas are characterized by dyspnea, syncope, arrhythmias, edema, hemoptysis, and sudden death. Some of the systemic characteristics of myxoma include embolic phenomena in 30% to 40% of patients. Approximately 10% to 15% of patients are asymptomatic and the myxoma is found accidentally during imaging studies [16]. Transthoracic or transesophageal echocardiography and MRI are the most common diagnostic tools for neoplasms of the heart [14]. In our case, the patient reported tachycardia, which led to the discovery of the myxoma by means of transesophageal echocardiography.

Surgery is the election treatment for myxoma; it must be performed without delay because of the high risk of sudden death from thromboembolism or valvular obstruction; resection of the tumor must be total [14, 17].

Macroscopically, myxomas are pedunculated and gelatinous, and their surface can be smooth, villous, or friable and, in some cases, they show areas of hemorrhage. Their diameter ranges from 1 to 15 cm, and their weight ranges between 15 and 180 grams [5, 18].

Histologically, myxomas are made up of stellate and polyhedral (lepidic) cells. These tumor cells have small round or oval nuclei and variable amounts of cytoplasm. Myxoma cells can appear singly or in small clusters or chords, and when grouped around small spaces they can simulate glandular structures; they rarely show mitotic activity. Myxomas have abundant, fibrillary, slightly basophilic, mucoid matrix [19]. These tumors may form large and small fibrin-platelet thrombi, which may be an additional source of emboli [19].

Myxomas show a diffuse positive reaction for the immunohistochemical marker Vimentin and focal expression of CD34, CD68, and SMA [20]. They also have variable positivity for cytokeratin, S100, factor VIII, and Calretinin [5, 20].

The IMMUNEPOTENT CRP (bovine dialyzable leukocyte extract) is a mixture of low molecular weight substances and is a drug capable of modulating the immune response. It has been used for years in clinical trials of multiple types of diseases such as cancer, toxic shock, and postoperative recovery, as in the clinical case presented here, increasing the quality of life of the patients [21, 22].

Synchronous tumors are rare and the coexistence of malignant and benign tumors is rarer still. Additionally, the association of fibrolamellar hepatocellular carcinoma and auricular myxoma is scarcely reported in the literature. In our case, our patient was treated in accordance with the established surgical procedures, received oral doses of IMMUNEPOTENT CRP, and, as of this writing, is completely asymptomatic.

Conflict of Interests

The authors declare that there is no conflict of interests regarding the publication of this paper.

Acknowledgments

The authors wish to thank the Laboratorio de Inmunología y Virología (Facultad de Ciencias Biológicas, Universidad Autónoma de Nuevo León) for the economic support. They also thank MSc. Alejandra Arreola-Triana for her editorial work on this paper.

References

[1] A. M. Anwar, Y. F. M. Nosir, M. A. R. Chamsi-Pasha, A. Ajam, and H. Chamsi-Pasha, "Right atrial metastasis mimicking myxoma in advanced hepatocellular carcinoma," *Echocardiography*, vol. 27, no. 1, pp. 80–83, 2010.

[2] T. Eggert, K. A. McGlynn, A. Duffy, M. P. Manns, T. F. Greten, and S. F. Altekruse, "Fibrolamellar hepatocellular carcinoma in the USA, 2000–2010: a detailed report on frequency, treatment and outcome based on the surveillance, epidemiology, and end Results database," *United European Gastroenterology Journal*, vol. 1, no. 5, pp. 351–357, 2013.

[3] P. Herman, A. L. Chagas, M. V. Perini et al., "Surgical treatment of fibrolamellar hepatocellular carcinoma: an underestimated malignant tumor?" *Hepatobiliary & Pancreatic Diseases International*, vol. 13, no. 6, pp. 618–621, 2014.

[4] I. I. P. Lim, B. A. Farber, and M. P. LaQuaglia, "Advances in fibrolamellar hepatocellular carcinoma: a review," *European Journal of Pediatric Surgery*, vol. 24, no. 6, pp. 461–466, 2014.

[5] Y. Wang and F. E. Sharkey, "Myxoma of the small bowel in a 47-year-old woman with a left atrial myxoma," *Archives of Pathology and Laboratory Medicine*, vol. 127, no. 4, pp. 481–484, 2003.

[6] N. Barbetakis, T. Xenikakis, A. Efstathiou, G. Samanidis, C. Tsilikas, and I. Fessatidis, "Synchronous left ventricular myxoma and malignant fibrous histiocytoma: simultaneous surgical management," *Hellenic Journal of Cardiology*, vol. 49, no. 5, pp. 371–373, 2008.

[7] M. Fernández-Ruiz, J.-M. Guerra-Vales, F.-J. Castelbón-Fernández, J. Llenas-García, L. Caurcel-Díaz, and F. Colina-Ruizdelgado, "Multiple primary malignancies in Spanish patients with hepatocellular carcinoma: analysis of a hospital-based tumor registry," *Journal of Gastroenterology and Hepatology*, vol. 24, no. 8, pp. 1424–1430, 2009.

[8] S. J. Oh, D. S. Bae, and B. J. Suh, "Synchronous triple primary cancers occurring in the stomach, kidney, and thyroid," *Annals of Surgical Treatment and Research*, vol. 88, no. 6, pp. 345–348, 2015.

[9] M. L. Ochoa, A. G. C. Gordillo, and M. M. Pérez, "Carcinoma hepatocelular sincrónico con mixoma auricular. Informe de un caso," *Investigación Clínica*, vol. 52, no. 2, 2011.

[10] E. Maffei, T. Arcadi, and F. Cademartiri, "Hepatocellular carcinoma mimicking an atrial mixoma," *European Heart Journal*, vol. 35, no. 13, p. 876, 2014.

[11] D. Castro-Villabón, L. E. Barrera-Herrera, P. A. Rodríguez-Urrego et al., "Hepatocellular carcinoma with both fibrolamellar and classical components: an unusual morphological pattern," *Case Reports in Pathology*, vol. 2015, Article ID 609780, 5 pages, 2015.

[12] S. Kakar, L. J. Burgart, K. P. Batts, J. Garcia, D. Jain, and L. D. Ferrell, "Clinicopathologic features and survival in fibrolamellar carcinoma: comparison with conventional hepatocellular carcinoma with and without cirrhosis," *Modern Pathology*, vol. 18, no. 11, pp. 1417–1423, 2005.

[13] V. B. Weeda, M. Murawski, A. J. McCabe et al., "Fibrolamellar variant of hepatocellular carcinoma does not have a better survival than conventional hepatocellular carcinoma—results and treatment recommendations from the Childhood Liver Tumour Strategy Group (SIOPEL) experience," *European Journal of Cancer*, vol. 49, no. 12, pp. 2698–2704, 2013.

[14] K. Durgut, N. Görmüs, M. Ozulku, U. Özergin, and C. Özpinar, "Clinical features and surgical treatment of cardiac myxoma: report of 18 cases," *Asian Cardiovascular and Thoracic Annals*, vol. 10, no. 2, pp. 111–114, 2002.

[15] P. Becker R, A. Ramírez M, R. Zalaquett S et al., "Mixoma cardiaco: caracterización clínica, métodos diagnósticos y resultados alejados del tratamiento quirúrgico durante tres décadas de experiencia," *Revista Médica de Chile*, vol. 136, no. 3, pp. 287–295, 2008.

[16] S. Mehra, Y. Parviz, and A. Al-Mohammad, "Left atrial myxoma with concurrent saddle pulmonary embolism and duke's B colorectal adenocarcinoma," *Journal of Medical Cases*, 2013.

[17] G. Samanidis, K. Perreas, P. Kalogris et al., "Surgical treatment of primary intracardiac myxoma: 19 years of experience," *Interactive Cardiovascular and Thoracic Surgery*, vol. 13, no. 6, pp. 597–600, 2011.

[18] R. Cohen, G. Singh, D. Mena, C. A. Garcia, P. Loarte, and B. Mirrer, "Atrial myxoma: a case presentation and review," *Cardiology Research*, vol. 3, no. 1, pp. 41–44, 2012.

[19] L. E. Wold and J. T. Lie, "Cardiac myxomas: a clinicopathologic profile," *The American Journal of Pathology*, vol. 101, no. 1, pp. 219–240, 1980.

[20] J.-G. Wang, Y.-J. Li, H. Liu, N.-N. Li, J. Zhao, and X.-M. Xing, "Clinicopathologic analysis of cardiac myxomas: Seven years' experience with 61 patients," *Journal of Thoracic Disease*, vol. 4, no. 3, pp. 272–283, 2012.

[21] M. A. Franco-Molina, "Anti-inflammatory and antioxidant effects of IMMUNEPOTENT CRP in Lipopolysaccharide (LPS)-stimulated human macrophages," *African Journal of Microbiology Research*, vol. 5, no. 22, 2011.

[22] H. H. Lara, L. I. Turrent, E. N. Garza-Treviño, R. Tamez-Guerra, and C. Rodriguez-Padilla, "Clinical and immunological assessment in breast cancer patients receiving anticancer therapy and bovine dialyzable leukocyte extract as an adjuvant," *Experimental and Therapeutic Medicine*, vol. 1, no. 3, pp. 425–431, 2010.

35

An Isolated Phlebolith on the Lip: An Unusual Case and Review of the Literature

Gabriela de Morais Gouvêa Lima, Renata Mendonça Moraes, Ana Sueli Rodrigues Cavalcante, Yasmin Rodarte Carvalho, and Ana Lia Anbinder

Department of Bioscience and Oral Diagnosis, Institute of Science and Technology, Campus São José dos Campos, Univ. Estadual Paulista (UNESP), Engenheiro Francisco José Longo Avenida 777, 12245-000 São José dos Campos, SP, Brazil

Correspondence should be addressed to Ana Lia Anbinder; ana.anbinder@ict.unesp.br

Academic Editor: Hiroko Kuwabara

Background. Calcified thrombi are a common finding, especially in the pelvic veins. There are generally multiple thrombi, and they are generally associated with vascular malformations. *Design.* Herein we report a rare case of a single labial phlebolith, not associated with any other vascular lesion. We aim to alert clinicians to the possibility of the occurrence of vascular thrombi in the mouth and to describe the clinical and histological characteristics of such lesions in order to simplify the diagnosis and treatment. Furthermore, we have reviewed the English-language literature published since 1970 reporting oral (including masticatory muscles) phleboliths. *Results.* Twenty-nine cases of phleboliths have been reported in the literature since 1970. Only three of the reported phleboliths were solitary and not associated with other vascular lesions, as in the case presented here. *Conclusion.* Although phleboliths not associated with other vascular lesions are not common, clinicians should be aware of the existence of this pathology and include it as differential diagnosis of oral lesions.

1. Introduction

Phleboliths are calcified thrombi usually associated with other vascular lesions, as vascular malformations (VM), and are caused by blood stasis [1] or even trauma [2].

In the literature, they are commonly found on routine radiographs of cases diagnosed as VM or hemangiomas, although they are better detected by computerized tomography [1, 3, 4]. Radiographically, they present as oval structures with concentric radiolucent or radio-opaque laminations. They can be found in periapical regions near dental structures in a plain radiograph [5, 6]. Nonionizing techniques, such as magnetic resonance imaging and ultrasound, can provide good images demonstrating the location and extent of the lesions [6, 7].

The pelvic area is the most common area affected by phleboliths, which can occur within prostatic, uterine, or intestine veins. Phleboliths are not unusual in the head and neck, but there are few cases in the literature of phleboliths not associated with other vascular anomalies [8–10]. When a phlebolith is located in salivary gland regions, it can be clinically misdiagnosed as a sialolith or salivary gland disease, especially when there is intermittent swelling, despite not being associated with food intake. In these cases, sialography can be used as diagnostic tool [11–13].

Besides imaging exams, biopsy followed by microscopic examination can help in the final diagnosis. Histologically, a phlebolith is seen as concentric calcifications with an onion-like appearance inside a vessel, caused by repetitive mineral deposition on a thrombus and secondary lamellar fibrosis [2, 7, 13]. Commonly, hematoxylin and eosin (HE) and immunohistochemistry are used [10, 14, 15], but use of electron microscopy and X-ray microdiffraction has also been reported [14].

We report herein an unusual case of a phlebolith presenting as a single lesion, not associated with a VM and clinically misdiagnosed as a neurofibroma. In describing this case, we aim to help clinicians to deal with this uncommon but simple lesion. We have also reviewed the literature of oral/masticatory muscle phleboliths.

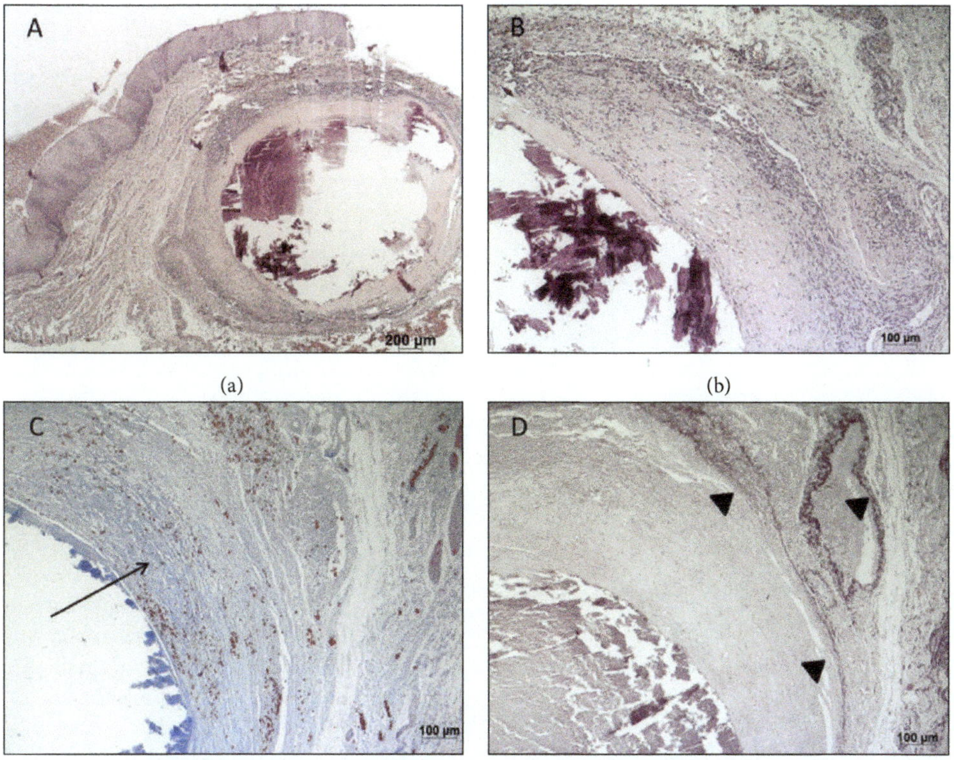

(a) (b) (c) (d)

FIGURE 1: Microscopic aspect of the lesion showing the vascular structures ((a) and (b) hematoxylin and eosin stain), collagen (Masson's Trichrome (c)), and elastic fibers (Weigert stain (d)).

2. Report of Case

A 56-year-old woman was referred to our institution presenting with a white-yellow painless papule in the right labial commissure. It was approximately 3 mm in diameter and firm to palpation and had been growing slowly for approximately one year, following trauma. The patient reported swelling after trauma with subsequent diminution and then a recent increase in volume. Her previous medical history was unremarkable.

No radiograph was performed, and the clinical diagnostic hypothesis was neurofibroma and pleomorphic adenoma. An excisional biopsy was performed followed by histopathological examination.

Microscopic examination revealed a submucous dilated vessel filled by a calcified thrombus with a concentric pattern of mineralization and surrounded by granulation tissue and small capillaries under a hyaline layer. The covering mucosa was intact and presented no alterations (Figure 1).

The diagnosis of phlebolith was confirmed by histochemical Weigert's and Masson's Trichrome staining and by immunohistochemistry with anti-CD34 and anti-smooth muscle actin (SMA) (Table 1; Figure 2), as evidenced by the vascular endothelium (CD34-positive), smooth muscle wall (SMA-positive), tunica intima elastic fibers (Weigert's elastic stain), and surrounding collagen fibers (Masson's Trichrome) of the vessel filled with the calcified thrombus.

TABLE 1: Antibodies and protocol used for immunohistochemistry.

Antibody	Antigen retrieval	Concentration
SMA (Dako)	No retrieval	1:100
CD34 (Dako)	Dako Target Retrieval Solution, pH 9	1:100

Complementary electron microscopy with energy dispersive X-ray spectrometry (EDS) revealed the presence of calcium (Ca), carbon (C), silicon (Si), and magnesium (Mg) (Figure 3), compatible with a phlebolith. The patient was followed without any complication after surgery.

3. Review of the Literature

Medline and Web of Science databases were searched using the descriptors "oral phlebolith" and "phleboliths," "phlebolith," "oral thrombus [case report]," and "lip and thrombus." Table 2 shows all cases of phleboliths in the oral region (including masticatory muscles) reported in the English literature from 1970 to 2013.

We found 29 cases of phleboliths. In five cases, there were multiple phleboliths not associated with other vascular lesions (16.13%), and, in four cases (12.90%), there was a solitary phlebolith, but only one was associated with a lesion diagnosed as hemangioma. Only three reported phleboliths

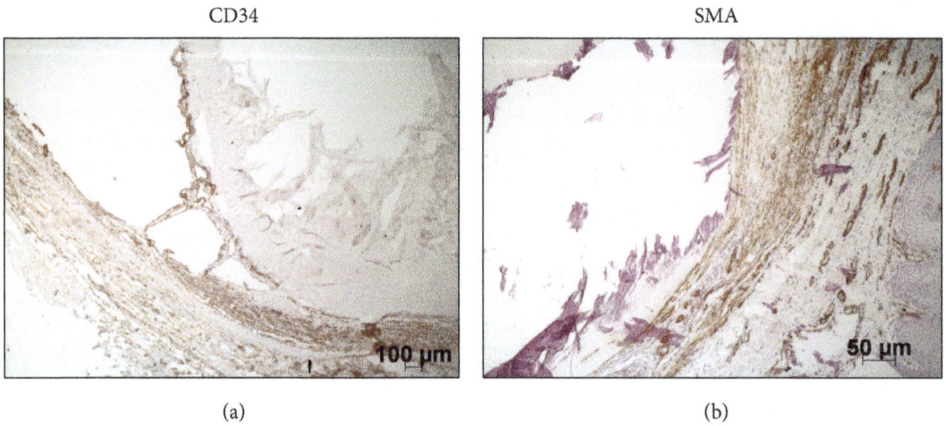

FIGURE 2: Immunohistochemistry showing vascular endothelium stained with anti-CD34 (a) and smooth muscle wall stained with anti-SMA (b).

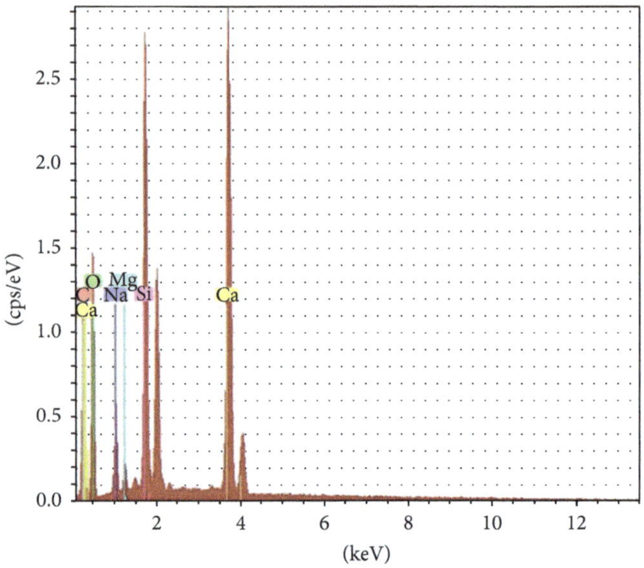

FIGURE 3: Energy dispersive X-ray spectrometry (EDS), results in graphic, with peaks of calcium, carbon, silicon, and magnesium.

were solitary and not associated with other vascular lesions, as in the case presented here.

Based on the reviewed literature, phleboliths of the oral region can be found in infants to elderly individuals, but mainly between the first and third decades of life (55.2%), with no sex predilection (48.28% female: 51.72% male), and are sometimes associated with masticatory muscles (27.6%).

4. Discussion

Phleboliths are calcified thrombi that commonly appear as multiple calcifications related to lesions diagnosed as VM or hemangiomas [1–4, 6, 7, 11–21]. They are rarely reported as solitary calcifications and/or not associated with a vascular lesion [8–10], as in the case reported here. We have reported herein a case of a single phlebolith on the lip, probably caused by trauma. The clinical appearance of a white-yellow color papule, without a calcified aspect or consistency, led us to suspect a neurofibroma or a small salivary gland lesion; therefore, we did not radiograph the lesion, which could have helped us with an accurate diagnosis.

The diagnosis of a phlebolith is commonly made by physical and imaging examinations and confirmed by microscopy (HE stain). In some cases, immunohistochemistry or even electron microscopy [10, 14, 15] is used. In our case, we reached the final diagnosis only after biopsy, and it was confirmed by histochemistry (Weigert's elastic stain and Masson's Trichrome), immunohistochemistry (CD34 and SMA), and EDS.

The EDS showed peaks of C, Ca (interpreted as calcium carbonate), Mg, and Si. A study of arterial biomineralization in autopsies found both apatitic and nonapatitic calcifications in different zones of the arterial wall [22]. The literature shows that the calcified crystals are mainly composed of phosphate and calcium carbonate, components of apatite. Minor crystals of Mg can be present in the hydroxyapatite [11, 17], and even Si may be present. Studies have shown that Si is a component of biomineralization [22], which was recently described as being involved in the early stages of this process [23]. The mineral composition, though phosphorus was missing, is intriguing; however, the components that should be present in a phlebolith are not well established, and the area we analyzed using EDS may not have been a representative area of apatitic calcification.

Cases of phleboliths not associated with other vascular lesions are rarely reported in the literature, especially as solitary nodules [8–10]. Trauma may have caused the slow flow, thrombus development, and consequent mineral deposition in this case.

5. Conclusion

Despite the rarity of this condition, clinicians should be aware of the existence of single phleboliths not associated with other vascular lesions when facing a submucous lesion on the lip or

Table 2: Cases of phleboliths in the oral region (including masticatory muscles) reported in the English literature from 1970 to 2013.

Author	Year	Location	Multiple	Other vascular lesions	Sex	Age
O'Riordan [11]	1974	Lower lip/neck	Yes	Yes	Female	23
O'Riordan [11]	1974	Buccal soft tissue	Yes	Yes	Male	43
O'Riordan [11]	1974	Mandible	Yes	Yes	Female	27
O'Riordan [11]	1974	Buccal soft tissue	Yes	Yes	Female	47
Keathley et al. [12]	1983	Submandibular	Yes	Yes	Male	23
Ikegami and Nishijima [16]	1984	Buccal soft tissue	Yes	Yes	Male	23
Gunge et al. [14]	1987	Buccinator muscle	Yes	Yes	Female	41
Sano et al. [17]	1988	Buccal soft tissue	Yes	Yes	Male	17
Sano et al. [17]	1988	Buccal soft tissue	Yes	Yes	Female	37
Hupp [18]	1989	Maxilla	Yes	Yes	Male	20
Zachariades et al. [8]	1991	Masseteric muscle	Yes	No	Male	8
Zachariades et al. [8]	1991	Masseteric muscle	Yes	No	Female	9
Zachariades et al. [8]	1991	Maxillary antrum	No	No	Male	42
Kurita et al. [9]	1994	Tongue	No	No	Female	69
Scolozzi et al. [13]	2003	Retromolar region	Yes	Yes	Female	92
Çankaya et al. [19]	2003	Submental	Yes	Yes	Male	18
Chuang et al. [3]	2005	Submandibular	Yes	Yes	Male	65
Altuğ et al. [1]	2007	Masseteric muscle	No	Yes	Male	21
Altuğ et al. [1]	2007	Buccal soft tissue	Yes	Yes	Male	22
Altuğ et al. [1]	2007	Submental/submandibular/neck	Yes	Yes	Male	21
Kanaya et al. [7]	2008	Masseteric muscle	Yes	Yes	Female	14
Su et al. [20]	2009	Submandibular	Yes	Yes	Female	26
Mandel and Perrino [2]	2010	Buccinator/masseter	Yes	Yes	Female	56
Mandel and Perrino [2]	2010	Tongue	Yes	Yes	Female	64
Gharaibeh et al. [15]	2010	Floor of the mouth	Yes	Yes	Male	11
Orhan et al. [4]	2012	Lower and upper lip/buccal soft tissue	Yes	Yes	Male	20
Kato et al. [10]	2012	Buccal soft tissue	No	No	Female	17
Zengin et al. [6]	2013	Masseteric muscle	Yes	Yes	Female	21

other regions susceptible to trauma and should include them in the differential diagnosis.

Conflict of Interests

The authors declare that there is no conflict of interests regarding the publication of this paper.

References

[1] H. A. Altuğ, V. Büyüksoy, K. M. Okçu, and N. Doğan, "Hemangiomas of the head and neck with phleboliths: clinical features, diagnostic imaging, and treatment of 3 cases," *Oral Surgery, Oral Medicine, Oral Pathology, Oral Radiology and Endodontology*, vol. 103, no. 3, pp. e60–e64, 2007.

[2] L. Mandel and M. A. Perrino, "Phleboliths and the vascular maxillofacial lesion," *Journal of Oral and Maxillofacial Surgery*, vol. 68, no. 8, pp. 1973–1976, 2010.

[3] C.-C. Chuang, H.-C. Lin, and C.-W. Huang, "Submandibular cavernous hemangiomas with multiple phleboliths masquerading as sialolithiasis," *Journal of the Chinese Medical Association*, vol. 68, no. 9, pp. 441–443, 2005.

[4] K. Orhan, M. Icen, S. Aksoy, H. Avsever, and G. Akcicek, "Large arteriovenous malformation of the oromaxillofacial region with multiple phleboliths," *Oral Surgery, Oral Medicine, Oral Pathology and Oral Radiology*, vol. 114, no. 4, pp. e147–e158, 2012.

[5] L. A. Parker Jr. and H. H. Frommer, "Phleboliths. Report of a case," *Oral Surgery, Oral Medicine, Oral Pathology*, vol. 18, no. 4, pp. 476–480, 1964.

[6] A. Z. Zengin, P. Celenk, and A. P. Sumer, "Intramuscular hemangioma presenting with multiple phleboliths: a case report," *Oral Surgery, Oral Medicine, Oral Pathology and Oral Radiology*, vol. 115, no. 1, pp. e32–e36, 2013.

[7] H. Kanaya, Y. Saito, N. Gama, W. Konno, H. Hirabayashi, and S.-I. Haruna, "Intramuscular hemangioma of masseter muscle with prominent formation of phleboliths: a case report," *Auris Nasus Larynx*, vol. 35, no. 4, pp. 587–591, 2008.

[8] N. Zachariades, G. Rallis, J. Papademetriou, E. Konsolaki, S. Markaki, and M. Mezitis, "Phleboliths. A report of three unusual cases," *British Journal of Oral and Maxillofacial Surgery*, vol. 29, no. 2, pp. 117–119, 1991.

[9] H. Kurita, M. Chino, K. Kurashina, and A. Kotani, "Phlebothrombosis with phlebolith of the tongue," *Oral Surgery, Oral Medicine, Oral Pathology*, vol. 77, no. 6, p. 552, 1994.

[10] H. Kato, Y. Ota, M. Sasaki, T. Arai, Y. Sekido, and K. Tsukinoki, "A phlebolith in the anterior portion of the masseter muscle," *Tokai Journal of Experimental and Clinical Medicine*, vol. 37, no. 1, pp. 25–29, 2012.

[11] B. O'Riordan, "Phleboliths and salivary calculi," *British Journal of Oral Surgery*, vol. 12, no. 2, pp. 119–131, 1974.

[12] C. J. Keathley, R. L. Campbell, and J. W. Isbell, "Arteriovenous malformation and associated phleboliths. Report of a case," *Oral Surgery, Oral Medicine, Oral Pathology*, vol. 56, no. 2, pp. 132–135, 1983.

[13] P. Scolozzi, F. Laurent, T. Lombardi, and M. Richter, "Intraoral venous malformation presenting with multiple phleboliths," *Oral Surgery, Oral Medicine, Oral Pathology, Oral Radiology, and Endodontics*, vol. 96, no. 2, pp. 197–200, 2003.

[14] M. Gunge, H. Yamamoto, T. Sakae, T. Katoh, and H. Izumi, "Venous hemangioma with phleboliths—a case study using immunohistochemistry, scanning electron microscopy and x-ray microdiffraction," *The Journal of Nihon University School of Dentistry*, vol. 29, no. 3, pp. 211–220, 1987.

[15] T. M. Gharaibeh, R. A. Safadi, M. A. Rawashdeh, and H. M. Hammad, "Plunging arteriovenous malformation in the floor of the mouth: a case report," *British Journal of Oral and Maxillofacial Surgery*, vol. 48, no. 8, pp. e35–e37, 2010.

[16] N. Ikegami and K. Nishijima, "Hemangioma of the buccal pad with phlebolithiasis: report of a case," *Acta Medica Okayama*, vol. 38, no. 1, pp. 79–87, 1984.

[17] K. Sano, A. Ogawa, T. Inokuchi, H. Takahashi, and K. Hisatsune, "Buccal hemangioma with phleboliths. Report of two cases," *Oral Surgery, Oral Medicine, Oral Pathology*, vol. 65, no. 2, pp. 151–156, 1988.

[18] J. R. Hupp, "Facial phleboliths," *Oral Surgery, Oral Medicine, Oral Pathology*, vol. 67, no. 3, p. 361, 1989.

[19] H. Çankaya, Ö. Ünal, S. Ugras, K. Yuca, and M. Kiriş, "Hemangioma with phleboliths in the sublingual gland: as a cause of submental opacity," *Tohoku Journal of Experimental Medicine*, vol. 199, no. 3, pp. 187–191, 2003.

[20] Y.-X. Su, G.-Q. Liao, L. Wang, Y.-J. Liang, M. Chu, and G.-S. Zheng, "Sialoliths or phleboliths?" *Laryngoscope*, vol. 119, no. 7, pp. 1344–1347, 2009.

[21] H. J. Choi, J. C. Lee, J. H. Kim, Y. M. Lee, and H. J. Lee, "Cavernous hemangioma with large phlebolith of the parotid gland," *The Journal of Craniofacial Surgery*, vol. 24, no. 6, pp. e621–e623, 2013.

[22] A. G. Leyva, S. L. Maguid, M. A. R. de Benyacar, M. A. Lazaro, J. M. Cocco, and G. Citera, "Pathological mineralizations: calcifications and Si-bearing particles in soft tissues and their eventual relationship to different prostheses," *Artificial Organs*, vol. 24, no. 3, pp. 179–181, 2000.

[23] N. B. Matsko, N. Žnidaršič, I. Letofsky-Papst et al., "Silicon: the key element in early stages of biocalcification," *Journal of Structural Biology*, vol. 174, no. 1, pp. 180–186, 2011.

36

Anaplastic Transformation of Papillary Thyroid Cancer in the Retroperitoneum

James P. Solomon,[1] Fang Wen,[1] and Lily J. Jih[1,2]

[1]*Department of Pathology, University of California, San Diego, 9500 Gilman Drive, La Jolla, CA 92093, USA*
[2]*Department of Pathology, Veteran Administration Medical Center, La Jolla, 3350 La Jolla Village Drive (113), San Diego, CA 92161, USA*

Correspondence should be addressed to Lily J. Jih; lily.jih@va.gov

Academic Editor: Prashant Bavi

Anaplastic thyroid carcinoma is an aggressive variant of thyroid cancer that in most cases arises from anaplastic transformation of terminally differentiated thyroid carcinomas. This process usually occurs in the thyroid or cervical lymph nodes. Anaplastic transformation in distant metastatic sites is exceedingly rare, only previously documented in a few case reports. We report a rare case of anaplastic transformation of papillary thyroid carcinoma within a large retroperitoneal metastasis in a 64-year-old male 30 years after the initial diagnosis.

1. Introduction

Anaplastic thyroid carcinoma (ATC) is a rare form of thyroid carcinoma that is associated with an extremely poor prognosis. Most ATCs arise in the thyroid itself or in cervical lymph node metastases from anaplastic transformation of preexisting terminally differentiated thyroid carcinomas such as papillary or follicular thyroid carcinoma [1]. While terminally differentiated thyroid cancer can metastasize to distant sites, anaplastic transformation occurring within a distant metastatic site is a very rare phenomenon, with only a few reported cases in the literature [2–8]. Here, we report a rare case of anaplastic transformation of papillary thyroid carcinoma (PTC) in a retroperitoneal metastasis in a patient who underwent total thyroidectomy almost 30 years earlier.

2. Case Presentation

A 64-year-old male presented with persistent abdominal pain, and on imaging, he was found to have a 20 cm abdominal mass causing mass effect on the stomach, pancreas, left adrenal gland, and kidney (Figure 1). The patient had a history of PTC that was initially discovered in 1985, and at that time, he underwent total thyroidectomy and had postoperative radioactive iodine treatment. In 1999, he was found to have metastatic disease to the cervical lymph nodes and underwent a second round of radioactive iodine therapy. In 2005, he developed metastatic disease to the left axilla and was treated with local resection. In 2013, the patient presented with abdominal pain and was found to have a large retroperitoneal tumor that demonstrated strong FDG uptake on PET-CT, but radioactive iodine testing was not performed. Fine needle aspiration of the retroperitoneal mass performed at an outside institution showed a papillary neoplasm that was positive for TTF-1 and thyroglobulin, consistent with metastatic PTC. The patient was referred to our institution six months later for palliative resection of the tumor. His postoperative course was complicated by large bowel obstruction and sepsis. The patient expired 3 weeks after surgery.

Histological Findings. Grossly, the resected retroperitoneal mass measured 37 cm in greatest dimension and it was mostly necrotic with minimal viable areas. Extensive sampling showed sheets of pleomorphic cells with rhabdoid features including abundant granular eosinophilic cytoplasm and eccentric, vesicular nuclei with prominent nucleoli. Mitoses were readily identified (Figure 2). Due to

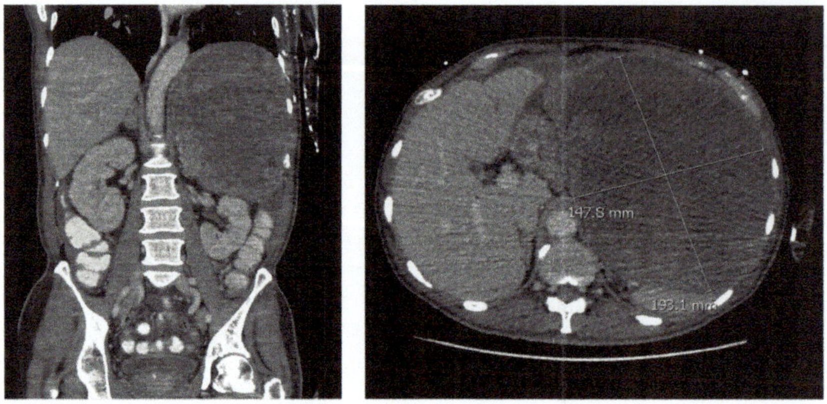

FIGURE 1: Abdominal CT scans demonstrating a 20 cm mass in the left upper quadrant retroperitoneum.

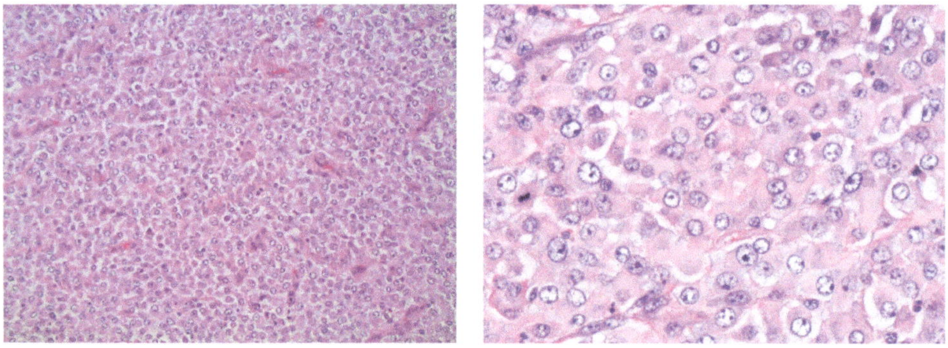

(a) (b)

FIGURE 2: Microscopic examination of the retroperitoneal mass. There were sheets of undifferentiated cells with no papillary architecture seen ((a) 100x). The malignant cells had rhabdoid features with abundant granular eosinophilic cytoplasm, eccentric, vesicular nuclei, and prominent nucleoli. Mitoses were readily identified ((b) 400x).

the unusual morphology and location, immunohistochemical stains were performed. The tumor cells were strongly positive for AE1/AE3, galectin-3, PAX8 (Figures 3(a)–3(c)), and vimentin, with patchy positivity for p53 (Figure 3(d)). There was focal weak staining for TTF-1 (Figure 3(e)), CK7, CK19, and S100. Thyroglobulin (Figure 3(f)), HBME-1, CK20, OCT3/4, CD117, CD45, and HMB45 were negative (Ventana Medical Systems, Tucson, AZ). Given the patient's long standing history of recurrent and metastatic PTC and the overall immunohistochemical profile, the findings were consistent with anaplastic transformation in a metastatic PTC.

3. Discussion

The retroperitoneal mass showed an undifferentiated tumor composed of sheets of malignant cells with eccentric nuclei, prominent nucleoli, and abundant eosinophilic cytoplasm. Although prior fine needle aspiration from an outside institution revealed tumor cells with papillary architecture consistent with metastatic PTC, no PTC component was identified in the resected specimen despite extensive sampling. Given the history of recurrent and metastatic PTC, anaplastic transformation of PTC was considered at the top of the differential diagnosis. However, because of the unusual location and the lack of identifiable PTC component in the resected retroperitoneal mass, other tumors were also considered. Differential diagnosis at this site included high-grade sarcoma, metastasis from other unknown primary, high-grade lymphoma, and melanoma. Additional immunohistochemistry was therefore performed for further characterization. The presence of strong and diffuse positivity for AE1/AE3 confirmed carcinoma. The tumor cells were negative for thyroglobulin and showed only focal staining for TTF-1, which often occurs in anaplastic transformation, as studies have demonstrated loss of thyroglobulin and TTF-1 expression in ATC [9]. The tumor cells were also positive for PAX-8, which is a transcription factor expressed in both normal and neoplastic thyroid, kidney, and female genital tract [10]. PAX-8 has been reported to be a reliable marker of thyroid origin, even after anaplastic transformation [11]. The tumor cells also expressed galectin-3 and focally expressed CK19, additional markers that have been shown to be positive in PTC [12]. Positivity for p53, which is correlated with mutations in the gene that expresses the protein, is also often seen

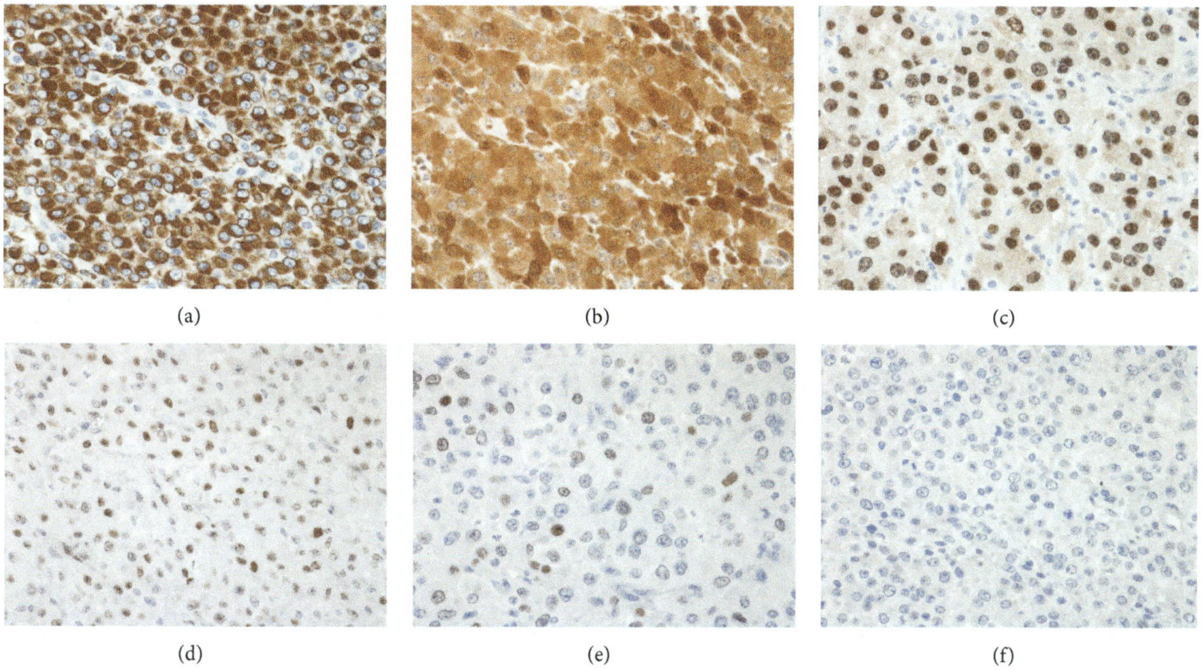

FIGURE 3: Immunohistochemical features of the tumor cells. The tumor cells showed diffuse positivity for AE1/AE3 (a), galectin-3 (b), and PAX-8 (c). There was patchy positivity for p53 (d). The tumor cells showed only weak focal positivity for TTF-1 (e) and were negative for thyroglobulin (f). All photographs at 400x magnification.

in a majority of ATC [6]. The overall immunohistochemical profile supported the diagnosis of anaplastic transformation of PTC.

ATC is the most aggressive type of thyroid neoplasm, with a 5-year survival rate of less than 10% and a mean survival time of six months after diagnosis [13]. Most patients present with rapidly enlarging neck mass and at least 40% of the patients have distant metastases at the time of diagnosis. Poor prognostic factors include higher age at diagnosis, male gender, leukocytosis, tumor size, extrathyroidal invasion, and presence of distant metastases [14]. While surgical treatment and radiotherapy have been shown to improve survival, the prognosis remains dismal [14].

Most cases of ATC are thought to arise from preexisting differentiated thyroid carcinoma. Some cases may develop de novo from preexisting multinodular goiter. Anaplastic transformation typically occurs within the thyroid gland and the cervical lymph nodes, and foci of ATC can occasionally be seen in these locations at the time of initial surgical management for differentiated thyroid carcinoma [1, 2]. Autopsy studies have demonstrated that ATC is often widely metastatic at the time of death, with two or more metastatic sites found in the vast majority of cases. The metastatic sites include the lungs, intrathoracic lymph nodes, cervical lymph nodes, pleura, adrenal glands, liver, brain, heart, and retroperitoneal lymph nodes [1].

Anaplastic transformation of a differentiated thyroid carcinoma at the distant site is exceedingly rare, only previously documented in a few case reports [2–8]. Only one of these reports described anaplastic transformation in a retroperitoneal metastasis [5], with other reported sites including the liver [6], pelvis [8], soft tissue of the shoulder [4], submandibular gland [7], and the lungs [2, 3]. The anaplastic transformation at the metastatic site can occur many years after the initial diagnosis and surgical treatment for the initial differentiated PTC; in these reported cases, the time from initial thyroidectomy to identification of anaplastic thyroid carcinoma at the metastatic site ranged from 7 to 17 years [2–8]. In many of these cases, the patients often have widespread metastatic PTC, and anaplastic transformation in distant metastases was identified on autopsy studies.

In the current case, the patient had a known history of metastatic PTC to cervical and axillary lymph nodes before presenting with a large retroperitoneal mass 30 years later. The retroperitoneal mass had evidence of PTC by cytological examination, suggesting that anaplastic transformation had occurred in the retroperitoneal mass. In addition, it has been proposed that postoperative radioactive iodine therapy can contribute to anaplastic transformation of PTC [6, 15], and in this case, the patient had two separate rounds of radioactive iodine therapy approximately 15 years apart.

In conclusion, this case demonstrates the rare occurrence of anaplastic transformation of PTC in an unusual distant site 30 years after the initial presentation. To our knowledge, this is the second reported case of anaplastic transformation of PTC within a retroperitoneal metastasis. As ATC has a much poorer prognosis than other types of thyroid carcinoma, its presence should always be reported. While it is known that thorough sampling and examination of thyroidectomy specimens and regional lymph node dissections should be performed, this case emphasizes that anaplastic transformation can occur even in distant metastases. It is therefore recommended that all resection specimens in patients with a history of thyroid carcinoma, including distant metastases, should be thoroughly sampled for the presence of ATC.

Conflict of Interests

The authors declare that there is no conflict of interests regarding the publication of this paper.

References

[1] N. Besic and B. Gazic, "Sites of metastases of anaplastic thyroid carcinoma: autopsy findings in 45 cases from a single institution," *Thyroid*, vol. 23, no. 6, pp. 709–713, 2013.

[2] W. Al-Qsous and I. D. Miller, "Anaplastic transformation in lung metastases of differentiated papillary thyroid carcinoma: an autopsy case report and review of the literature," *Annals of Diagnostic Pathology*, vol. 14, no. 1, pp. 41–43, 2010.

[3] M. E. Costaldi and Z. R. Zhou, "Case report: different metastatic components from anaplastic thyroid carcinoma in mediastinal and neck lymph nodes simultaneously diagnosed by FNA," *Diagnostic Cytopathology*, vol. 42, no. 8, pp. 694–699, 2014.

[4] S. Kaushal, M. C. Sharma, S. R. Mathur, S. Rastogi, C. S. Bal, and S. Chumber, "Anaplastic transformation of metastatic papillary thyroid carcinoma at shoulder mimicking soft tissue sarcoma," *Indian Journal of Pathology and Microbiology*, vol. 54, no. 4, pp. 796–799, 2011.

[5] K. Sotome, T. Onishi, A. Hirano et al., "A rare case of anaplastic transformation within the metastatic site of the retroperitoneal region in a patient 17 years after total thyroidectomy for papillary carcinoma of the thyroid beginning with multiple bone metastases," *Thyroid*, vol. 17, no. 12, pp. 1309–1311, 2007.

[6] Y. Takeshita, T. Takamura, H. Minato et al., "Transformation of p53-positive papillary thyroid carcinoma to anaplastic carcinoma of the liver following postoperative radioactive iodine-131 therapy," *Internal Medicine*, vol. 47, no. 19, pp. 1709–1712, 2008.

[7] T. Sumida, H. Hamakawa, M. Imaoka et al., "A case of submandibular malignant rhabdoid tumor transformed from papillary thyroid carcinoma," *Journal of Oral Pathology and Medicine*, vol. 30, no. 7, pp. 443–447, 2001.

[8] R. Nakayama, K. Horiuchi, M. Susa et al., "Anaplastic transformation of follicular thyroid carcinoma in a metastatic skeletal lesion presenting with paraneoplastic leukocytosis," *Thyroid*, vol. 22, no. 2, pp. 200–204, 2012.

[9] M. Miettinen and K. O. Franssila, "Variable expression of keratins and nearly uniform lack of thyroid transcription factor 1 in thyroid anaplastic carcinoma," *Human Pathology*, vol. 31, no. 9, pp. 1139–1145, 2000.

[10] D. Tacha, D. Zhou, and L. Cheng, "Expression of PAX8 in normal and neoplastic tissues: a comprehensive immunohistochemical study," *Applied Immunohistochemistry & Molecular Morphology*, vol. 19, no. 4, pp. 293–299, 2011.

[11] J. A. Bishop, R. Sharma, and W. H. Westra, "PAX8 immunostaining of anaplastic thyroid carcinoma: a reliable means of discerning thyroid origin for undifferentiated tumors of the head and neck," *Human Pathology*, vol. 42, no. 12, pp. 1873–1877, 2011.

[12] M. F. Beesley and K. M. McLaren, "Cytokeratin 19 and galectin-3 immunohistochemistry in the differential diagnosis of solitary thyroid nodules," *Histopathology*, vol. 41, no. 3, pp. 236–243, 2002.

[13] M. Ragazzi, A. Ciarrocchi, V. Sancisi, G. Gandolfi, A. Bisagni, and S. Piana, "Update on anaplastic thyroid carcinoma: morphological, molecular, and genetic features of the most aggressive thyroid cancer," *International Journal of Endocrinology*, vol. 2014, Article ID 790834, 13 pages, 2014.

[14] J. Akaishi, K. Sugino, W. Kitagawa et al., "Prognostic factors and treatment outcomes of 100 cases of anaplastic thyroid carcinoma," *Thyroid*, vol. 21, no. 11, pp. 1183–1189, 2011.

[15] N. Sera, K. Ashizawa, T. Ando et al., "Anaplastic changes associated with p53 gene mutation in differentiated thyroid carcinoma after insufficient radioactive iodine (1-31I) therapy," *Thyroid*, vol. 10, no. 11, pp. 975–979, 2000.

37

A Large Extragnathic Keratocystic Odontogenic Tumour

Soumya Makarla,[1] Radhika M. Bavle,[1] Sudhakara Muniswamappa,[1] and Srinath Narasimhamurthy[2]

[1]*Department of Oral Pathology, Krishnadevaraya College of Dental Sciences, Bangalore 562157, India*
[2]*Department of Oral Surgery, Krishnadevaraya College of Dental Sciences, Bangalore 562157, India*

Correspondence should be addressed to Soumya Makarla; soumyamakarla@gmail.com

Academic Editor: Tanja Batinac

Odontogenic keratocysts (OKCs) are developmental cysts which occur typically in the jawbones. They present more commonly in the posterior mandible of young adults than the maxilla. OKCs have been reclassified under odontogenic tumours in 2005 by the WHO and have since been termed as keratocystic odontogenic tumours (KCOTs). Here we report a case of a recurrent buccal lesion in a 62-year-old man which was provisionally diagnosed as a space infection (buccal abscess) but surprisingly turned out to be a soft tissue KCOT in an unusual location on histopathologic examination.

1. Introduction

Odontogenic keratocysts are developmental odontogenic cysts which were reclassified as tumours in 2005 by the WHO on account of their aggressive behavior and recurrence potential [1]. They are most commonly gnathic lesions, meaning that they arise within the jaws, that is, the mandible and maxilla. Occasionally they have been found to arise in a peripheral location especially in the gingiva which has earned them the term "peripheral KCOTs" [1].

The histogenesis of intraosseous KCOT can be attributed to the sources of odontogenic epithelium, that is, dental lamina and its remnants and the extensions of basal cells from the overlying epithelium [2]. The involvement of the Hedgehog signaling pathway due to PTCH-1 inactivation has been suggested and accepted as the underlying cause in the pathogenesis of this cystic tumour [2].

Cysts and tumours which arise from the epithelium and its remnants associated with tooth development are termed as "odontogenic." These lesions typically occur centrally within the bone. However, occasional reports exist concerning those odontogenic lesions having occurred in the soft tissues overlying the alveolar bone. These have been aptly termed "peripheral" or "extragnathic" [3].

Rare cases of parakeratinized cysts in the facial soft tissues, skin, muscles of mastication, and also temporomandibular joint, which histopathologically resemble intraosseous KCOT, have been reported. Owing to the rarity of these loci, variants of KCOT can be described and further discussed as intraosseous, solid-cystic, and peripheral types [2].

2. Case Report

A 62-year-old male reported to our hospital with an asymptomatic swelling in the right lower half of the face with reduced mouth opening since two weeks. History revealed that this was the 3rd time that such a swelling had appeared in the buccal region over a span of 8 years. The first episode 5 years before involved a previous history of pus discharge with a diagnosis of buccal space infection treated by incision and drainage. The buccal swelling had regressed on its own upon a second occurrence 2 years back. The patient has been a known diabetic since a year and on regular medication. A detailed medical examination was performed in which the patient was screened for anomalies of the skin, eyes, skeletal system, endocrine system, nervous system, and any other developmental disorders, ruling out any syndromic association.

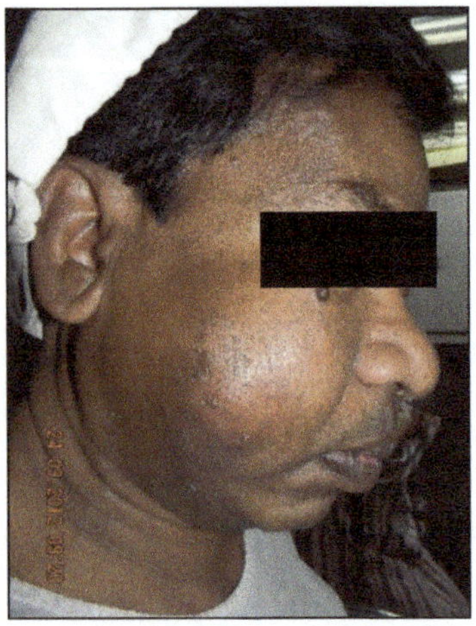

Figure 1: Clinical image showing right side of the face with a solitary mass extending from posterior ala region to preauricular area. Superiorly, it extends till infraorbital margin to angle of the mouth inferiorly.

On examination, gross asymmetry on the right side of the face was evident. A large ovoid submucosal swelling (6 × 6 cm in size) was observed extraorally, extending superoinferiorly from the level of the right lateral canthus of the eye to 1 cm below the corner of the mouth and anteroposteriorly from the corner of the mouth to the mandibular ramus (Figure 1). The borders of the lesion were ill-defined on palpation. The consistency of the swelling varied from being soft to firm. Overlying skin was normal. There was no history of any pain, fever associated with the swelling. Submandibular and cervical lymphadenopathy was absent. Paresthesia or palsy of the right side of the face or swelling of the right parotid gland was not noted.

Intraorally, the ovoid swelling presented as a slight elevation of the buccal mucosa without any obliteration of the buccal vestibule. It extended from 1 cm from the commissure of lip to 1 cm short of the pterygomandibular raphae. The buccal mucous membrane appeared stretched and glistening without any signs of inflammation. Mouth opening was restricted due to the size of the lesion.

Computed tomography revealed a well-defined lesional mass with cystic areas involving the buccal space. Intracystic loculation was visible with a pus-like dense cystic content. Erosion of the posterior buccal cortex was evident with no perforation of the maxillary bone. The maxillary antral wall was compressed (Figures 2(a)–2(d)).

A clinical diagnosis of a nonspecific chronic abscess with spread of infection was made and the lesion was treated under GA through an intraoral approach. An incision was made on the buccal mucosa and the lesion was excised in toto along with a safe margin of a fibrous tissue cuff. The lesion shelled out easily without any involvement of the buccinator muscle nor of any bony component. On surgical exposure, the lesional mass was well circumscribed with a fibrous outer covering. The lesion looked lobulated as the mass had herniated into the pterygomaxillary space (Figures 3(a) and 3(b)).

The excised lesion resembling a leathery pouch was present completely within the soft tissue in the buccal space. It was not attached to the buccinator muscle nor was it attached to any bony component of the maxilla or related to the parotid gland or duct.

The specimen obtained was 4.8 × 4.5 cm in size, creamish brown in colour with a firm consistency with an irregular surface. Multiple samples were routinely processed and stained with hematoxylin and eosin (Figure 4).

A differential of a large dermoid or epidermoid cyst, a parasitic cyst, and a cyst of inflammatory origin was considered.

Microscopically, the tissue sections showed a cystic lumen lined by parakeratinized epithelium of uniform thickness. The basal cells were cuboidal to columnar in shape exhibiting nuclear palisading. The spinous layer was thin and the parakeratin layer showed surface corrugations. Some areas were lined by flattened, stretched epithelium whereas other areas exhibited numerous infoldings of the epithelium into the connective tissue wall. The epithelium connective tissue interface was smooth and flat with no rete ridges. Underlying fibrous connective tissue was thin and mature with fibrocytes and fibroblasts with few odontogenic rests. Areas of haemorrhage and blood vessels were evident in the stroma. No daughter cysts, epithelial islands, skeletal muscle tissue, or any appendages were present in the connective tissue wall (Figures 5(a) and 5(c)).

A diagnosis of an *extragnathic KCOT of the buccal region* was made taking into account mainly the histologic features supported by the clinical and CT (radiologic features). Regular patient follow-up is carried out every 6 months with no evidence of recurrence in 24 months.

The lesional tissue was immunostained with Ki-67 (Biogenex) to assess the mitotic activity of the cystic lining to reveal the proliferative potential of the lesion as compared to conventional intraosseous KCOT. An interesting finding was that almost all the basal cells and only few suprabasal cell nuclei stained positive for Ki-67. A converse of this finding is generally observed in most conventional intraosseous KCOTs wherein a larger number of suprabasal cell nuclei stain positive for Ki-67 as opposed to the nuclei of the palisading basal cells (Figures 5(b) and 5(d)).

3. Review of Literature

A PubMed search of the English literature of all the cases of KCOT occurring in the buccal region has been compiled in a chronological order in Table 1.

4. Discussion

KCOTs are cystic odontogenic lesions arising in the gnathic skeleton. KCOT has been defined by the latest WHO classification of tumours of head and neck as "a benign uni- or multicystic, intraosseous tumour of odontogenic origin, with characteristic lining of parakeratinized stratified squamous epithelium and potential aggressive, infiltrative behaviour" [6]. KCOTs have a distinct pattern of growth, that is, by

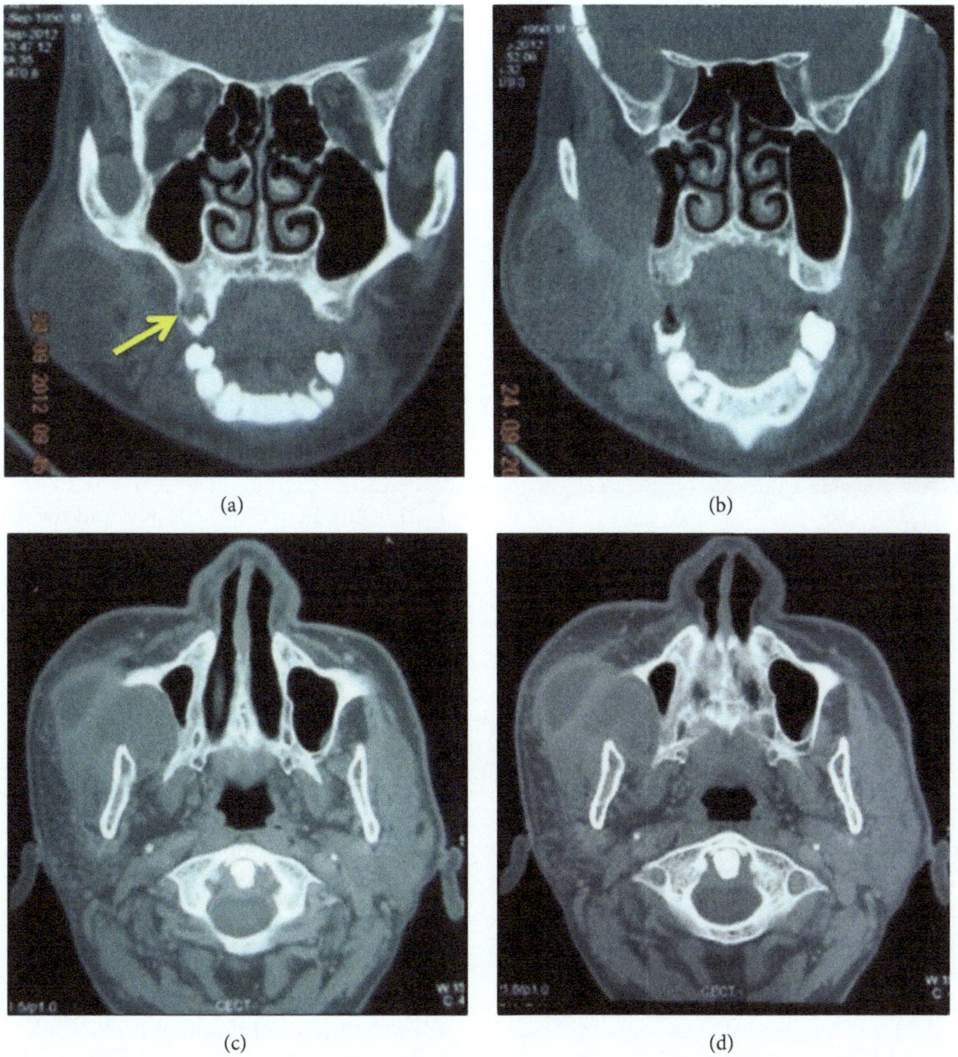

(a) (b) (c) (d)

Figure 2: ((a) and (b)) Posteroanterior view; ((c) and (d)) transverse CT at C 6 level: CT scan showing a well-defined loculated soft tissue mass in the buccal space. The lesion shows multilocularity with gel or fluidic content. The lesion is seen compressing the maxillary bone in the area of antral wall laterally.

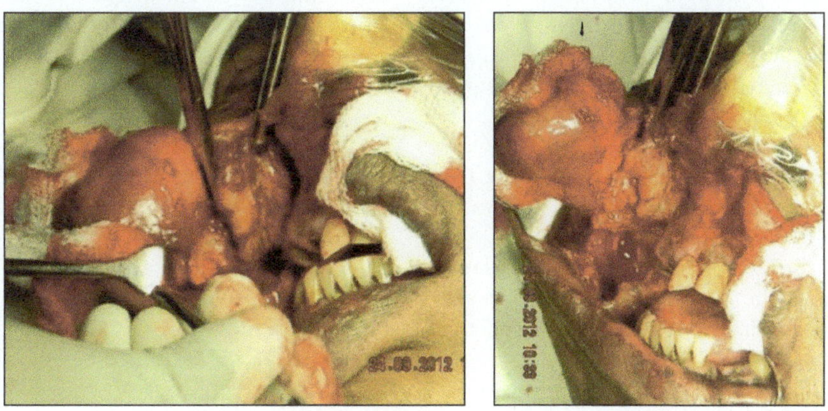

(a) (b)

Figure 3: ((a) and (b)) Surgical image showing a capsulated enmasse of lesion which was easily dissected out, devoid of any muscle or bone involvement.

TABLE 1: List of all the reported cases of KCOT in the buccal mucosa.

Case number	Age/sex	Treatment	Recurrence	Reference
1	59/M	Excision	—	Precheur and Krolls, 2009 [4]
2	60/M	Enucleation	No	Ide et al., 2010 [3]
3	16/M	—	—	Ide et al., 2010 [3]
4	74/M	Extirpation	No (4 yrs)	Yamamoto et al., 2013 [1]
5	37/M	Excision	No (12 mo)	Kaminagakura et al., 2013 [2]
6	52/M	Excision	No	Grobe et al., 2012 [5]
7	62/M	Excision in toto	No (2 yrs)	Present case

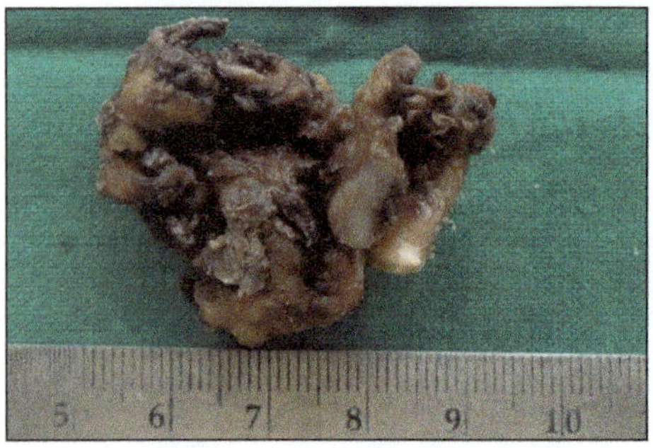

FIGURE 4: Gross image of a 4.5 × 4.8 cm lobulated soft tissue mass.

traversing through the marrow spaces of the jaws, and also have a high recurrence rate of 23.15% [7].

Though KCOTs conventionally occur in an intraosseous location; reports of odontogenic tumours like ameloblastoma, CEOT, and AOT including KCOT arising in a peripheral location exist in literature [8]. The location of these peripheral counterparts has most commonly been in the gingiva. Therefore the term "peripheral" has come to depict a primarily intraosseous lesion occurring in the gingival soft tissues.

However, KCOTs of the soft tissue have been reported in other anatomic sites like the buccal mucosa and masticatory muscles apart from the gingiva. A review of the English literature revealed 25 cases of peripheral (soft tissue) KCOTs. Of the 25, 17 of them were found in the gingiva, 6 in the buccal mucosa, and 2 cases intramuscularly [1], the details of which are listed in Table 1. Therefore the terms "extraosseous" or "extragnathic" would be more apt in referring to those lesions occurring in the soft tissues other than gingiva. Ours will hence be the 7th reported case of a soft tissue KCOT occurring in the buccal mucosa and the 26th case of a peripheral KCOT [2, 9].

Generally KCOTs of the jawbone do not produce a large expansion of the cortex as the cyst proliferates within the marrow spaces, thus growing in a longitudinal manner. But when it occurs in the buccal soft tissues, it tends to grow in a centrifugal direction, therefore causing the cyst to expand uniformly on all sides, resulting in a large buccal swelling as the main clinical presentation. The cyst also simulated spread of infection as it had extended into the pterygomandibular space and infratemporal space but could be easily dissected during surgery.

Plain radiographs play a very limited role in the detection of a soft tissue lesion. However, studies prove that the positive rate of computed tomography (CT) in the diagnosis of PKCOT (peripheral KCOTs) is 100%. CT can reveal the relationship between the lesion and the adjacent hard or soft tissues. By measuring the CT value, the lesion can be defined as cystic [10]. These features concur with the CT findings in our case of a well-defined cystic mass involving the buccal space. Intracystic loculation could also be appreciated with cystic content. The bony findings of erosion of the posterior buccal cortex with no perforation of the maxillary bone also provided more clarity in diagnosing the lesion being situated in the buccal space.

Though an organising abscess with buccal space infection can give a similar picture, absence of signs of inflammation ruled out this possibility.

KCOT is a distinct lesion, owing to its unique histopathology. The cystic lining is characterized by a parakeratinized stratified squamous epithelium of uniform thickness, with a corrugated surface and a palisaded and polarized basal layer with "picket fence" or "tombstone" appearance, devoid of rete ridges. Numerous infoldings of the epithelium are a common finding. The cystic lumen generally contains a straw colored fluid or a thick creamy material which may represent keratin [11].

Our case also exhibited a cystic epithelium comprising of numerous folds and a benign fibrous connective tissue wall. The lining was characterized by 5-6-cell layer uniformly thick epithelium with parakeratinization and surface corrugation, basal cell palisading and devoid of rete pegs which conforms to the typical descriptive diagnosis of an intraosseous KCOT.

The main histopathologic differentials for a soft tissue KCOT include epidermoid cyst, cutaneous keratocyst (CKC) ectopic occurrence of keratocyst of skin adnexa in buccal mucosa (hair follicles, sebaceous glands), trichilemmal cyst, and steatocystoma.

Epidermoid cysts are developmental pathologies occurring in the head and neck region almost always found in the regions of embryonic fusion with an intraoral incidence of less than 0.01% [12]. Histologically, epidermoid cysts reveal a cystic cavity filled with large amounts of keratin flakes lined by orthokeratinized stratified squamous epithelium with prominent stratum granulosum. Surface corrugations are seen in few areas which may resemble KCOT. KCOTs may be distinguished by the presence of parakeratinization and absence of a prominent stratum granulosum. Their basal cell

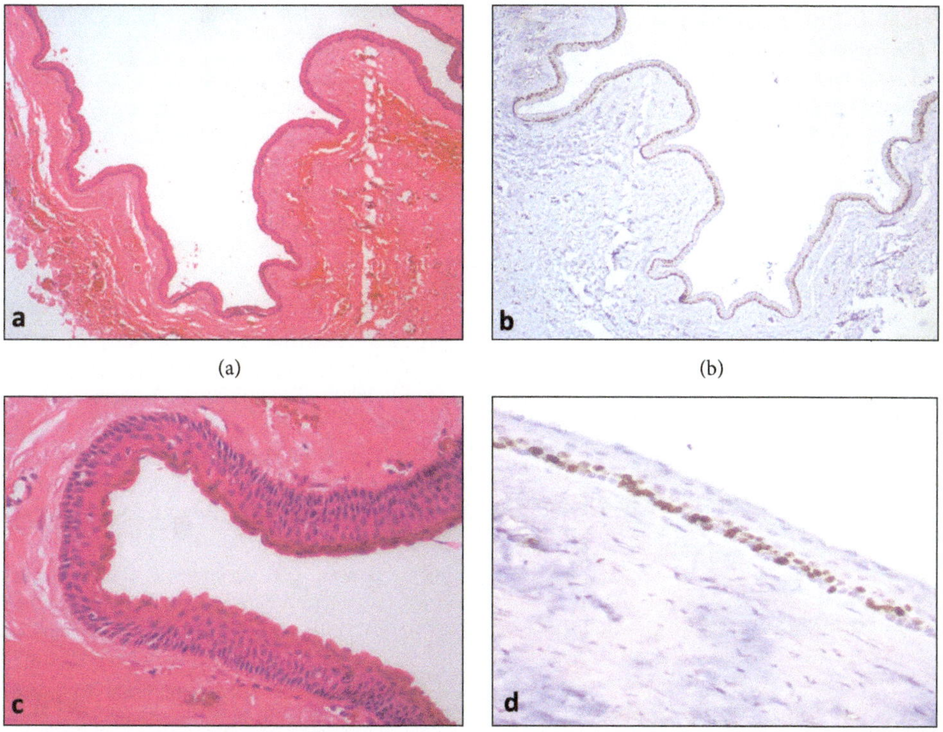

(a) (b) (c) (d)

FIGURE 5: (a) Hematoxylin and eosin stained histopathological section of the lesion showing cystic epithelium of odontogenic keratocyst with numerous infoldings (×40). (b) Corresponding IHC image showing nuclear expression of Ki-67 seen continuously in the basal layer (×40). (c) High power view showing 5–7 cell layer thick, corrugated parakeratinized cystic epithelium with columnar basal cells exhibiting palisading nuclear polarity (H&E stain, ×200). (d) Corresponding IHC image showing nuclear expression of Ki-67 continuously in the basal layer and sparsely in the parabasal layer. Superficial layers are completely free of Ki-67 expression (×200).

layer shows prominent palisading nuclei which is lacking in an epidermoid cyst.

CKCs were first reported by Barr et al. as subcutaneous cysts in 1986 [13]. CKCs are highly correlated with nevoid basal cell carcinoma syndrome (NBCCS), 91.7% [13–16]. But there are reports of cases of CKCs having risen independent of the syndrome. They most commonly occur in the extremities and their cystic content resembles a brown grumous substance [17].

The lining epithelium comprises several layers of squamous epithelial cells without a granular cell layer and skin appendages. The cystic epithelium appears wavy or festooned with normal maturation [17]. Presence of mural daughter cysts is a common finding [9, 13]. Distinguishing these CKCs from KCOT is difficult as the corrugated anagen-like lining of these cysts resembles that of a KCOT. Therefore the possibility of a CKC arising ectopically in the buccal mucosa in such cases cannot be completely omitted [1].

Steatocystoma simplex is an uncommon benign cutaneous hamartomatous malformation arising from the pilosebaceous duct junction [17, 18]. It generally occurs on the trunk, axilla, scalp, and neck. Their cystic lumen consists of an oily sebaceous material [19]. Steatocystoma simplex is found as a solitary cystic nodule. The cyst exhibits folds of stratified squamous epithelium, basal layer palisading, and absence of granular layer with a characteristic dense eosinophilic hyaline layer/cuticle present on the epithelium. Lobules of sebaceous glands are evident in its connective tissue wall [20, 21]. It can be distinguished from KCOT by the presence of the flattened sebaceous structures.

Trichilemmal cysts mainly occur on the scalp and their cystic content comprises a cheesy, foul smelling thick material [17]. The cyst walls are composed of epithelial cells with no clearly distinguishable intercellular bridges. The peripheral cells show a distinct palisade arrangement. Epithelial cells close to the lumen are swollen and eosinophilic and a distinct granular layer is absent. The lumen is filled with eosinophilic homogenous material (trichilemmal keratinization) [22].

The mechanism of KCOT development in the soft tissues especially the buccal mucosa is yet to be established. It is common knowledge that the KCOT is considered to originate from the remnants of dental lamina. Therefore, to have occurred in the buccal soft tissues, these cells should have been displaced into the buccal mucosa and persisted during embryogenesis [23]. Recent reports may provide important clues in understanding the relationship between deciduous dentition and the oral vestibule during embryological development. According to them the primitive vestibular lamina involved in the formation of the future oral vestibule and the buccal mucosa reiteratively intermigrated with the dental epithelium around the maxillary molar areas during tooth formation [24, 25].

These findings suggest that the remnants of the dental lamina entrapped in the buccal tissues during embryogenesis may be triggered to form a keratocyst with the features of KCOT. Other odontogenic lesions such as ameloblastoma and odontoma developed in the buccal mucosa have also been reported in the English literature [26, 27].

It is also established that KCOTs may originate from the basal cells of the oral epithelium [4]. Therefore, the prospect of an extraosseous KCOT developing from the basal epithelial cell cannot be completely discarded. Surgical implantation of the cyst on account of the recurrent nature of the lesion should also be considered as a probable reason for occurrence.

In the statistics of soft tissue KCOT given by Abé et al., the recurrence rate of 21 cases was 13.6%, which is in close proximity to the recurrence rate of jawbone KCOTs [9, 28].

In this case, as the cyst was present in an unusual location, that is, the buccal soft tissue, IHC was applied to compare intraosseous KCOT and extraosseous KCOT in its Ki-67 staining properties.

Previous reports and observations reveal that, in conventional intraosseous KCOT, a larger number of suprabasal cells and very few basal cells take up the stain. But, in our case, a larger number of basal cells as compared to suprabasal cells showed positivity for anti-Ki-67 antibody.

This finding may question the general assumption that peripheral counterparts of central odontogenic lesions may exhibit less aggressive behaviour and may show lesser rates of recurrence. A larger number of cases need to be included to test this premise. Until then this will remain as a topic of speculation.

5. Conclusion

The diagnosis of KCOT of the jawbone is based purely on its characteristic histologic picture. However, in our case, similar findings were associated with a keratinizing cyst of the buccal mucosa. The locale for the predilection of this site is extremely rare, but the rationale for this topographic location can be explained by a theory of displaced and persistent dental lamina rests in the buccal mucosa during odontogenesis in the embryo. Therefore, though KCOT of the buccal mucosa represents an example of heterotopia, it is to be noted that the frequency of detection and identification of the peripheral variant of this pathology has risen. As our case is the 7th one to be reported till date, we propose that PKCOT deems recognition as a separate entity or as an extragnathic (soft tissue/mucosal) counterpart of the central (intraosseous) KCOT.

Conflict of Interests

The authors declare that there is no conflict of interests regarding the publication of this paper.

References

[1] K. Yamamoto, Y. Matsusue, M. Kurihara, Y. Takahashi, and T. Kirita, "A keratocyst in the buccal mucosa with the features of keratocystic odontogenic tumor," *The Open Dentistry Journal*, vol. 7, no. 1, pp. 152–156, 2013.

[2] E. Kaminagakura, J. D. Almeida, Y. R. Carvalho et al., "Keratocyst of the buccal mucosa: case report and immunohistochemical comparative study with sporadic intraosseous keratocystic odontogenic tumor," *Oral Surgery, Oral Medicine, Oral Pathology and Oral Radiology*, vol. 116, no. 5, pp. e387–e392, 2013.

[3] F. Ide, K. Kikuchi, Y. Miyazaki, K. Mishima, I. Saito, and K. Kusama, "Keratocyst of the buccal mucosa: is it odontogenic?" *Oral Surgery, Oral Medicine, Oral Pathology, Oral Radiology and Endodontology*, vol. 110, no. 5, pp. e42–e47, 2010.

[4] H. V. Precheur and S. O. Krolls, "An unusual presentation of an odontogenic keratocyst in the buccal space: case report," *Journal of Oral and Maxillofacial Surgery*, vol. 67, no. 11, pp. 2513–2515, 2009.

[5] A. Grobe, H. Hanken, M. Blessmann, J. Zustin, M. Heiland, and A. Al-Dam, "An odontogenic keratocystic tumour in the buccal space: an unusual site of origin and a review of literature," *In Vivo*, vol. 26, pp. 847–851, 2012.

[6] L. Barnes, J. W. Everson, P. Reichart, and D. Sidransky, *WHO Classification of Tumours, Pathology and Genetics of Head and Neck Tumours*, IARC Press, Lyon, France, 2005.

[7] T. Kaczmarzyk, I. Mojsa, and J. Stypulkowska, "A systematic review of the recurrence rate for keratocystic odontogenic tumour in relation to treatment modalities," *International Journal of Oral and Maxillofacial Surgery*, vol. 41, no. 6, pp. 756–767, 2012.

[8] A. E. Curran, "Peripheral odontogenic tumors," *Oral and Maxillofacial Surgery Clinics of North America*, vol. 16, no. 3, pp. 399–408, 2004.

[9] T. Abé, S. Maruyama, M. Yamazaki et al., "Intramuscular keratocyst as a soft tissue counterpart of keratocystic odontogenic tumor: differential diagnosis by immunohistochemistry," *Human Pathology*, vol. 45, no. 1, pp. 110–118, 2014.

[10] L. Zhu, J. Yang, and J.-W. Zheng, "Radiological and clinical features of peripheral keratocystic odontogenic tumor," *International Journal of Clinical and Experimental Medicine*, vol. 7, no. 1, pp. 300–306, 2014.

[11] W. G. Shafer, M. K. Hine, and B. M. Levy, "Cysts and tumours of odontogenic origin," in *A Textbook of Oral Pathology*, W. G. Shafer, M. K. Hine, and B. M. Levy, Eds., W.B. Saunders Company, Philadelphia, Pa, USA, 4th edition, 1983.

[12] F. Ozan, H. B. Polat, S. Ay, and F. Goze, "Epidermoid cyst of the buccal mucosa: a case report," *Journal of Contemporary Dental Practice*, vol. 8, no. 3, pp. 90–96, 2007.

[13] R. J. Barr, J. L. Headley, J. L. Jensen, and J. B. Howell, "Cutaneous keratocysts of nevoid basal cell carcinoma syndrome," *Journal of the American Academy of Dermatology*, vol. 14, no. 4, pp. 572–576, 1986.

[14] A. F. Hamel, W. F. A. den Dunnen, and A. J. H. Suurmeijer, "The cutaneous keratocyst: a rare hallmark of the nevoid basal cell carcinoma syndrome," *International Journal of Surgical Pathology*, vol. 11, article 36, 2003.

[15] H. S. Zackheim, J. B. Howell, and A. V. Loud, "Nevoid basal cell carcinoma syndrome," *Archives of Dermatology*, vol. 93, pp. 317–323, 1966.

[16] B. J. Leppard, "Skin cysts in the basal cell naevus syndrome," *Clinical and Experimental Dermatology*, vol. 8, no. 6, pp. 603–612, 1983.

[17] H. W. Lee, J. Y. Park, S. H. Kang, and M. Choe, "Sporadic cutaneous keratocyst without nevoid basal cell carcinoma

syndrome: report of 1 case," *The Korean Journal of Pathology*, vol. 45, no. 3, pp. 322–325, 2011.

[18] F. Procianoy, M. B. Golbert, L. Golbspan, K. M. Duro, and F. J. L. Bocaccio, "Steatocystoma simplex of the eyelid," *Ophthalmic Plastic and Reconstructive Surgery*, vol. 25, no. 2, pp. 147–148, 2009.

[19] M. Sunohara, T. Ozawa, K. Morimoto, C. Tateishi, and M. Ishii, "Two cases of steatocystoma simplex in infants," *Dermatology Online Journal*, vol. 18, no. 7, p. 2, 2012.

[20] M. Varshney, M. Aziz, V. Maheshwari et al., "Steatocystoma multiplex," *BMJ Case Reports*, 2011.

[21] D. S. Cassarino, K. G. Linden, and R. J. Barr, "Cutaneous keratocyst arising independently of the nevoid basal cell carcinoma syndrome," *The American Journal of Dermatopathology*, vol. 27, no. 2, pp. 177–178, 2005.

[22] N. Kirkham, "Tumours and cysts of the epidermis," in *Lever's Histopathology of the Skin*, D. E. Elder, R. Elenitsas, B. L. Johnson, and G. F. Murphy, Eds., pp. 815–816, Lippincott Williams & Wilkins, Philadelphia, Pa, USA, 9th edition, 2005.

[23] F. Ide, N. Horie, T. Shimoyama, I. Saito, A. Tanaka, and K. Kusama, "Infrequent clinicopathologic features of keratocystic odontogenic tumour: a 29-year multi-institutional retrospective review," *Oral Surgery*, vol. 2, no. 1, pp. 1–9, 2009.

[24] M. Hovorakova, H. Lesot, M. Peterka, and R. Peterkova, "The developmental relationship between the deciduous dentition and the oral vestibule in human embryos," *Anatomy and Embryology*, vol. 209, no. 4, pp. 303–313, 2005.

[25] M. Hovorakova, H. Lesot, J.-L. Vonesch, M. Peterka, and R. Peterkova, "Early development of the lower deciduous dentition and oral vestibule in human embryos," *European Journal of Oral Sciences*, vol. 115, no. 4, pp. 280–287, 2007.

[26] E. T. Isomura, M. Okura, S. Ishimoto et al., "Case report of extragingival peripheral ameloblastoma in buccal mucosa," *Oral Surgery, Oral Medicine, Oral Pathology, Oral Radiology, and Endodontology*, vol. 108, no. 4, pp. 577–579, 2009.

[27] N. El Sedfy Bakry, "An ectopic odontome in the cheek," *Oral Surgery, Oral Medicine, Oral Pathology*, vol. 43, no. 4, pp. 583–584, 1977.

[28] B. W. Neville, D. D. Damm, C. M. Allen, and J. E. Bouquot, "Follicular cysts of the skin," in *Oral and Maxillofacial Pathology*, B. W. Neville, D. D. Damm, C. M. Allen, and J. E. Bouquot, Eds., pp. 32–34, Saunders, Philadelphia, Pa, USA, 3rd edition, 2008.

38

Desmoplastic Small Round Cell Tumor, a "Floating Island" Pattern in Pleural Fluid Cytology: A Case Report and Review of the Literature

Hui Zhu, Emily Marie McMeekin, and Charles D. Sturgis

Pathology and Laboratory Medicine Institute, Cleveland Clinic, 9500 Euclid Avenue, Cleveland, OH 44195, USA

Correspondence should be addressed to Charles D. Sturgis; sturgic@ccf.org

Academic Editor: Zsuzsa Schaff

Desmoplastic small round cell tumor (DSRCT) is a rare aggressive sarcoma with characteristic clinical and pathologic features. It typically involves pelvic and abdominal organs of young male patients, and patients usually present at advanced stage with poor prognosis. A few reports are available describing the cytopathologic features of DSRCT in serous effusions, with the majority of published cases depicting undifferentiated small blue cells that need to be distinguished from other small blue cell tumors. We report an interesting case of DSRCT involving a pleural effusion with a "floating island" pattern that has been described in hepatocellular carcinoma, renal cell carcinoma, and adrenal cortical carcinoma. In our case, the epithelioid tumor cells form cohesive aggregates surrounded by a single layer of spindle cells, mimicking the "endothelial wrapping" in other tumors with "floating island" patterns. We demonstrate, by ancillary testing, that these peripheral spindle cells are tapered/flattened DSRCT cells, in contrast to endothelial wrapping cells, as seen in other tumors with this unique cytomorphology. To our knowledge, this is the first case report describing DSRCT showing a "floating island" pattern that needs to be differentiated from metastatic hepatocellular carcinoma, renal cell carcinoma, and adrenal cortical carcinoma in effusion cytology.

1. Introduction

Desmoplastic small round cell tumors (DSRCTs) are aggressive malignancies with characteristic clinical presentations, pathological findings, and specific associated chromosomal translocations t(11;22) (p13;q12) involving EWSR1 and WT1 genes. These tumors most commonly present with pelvic and abdominal organ involvement in male patients less than 40 years of age. DSRCTs usually present at advanced stages, are resistant to treatment, and pursue aggressive clinical courses with average survival of 3 years or less [1]. Histopathologic findings are specific. The tumors present as nests or cords of undifferentiated small blue tumor cells surrounded by dense fibrous stroma. Immunohistochemically, the tumor cells express cytokeratins and EMA (>90% of cases), desmin (90% of cases), and variable neural markers [2, 3]. The characteristic translocations [t(11;22)] with resultant EWSR1-WT1 fusions can be detected by fluorescence in situ hybridization (FISH) or reverse transcriptase-polymerase chain reaction (RT-PCR) technology. Confirmatory cytogenetic and/or molecular testing is often pursued, as DSRCTs are rare malignancies and are often associated with poor clinical outcomes.

Cells of metastatic sarcoma are rarely diagnosed in cytologic preparations of serous effusions, and involvement of effusion fluid by DSRCT is extremely uncommon, with fewer than 15 cases reported in the literature. The largest case series of DSRCT involving fluids contained seven cases from five patients [4]. All reported fluid cytology cases of DSRCT describe characteristic morphology of DSRCT including dyshesive small blue cells with high nuclear/cytoplasmic ratios, scant to moderate cytoplasm, granular chromatin, and at least moderate nuclear atypia with frequent molding and mitotic activity. Dense fibrous stromal fragments may be present and are an important clue to the correct diagnosis. In the majority of cases, in the absence of fibrous stroma, the cytomorphologic features of DSRCT are difficult to distinguish from other small round blue cell tumors such as lymphoma, neuroblastoma, Ewing's sarcoma, primitive neuroectodermal tumor (PNET), and small cell carcinoma. Most patients with serous effusion involvement will have a known history of DSRCT. Immunocytochemical studies confirming characteristic cytokeratin and desmin positivity and molecular/genetic testing confirming a characteristic t(11;22)(p13;q12) translocation will prove useful in challenging cases.

In this study we report a case of DSRCT involving a pleural effusion with the lesional cells appearing in "floating island" patterns. The groups of lesional cells are comprised of cohesive, epithelioid tumor cells with moderately abundant cytoplasm and slight nuclear atypia. In some areas, the peripheries of the cohesive cell groups have a thin and incomplete layer of adherent flattened/spindled cells. Similar "floating island" cytomorphologies have been described in cytology specimens obtained from primary and metastatic hepatocellular carcinomas, adrenal cortical carcinomas, and renal cell carcinomas, in which tumor cell nests may be intimately associated with investing outer single layers of endothelial cells [5, 6]. We demonstrate, by immunohistochemical and special staining methods, that the spindle cells at the peripheries of the "floating islands" of DSRCT in serous effusions appear more likely to be spindled forms of the neoplastic cells proper, rather than investing types of nonneoplastic endothelial or mesenchymal cells.

2. Case Presentation

Three years prior to the development of the current thoracic effusion, a 35-year-old man with a past medical history of hypertension, hydronephrosis, kidney stones, and desmoid tumor of the knee presented with fatigue, weakness, an unintentional 14-kilogram weight loss, and left supraclavicular lymphadenopathy. Excisional biopsy of a left supraclavicular lymph node showed replacement of the node by small round cells with intervening dense fibrous stroma (Figure 1). Immunohistochemical studies performed at an outside hospital showed that the tumor cells were positive for AE1/AE3, CK8, CAM 5.2, and CD99. The lesional cells were negative for desmin, EMA, and S-100. Germ cell markers including PLAP, HCG, and AFP were also negative. Markers of neuroendocrine differentiation including chromogranin and synaptophysin were negative, and lymphocytic markers including CD45, CD30, CD3, CD5, CD20, CD138, BCL2, and BCL6 were also nonreactive. The case was then sent to Cleveland Clinic for an expert soft tissue tumor second opinion consultation, as the immunopattern did not exactly fit what was expected for DSRCT by the referring pathologist. The clinical presentation and histologic findings were felt to be diagnostic of DSRCT by two experienced soft tissue pathologist consultants at our center, and the consultants noted that, like all malignant neoplasms, not all examples of DSRCT show "classical" patterns of immunoreactivity. The expert consultants at Cleveland Clinic pursued FISH for the EWSR1 gene (22q12) break-apart, which was positive, confirming the diagnosis of metastatic DSRCT. A definitive diagnosis of DSRCT was rendered, and the patient was managed based upon this diagnosis. Staging by CT scan showed extensive

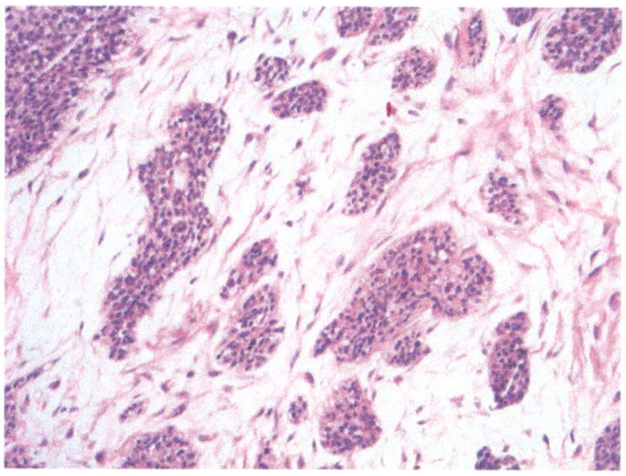

FIGURE 1: The excised supraclavicular lymph node showed the characteristic morphology of DSRCT. Cohesive nests of undifferentiated small blue cells with some degree of nuclear atypia were seen embedded within moderately cellular fibrous stroma (histopathology, hematoxylin and eosin stain, 100x).

intra-abdominal disease (including liver lesions) and mediastinal lymphadenopathy. With the bulk of the disease being present in the mesentery, an abdominal primary site was favored. The patient was treated with seven cycles of combination chemotherapy (including cyclophosphamide, doxorubicin, ifosfamide, and etoposide). He experienced a partial radiologic and clinical response with diminution of liver, abdominal, and mediastinal lesions. After combination chemotherapy, it was noted that not all of his abdominal lesions could be surgically resected, so he began second-line combination chemotherapy including vincristine and cyclophosphamide. He tolerated the second-line treatment well with stable disease for 21 months, until he was found to have disease progression in the liver and began pazopanib (oral multityrosine kinase inhibitor) therapy. He did well for another 14 months on pazopanib until he presented with bowel microperforation. Biopsy of a mesenteric nodule confirmed persistent abdominal DSRCT. Subsequent CT examination demonstrated progressive disease involving the liver, peritoneum, and abdominal lymph nodes. In addition, enlarged supradiaphragmatic lymph nodes, multiple small bilateral lungs nodules, and a right pleural effusion were noted (Figure 2). Thoracentesis was performed, and the collected right pleural fluid was sent to cytology for morphologic examination as well as to microbiology for exclusion of an infectious etiology. The microbiologic studies of the pleural fluid proved negative. After empiric antibiotic treatment for the bowel microperforation, the patient was hospitalized to begin salvage chemotherapy with etoposide and ifosfamide.

The cytology sample (1,000 mL of transparent, nonturbid, yellow fluid) was accessioned and routinely processed with an aliquot of fluid used to create Papanicolaou stained ThinPrep slides. An additional portion of the body fluid was used to create a Cellient cell block that was fixed in 10% neutral buffered formalin and yielded hematoxylin and eosin stained histologic sections. The ThinPrep slides of the pleural fluid showed predominantly a mixture of reactive mesothelial cells, macrophages, lymphocytes, and a few neutrophils. Rare groups of lesional cells were also noted (Figure 3). These groups of cells were cohesive with some degree of cell

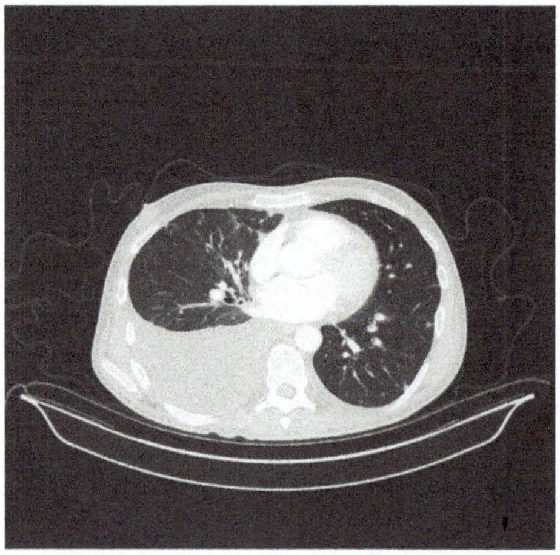

FIGURE 2: CT examination confirmed a unilateral right pleural effusion and small lung nodules (transverse computed tomographic image of patient's chest demonstrating posterior right chest effusion).

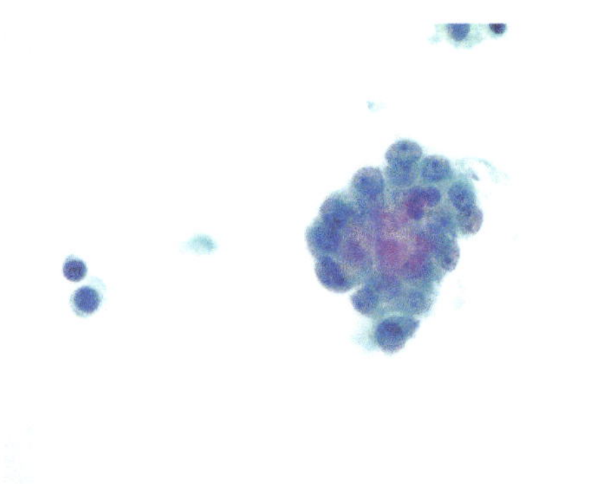

FIGURE 3: Liquid-based cytology slides contained rare crowded groups of lesional cells with nuclear overlapping, high nuclear/cytoplasmic ratios, open chromatin, and small but discernible nucleoli. These cells were difficult to differentiate from reactive mesothelial cells by microscopy (ThinPrep, Papanicolaou stain, 600x).

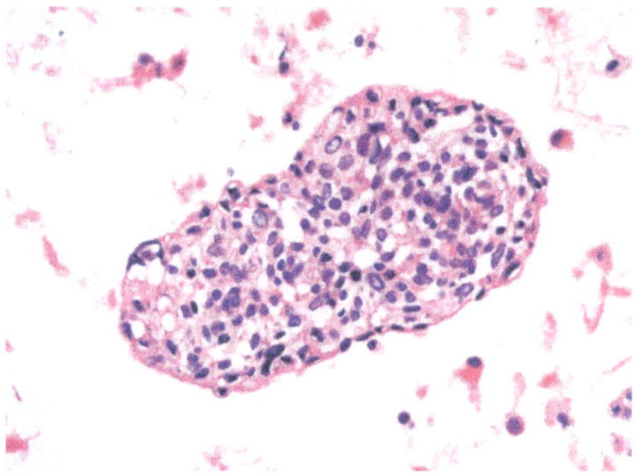

FIGURE 4: A cohesive and crowded group of metastatic DSRCT cells in pleural fluid with central epithelioid forms having minimal to moderate eosinophilic cytoplasm and open chromatin. Some cells at the tumor group margin have elongated/spindled morphologies with more dense chromatin (cell block, hematoxylin and eosin stain, 400x).

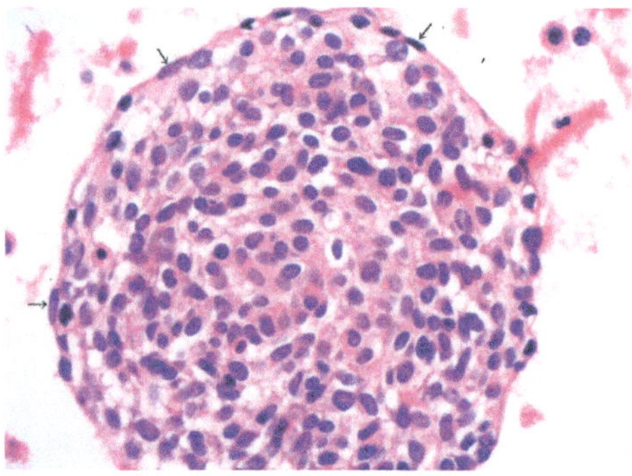

FIGURE 5: A higher magnification view of DSRCT involving fluid. The image shows a cohesive and crowded group of lesional cells from the pleural fluid with central epithelioid forms. Small arrows mark peripheral elongated/spindled forms. Some of these cells have more dense chromatin, while others have chromatin that is similar to that seen in the epithelioid cells within the body of the island (cell block, hematoxylin and eosin stain, 600x).

crowding and nuclear overlapping. An experienced cytotechnologist interpreted these rare lesional cell groups as reactive mesothelial cells. Hematoxylin and eosin stained sections prepared from the cell block showed cohesive groupings of metastatic tumor cells with a "floating island" morphology (Figures 4 and 5). The more central and epithelioid-appearing tumor cells in these groups had bland oval nuclei that were about the same size as mesothelial cell nuclei. The cytoplasm of the lesional cells was minimally to moderately abundant, eosinophilic, and focally vacuolated. Mitoses were infrequent to absent. While no fibrous stromal cell groups were identified in the liquid-based cytology or cell block slides, some of the cell groups in the cell block showed an incomplete single layer of bland elongated/spindled cells intimately applied to the periphery of the tumor cell aggregates. In some areas these peripheral spindled cells were hyperchromatic with dense chromatin, while, in other areas, the nuclear chromatin of these more elongated and less epithelioid cells was better preserved and more similar in tinctorial appearance to that seen in the nuclei of the cells within the intrinsic regions of the cohesive lesional cell groups.

Because of the patient's well-documented history of DSRCT and the availability of histologic materials for cytohistologic correlation, the effusion sample was diagnosed as metastatic DSRCT without a need for ancillary immunohistochemistry or molecular testing.

3. Discussion

We report a case of DSRCT in a serous effusion with tumor cells showing "floating island" patterns. Only a few case reports and small case series pertaining to DSRCT involving serous effusions have been published [4, 7–11]. Various morphologic features have been set forth as being of value in diagnosing DSRCT in serous fluids. The majority of

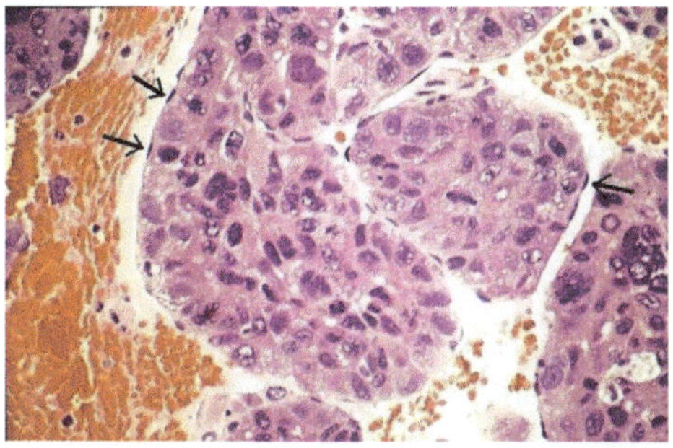

FIGURE 6: The "floating island" pattern of hepatocellular carcinoma. This image is used to illustrate the unique tumoral growth pattern of cohesive sheets of lesional epithelial cells that are intimately invested by a delicate outer layer of flattened endothelial cells. Arrows mark some of the peripheral wrapping endothelial cell nuclei (cell block, hematoxylin and eosin stain, 400x). This photomicrograph comes from a metastatic moderately differentiated hepatocellular carcinoma in a 64-year-old female and is not from the index patient in the current case report. It is presented for comparison as an example of a morphologic differential diagnosis with some overlapping features with the current unique example of metastatic DSRCT.

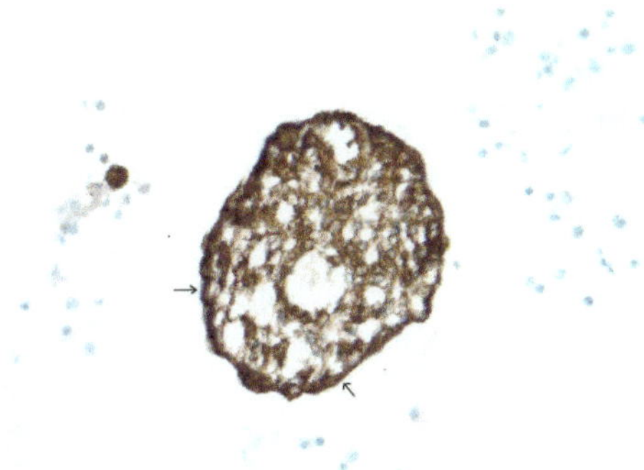

FIGURE 7: A cohesive group of metastatic DSRCT cells in pleural fluid with central epithelioid forms and a few flattened/elongated cell forms at the periphery of the island, marked with small arrows. The lesional central epithelioid cells are diffusely immunoreactive with cytokeratin AE1/AE3, and the peripheral spindled forms show the same pattern of reactivity with strong cytoplasmic staining (cell block, AE1/AE3 immunohistochemistry, 400x).

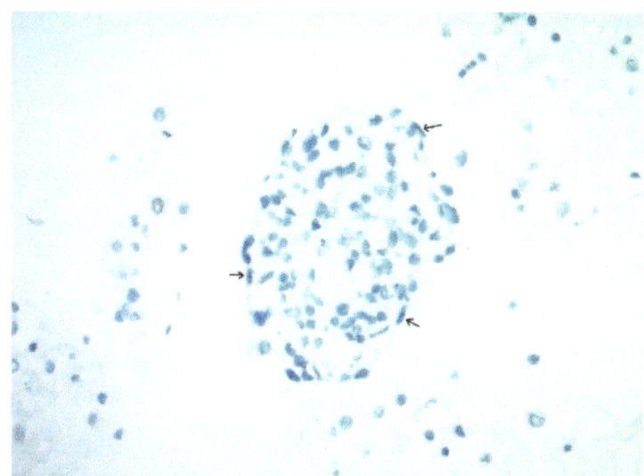

FIGURE 8: A cohesive group of metastatic DSRCT cells in pleural fluid with central epithelioid forms and a few flattened/elongated cell forms at the periphery of the island, marked by small arrows. The lesional epithelioid cells are nonreactive with smooth muscle actin (SMA), and the peripheral spindled forms show the same pattern of reactivity with no cytoplasmic staining (cell block, SMA immunohistochemistry, 400x).

existing reports emphasize the presence of lesional undifferentiated small blue cells that are difficult to distinguish from other small blue cell tumors such as lymphomas, small cell carcinomas, neuroblastomas, and other blastemal neoplasms of adolescence and young adulthood. Some citations have also raised the differential diagnostic consideration that prominent cytoplasmic vacuoles and cohesion in cases of DSRCT involving serous effusions may mimic metastatic adenocarcinoma [4, 12, 13]. To our knowledge, our report is the first in the literature in which a case of DSRCT has been recognized to display a "floating island" pattern that might raise the differential diagnosis of metastatic hepatocellular carcinoma, adrenal cortical carcinoma, or possibly renal cell carcinoma.

The moniker of "floating islands" has been previously applied by authors such as Bibbo and de Boer to cohesive aggregates of lesional epithelioid cells surrounded by delicate layers of spindled cells [5, 6]. In cytologic preparations of primary and metastatic adrenal cortical carcinomas, hepatocellular carcinomas, and some renal cell carcinomas, this morphology correlates to cohesive groups of lesional epithelial cells rimmed by variably complete, delicate, outer endothelial wrapping (Figure 6). To our knowledge, an outer incomplete layer of tapered cells has not been previously described in "floating islands" of DSRCTs involving fluids. Ancillary testing confirmed these peripheral spindle cell forms to have the same patterns of cell block immunoreactivity as the epithelioid central cells in the DSRCT cell groups. The peripheral flattened cells were immunoreactive with cytokeratin AE1/AE3 and were negative for smooth muscle actin (Figures 7 and 8). In addition, a trichrome stain performed on the cell block showed no adherent mesenchymal cells. Based upon light microscopy and results of ancillary testing, we conclude that the partially ringing spindled cells in the "floating islands" of metastatic DSRCT represent tapered/flattened malignant cells (tumor cells proper), in contrast to the endothelial wrapping documented by others in adrenal cortical carcinomas and hepatocellular carcinomas.

EWSR1 rearrangements have been documented in many soft tissue neoplasms, including Ewing's sarcoma/primitive neuroectodermal tumor (EW/PNET), DSRCT, low grade myoid tumor, myxoid liposarcoma, extraskeletal myxoid chondrosarcoma, sclerosing epithelioid fibrosarcoma, myoepithelial tumor, angiomatoid fibrous histiocytoma, clear cell sarcoma of soft tissue, clear cell sarcoma-like tumor of gastrointestinal tract, and primary pulmonary myxoid sarcoma. Each of these soft tissue tumors with EWSR1 rearrangements is associated with characteristic clinical presentations and histopathologic findings. The only EWSR1 rearranged tumor that is likely to show overlapping clinical presentation and immunohistochemical features with DSRCT is EW/PNET. However, EW/PNET and DSRCT have differing histologic findings. EW/PNET cases usually show monotonous tumor cells with fine chromatin and extensive necrosis, while DSRCT cases may demonstrate more pleomorphism. In addition, dense fibrous stroma is a characteristic intrinsic feature of DSRCT, but not EW/PNET. By combining clinical setting, disease presentation, histologic/cytologic features, immunohistochemistry, and fluorescence in situ hybridization studies (using dual color, break-apart probes for the EWSR1 gene) it is possible to specifically diagnose DSRCT and to exclude EW/PNET, as was historically done in this case [2].

DSRCTs are aggressive sarcomas with characteristic clinical and pathologic features. These tumors typically involve pelvic and abdominal organs of young patients and show a male predominance [2]. Patients usually present at advanced stage, and prognoses are generally poor. Curative drug therapies are not available, and the best treatments seem to be complete surgical resections, when possible [1]. Cases of DSRCT typically harbor the unique t(11;22) (p13;q12) translocation, which may be confirmed by FISH and/or PCR studies. While sarcomas rarely involve serous cavities, DSRCT has been described in peritoneal fluid cytology cases [14]. The number of cases in the literature is small (fewer than 15 patients described, to our knowledge). It is possible that chemotherapy may change the morphology of tumors with resultant therapy related atypias and degenerative changes being previously reported [15]. Cytologic studies in the current case showed most of the lesional cell groups to be present in the cell block slides rather than the liquid-based cytology preparations, and these studies revealed the unique appearance of "floating island" patterns of lesional cells. (One speculation as to why the ThinPrep slide showed fewer lesional cell groups than the cell block may be that ThinPrep processing includes a proprietary filtering step, and the comparatively large sized "floating islands" of tumor in the fluid may be one explanation for lower cellularity in the liquid-based slide.)

Recognition of islands of cohesive small lesional cells with minimal to moderate cytoplasm and some vacuolization with patchy peripheral spindled forms may be of value in establishing a correct diagnosis and/or in formulating appropriate differential diagnoses and selecting ancillary testing. The flattened cells at the periphery of the "floating islands" in DSRCT appear to be true tumor cells and not investing mesenchymal or endothelial wrapping cells.

Conflict of Interests

The authors declare that there is no conflict of interests regarding the publication of this paper.

References

[1] I. Hassan, R. Shyyan, J. H. Donohue et al., "Intraabdominal desmoplastic small round cell tumors: a diagnostic and therapeutic challenge," *Cancer*, vol. 104, no. 6, pp. 1264–1270, 2005.

[2] J. R. Goldblum, A. L. Folpe, and S. W. Weiss, "Malignant soft tissue tumors of uncertain type," in *Enzinger and Weiss's Soft Tissue Tumors*, chapter 37, pp. 1203–1208, Elsevier, 2013.

[3] D. M. Fletcher, K. K. Unni, and F. Mertens, "Tumors of uncertain differentiation," in *WHO Classification of Tumors of Soft Tissue and Bone*, chapter 12, pp. 225–227, IRAC Press, 2013.

[4] J. P. Crapanzano, M. Cardillo, O. Lin, and M. F. Zakowski, "Cytology of desmoplastic small round cell tumor: a series including findings in ThinPrep," *Cancer*, vol. 96, no. 1, pp. 21–31, 2002.

[5] M. Bibbo and D. Wilbur, "Kidneys, adrenals and retroperitoneum," in *Comprehensive Cytopathology*, chapter 28, pp. 703–712, Elsevier, 2015.

[6] W. B. de Boer, A. Segal, F. A. Frost, and G. F. Sterrett, "Cytodiagnosis of well differentiated hepatocellular carcinoma: can indeterminate diagnoses be reduced?" *Cancer*, vol. 87, no. 5, pp. 270–277, 1999.

[7] S. Z. Ali, T. L. Nicol, J. Port, and G. Ford, "Intraabdominal desmoplastic small round cell tumor: cytopathologic findings in two cases," *Diagnostic Cytopathology*, vol. 18, no. 6, pp. 449–452, 1998.

[8] R. P. Perez and P. J. L. Zhang, "Detection of EWS-WT1 fusion mRNA in ascites of a patient with desmoplastic small round cell tumor by RT-PCR," *Human Pathology*, vol. 30, no. 2, pp. 239–242, 1999.

[9] J. R. Hallman and K. R. Geisinger, "Cytology of fluids from pleural, peritoneal and pericardial cavities in children: a comprehensive survey," *Acta Cytologica*, vol. 38, no. 2, pp. 209–217, 1994.

[10] Y. Bian, A. G. Jordan, M. Rupp, H. Cohn, C. J. McLaughlin, and M. Miettinen, "Effusion cytology of desmoplastic small round cell tumor of the pleura: a case report," *Acta Cytologica*, vol. 37, no. 1, pp. 77–82, 1993.

[11] I. El-Kattan, R. W. Redline, A. K. El-Naggar, M. C. Grimes, and F. W. Abdul-Karim, "Cytologic features of intraabdominal desmoplastic small round cell tumor: a case report," *Acta Cytologica*, vol. 39, no. 3, pp. 514–520, 1995.

[12] N. Dutt, M. T. Sheaff, and R. M. Feakins, "Intraabdominal desmoplastic small cell tumor mimicking adenocarcinoma: a case report," *Acta Cytologica*, vol. 45, no. 1, pp. 82–85, 2001.

[13] Y. Hattori, A. Yoshida, N. Sasaki, Y. Shibuki, K. Tamura, and K. Tsuta, "Desmoplastic small round cell tumor with sphere-like clusters mimicking adenocarcinoma," *Diagnostic Cytopathology*, vol. 43, no. 3, pp. 214–217, 2014.

[14] R. M. DeMay, "Fluid," in *The Art and Science of Cytopathology*, vol. 1, chapter 2, p. 312, ASCP Press, 2012.

[15] A. E. Presley, C. S. Kong, D. M. Rowe, and K. A. Atkins, "Cytology of desmoplastic small round-cell tumor: comparison of pre- and post-chemotherapy fine-needle aspiration biopsies," *Cancer*, vol. 111, no. 1, pp. 41–46, 2007.

An Uncommon Case of Chronic Tubercular Appendicitis

Sushna Maharjan

Department of Pathology, Chitwan Medical College Teaching Hospital, P.O. Box 42, Bharatpur-10, Chitwan, Nepal

Correspondence should be addressed to Sushna Maharjan; sushnamaharjan74@gmail.com

Academic Editor: Dimosthenis Miliaras

Tuberculosis (TB) is a common disease that ranks as the second leading cause of death from an infectious disease worldwide, after the human immunodeficiency virus (HIV). However, primary TB of the appendix is rare and may or may not be associated with specific clinical features. Thus, diagnosis is made only after histopathological examination. It suggests that all surgically removed appendices should be subjected to histopathological examination. This reported case is an uncommon case of chronic tubercular appendicitis.

1. Introduction

Tuberculosis (TB) is a major global health problem. The current global scenario of TB shows an estimated 9.0 million incident cases of TB and 1.5 million people who died of the disease in 2013. Among 9.0 million of cases, more than half (56%) were in the Southeast Asia and Western Pacific Regions. Another one-quarter was in the African Region. It accounted for 24% and 11% of total cases, respectively, in India and China alone. In 2013, an estimated 13% of new TB cases were HIV-positive [1]. The incidence of TB is rising in developed countries because of acquired immune deficiency syndrome (AIDS) and it indicates a global comeback of TB in combination with AIDS [2].

Terminal ileum [3, 4], ileocaecal junction [5], and peritoneum [2] are the most common sites of TB in abdomen. It is quite interesting that involvement of the appendix is very rare although it lies so close to ileocecal region. Primary appendicular TB as isolated form is even rarer [6].

Most of the patients with gastrointestinal (GI) TB commonly present with the clinical features of abdominal pain, fever, and weight loss [2]. However, the diagnosis may be difficult due to nonspecific clinical presentation. Patients who have appendicular TB may present with signs and symptoms similar to acute appendicitis and make it difficult for a correct diagnosis [6, 7]. Thus, the diagnosis of appendicular TB is usually made on histopathological examination which delays treatment of the patient.

2. Case Report

A 40-year-old male presented with chronic abdominal pain for 2 weeks with history of diarrhea and weakness. Ultrasonogram of abdomen diagnosed the case as inflamed appendix. On examination of abdomen, there was tenderness in right iliac fossa with rebound localized to McBurney's point. Total leucocyte count was raised to 16,000/cu mm. Other routine biochemical and hematological investigations were normal. Clinical diagnosis was made as chronic appendicitis and appendectomy was performed. Peroperative findings were inflamed appendix studded with few tubercles. Thus, appendix and mesenteric lymph node were sent for histopathological examination for definite diagnosis.

Grossly, appendix measured 4.5 × 1 cm. External surface was congested and tubercles were present on the serosal surface and periappendiceal fat (Figure 1). Cut section of appendix showed yellowish foci of caseous necrosis in the wall. Lymph node measured 0.8 × 0.5 cm with focal yellowish area of caseous necrosis likewise in appendix. Histopathological examination revealed transmural inflammation of appendicular wall and also lymph node composed of caseating granulomas with epithelioid histiocytes, Langhans' giant cells, and lymphocytes (Figures 2, 3, and 4). However, tubercle bacilli were not detected by Ziehl-Neelsen (ZN) stain. Diagnosis of tuberculous appendicitis with mesenteric lymph node involvement was given. He was treated with antitubercular therapy in directly observed treatment short course

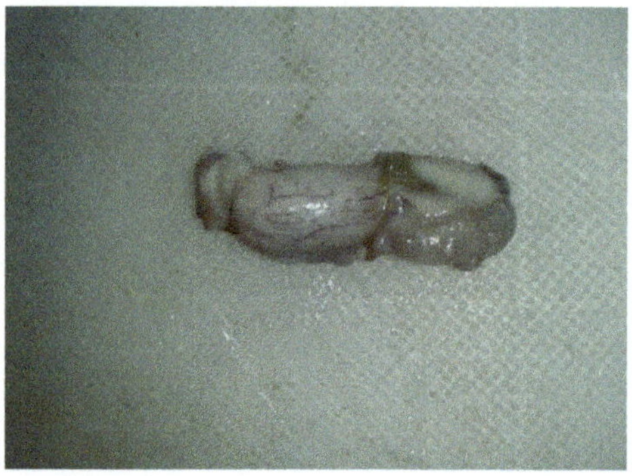

FIGURE 1: Gross specimen of appendix showing multiple tubercles in periappendiceal fat and surface.

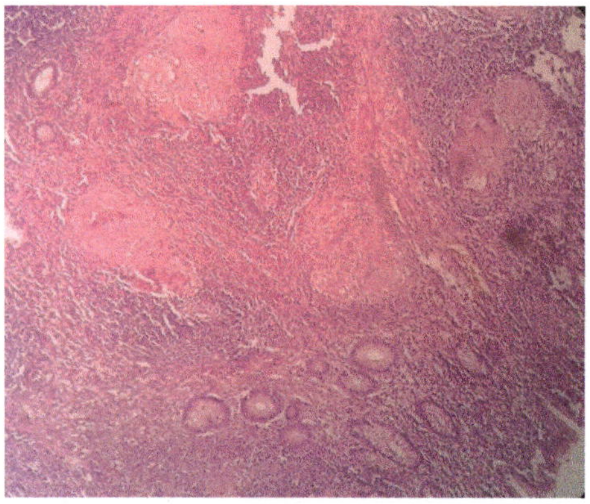

FIGURE 2: Histopathological examination of appendix showing numerous granulomas in the wall at low power.

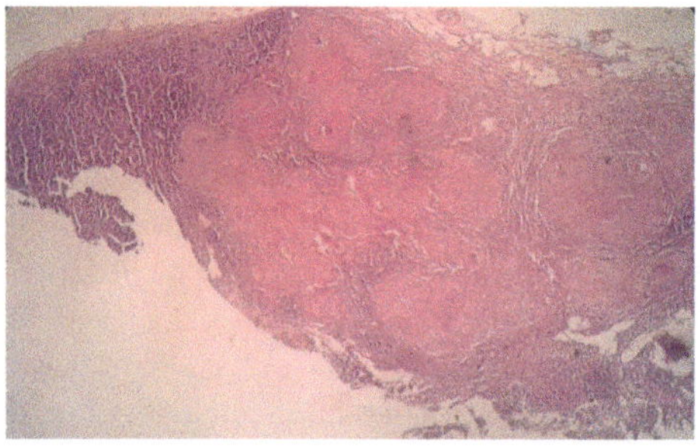

FIGURE 3: Histopathological examination of mesenteric lymph node with multiple granulomas at low power.

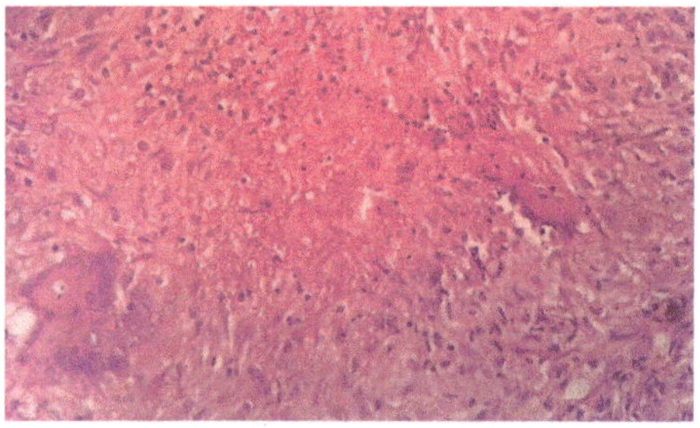

FIGURE 4: Histopathological examination of appendix showing caseation in the centre with surrounding multinucleated giant cells and epithelioid histiocytes at high power.

centre (DOTs). The patient was doing well and showed clinical recovery on follow-up in regular intervals. Primary focus was not detected on further investigations of TB involving other organs. HIV was also nonreactive.

3. Discussion

Infection of hollow or solid abdominal organs, peritoneum, and abdominal lymphatics with *Mycobacterium tuberculosis* bacilli is known as abdominal TB. The isolated form is less observed than combination of two or more sites [2]. The present case was a combination of GI TB involving appendix and mesenteric lymph node.

Among the abovementioned sites of abdomen (hollow organs), GI TB in patients with active pulmonary TB before the advent of specific antitubercular treatment had been reported as high as 55–90%, but the cases decreased to 25% after specific drugs developed [8]. The success rate of treatment was 86% among all new TB cases globally in 2012 [1].

The estimated incidence of abdominal TB among all cases of TB is 1–3% worldwide [9]. GI TB is more common in developing countries like Nepal [2]. Demographically the incidence of TB appendicitis has also shown variation in different countries. In Brunei Darussalam, it comprised 0.2% of all TB cases and 8.6% of abdominal TB cases among 6,593 appendectomies performed [7]. A study conducted in Nepal reported that cases of granuloma consistent with TB constituted 0.58% of total 518 appendectomy specimens [10]. In a tertiary centre in India, 2.3% of cases of TB appendicitis among 2921 appendectomies were diagnosed, being much higher than the reported cases in Nepal [11]. Tuberculous peritonitis was diagnosed in 2 cases among total cases of 177 abdominal surgeries in the other study of Nepal. It was not explained how tuberculous peritonitis occurred, whether it was manifestations of disseminated TB or if there was perorated GI TB [12].

It was thought that ingestion of milk contaminated with TB bacilli, *Mycobacterium bovis*, was the reason behind primary GI TB but boiled milk is usually consumed in developing countries and pasteurized milk in the west which makes it unlikely for ingestion of bacilli [2]. The reason behind rare involvement of the isolated appendix in spite of the ileocaecal junction being the common site of involvement in intestinal

TB is that luminal mucosa of the appendix has minimal exposure with the intestinal contents [13, 14].

Secondary appendicular TB is spread through hematogenous route or swallowing of infected sputum from primary pulmonary TB or direct contact through the infected lymph nodes and retrograde spread via fallopian tube infection [2].

Abdominal TB is common between 25 and 45 years of age [15]. Similarly other studies also found that young adults of 21–40 years are most commonly affected by abdominal TB [3–5]. TB appendix was found in age group of 25–48 years in a study conducted by Chong et al. [7].

Patients present with a vague clinical presentation in GI TB. Abdominal pain, weight loss, diarrhea, and intermittent constipation associated with worsening of the pain were common in a study of Nepal by Gautam et al. [2]. Abdominal pain was the most common presenting symptom followed by fever and weight loss [16] similar to the triad of symptoms in a study of Nepal. Patients also may present with constitutional symptoms. Symptoms of intestinal obstruction such as abdominal pain, constipation, and vomiting are usually seen in intestinal TB [15].

Chong et al. found that majority of patients with TB appendix had symptoms consistent with acute appendicitis [7]. Other symptoms such as localized or generalized ascites, abdominal distention, diarrhea, melaena, and anemia may be seen [16]. Hence, we cannot point out specific clinical features that are pathognomonic of appendicular TB.

Granulomatous appendicitis has other differential diagnoses such as parasite-related appendicitis, Crohn's disease, sarcoidosis, and foreign body-induced inflammation [11]. Differentiation between Crohn's disease and TB is very important among these conditions because of different approach to the management of these two diseases. Glucocorticosteroid is the main choice of drug for the treatment in Crohn's disease [2]. However, use of steroid therapy for patients with TB was hazardous without antituberculous therapy [17], but utility of adjunctive corticosteroid therapy in the management of TB with effective antituberculous drugs could improve outcomes [18–20]. It has proved to be beneficial in miliary TB, tuberculous meningitis, tuberculous pericarditis, tuberculous pleurisy, and endobronchial TB [21, 22]. The improvement of the outcome in TB patients with corticosteroids therapy is by suppressing the host mediated inflammation. When steroid therapy is given to patients with untreated or unrecognized TB, it results in overwhelming disease and death. Hence, clinicians must closely observe such patients and one should always remember drug interactions that may occur during treatment [22].

4. Conclusion

The present case was not suspected as TB of appendix unless laparotomy was performed and suspected tubercles were noticed. Diagnosis was made only after histopathological examination. Hence, it suggests that all surgically removed appendices should be subjected to histopathological examination.

Conflict of Interests

The author declares that there is no conflict of interests regarding the publication of this paper.

Acknowledgment

The author would like to thank Mr. Manohar Shrestha, the staff of histopathology department, for his technical assistance.

References

[1] WHO, *Global Tuberculosis Report 2014*, World Health Organization, Geneva, Switzerland, 2014, http://www.who.int/tb/publications/global_report/en/.

[2] M. P. Gautam, P. Karki, and S. Rijal, "Abdominal tuberculosis," *Journal of Nepal Medical Association*, vol. 43, pp. 40–48, 2004.

[3] S. K. Bhansali, "Abdominal tuberculosis. Experiences with 300 cases," *American Journal of Gastroenterology*, vol. 67, no. 4, pp. 324–337, 1977.

[4] R. K. Tandon, S. K. Sarin, S. L. Bose, M. Berry, and B. N. Tandon, "A clinico-radiological reappraisal of intestinal tuberculosis—changing profile?" *Gastroenterologia Japonica*, vol. 21, no. 1, pp. 17–22, 1986.

[5] K. R. Palmer, D. H. Patil, G. S. Basran, J. F. Riordan, and D. B. A. Silk, "Abdominal tuberculosis in urban Britain: a common disease," *Gut*, vol. 26, no. 12, pp. 1296–1305, 1985.

[6] S. Gupta, R. Kaushik, A. Kaur, and A. K. Attri, "Tubercular appendicitis—a case report," *World Journal of Emergency Surgery*, vol. 1, article 22, 2006.

[7] V. H. Chong, P. U. Telisinghe, S. K. S. Yapp, and C. F. Chong, "Tuberculous appendix: a review of clinical presentations and outcomes," *Singapore Medical Journal*, vol. 52, no. 2, pp. 90–93, 2011.

[8] P. J. Dolin, M. C. Raviglione, and A. Kochi, "Global tuberculosis incidence and mortality during 1990–2000," *Bulletin of the World Health Organization*, vol. 72, no. 2, pp. 213–220, 1994.

[9] T. A. Sheer and W. J. Coyle, "Gastrointestinal tuberculosis," *Current Gastroenterology Reports*, vol. 5, no. 4, pp. 273–278, 2003.

[10] R. Makaju, A. Mohammad, and A. Shakya, "Acute appendicitis: analysis of 518 histopathologically diagnosed cases at the Kathmandu University Hospital, Nepal," *Kathmandu University Medical Journal*, vol. 8, no. 30, pp. 227–230, 2010.

[11] S. C. Gupta, A. K. Gupta, N. K. Keswani, P. A. Singh, A. K. Tripathi, and V. Krishna, "Pathology of tropical appendicitis," *Journal of Clinical Pathology*, vol. 42, no. 11, pp. 1169–1172, 1989.

[12] S. Khan, I. U. Khan, S. Aslam, and A. Haque, "Retrospective analysis of abdominal surgeries at Nepalgunj Medical College (NGMC), Nepalgunj, Nepal: 2 year's experience," *Kathmandu University Medical Journal*, vol. 2, no. 4, pp. 336–343, 2004.

[13] M. K. Singh, Arunabh, and V. K. Kapoor, "Tuberculosis of the appendix—a report of 17 cases and a suggested aetiopathological classification," *Postgraduate Medical Journal*, vol. 63, no. 744, pp. 855–857, 1987.

[14] R. C. Shah, K. N. Mehta, and J. M. Jalundhwala, "Tuberculosis of the appendix," *Journal of the Indian Medical Association*, vol. 49, no. 3, pp. 138–140, 1967.

[15] I. Wani, R. A. Wani, A. A. Malik et al., "Abdominal tuberculosis," *OA Case Reports*, vol. 3, no. 5, p. 45, 2014.

[16] A. R. Miah, Y. R. Sharma, M. T. Rahman, A. Raihan, P. K. Roy, and M. Hasan, "Clinicopathological profile of patients with abdominal tuberculosis," *Journal of Nepal Health Research Council*, vol. 9, no. 2, pp. 169–175, 2011.

[17] J. Ilavsky and E. J. Foley, "Studies on the effect of cortisone with chemotherapeutic agents on tuberculous peritonitis in mice," *Antibiotics & Chemotherapy*, vol. 4, no. 10, pp. 1068–1074, 1954.

[18] J. R. Johnson and W. N. Davey, "Cortisone, corticotropin, and antimicrobial therapy in tuberculosis in animals and man: a review," *American Review of Tuberculosis*, vol. 70, no. 4, pp. 623–636, 1954.

[19] G. Favez, F. Aguet, P. Sourdat, P. Magnenat, and A. Brinsmade, "The treatment of certain forms of tuberculosis with a combination of prednisone (or hydrocortisone) and antibiotics," *Diseases of the Chest*, vol. 32, no. 1, pp. 70–82, 1957.

[20] R. M. Des Prez and A. Organick, "Corticotropin and corticosteroid therapy in tuberculosis," *Archives of Internal Medicine*, vol. 101, pp. 1129–1142, 1958.

[21] J. R. Cisneros and K. M. Murray, "Corticosteroids in tuberculosis," *Annals of Pharmacotherapy*, vol. 30, no. 11, pp. 1298–1303, 1996.

[22] N. Chhabra, R. Dixit, and M. L. Aseri, "Adjunctive corticosteroid therapy in tuberculosis management: a critical reappraisal," *International Journal of Pharmaceutical Sciences and Research*, vol. 2, pp. 10–15, 2011.

Clonal CD8+ T Lymphocytic Proliferation and Karyotypical Abnormalities in an EBV Associated Hemophagocytic Lymphohistiocytosis

Jiehao Zhou,[1] Dehua Wang,[2] and Mehdi Nassiri[1]

[1]*Department of Pathology and Laboratory Medicine, Indiana University, Indianapolis, IN 46202, USA*
[2]*Department of Pathology and Laboratory Medicine, Cincinnati Children's Hospital and Medical Center, Cincinnati, OH 45229, USA*

Correspondence should be addressed to Jiehao Zhou; zhouji@iupui.edu

Academic Editor: Dimosthenis Miliaras

EBV associated hemophagocytic lymphohistiocytosis and EBV-positive T cell lymphoproliferative disease of childhood share many histologic and clinical features, which sometimes makes it very difficult to render a definitive diagnosis. In this report, we present a 16-year-old male who developed symptoms clinically consistent with EBV associated hematophagocytic lymphohistiocytosis including fulfilling most of HLH diagnostic criteria and responding promptly to HLH targeted therapy. However, histologic and cytogenetics features of this case are very concerning for EBV-positive T cell lymphoproliferative disease of childhood. This case demonstrates an ambiguous boundary of these two disease entities and emphasizes the importance of comprehensive evaluation and clinical correlation with cases suspicious of EBV driven hemophagocytic or lymphoproliferative process.

1. Introduction

Hemophagocytic lymphohistiocytosis (HLH) is clinical syndrome characterized by fever, splenomegaly, pancytopenia, liver dysfunction, and coagulopathy. It is believed that there is an uncontrolled hyperinflammatory process associated with proliferation of activated lymphocytes and histiocytes which secrete excessive amount of proinflammatory cytokines. Histologically, proliferation of lymphocytes, histiocytes, and often hemophagocytosis are seen in bone marrow, spleen, and lymph nodes. There are two forms of HLH: primary HLH and secondary HLH. Primary HLH is an autosomal recessive disease featured by defects in a set of genes including PRF1, UNC13D, or STX11 [1]. Secondary HLH occurs after a strong immunologic activation, such as systemic infection, immunodeficiency, or malignancy. Epstein-Barr virus (EBV) is the most common infectious etiology for development of secondary HLH (EBV-HLH) usually following a primary EBV infection in adolescents. The EBV infests T cells, leading to monoclonal/oligoclonal expansion of T cells. Immunochemotherapy is most common treatment and consists of corticosteroid, etoposide, and cyclosporin [2]. The prognosis is guarded with an overall mortality of ~50%. On the other hand, EBV infection in adolescents can rarely evolve to a malignant T cell proliferative process known as EBV-positive T cell lymphoproliferative disease of childhood as described in WHO hematopoietic disorder classification [3]. This disease is characterized by an extremely high mortality rate despite aggressive management. However, it has significant overlapping features with EBV associated HLH including T cell immunophenotypic aberrancy and T cell clonality, which pose a diagnostic difficulty [4].

Herein, we report a case with clinical features of EBV associated HLH which was associated with a rather abundant clonal CD8+ T cell expansion. These T cells demonstrated aberrant antigen expression and harbored EBV. Cytogenetics study demonstrated abnormal karyotype. These features raised a concern for EBV driven neoplastic process. However, the overall clinical course was more in line with a reactive process.

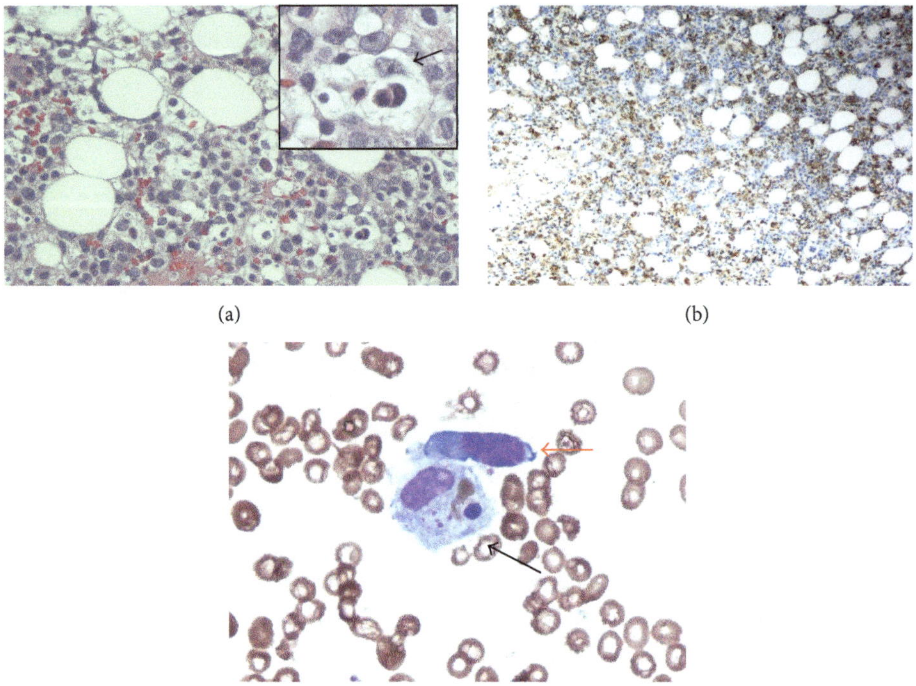

(a) (b) (c)

FIGURE 1: Histologic features of bone marrow. (a) Bone marrow biopsy demonstrated hypocellular marrow with prominent lymphohistiocytic infiltrates. Black arrow in the inset pointed to a histiocyte with engulfed hematopoietic elements. (b) Immunohistochemical stain of CD68 showed increased histiocytes. (c) Bone marrow aspirate smears highlighted hemophagocytosis (black arrow) and atypical lymphoid cell (red arrow).

2. Case Presentation

2.1. Initial Clinical Presentation. A 16-year-old previously healthy white male initially presented with fever, sore throat, and skin rash involving upper arms and face. A diagnosis of infectious mononucleosis was rendered based on the clinical symptoms and apositive EBV-VCA IgM titer at an outside institute. He was managed by supportive measurements. However, his symptom was worsening and subsequent laboratory studies showed thrombocytopenia with platelets at 56,000 k/μL. Serum transaminases elevated to the ~220 IU/L, and LDH was in the range of 500s IU/L. He was hospitalized and received IV fluids and antibiotics. Nevertheless, his symptoms were further worsening. CBC evaluation showed leukopenia with WBC at 1.5 k/μL and thrombocytopenia with platelets at 36,000 k/μL. In addition, peripheral blood smear showed atypical lymphoid cells. CT study demonstrated hepatosplenomegaly and lymphadenopathy. The patient was transferred to our hospital for further evaluation approximately 6 weeks after initial symptoms.

At the time of transfer, the patient demonstrated profound pancytopenia with white blood cell count at 0.6 k/μL, hemoglobin at 9 g/dL, and platelets at 14 k/μL. Patient also showed renal insufficiency. His creatinine was elevated to 3.2 mg/dL. Additional laboratory studies revealed hyperferritinemia (~48000 μg/L), hypofibrinogenemia (63 mg/dL), markedly elevated soluble IL-2 receptor (~57000 pg/mL), high LDH (2154 IU/L), and mildly increased serum triglyceride. Both EBV-VCA IgM and IgG were positive. PCR study of EBV titer was marked elevated, >7 million copies/mL. Peripheral blood smear showed atypical lymphoid cells with large size, mature chromatin, distinct nucleolus, and basophilic cytoplasm. Molecular genetic testing for familial HLH including SH2D1A, BIRC4, and STXBP2 gene was all normal. The clinical impression was EBV associated secondary hemophagocytic lymphohistiocytosis. A bone marrow evaluation was performed to further characterize the disease.

2.2. Pathological, Immunophenotypic, Molecular, and Cytogenetics Findings. Bone marrow evaluation showed hypocellular bone marrow with decreased trilineage hematopoiesis and diffuse lymphohistiocytic infiltrates (Figure 1(a)). Increased histiocytes were seen by H&E and immunohistochemical stain of CD68 (Figure 1(b)). Histiocytes with evident phagocytosis were present in both biopsy (Figure 1(a) and inset) and bone marrow aspirate (Figure 1(c)). In addition, there was a very prominent atypical lymphoid cell infiltration composed of lymphoid cells with medium to large size, irregular nuclear contour, and visible nucleolus (Figure 1(a)). Concurrent immunophenotyping by flow cytometric analysis of marrow aspirate also revealed a prominent atypical T cell population which was positive for CD2, CD3, and

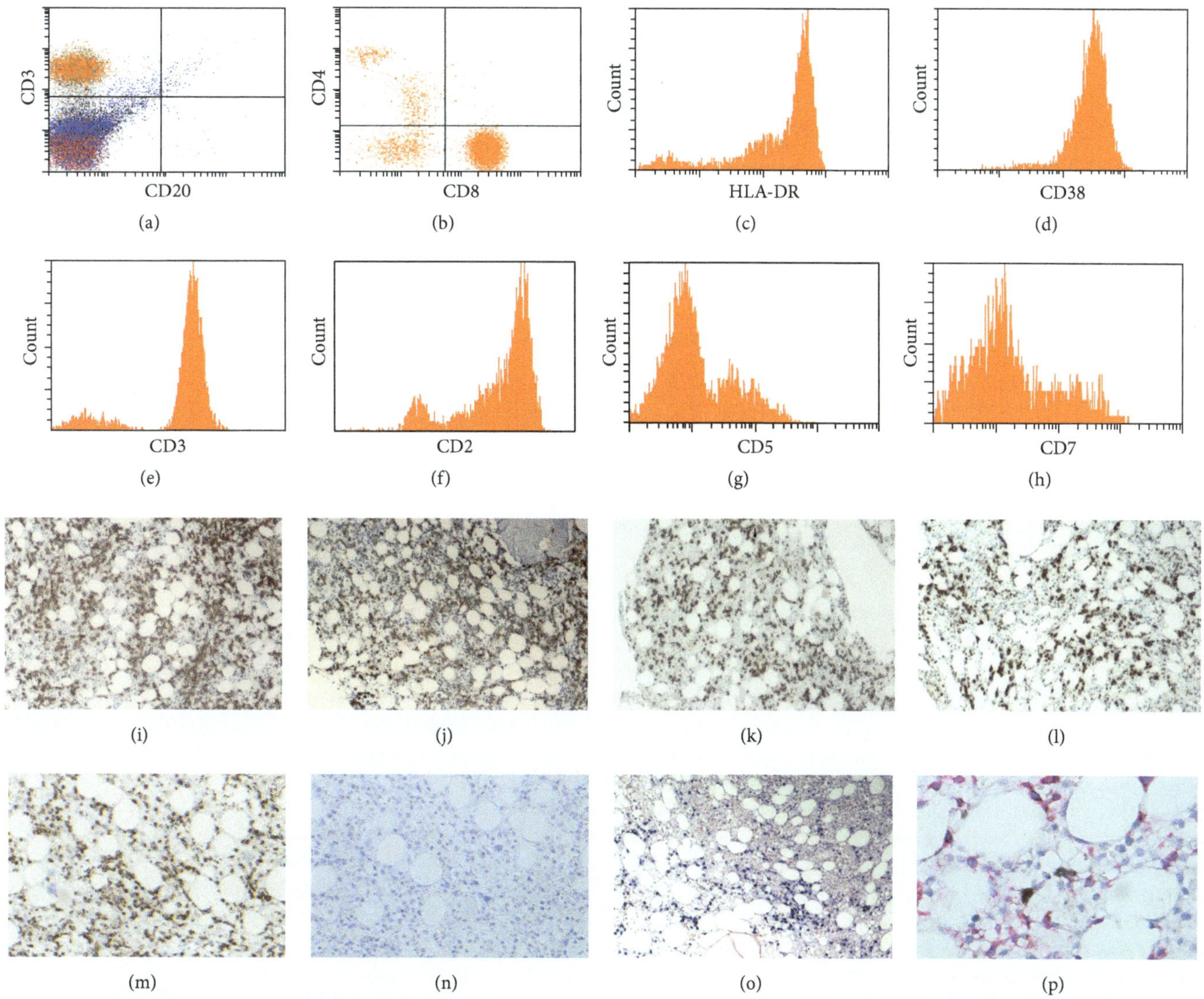

FIGURE 2: Immunophenotypic features of atypical lymphoid infiltrates. (a)–(h) Flow cytometry analysis of bone marrow showed most of lymphoid infiltrates were CD3+ (a and e), CD2+ (f), CD8+ (b) positive T cells with few CD4+ (b) T cells, and rare CD20+ (a) B cells. These T cells have bright HLA-DR (c) and CD38 (d) expression. Loss of CD5 (g) and CD7 (h) in T cells was evident. (i)–(n) Immunohistochemical stains of bone marrow showed a prominent CD3+ (i) and CD8+ (j) T cell infiltration. These T cells are positive for cytotoxic markers perforin (k), granzyme B (l), and TIA-1 (m) and negative for CD56 (n). (o) In situ hybridization of EBER showed diffuse EBER positive cells in the bone marrow biopsy. (p) Double immunohistochemical stains of CD3 (red) and EBV-LMP (brown) demonstrated colocalization of EBV and CD3.

CD8, with uniformly bright CD38 and HLA-DR expression (Figures 2(a)–2(f)). Loss of CD5 and CD7 antigen expression in these T cells was easily appreciated (Figures 2(g)-2(h)). Immunohistochemical work-up on bone marrow biopsy confirmed that these atypical lymphoid cells are predominant CD3+/CD8+ T cells (Figures 2(i) and 2(j)) with loss of CD5 and CD7 antigen expression. In addition, these atypical lymphoid cells were positive for cytotoxic markers including perforin, granzyme B, and TIA-1 and negative for CD56 (Figures 2(k)–2(n)). These atypical lymphoid cells were also positive for EBV as demonstrated by positive EBV LMP immunohistochemical stain (not shown) and by in situ hybridization of EBER (Figure 2(o)). Double stain of CD3 and EBV LMP demonstrated colocalization of EBV and CD3 (Figure 2(p)).

In order to further characterize this atypical T cell infiltration, PCR of T cell receptor gamma chain gene rearrangement was performed on DNA extracted from bone marrow aspirate. Two clonal TCR-gamma gene PCR products of ~62 and ~185 bp were identified with Vγ 1-8,9/Jγ1/2 primer set (Figure 3(a)) and one clonal TCR-gamma PCR product of ~244 bp was identified with Alt. Vγ/Jγ1/2 primer sets (Figure 3(b)). Therefore, T cell gene rearrangement study showed a clonal TCR-gamma gene PCR product.

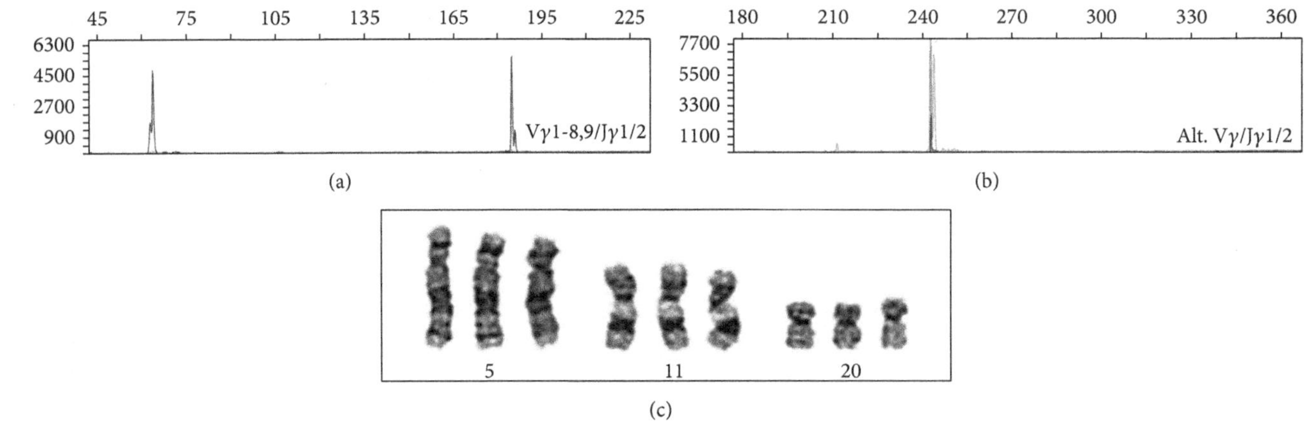

FIGURE 3: Molecular and cytogenetics findings in the bone marrow. (a) and (b) Assessment of TCR gamma receptor gene rearrangement by PCR on formalin-fixed, paraffin-embedded tissue sections from bone marrow clot demonstrated biclonal PCR product using Vγ 1-8,9/Jγ1/2 primer set (a) and monoclonal PCR product using Alt. Vγ/Jγ1/2 primer sets (b). (c) G-band karyotypic study on bone marrow aspirate demonstrated an abnormal karyotype in all 20 dividing cells examined: 49,XY,+5,+11,+20/[20].

Cytogenetics study on bone marrow aspirate showed an abnormal karyotype on all metaphases examined: 49,XY,+5, +11,+20/[20] (Figure 3(c)).

2.3. Treatment and Posttreatment Clinical Findings. Since patient met the proposed diagnostic criteria for HLH, he was started on etoposide, dexamethasone, and Rituxan in addition to supportive care. Cyclosporin administration was initially held due to renal insufficiency. The patient responded to the therapy very well. He was discharged to an outside hospital one week after start of therapy. By the end of 6-week therapy, he was reported to have normal WBC count, mild anemia, mild thrombocytopenia, normal ferritin, fibrinogen, and sIL-2R values. The EBV titer by PCR fell to undetectable level. Posttherapy bone marrow evaluation demonstrated hypocellular bone with trilineage hypoplasia. Neither abnormal lymphoid infiltrates nor overt hemophagocytic activities were identified. Cytogenetic study on the post treatment marrow showed a normal karyotype [46, XY].

The patient was gradually taken off chemotherapy and was followed up clinically. Currently, the patient has been off treatment for three years. He has normal CB except a persistent borderline thrombocytopenia (platelet count is in low 100s). There is no clinical concern of HLH or lymphomatous process.

3. Discussion

Primary infection with the EBV in immunocompetent individuals is characterized by the infection of B lymphocytes by virus via CD21 antigens on the B cells. Usually it is asymptomatic. Some of infected patients develop infectious mononucleosis which is a self-limited disease characterized as strong antibody reaction associated with polyclonal B cell proliferation as well as a robust cytotoxic T cell response which is often monoclonal or oligoclonal [5]. Uncommonly, acute EBV infection leads to the development of hemophagocytic lymphohistiocytosis (HLH), with unregulated activation of histiocytes and often a clonal cytotoxic lymphocyte expansion. Clinical and morphology evaluations demonstrate high fever, hepatosplenomegaly, lymphadenopathy pancytopenia, hemophagocytosis, hypercytokinemia, and multiorgan system failure. Although EBV-HLH is associated with substantial morbidity and mortality, early recognition and prompt immunochemotherapy, such as HLH 2004 protocol, result in successful treatment of EBV-induced HLH. Very rarely, EBV infection results in EBV positive T cell lymphoproliferative disorder of childhood with overt monoclonal T cell proliferation and similar symptoms as those of EBV-HLH. Most of patients with this disease have a fulminant clinical course and extremely high mortality despite aggressive management.

The clinical course and laboratory findings of current case are compatible with EBV associated HLH. For diagnosis of HLH, at least 5 out of 8 findings are required [6]. These findings include (1) persistent fever; (2) splenomegaly; (3) cytopenias in 2 or more cell lines; (4) hypertriglyceridemia (triglyceride level ≥265 mg/dL) or hypofibrinogenemia (fibrinogen level ≤150 mg/dL); (5) hemophagocytosis in the bone marrow, spleen, or lymph nodes; (6) hyperferritinemia (ferritin level ≥500 ng/mL); (7) impaired NK cell function; and (8) elevated soluble IL2 receptor. In our case, seven out of eight findings are identified except for impaired NK cell function which was not performed due to low WBC count in the peripheral blood. Given patient's high EBV titer and negative molecular study result for primary HLH, it is compatible with EBV associated secondary HLH.

In addition to these findings consistent with EBV associated HLH, evaluation of marrow demonstrated a rather abundant abnormal CD3+/CD8+ T cell population which was clonal by TCR gene rearrangement testing. This population was composed of EBV positive and cytotoxic CD8+ T cells with evident aberrant loss of CD5 and CD7 antigen expression. More interestingly, cytogenetic studies of marrow demonstrated a hyperploid karyotype in all cells examined, 49,XY,+5,+11,+20. These findings are highly suspicious for a neoplastic process, particularly systemic EBV-positive T cell lymphoproliferative disorder of childhood as defined in the current WHO classification [3].

Systemic EBV-positive T cell lymphoproliferative disorder of childhood is a rare clonal T cell neoplasm development shortly after primary acute EBV infection in previously healthy children and young adults. Sometimes this entity can arise in a setting of severe chronic active EBV infection. Most of cases were reported in immunocompetent Asians and Native Americans with a very aggressive clinical course and very high mortality. The most classical immunophenotype of this entity is CD3+/CD2+/CD8+ T cells with expression of selective cytotoxic markers including positive for TIA-1 and negative for CD56. Loss of CD5 and CD7 antigen expression in neoplastic T cells is very common. Cases arising in the setting of severe chronic active EBV infection are usually CD4+. Rare cases show neoplastic CD4+/CD8+ double positive T cells. Most of neoplastic cells have clonally rearranged TCR gene and are positive for EBER/EBV-LMP [3].

Although the morphology and immunohistochemical cytogenetics/molecular findings in the bone marrow made us concerned with the diagnosis of EBV-positive T cell lymphoproliferative disease of childhood, our case presented with a few unusual characteristics when compared to the more typical case of EBV-positive T cell lymphoproliferative disorder of childhood. First of all, typical EBV-positive T cell lymphoproliferative disorder of childhood is usually found in children or adolescents of Asian or Native American origin [3]. It is hypothesized that a genetically determined susceptibility leads to an abnormal response to primary EBV infection. By contrast, our patient is a white male without known immunodeficiency. Secondly, a relatively common finding in typical EBV-positive T cell lymphoproliferative disease of childhood is the absence of serologic response to EBV. EBV anti-VCA IgM was negative in the majority of reported typical cases whereas EBV anti-VCA IgG is either absent or only moderately elevated [7]. Sometimes, the negative EBV serology result may be clinically misleading since it does not indicate an ongoing EBV infection, which may lead to a wrong diagnosis path. It has been speculated that the lack of humoral response to EBV results in virus proliferation in T cells and subsequently development of clonal expansion of EBV positive T cells. In contrast, our patient demonstrated a relatively robust antibody response to EBV with both positive EBV anti-VCA IgG and IgM (titer up to 1:1280). Ultimately, systemic EBV-positive T cell lymphoproliferative disorder of childhood has a very aggressive clinical course with extremely high mortality which is thought to be related with uncontrolled HLH. Most of cases have a fulminant course resulting in death in days to month. Only extremely rare cases showed clinical remission after aggressive chemotherapy. Our patient had a very good response to HLH 2004 protocol treatment. Liver function, hematology index, and viral titers all recovered following treatment. Bone marrow examination ~2 months after treatment showed no evidence of clonal T cell infiltration and normal cytogenetics. Overall these findings are more compatible with self-limited clonal T cell proliferation associated with EBV associated HLH.

Aberrant antigen expression in T cells and monoclonal and oligoclonal T cell expansion in infectious mononucleosis and EBV associated HLH has been reported previously. Weisberger et al. [8] demonstrated that acute infectious mononucleosis is featured by expansion of activated CD8+ cytotoxic T cells with frequent downregulation of CD7 antigen. Bright CD38 and HLA-DR antigen expression in T cells are noted. Not uncommonly, molecular studies demonstrated clonal T cell population. Weisberger et al. [8] had proposed that the bright expression of activation marker of HLA-DR served as a clue of reactive nature as most of peripheral T cell neoplasms often have absent to heterogenous expression of HLA-DR. On the other hand, Toga et al. [9] reported expanded CD8+ cytotoxic T cells in peripheral blood of six EBV associated HLH pediatric patients in Japan. Different from T cells in infectious mononucleosis, these T cells demonstrated more evident downregulation of CD5 antigen in addition to loss of CD7 and bright HLA-DR expression by immunophenotyping. Flow cytometry analysis of TCR Vβ and PCR analysis of TCR beta gene rearrangement analysis demonstrated T cell clonality in the majority of patients. Moreover, immunohistochemical studies revealed that these CD8+ T cells were cellular target of EBV infection as compared to the B cells which were target of EBV infection in infectious mononucleosis. Toga proposed that clonal expansion of CD8+ T cells with CD5 downregulation as characteristic immunophenotypic features of EBV associated HLH as a tool to distinguish patients with infectious mononucleosis since no such population was identified in patients with infectious mononucleosis.

Cytogenetics abnormalities have been reported sporadically in EBV associated HLH [10–12]. Imashuku et al. [11] showed that the EBV associated HLH with abnormal karyotype is comprised of ~20% case in a retrospective cohort of 32 EBV associated HLH cases and was invariably fatal with a 3-year survival of 14%. The majority of cytogenetically abnormal clone demonstrated hyperdiploid. However, no recurrent clonal chromosomal abnormality has been documented in HLH cases with cytogenetics abnormalities in their series [11]. A separate study led by Chen et al. [12] showed 3 cases of EBV-HLH with cytogenetics abnormality at a single medical center. There is a recurrent karyotypic abnormality of add(9)(p24) in two of them. Our patient demonstrated a nonrandom hyperploid karyotype 49, XY,+5,+11,+20 in all 20 metaphases examined. Usually, clonal karyotypic abnormality in this clinical setting is an indication of neoplastic process. However, our patient recovered rather promptly after typical courses of immunochemotherapy for HLH. Posttreatment study demonstrates normal karyotype and the long term follow-up (3-year) showed no evidence of reoccurrence of disease.

In summary, we report a rare case of EBV-HLH associated with evident clonal CD8+ T cell expansion. The abundance of T cell infiltration in the bone marrow, aberrant immunophenotypic features, clonality by TCR gamma gene rearrangement, and abnormality by karyocytic cytogenetics study are highly suspicious for EBV-positive T cell lymphoproliferative disorder of childhood. However, the clinical course and responsiveness to the immune chemotherapy are more in line with a reactive process. This case further highlights the diagnostic difficulties to distinguish EBV driven reactive versus malignant process. Comprehensive evaluation including morphological, immunophenotypic, molecular, and karyotypical studies is important. Clinical correlation, prompt treatment, and posttreatment follow-up are essential.

Conflict of Interests

The authors declare that there is no conflict of interests regarding the publication of this paper.

References

[1] J.-I. Henter, M. Arico, G. Elinder, S. Imashuku, and G. Janka, "Familial hemophagocytic lymphohistiocytosis. Primary hemophagocytic lymphohistiocytosis," *Hematology/Oncology Clinics of North America*, vol. 12, no. 2, pp. 417–433, 1998.

[2] S. Imashuku, "Treatment of Epstein-Barr virus-related hemophagocytic lymphohistiocytosis (EBV-HLH); update 2010," *Journal of Pediatric Hematology/Oncology*, vol. 33, no. 1, pp. 35–39, 2011.

[3] L. Quintanilla-Martinez, H. Kimura, and E. S. Jaffe, "EBV-positive T-cell lymphoproliferative disorders of childhood," in *WHO Classification of Tumours of Haematopoietic and Lymphoid Tissues*, S. H. Swerdlow, E. Campo, N. L. Harris et al., Eds., pp. 278–280, IARC Press, Lyon, France, 2008.

[4] M. C. Smith, D. N. Cohen, B. Greig et al., "The ambiguous boundary between EBV-related hemophagocytic lymphohistiocytosis and systemic EBV-driven T cell lymphoproliferative disorder," *International Journal of Clinical and Experimental Pathology*, vol. 7, no. 9, pp. 5738–5749, 2014.

[5] M. F. C. Callan, N. Steven, P. Krausa et al., "Large clonal expansions of $CD8^+$ T cells in acute infectious mononucleosis," *Nature Medicine*, vol. 2, no. 8, pp. 906–911, 1996.

[6] J.-I. Henter, A. Horne, M. Aricó et al., "HLH-2004: diagnostic and therapeutic guidelines for hemophagocytic lymphohistiocytosis," *Pediatric Blood and Cancer*, vol. 48, no. 2, pp. 124–131, 2007.

[7] L. Quintanilla-Martinez, S. Kumar, F. Fend et al., "Fulminant EBV^+ T-cell lymphoproliferative disorder following acute/chronic EBV infection: a distinct clinicopathologic syndrome," *Blood*, vol. 96, no. 2, pp. 443–451, 2000.

[8] J. Weisberger, D. Cornfield, W. Gorczyca, and Z. Liu, "Down-regulation of pan-T-cell antigens, particularly CD7, in acute infectious mononucleosis," *American Journal of Clinical Pathology*, vol. 120, no. 1, pp. 49–55, 2003.

[9] A. Toga, T. Wada, Y. Sakakibara et al., "Clinical significance of cloned expansion and CD5 down-regulation in epstein-barr virus (EBV) infected $CD8^+$ T lymphocytes in EBV-Associated hemophagocytic lymphohistiocytosis," *Journal of Infectious Diseases*, vol. 201, no. 12, pp. 1923–1932, 2010.

[10] Y. Kaneko, N. Maseki, M. Sakurai et al., "Clonal and non-clonal karyotypically abnormal cells in haemophagocytic lymphohistiocytosis," *British Journal of Haematology*, vol. 90, no. 1, pp. 48–55, 1995.

[11] S. Imashuku, S. Hibi, Y. Tabata et al., "Outcome of clonal hemophagocytic lymphohistiocytosis: analysis of 32 cases," *Leukemia & Lymphoma*, vol. 37, no. 5-6, pp. 577–584, 2000.

[12] J.-S. Chen, C.-C. Tzeng, C.-J. Tsao et al., "Clonal karyotype abnormalities in EBV-associated hemophagocytic syndrome," *Haematologica*, vol. 82, no. 5, pp. 572–576, 1997.

Spindle Cell Lipoma Occurring in the Buccal Mucosa: An Unusual Location of This Benign Lipomatous Neoplasm

Noala Vicensoto Moreira Milhan, Ana Sueli Rodrigues Cavalcante, Yonara Maria Freire Soares Marques, Yasmin Rodarte Carvalho, and Ana Lia Anbinder

Department of Bioscience and Oral Diagnosis, Institute of Science and Technology (ICT), Universidade Estadual Paulista (UNESP), Avenida Engenheiro Francisco José Longo 777, 12245-000 São José dos Campos, SP, Brazil

Correspondence should be addressed to Ana Lia Anbinder; ana.anbinder@fosjc.unesp.br

Academic Editor: Marco Mazzocchi

Spindle cell lipoma is a benign lipomatous neoplasm, which rarely occurs in the oral cavity. The aims of this paper are to report a case of spindle cell lipoma located in buccal mucosa and discuss the main clinical, histological, and immunohistochemical findings of this entity. Thus, we report a 4-year history of an asymptomatic smooth surface nodule in an elderly Caucasian man with clinical hypothesis of fibroma. The histopathological examination showed spindle cells, mature adipose tissue, and many mast cells in a stroma of connective tissue presenting ropey collagen fibers bundles. After immunohistochemical analysis, the final diagnosis was spindle cell lipoma.

1. Introduction

Spindle cell lipoma (SCL) is a histological variant of lipoma that often occurs in the neck, back, and shoulder [1]. It is rare in the oral cavity [2] and only 35 well-documented cases were published between 1984 and 2012 in the oral region [3]. Usually SCL is less than 5 cm in size, affects mainly elderly men [1, 3], and has a benign clinical course [1]. Generally, SCL is removed without imaging examination because it is usually found in superficial locations and is small in size [4].

In this paper, we report a case of a spindle cell lipoma located in the buccal mucosa and discuss important features of this rare oral lesion.

2. Case Report

A 64-year-old Caucasian man presented with a 4-year history of an asymptomatic nodular soft tissue mass located in the right buccal mucosa. Clinical examination of oral mucosa revealed a pedunculated and well-circumscribed nodule with about 1 cm in diameter. The nodule had fibrous consistency, smooth surface and it was covered by undamaged mucosa. The clinical hypothesis was traumatic fibroma.

Excisional biopsy of the nodule was performed and histopathological examination revealed connective tissue fragments presenting spindle cells in a background with ropey collagen fibers bundles. A diffuse infiltrate of mast cells was observed. In some slices, a central area of mature adipose tissue, with normal aspect, was noted. The lesion was well vascularized and covered by stratified squamous epithelium with areas of acanthosis, hyperplasia, duplication of basal cell layer, and hydropic degeneration (Figures 1(a)–1(d)).

After initial microscopic examination, the diagnoses hypothesis included traumatic fibroma, neurofibroma, and SCL. Immunostaining of the specimen with primary antibodies against vimentin (VIM, Clone V9-Dako), CD-34 (Clone QBEnd10-Dako), S-100 (Clone S100-Dako), Bcl-2 (Clone 124-Dako), smooth muscle actin (SMA, Clone 1A4-Dako), and mast cell (Clone AA1-Imgenex) was performed. The immunohistochemical reactions revealed negativity of spindle cells for S-100 and SMA and positivity for CD-34 (Figure 1(e)), Bcl-2 (Figure 1(f)), and VIM

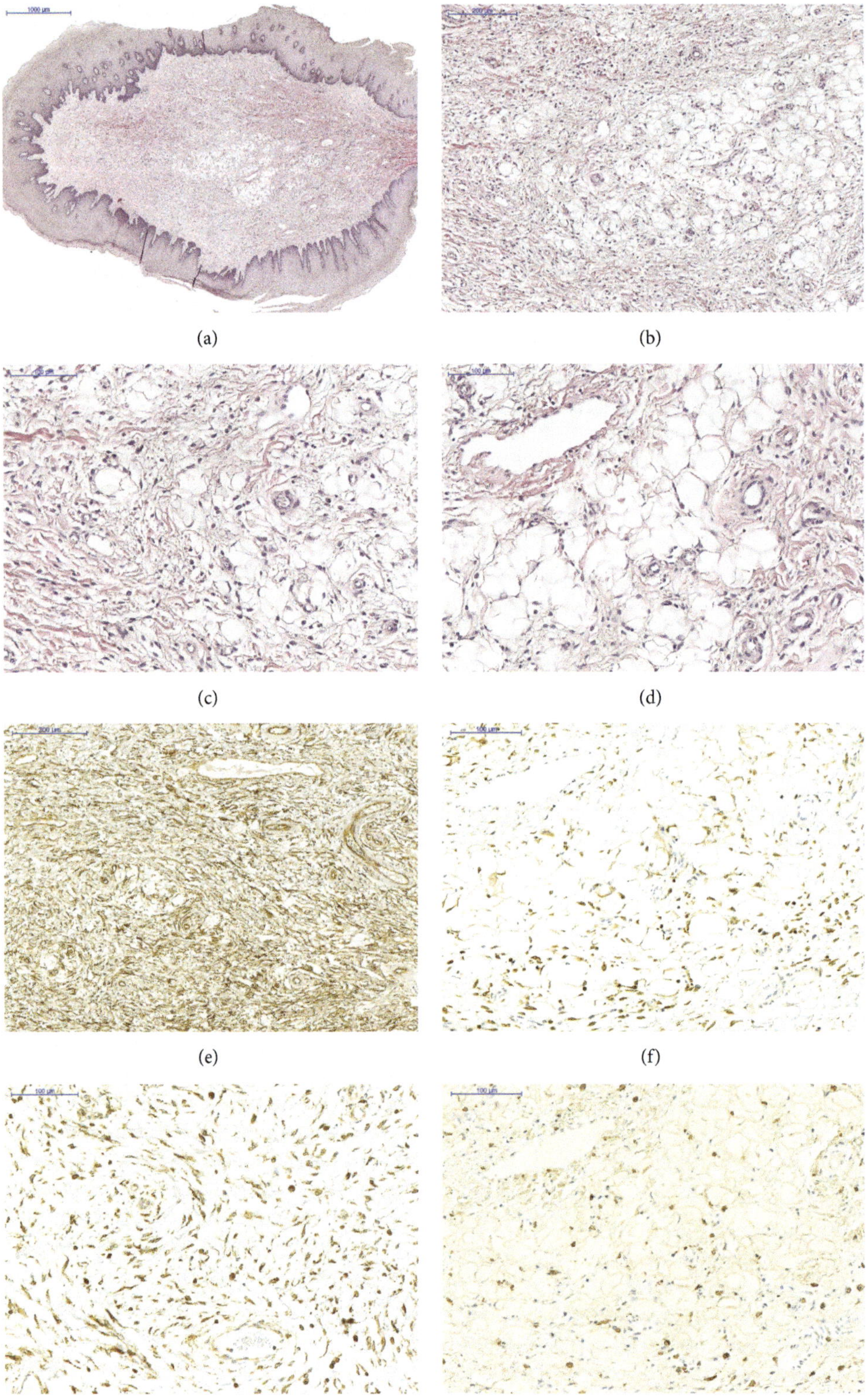

(a) (b) (c) (d) (e) (f) (g) (h)

FIGURE 1: A circumscribed fibrous lesion covered by acanthotic epithelium showing lipomatous content at the centre of connective tissue (a). Mature adipose tissue in a background presenting ropey collagen fibers bundles (b). Spindle cells, vessels, and mast cells near lipomatous content ((c)-(d)). Spindle cells were strongly positive for CD-34 antibody (e) and positive for Bcl-2 (f) and vimentin antibodies (g). The great number of mast cells was demonstrated by mast-cell staining (h). ((a) to (d)) Hematoxylin and eosin stain; ((d) to (h)) immunohistochemistry stain.

(Figure 1(g)). Moreover, mast-cell immunohistochemistry staining was performed and confirmed the presence of these cells (Figure 1(h)). These findings were consistent with the diagnosis of SCL. The patient has been followed up and no recurrence occurred after one year.

3. Discussion

The World Health Organization (WHO) categorizes benign lipomatous entities into some distinct lesions: lipoma, lipoblastoma, lipomatosis, lipomatosis of a nerve, myolipoma of soft tissue, angiolipoma, spindle cell/pleomorphic lipoma, chondroid lipoma, and hibernoma [5].

SCL was first described by Enzinger and Harvey in 1975. This lesion is usually located in the subcutaneous tissues of the neck, back, and shoulder [1]. In contrast, SCL is rare in the oral region [3] and comprises only about 1,62% of intraoral lipomatous tumors [2]. SCL has been reported in the tongue, buccal mucosa, floor of the mouth, hard palate, lip, and alveolar ridge [3]. One case in the maxilla was also reported [6].

SCL has a male predilection (male : female, 10 : 1) and the mean age of occurrence is 56 years [1]. In oral cavity cases, the male predilection is 2 : 1, while the mean age of occurrence is about 55 [3]. Usually, SCL appears as a well-circumscribed and painless mass [1] that generally has less than 5 cm in diameter [1, 3], although it may reach more than 10 cm [1, 4].

When SCL occurs on the face it may be misdiagnosed as an atypical lipomatous tumor because in this area the infiltrative behavior of SCL is common, such as malignant tumors. This infiltration occurs probably due to facial anatomical features, which involve poorly demarcated fascial planes [7]. SCL is generally solitary, although patients with bilateral SCLs of the tongue [8, 9] and nose [7] and lesions located simultaneously in upper region of the back and axilla [10] have been reported. Multiple SCLs may be familial or nonfamilial [11]. The treatment for SCL is local excision, usually without local recurrence [1, 3].

Histologically, SCL is composed of spindle/fusiform cells that may present a parallel arrangement, showing nuclear palisading. The stromal background shows ropey collagen fibers bundles. This lesion may also have myxoid areas. In association with spindle cells, different amounts of adipose tissue are usually observed. Moreover, the presence of mast cells in SCL is common [1, 5]. The vascular pattern usually is inconspicuous but there are lesions with prominent vascular pattern [1].

SCL is also called pleomorphic lipoma because it may show pleomorphic or bizarre multinucleated giant cells, sometimes with floret-like arrangement of the nuclei. Moreover, fat cells with varying size may be observed in SCL [5].

Some SCLs show several histological differences from classic SCL and have been proposed as variants. SCL presenting prominent fibrous tissue was described as fibrous SCL. This feature may represent one end of the histopathological spectrum of SCL, once the spindle cells are able to produce significant amounts of collagen [12]. SCL showing irregular and sometimes cleft-like spaces and villiform projections was classified as angiomatous. The cells of these irregular spaces may present vascular-lymphatic differentiation; however lymphatic phenotype is more common than vascular one [13].

Spindle to stellate cells, with cytoplasmic dendritic processes, and adipose tissue in a myxoid background have been observed in a recently described lesion known as dendritic fibromyxolipoma. However, some studies have proposed that this lesion is just a variant of the SCL [14, 15]. Wong et al. [15] performed cytogenetic analysis and concluded that this lesion does not represent a separate entity.

In a classic SCL, the ratio of mature adipocytes and spindle cells is variable; however the majority of cases have high amounts of both components. There are low-fat and fat-free SCLs, but they are less common than classic SCLs. In a previous study that evaluated over 300 cases of SCLs, only 34 low-fat and fat-free SCLs were identified. Moreover, only 3 cases of low-fat and fat-free SCLs were considered as a diagnosis, showing that different proportions of histopathologic elements, especially adipose tissue, hamper the diagnosis [16].

The histological differential diagnosis of SCL depends on features that predominate in each lesion. It usually includes benign tumors such as classic lipoma, schwannoma, neurofibroma [7], leiomyoma [1], and solitary fibrous tumor [16]. However, atypical lipomatous tumors (ALT) may also represent a differential diagnosis of SCL [7]. Dermatofibrosarcoma protuberans and subconjunctival herniated orbital fat are malignant [17] and benign [18] lesions, respectively, which may be confused with SCL. However, subconjunctival herniated orbital is a specific eye condition and only 2 cases of intraoral dermatofibrosarcoma protuberans have been described in literature [17]. Then, these lesions usually are differential diagnosis of extraoral SCLs.

Less commonly, ALT, also known as well-differentiated liposarcoma, may also be a differential diagnosis of SCL [7, 19]. SCL may be confused with ALT; however there are histological components that may help to differentiate ALT from benign lesions: ALT presents fibrous septa with atypical stromal cells demonstrating nuclear hyperchromasia, significant variation in adipocyte shape and size, which includes enlarged and atypical adipocyte nuclei. Moreover, ropey collagen fibers have not been observed in ALT [7, 20]. In cases where the histological evaluation is not sufficient to differentiate SCL from ALT, the positive immunoreactivity for MDM2, CDK4, p16, and Rb in ALT and not in SCL may be helpful in the final diagnoses [21].

In this study, after initial microscopic evaluation the hypotheses were benign tumors, which included traumatic fibroma, neurofibroma, and SCL. SCL was the last one to be considered because the central area of adipose tissue was present only in some slices. Considering the proliferation of spindle cells in a collagenized background, traumatic fibroma was a hypothesis. The spindle cell component and the numerous mast cells contributed to the hypothesis of neurofibroma. When the slices showing adipose tissue were observed, SCL was also considered. However, we could not eliminate the hypotheses of traumatic fibroma and neurofibroma without immunohistochemical analysis. A previous study that evaluated 320 cutaneous neurofibromas showed that 6.9% presented intratumoral mature fat [22].

The immunohistochemical analysis was accomplished and the positivity of spindle cells for CD-34 excluded the possibility of a traumatic fibroma [23] while their negativity for S-100 excluded the possibility of a neurofibroma [22]. Furthermore, the spindle cells showed positivity for VIM and Bcl-2 and negativity for SMA which was compatible with the immunohistochemical panel of SCL [24]. The SMA negative staining excluded the muscular and myofibroblastic origin of spindle cells [25]. Thus, considering the histological and immunohistochemical findings, our diagnosis was classic SCL.

In spite of the fact that adipose tissue has been seen only in some areas, it was more than 5% of the lesion. Low-fat and fat-free SCL are considered to be tumors in which mature adipocytes are less than 5% of the tumor [16].

In summary, SCL is a rare lesion in the oral cavity that may be confused with other entities. In this report we presented a rare case of a classic SCL to make clinicians and pathologists aware of this lesion in the oral cavity and discussed the possible differential diagnoses.

Conflict of Interests

The authors declare that there is no conflict of interests regarding the publication of this paper.

References

[1] F. M. Enzinger and D. A. Harvey, "Spindle cell lipoma," *Cancer*, vol. 36, no. 5, pp. 1852–1859, 1975.

[2] N. Said-Al-Naief, F. R. Zahurullah, and J. J. Sciubba, "Oral spindle cell lipoma," *Annals of Diagnostic Pathology*, vol. 5, no. 4, pp. 207–215, 2001.

[3] E. Manor, N. Sion-Vardy, P. A. Brennan, and L. Bodner, "Spindle cell lipoma of the oral cavity: a clinico-pathologic analysis of 35 reported cases," *Surgical Science*, vol. 4, no. 3, pp. 196–201, 2013.

[4] A. Khashper, J. Zheng, A. Nahal, and F. Discepola, "Imaging characteristics of spindle cell lipoma and its variants," *Skeletal Radiology*, vol. 43, no. 5, pp. 591–597, 2014.

[5] C. D. M. Fletcher, J. A. Bridge, P. Hogendoorn, and F. Mertens, *World Health Organization Classification of Tumours. Pathology and Genetics. Tumours of Soft Tissue and Bone*, IARC Press, Lyon, France, 2013.

[6] S. M. Stokes, J. P. Wood, and J. T. Castle, "Maxillary intraosseous spindle cell lipoma," *Journal of Oral and Maxillofacial Surgery*, vol. 69, no. 6, pp. e131–e134, 2011.

[7] A. Cheah, S. Billings, J. Goldblum, J. Hornick, N. Uddin, and B. Rubin, "Spindle cell/pleomorphic lipomas of the face: an under-recognized diagnosis," *Histopathology*, vol. 66, no. 3, pp. 430–437, 2015.

[8] N. Kaku, K. Kashima, T. Daa et al., "Multiple spindle cell lipomas of the tongue: report of a case," *Acta Pathologica, Microbiologica, et Immunologica Scandinavica*, vol. 111, no. 5, pp. 581–585, 2003.

[9] T. Imai, M. Michizawa, H. Shimizu, N. Yamamoto, and Y. Yura, "Bilateral multiple spindle cell lipomas of the tongue," *Oral Surgery, Oral Medicine, Oral Pathology, Oral Radiology, and Endodontics*, vol. 106, no. 2, pp. 264–269, 2008.

[10] L. Wang, Y. Liu, D. Zhang, Y. Zhang, N. Tang, and E.-H. Wang, "A case of 'fat-free' pleomorphic lipoma occurring in the upper back and axilla simultaneously," *World Journal of Surgical Oncology*, vol. 11, article 145, 2013.

[11] J. C. Fanburg-Smith, K. O. Devaney, M. Miettinen, and S. W. Weiss, "Multiple spindle cell lipomas: a report of 7 familial and 11 nonfamilial cases," *American Journal of Surgical Pathology*, vol. 22, no. 1, pp. 40–48, 1998.

[12] C. Diaz-Cascajo, S. Borghi, and W. Weyers, "Fibrous spindle cell lipoma: report of a new variant," *The American Journal of Dermatopathology*, vol. 23, no. 2, pp. 112–115, 2001.

[13] M. Zamecnik and M. Michal, "Angiomatous spindle cell lipoma: report of three cases with immunohistochemical and ultrastructural study and reappraisal of former 'pseudoangiomatous' variant," *Pathology International*, vol. 57, no. 1, pp. 26–31, 2007.

[14] R. Z. Karim, S. W. McCarthy, A. A. Palmer, S. F. Bonar, and R. A. Scolyer, "Intramuscular dendritic fibromyxolipoma: myxoid variant of spindle cell lipoma?" *Pathology International*, vol. 53, no. 4, pp. 252–258, 2003.

[15] Y.-P. Wong, W. K. Chia, S. F. Low, N. H. Mohamed-Haflah, and N. A. Sharifah, "Dendritic fibromyxolipoma: a variant of spindle cell lipoma with extensive myxoid change, with cytogenetic evidence," *Pathology International*, vol. 64, no. 7, pp. 346–351, 2014.

[16] S. D. Billings and A. L. Folpe, "Diagnostically challenging spindle cell lipomas: a report of 34 'low-fat' and 'fat-free' variants," *The American Journal of Dermatopathology*, vol. 29, no. 5, pp. 437–442, 2007.

[17] D. Nemenqani, N. Yaqoob, H. Khoja, and A. A. Qurashi, "Dermatofibrosarcoma protuberance of the oral cavity: does it exist?" *Journal of the Pakistan Medical Association*, vol. 60, no. 3, pp. 234–236, 2010.

[18] I. Schmack, R. M. Patel, A. L. Folpe et al., "Subconjunctival herniated orbital fat: a benign adipocytic lesion that may mimic pleomorphic lipoma and atypical lipomatous tumor," *The American Journal of Surgical Pathology*, vol. 31, no. 2, pp. 193–198, 2007.

[19] B. M. Shmookler and F. M. Enzinger, "Pleomorphic lipoma: a benign tumor simulating liposarcoma. A clinicopathologic analysis of 48 cases," *Cancer*, vol. 47, no. 1, pp. 126–133, 1981.

[20] A. F. Nascimento, M. E. Mc Menamin, and C. D. M. Fletcher, "Liposarcomas/atypical lipomatous tumors of the oral cavity: a clinicopathologic study of 23 cases," *Annals of Diagnostic Pathology*, vol. 6, no. 2, pp. 83–93, 2002.

[21] D. Creytens, J. van Gorp, S. Savola, L. Ferdinande, T. Mentzel, and L. Libbrecht, "Atypical spindle cell lipoma: a clinicopathologic, immunohistochemical, and molecular study emphasizing its relationship to classical spindle cell lipoma," *Virchows Archiv*, vol. 465, no. 1, pp. 97–108, 2014.

[22] J. F. Val-Bernal and M. C. González-Vela, "Cutaneous lipomatous neurofibroma: characterization and frequency," *Journal of Cutaneous Pathology*, vol. 32, no. 4, pp. 274–279, 2005.

[23] F. Alawi and P. D. Freedman, "Sporadic sclerotic fibroma of the oral soft tissues," *The American Journal of Dermatopathology*, vol. 26, no. 3, pp. 182–187, 2004.

[24] J. C. Tardío, J. A. Aramburu, and C. Santonja, "Desmin expression in spindle cell lipomas: a potential diagnostic pitfall," *Virchows Archiv*, vol. 445, no. 4, pp. 354–358, 2004.

[25] W. Schurch, O. Skalli, T. A. Seemayer, and G. Gabbiani, "Intermediate filament proteins and actin isoforms as markers for soft tissue tumor differentiation and origin: i. Smooth muscle tumors," *American Journal of Pathology*, vol. 128, no. 1, pp. 91–103, 1987.

42

Follicular Thyroid Carcinoma Metastatic to the Kidney: Report of a Case with Cytohistologic Correlation

Vikas Nath,[1] Mithra Baliga,[1] Jack Lewin,[1] Frederico Souza,[2] and Israh Akhtar[1]

[1] *Department of Pathology, University of Mississippi Medical Center, 2500 North State Street, Jackson, MS 39216, USA*
[2] *Department of Radiology, University of Mississippi Medical Center, 2500 North State Street, Jackson, MS 39216, USA*

Correspondence should be addressed to Vikas Nath; vnath@umc.edu

Academic Editor: Ondrej Hes

Here we report a case of a 45-year-old female who underwent thyroidectomy for thyroid cancer and presented 20 years later with a left renal mass. CT-guided core biopsy was performed, and imprints and histologic sections of the biopsy showed cells resembling thyroid follicular cells with a background containing colloid. Immunohistochemistry revealed positivity for thyroglobulin and thyroid transcription factor 1, consistent with metastatic follicular thyroid carcinoma (FTC). The patient later underwent radical nephrectomy; histologic sections of the resected tumor revealed an encapsulated lesion morphologically similar to the biopsy specimen. Thyroid metastases to the kidney are extremely rare and are often detected during postthyroidectomy surveillance by elevation in thyroid hormone levels, ^{131}I scintigraphy, or ^{18}F-fluorodeoxyglucose uptake in positron emission tomography studies. Treatment involves total thyroidectomy, resection of the metastatic foci, and ^{131}I therapy. The differential diagnoses of renal metastasis of FTC include the encapsulated follicular variant of papillary thyroid carcinoma (PTC), which possesses some of the nuclear features seen in conventional PTC but may occasionally be indistinguishable from FTC in cytologic preparations, and renal lesions such as benign thyroidization of the kidney and thyroid-like follicular carcinoma of the kidney, which mimic FTC in histologic appearance but do not stain with thyroid markers.

1. Introduction

Follicular thyroid carcinoma (FTC) is the second most common type of thyroid cancer, after papillary thyroid carcinoma (PTC), accounting for approximately 10% of all malignant thyroid tumors. It has a predilection for women and is more common in areas of endemic goiter [1, 2]. FTC is defined as a malignant epithelial tumor with follicular differentiation that (1) lacks the nuclear features associated with PTC and (2) demonstrates capsular and/or vascular invasion, extrathyroidal extension, or lymphatic or distant metastases [1, 3–6]. FTC is considered a more aggressive tumor than PTC as it often presents at a higher stage, with distant metastases in 25 to 30% of cases [2, 7]. Unlike PTC, which tends to metastasize to cervical lymph nodes, FTC more commonly presents with hematogenous metastases to lung and bone [2, 7, 8]; however, other metastatic sites have been reported as well. We report a case of FTC metastatic to the kidney in a patient presenting with a left renal mass, which was diagnosed by touch imprint cytology and histologic sections of a CT-guided renal core biopsy.

2. Case Report

A 45-year-old African American female presented for evaluation of a left renal mass. She did not complain of any urinary symptoms such as flank pain or hematuria, and her past medical history was significant for type 2 diabetes mellitus, gastric bypass surgery, and thyroid cancer diagnosed at an outside hospital 20 years previously, which was treated by total thyroidectomy. However, the histologic type of the thyroid tumor was unknown, and neither the outside medical records nor histologic sections of the thyroid tumor were available for review. The patient's primary care physician had told her that imaging studies of her left kidney were suspicious for renal cell carcinoma and had suggested that she undergo nephrectomy. A CT of the abdomen and pelvis revealed a 7.5×6.8 cm, exophytic, homogeneously enhancing

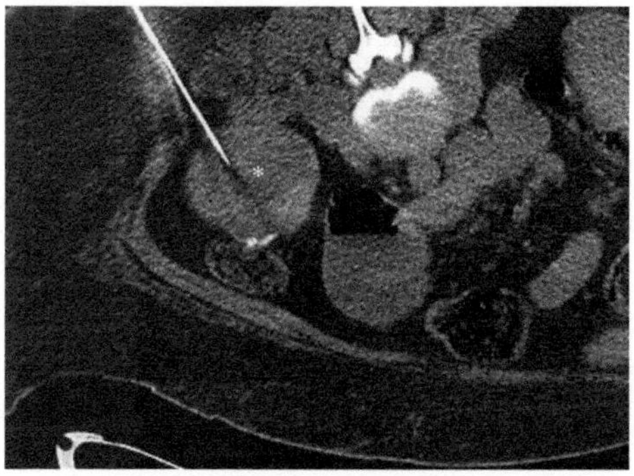

FIGURE 1: Axial noncontrast CT of the abdomen and pelvis demonstrated a 7.5 × 6.8 cm homogeneous, predominantly exophytic mass arising from the inferior pole of the left kidney. CT-guided biopsy of the left renal mass was performed with a large needle (18 G × 15 cm) (*asterisk*) with the patient in a prone position.

mass in the inferior pole of the left kidney. There was no evidence of hydronephrosis or nephrolithiasis, and the urinary bladder, ureters, and adrenal glands were all unremarkable. A percutaneous CT-guided core biopsy of the mass was performed (Figure 1), and imprints and histologic sections of the biopsy specimen were evaluated and deemed positive for metastatic FTC.

Nine months following biopsy, the patient underwent left radical nephrectomy, and examination of histologic sections of the resection specimen confirmed the cytologic diagnosis made on the core biopsy specimen. She did well in the immediate postoperative period, with no evidence of wound infection, and was discharged. Three years later, she was admitted for malnutrition and dehydration due to an anastomotic leak from her previous gastric bypass surgery. She was discharged after a 2-month inpatient stay, during which she underwent gastrostomy tube placement, and has not been hospitalized since. A repeat CT at that time showed several hypodense lesions in the right kidney, as well as one of intermediate density measuring up to 1 cm in greatest dimension that had remained stable since the previous CT, 3 years earlier. The patient was subsequently lost to follow-up.

3. Cytohistologic Findings

A CT-guided core biopsy of the renal mass was performed, and immediate assessment was done using Diff-Quik stain. Touch imprints of the mass showed numerous cells that were arranged in large sheets and cohesive clusters (Figure 2(a)), with proteinaceous material in the background; these features were highly suggestive of a thyroid origin. However, at the time when on-site evaluation of the imprints was performed, the patient's history of thyroid cancer was not known; therefore, a benign kidney lesion was the favored interpretation initially. Papanicolaou stain revealed sheets of monomorphic cells with round to oval nuclei, uniformly distributed chromatin, and inconspicuous nucleoli. Histologic sections of the biopsy specimen showed variably sized follicles lined by an attenuated layer of thyroid follicular cells and filled with colloid, closely resembling normal thyroid gland (Figure 2(b)). Immunohistochemistry (IHC) revealed positive cytoplasmic staining for thyroglobulin (Figure 2(c)) and positive nuclear staining for thyroid transcription factor 1 (TTF-1; Figure 2(d)) in the nuclei of the follicular cells, thus confirming a thyroid origin. Touch imprint cytology and histologic features showed that the cells had morphology compatible with FTC such as a repetitive microfollicular pattern, round nuclei with irregular chromatin, uniform nuclear membranes, and absent nucleoli. Features that were characteristic of PTC such as longitudinal grooves, nuclear membrane irregularities, nuclear clearing, or intranuclear pseudoinclusions were not seen. Due to these findings, a diagnosis of metastatic FTC was rendered. In the course of further workup of the patient, it was discovered that she had a history of thyroid cancer that was treated with total thyroidectomy at another institution; however, medical records and slides from the outside hospital were not available for review, and so the histology of her primary tumor was uncertain.

The surgical resection specimen consisted of a left radical nephrectomy that was bisected to reveal a large, well-circumscribed mass in the inferior pole with spongy pink-tan cut surfaces and areas of hemorrhage and cystic degeneration (Figure 3(a)). The mass abutted the renal capsule but did not invade into the perinephric fat; neither was there tumor involvement of the renal pelvis, renal vein, or adrenal gland. The uninvolved renal parenchyma was unremarkable. Examination of histologic sections of the tumor showed a mass composed of colloid-filled thyroid follicles lined by flattened cells with scant cytoplasm and small round nuclei, which was separated from the adjacent renal parenchyma by a fibrous capsule (Figure 3(b)). There was no evidence of lymphovascular invasion, and the surgical margin, renal vascular margin, and ureteral margin were all negative for tumor. IHC for thyroglobulin and TTF-1 showed the same pattern of expression in the malignant follicular cells as in the core biopsy specimen, thereby providing histologic confirmation of the cytologic diagnosis of metastatic FTC.

4. Discussion

Renal metastases of well-differentiated thyroid carcinoma are exceedingly rare, with fewer than 20 cases reported in the English-language literature [1, 8–11] and another 30 in the Japanese literature [1, 8]. By definition, FTC is a histologic diagnosis that requires demonstration of capsular and/or vascular invasion. This essentially precludes diagnosis of a thyroid nodule as FTC by fine-needle aspiration cytology [3, 4], which is why the Bethesda System for Reporting Thyroid Cytopathology allows a cytologic specimen of FTC to be categorized, at most, as a "follicular neoplasm/suspicious for a follicular neoplasm" [12]. Nevertheless, there are certain cytologic features that favor FTC over its benign counterpart, follicular adenoma (FA). For example, aspirate smears of FA have been shown to demonstrate cells in a follicular pattern and to contain colloid; indeed, the presence of a macrofollicular pattern coupled with abundant, watery colloid is a strong indicator that a thyroid nodule is benign. By contrast, FTC may demonstrate a repetitive microfollicular pattern or

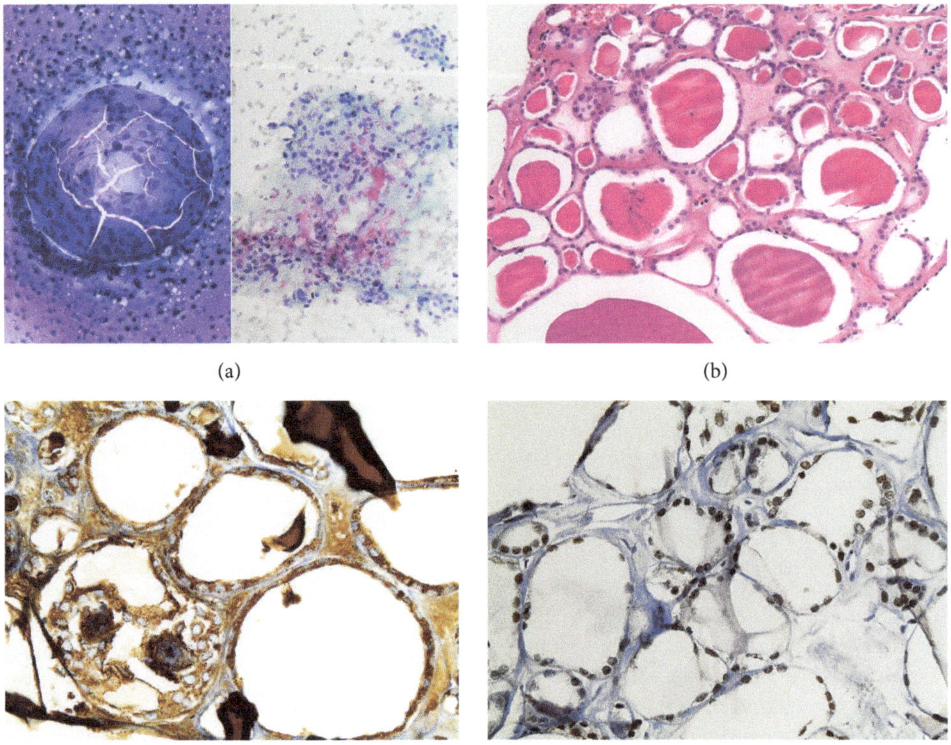

(a) (b)

(c) (d)

FIGURE 2: Core biopsy imprints of the left renal mass showed an abundance of cells that resembled thyroid follicular cells arranged in large sheets (a) in a background containing proteinaceous material (Diff-Quik, 200x) (*left*). The cells possessed round to oval nuclei, uniformly distributed chromatin, and inconspicuous nucleoli, without any nuclear features of PTC such as longitudinal grooves, nuclear clearing, or intranuclear pseudoinclusions (Papanicolaou, 200x) (*right*). Histologic sections of the biopsy specimen showed variably sized colloid-filled follicles lined by flattened follicular cells, resembling normal thyroid (H&E, 200x) (b). The thyroid origin of the tumor was confirmed by immunohistochemical stains that demonstrated positive cytoplasmic expression of thyroglobulin (400x) (c) and positive nuclear expression of TTF-1 (400x) (d).

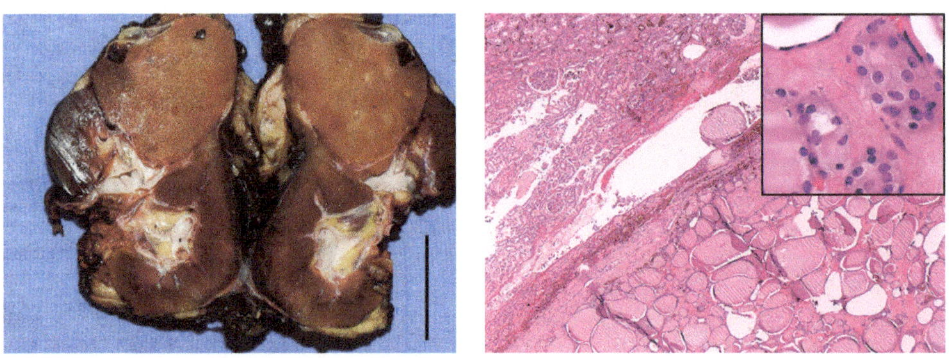

(a) (b)

FIGURE 3: The left radical nephrectomy specimen was bisected to reveal a pink-tan, well-circumscribed mass in the inferior pole (*bar*, 5 cm) (a). Histologic sections of the resection specimen showed follicles filled with colloid and lined by thyroid follicular cells, separated from the adjacent renal parenchyma by a fibrous capsule (H&E, 40x) (b). Higher magnification revealed monomorphic cells with bland nuclei, similar to those in the biopsy specimen, with none of the nuclear features associated with PTC (H&E, 400x) (*inset*).

some other cytologic architecture such as a solid, trabecular, or cribriform pattern; in addition, the presence of nuclear atypia, high nuclear/cytoplasmic ratio, and coarse chromatin suggests malignancy. If cytologic assessment of malignancy is to be performed on a follicular neoplasm, it is better done on poorly differentiated tumors, which possess more of the above-mentioned features, than on well-differentiated FTC, which may mimic FA or even normal thyroid [3].

A second, and more diagnostically challenging, lesion in the differential diagnosis of metastatic FTC is PTC, specifically the encapsulated follicular variant of PTC (FVPTC). This variant resembles FTC not only in the sense of being well circumscribed with a fibrous capsule, but also in its behavior of metastasizing to lung and bone by the hematogenous route, rather than the lymphatic route as is the case with conventional PTC [6]. In addition, it shares several genetic abnormalities with FTC, including *RAS* mutations and *PAX8/PPARγ* rearrangements [6, 13]. Diagnosis of FVPTC by fine-needle aspiration cytology is difficult, as this tumor possesses some, but not all, of the nuclear features associated with PTC. Classically, cytologic preparations of conventional PTC are characterized by papillary architecture with central fibrovascular cores; the accompanying nuclear features include nuclear enlargement, nuclear overlap, chromatin clearing ("Orphan Annie nuclei"), longitudinal grooves, and intranuclear pseudoinclusions [3]. In FVPTC, the most common features are nuclear overlap and chromatin clearing, which are seen in 80% of cases. By contrast, nuclear grooves are present in only 12% of cases and pseudoinclusions in only 5%. In some cases, cells with atypical nuclei are completely absent in cytologic preparations, and the diagnosis of FVPTC can only be made on the basis of histology; the most common cytologic pattern in these specimens is the microfollicular one [13], which, as previously mentioned, is also frequently present in aspirate smears of FTC. FVPTC cytologic specimens are frequently classified under either the "follicular neoplasm/suspicious for a follicular neoplasm" or "suspicious for PTC" category within the Bethesda System, depending on the degree of atypia present [12].

One method that may be used to evaluate diagnostically difficult specimens is IHC, as the triad of galectin-3, Hector Battifora mesothelial cell 1 (HBME-1), and cytokeratin 19 (CK19) is well established as a means of differentiating between various thyroid neoplasms [14, 15]. Galectin-3, a cytoplasmic stain, has high sensitivity and specificity for malignant tumors, particularly PTC and FVPTC, though it is frequently expressed in FTC as well; FA, however, is negative. HBME-1, a nuclear stain, likewise is highly sensitive and specific for thyroid carcinoma. CK19, a membranous stain, shows strong, diffuse positivity in PTC—which includes FVPTC [14]—and is either absent or only focally present in FA and FTC; however, exceptions to this rule do exist [14, 15], and for this reason a combination of immunostains is usually preferable to ordering any individual stain alone. In addition to the above three, several other immunostains have been cited as useful in distinguishing benign from malignant thyroid lesions. Among these is the CD44 isoform CD44v6, whose expression correlates with metastatic potential and which has been shown to be negative in follicular adenoma but positive in several thyroid malignancies; membranous and cytoplasmic CD44v6 positivity has been documented in PTC [14]. Fibronectin 1 and CITED-1 (CBP/p300-Interacting Transactivators with glutamic acid [E] and aspartic acid [D]-rich C-terminal domain) are two other markers that are more highly expressed in malignant thyroid lesions—particularly PTC—than in benign ones; the former shows membranous and cytoplasmic positivity and the latter nuclear and cytoplasmic positivity [16]. We did not order IHC other than thyroglobulin and TTF-1 in this case, as we were able to make the diagnosis of metastatic FTC purely on the basis of cytohistologic and clinical features.

In patients with FTC who have not undergone thyroidectomy, the primary thyroid tumor may present as a neck mass [9, 17]. Presenting symptoms of renal metastases vary, depending on whether the metastasis is isolated to the kidney or involves multiple organs. As a general rule, when tumors metastasize to the kidney, the lesions are multifocal and often bilateral. However, several case reports exist of metastatic FTC presenting as a solitary renal mass [1, 9, 10, 18, 19]; these patients may present with flank pain and/or microscopic hematuria [1, 7, 18]. In patients with an established diagnosis of FTC, postthyroidectomy surveillance is performed by measurement of serum thyroglobulin levels, ^{131}I scintigraphy, and positron emission tomography (PET) using an ^{18}F-fluorodeoxyglucose- (FDG-) labeled tracer for detection of metastatic foci. Case reports exist of renal metastases of FTC detected by a rise in serum thyroglobulin, areas of increased ^{131}I uptake, or FDG-avid foci on PET indicating increased metabolic activity [1, 9, 10, 17], in addition to the presence of a mass on conventional or contrast-enhanced CT. It is not unheard of for patients to present with metastases a decade or more after thyroidectomy [7, 18, 19]. Treatment of metastatic FTC consists of total thyroidectomy, regional lymph node dissection, surgical resection of the metastatic foci with clear margins, and ^{131}I radioablative therapy for removal of any residual disease or micrometastases [1, 8–10, 19]. Levothyroxine is also given, with the intent of both replacing thyroid hormone and suppressing thyroid-stimulating hormone levels [9, 17]. The prognosis of metastatic well-differentiated thyroid carcinoma is variable, but on average 50 to 75% of patients die within 5 years of diagnosis [9, 19]; however, younger patients may respond better, especially if aggressive surgical excision is combined with ^{131}I radioablation [19]. Radical, or at least partial, nephrectomy to reduce tumor burden is highly recommended to manage solitary late metastases of thyroid carcinoma to the kidney [9, 18].

5. Conclusion

Given the rarity of thyroid metastases to the kidney, this case was a diagnostic challenge. Her history of thyroid carcinoma, which was not known to us during our initial assessment of her renal core biopsy, later proved invaluable in directing our approach to formulate a diagnosis, along with the help of immunostains. The histologic appearance of the tumor was suggestive of metastatic thyroid carcinoma, which we were able to confirm using IHC for thyroglobulin and TTF-1. The nuclear features of PTC are readily appreciated on cytologic as well as histologic specimens and were not seen in our case; this was helpful in ruling out FVPTC, which was also in the differential diagnosis. Metastatic tumors in the kidney can be difficult to diagnose on cytologic specimens, and accordingly the differential diagnosis must be wide. Cytohistologic examination has certain limitations when it comes to rare lesions; however, an extensive clinical workup and ancillary studies are useful in formulating a diagnosis. Cases like this enrich the cytology literature by providing awareness of thyroid carcinomas metastasizing to the kidney.

Conflict of Interests

The authors declare that there is no conflict of interests regarding the publication of this paper.

References

[1] H. Xu, W. Zeng, and Y. Tang, "Metastatic thyroid follicular carcinoma presenting as a primary renal tumor," *Internal Medicine*, vol. 51, no. 16, pp. 2193–2196, 2012.

[2] A. D'Avanzo, P. Treseler, P. H. G. Ituarte et al., "Follicular thyroid carcinoma: histology and prognosis," *Cancer*, vol. 100, no. 6, pp. 1123–1129, 2004.

[3] J. Maruta, H. Hashimoto, Y. Suehisa et al., "Improving the diagnostic accuracy of thyroid follicular neoplasms: cytological features in fine-needle aspiration cytology," *Diagnostic Cytopathology*, vol. 39, no. 1, pp. 28–34, 2011.

[4] S. Sanii, H. Saffar, H. M. Tabriz, M. Qorbani, V. Haghpanah, and S. M. Tavangar, "Expression of matrix metalloproteinase-2, but not caspase-3, facilitates distinction between benign and malignant thyroid follicular neoplasms," *Asian Pacific Journal of Cancer Prevention*, vol. 13, no. 5, pp. 2175–2178, 2012.

[5] A. E. Romero-Rojas, J. A. Diaz-Perez, M. Mastrodimos, and S. I. Chinchilla, "Follicular thyroid carcinoma with signet ring cell morphology: fine-needle aspiration cytology, histopathology, and immunohistochemistry," *Endocrine Pathology*, vol. 24, no. 4, pp. 239–245, 2013.

[6] M. Sobrinho-Simões, C. Eloy, J. Magalhes, C. Lobo, and T. Amaro, "Follicular thyroid carcinoma," *Modern Pathology*, vol. 24, pp. S10–S18, 2011.

[7] H. Iwai, Y. Ohno, H. Ito, T. Kiyokawa, and N. Aoki, "Renal rupture associated with a poorly differentiated follicular thyroid carcinoma metastasizing to the thigh muscle, lung and kidney," *Internal Medicine*, vol. 44, no. 8, pp. 848–852, 2005.

[8] G. Cochetti, P. Puxeddu, M. Del Zingaro et al., "Laparoscopic partial nephrectomy of thyroid cancer metastasis: case report and review of the literature," *OncoTargets and Therapy*, vol. 6, pp. 355–360, 2013.

[9] L. García-Sanchis, D. Lopez-Aznar, A. Oltra et al., "Metastatic follicular thyroid carcinoma to the kidney: a case report," *Clinical Nuclear Medicine*, vol. 24, no. 1, pp. 48–50, 1999.

[10] M. Cheon, J. Y. Choi, H. K. Kim et al., "Renal metastasis from follicular thyroid carcinoma diagnosed by I-131 whole-body scan mimicking renal cell carcinoma on contrast-enhanced computed tomography," *Nuclear Medicine and Molecular Imaging*, vol. 45, no. 1, pp. 72–75, 2011.

[11] M. B. Amin, R. Gupta, H. Ondrej et al., "Primary thyroid-like follicular carcinoma of the kidney: report of 6 cases of a histologically distinctive adult renal epithelial neoplasm," *The American Journal of Surgical Pathology*, vol. 33, no. 3, pp. 393–400, 2009.

[12] S. Z. Ali and E. S. Cibas, Eds., *The Bethesda System for Reporting Thyroid Cytopathology*, Springer, New York, NY, USA, 2010.

[13] G. C. H. Yang, K. Fried, T. V. Yakoushina, and A. M. Schreiner, "Encapsulated follicular variant of papillary thyroid carcinoma: fine-needle aspiration with ultrasound and histologic correlation of 41 cases," *Acta Cytologica*, vol. 57, no. 1, pp. 26–32, 2013.

[14] S. Rezk and A. Khan, "Role of immunohistochemistry in the diagnosis and progression of follicular epithelium-derived thyroid carcinoma," *Applied Immunohistochemistry and Molecular Morphology*, vol. 13, no. 3, pp. 256–264, 2005.

[15] F. Barut, N. O. Kandemir, S. Bektas, B. Bahadir, S. Keser, and S. O. Ozdamar, "Universal markers of thyroid malignancies: galectin-3, HBME-1, and cytokeratin-19," *Endocrine Pathology*, vol. 21, no. 2, pp. 80–89, 2010.

[16] M. L. Prasad, N. S. Pellegata, Y. Huang, H. N. Nagaraja, A. de la Chapelle, and R. T. Kloos, "Galectin-3, fibronectin-1, CITED-1, HBME1 and cytokeratin-19 immunohistochemistry is useful for the differential diagnosis of thyroid tumors," *Modern Pathology*, vol. 18, no. 1, pp. 48–57, 2005.

[17] M. Djekidel, M. Gordon, R. B. Shah, M. D. Gross, and A. Avram, "Renal metastasis from hurthle cell thyroid carcinoma and its evaluation with hybrid imaging," *Thyroid*, vol. 20, no. 4, pp. 429–433, 2010.

[18] K. Y. Lam and W. K. Ng, "Follicular carcinoma of the thyroid appearing as a solitary renal mass," *Nephron*, vol. 73, no. 2, pp. 323–324, 1996.

[19] D. V. Matei, F. Verweij, E. Scardino et al., "Late solitary thyroid carcinoma metastasis to the kidney: a case report," *Anticancer Research*, vol. 23, no. 1, pp. 561–564, 2003.

An Unusual Location of Neuroendocrine Tumour: Primary Hepatic Origin

A. Bahar Ceyran,[1] A. Tarık Artış,[2] Serkan Şenol,[1] and Bengü Çobanoğlu Şimşek[1]

[1] *Department of Pathology, Medeniyet University Medical School Göztepe Research and Training Hospital, Kadıkoy, 34730 Istanbul, Turkey*
[2] *Department of General Surgery, Medeniyet University Medical School Göztepe Research and Training Hospital, Kadıkoy, 34730 Istanbul, Turkey*

Correspondence should be addressed to A. Bahar Ceyran; baharceyran@gmail.com

Academic Editor: Peter Kornprat

Although neuroendocrine tumours (NETs) of primary hepatic origin are extremely rare, most of NETs present with liver metastasis. When a NET is found in the liver, it must be treated to exclude metastasis from extrahepatic primary sites. The patient was a 38-year-old female. Abdominal ultrasound showed an 8 cm tumour in liver during a routine examination. Liver biopsy was done. The tumour was first considered a metastatic hepatic tumour on histopathological examination. No clues to the origin of a primary tumour were found. Upper and lower endoscopy of the GI tract and chest CT were performed to search for a primary tumour and were negative for any tumour. One month later, more extensive areas of the tumour were seen on histopathological examination of second liver biopsy with the same morphologic characteristics as the first biopsy. Immunohistochemically, there was positive staining for synaptophysin, CD 56, and S-100 in the tumour cells. These findings suggested the diagnosis of NET. The diagnosis of primary liver NET was considered in a multidisciplinary meeting. Then, left hepatectomy was performed. The final pathologic diagnosis of the tumour in the resected liver specimen was Grade II NET. The patient was doing well at postoperative 28-month follow-up.

1. Introduction

Neuroendocrine tumours (NETs) are rare tumours that originate from dispersed neuroendocrine cells distributed throughout the body. NETs can be either functioning or nonfunctioning. Functioning NETs produce vasoactive hormones such as serotonin, gastrin, insulin, glucagon, and somatostatin, which may cause carcinoid syndrome [1].

NETs are also called carcinoid tumours. According to the World Health Organisation (WHO) 2000 classification, classic carcinoids were classified as well-differentiated endocrine tumours; however, in the WHO 2010 classification, they were classified as NET Grade I. Well-differentiated endocrine carcinomas were classified as NET Grade II, and poorly differentiated endocrine carcinomas were classified as neuroendocrine carcinomas (NECs), large-cell or small-cell type [2].

NETs are seen most frequently in the bronchopulmonary tree or gastrointestinal tract, but they may be seen in nearly every organ [3, 4]. Primary NETs are most commonly seen in the lung, stomach, ileum, duodenum, jejunum, pancreas, Meckel, appendix, rectum, colon, breast, and ovaries [5]. Gastroenteropancreatic (GEP) NETs are the largest group, accounting for 2% of all gastrointestinal tumours [3, 5].

The incidence of NETs in the United States is 2-3/100.000 per year [3, 5, 6]. However, the majority of NETs are clinically silent, so the real incidence might be higher [3]. Primary hepatic NETs are extremely rare [1, 3]. According to our literature search, fewer than 100 primary hepatic NET cases were reported, mostly as case reports [7]. The largest reported groups included 11, 9, and 8 patients, respectively [1, 7]. In addition, most NET cases present with liver metastasis. Therefore, when an NET is found in the liver, it must be

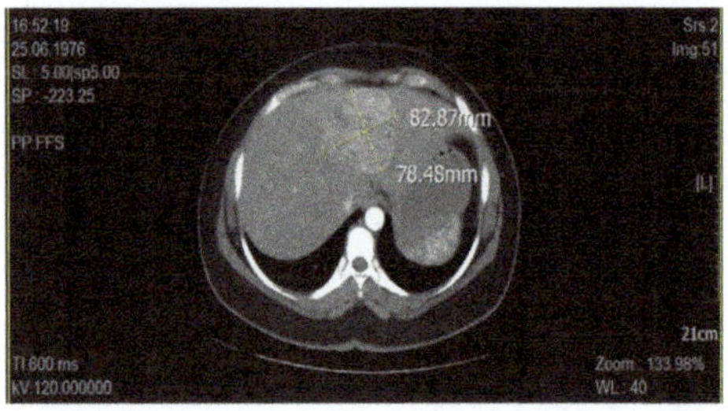

FIGURE 1: CT appearance of the tumor in the liver (CT image of hepatic mass).

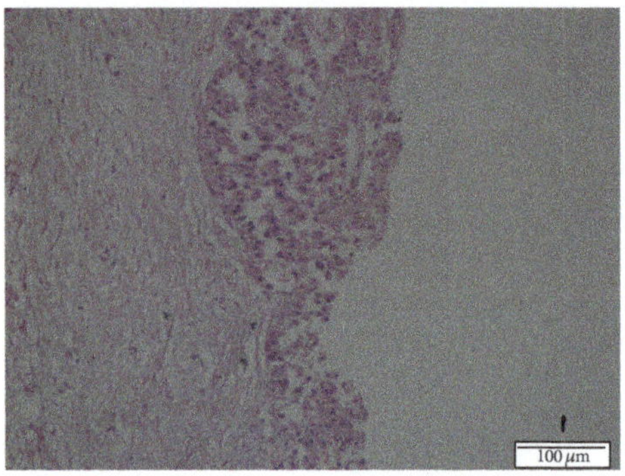

FIGURE 2: Histopathologic appearance of tumoral lesion in first Tru-Cut biopsy. Microscopically, a tumor consists of epithelial cells with round, basophilic, uniform nucleus, inconspicuous nucleoli, and pale eosinophilic granulated cytoplasm. The architectural pattern was trabecular, ribbonlike, and partly acinar. No significant cytologic atypia, mitosis, and necrosis were present. H.E. ×200.

treated with great care to exclude metastasis from extrahepatic primary sites, as there is much more common occurrence [1, 3, 5, 7]. In the literature, the first primary hepatic NET was reported by Edmonson in 1958 [3]. Herein, we report a new case of primary hepatic NET.

2. Case Report

A 38-year-old female complained of abdominal discomfort and pain. Her past medical history was not significant. Physical examination and all biochemical laboratory results were within normal limits, including liver function tests, tumour markers (CA19-9, CEA, AFP, and CA15-3), and chromogranin A. Abdominal ultrasound showed an 8 cm tumour in liver segment IV. Characteristics of abdominal CT (Figure 1) and MRI led to a diagnosis of either fibrolamellar hepatocellular carcinoma (HCC) or focal nodular hyperplasia (FNH).

Liver biopsy was done. Histopathological examination revealed a tumour that consisted of epithelial cells with round basophilic uniform nuclei, inconspicuous nucleoli, and pale eosinophilic granulated cytoplasm. The architectural pattern was trabecular, ribbonlike, and partly acinar. No significant cytologic atypia, mitosis, or necrosis was present (Figure 2). Immunohistochemically, there was negative staining for Heppar-1, CK 19, and CK 20.

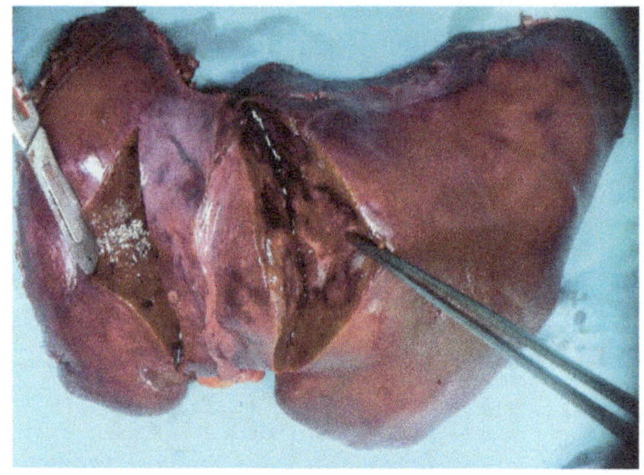

FIGURE 3: Gross appearance of the resected liver specimen.

Morphology was not characteristic for HCC, and at first the tumour was considered a metastatic hepatic tumour. No clues to the origin of a primary tumour were found. Further evaluations and examinations were undertaken to search for a primary tumour. Chest CT and upper and lower endoscopy of the GI tract were performed and were negative for any tumour.

One month later, a second liver biopsy was done, and histopathological examination showed the same morphologic characteristics as the first biopsy, but more extensive areas of the tumour were seen. Immunohistochemically, there was diffuse and strongly positive staining for synaptophysin, CD 56, and S-100 in the tumour cells. These findings supported the diagnosis of NET. Additionally, there was negative staining for Heppar-1, AFP, pCEA, and TTF-1 and positive staining for CK 8/18, and the Ki 67 proliferation index was 5-6%.

Given these findings, the pathological diagnosis was Grade II NET. At first, it was considered a metastatic NET, so Gallium 68 peptide PET scintigraphy was done to search for a primary tumour. But this test was negative, and another tumour could not be detected. A multidisciplinary meeting confirmed the diagnosis of primary liver NET, and laparotomy was decided upon for surgical resection.

The patient underwent laparotomy, and, during the exploration, intraoperative ultrasound was done, finding no other tumour. An anatomical left hepatectomy was performed. The patient's postoperative course was uneventful, and she was discharged on postoperative day 10.

An 8 cm tumour was found upon macroscopic evaluation of the specimen (Figure 3). The tumour was strongly and diffusely positive for chromogranin A. Three mitoses were present per 10 high power fields.

The final pathologic diagnosis was Grade II NET (Figures 4–8). Surgical margins were free of tumour. Adjuvant therapy was not indicated by the oncological consultation. Recently, the patient was doing well at her 28-month postoperative follow-up.

3. Discussion

Primary hepatic NETs characteristically grow slowly and become clinically evident only at an advanced stage [8].

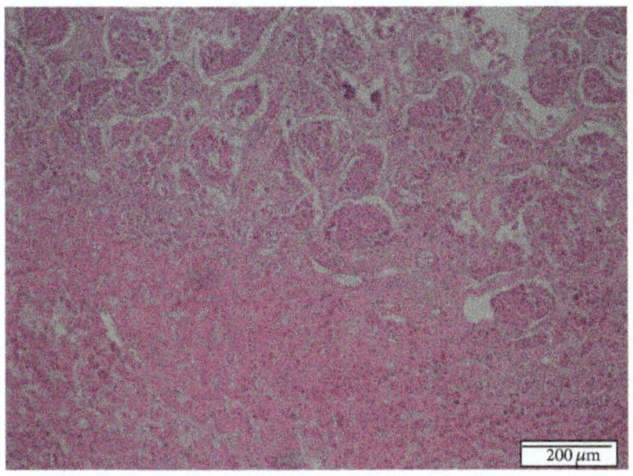

FIGURE 4: Histopathologic appearance of tumoral lesion in the resected liver specimen. Microscopic characteristics are similar in first and second Tru-Cut biopsies. H.E. ×100.

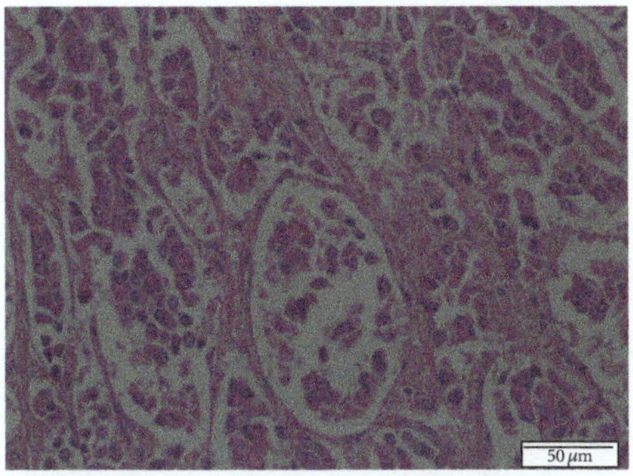

FIGURE 5: Microscopic appearance of tumoral lesion in the resected liver specimen at higher magnification. H.E. ×400.

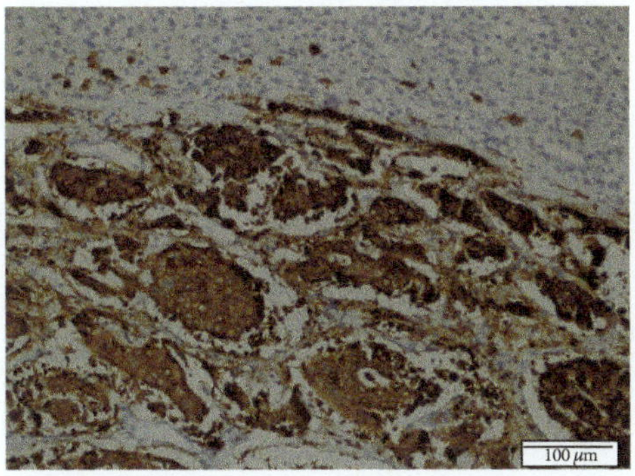

FIGURE 6: Diffuse, strong immunoreactivity for synaptophysin in tumor cells in the resected liver specimen. Immunohistochemical (IHC) staining, ×200.

In most cases, they are incidentally detected, as they are nonfunctional [3]. Mean age is 49.8, with a slight female predominance [3, 7]. In a group of 53 primary hepatic NETs, the male/female ratio was 20/33 [9]. In general, such tumours are located in the central liver. Our patient was 38-year-old female and had nonspecific symptoms regarding the liver tumour, which was centrally located in the liver and found incidentally, as reported in the literature.

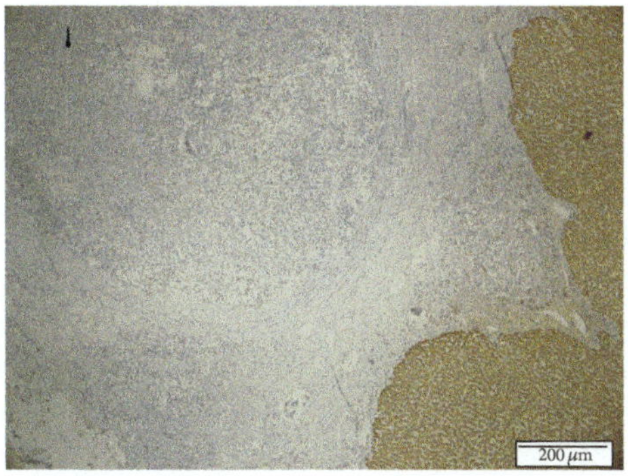

FIGURE 7: Negative immunoreactivity for Heppar-1 in tumor cells; in contrast positive immunoreactivity occurs in normal liver cells in the resected liver specimen. IHC staining, ×40.

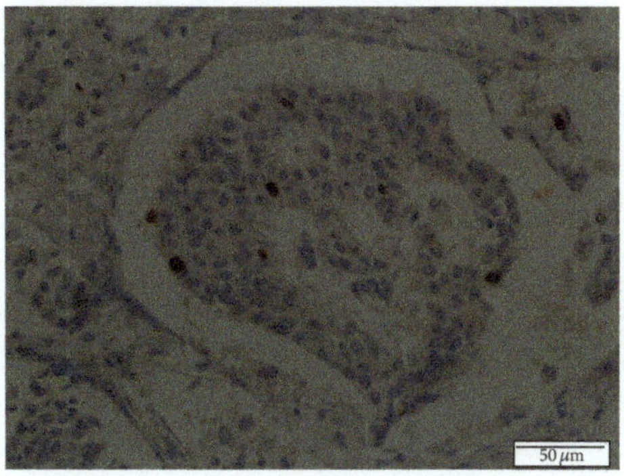

FIGURE 8: Ki 67 proliferation index is 5-6% in tumor cells. IHC staining, ×400.

The histogenesis of primary hepatic NET is not clear. According to one theory, it originates from neuroendocrine cells scattered in the intrahepatic biliary epithelium. A second theory speculates that chronic inflammation in the biliary system causes intestinal metaplasia and NET [3]. In our case, there is no chronic liver or biliary disease or history of chronic inflammation. Therefore, this case does not correlate with the second theory.

Symptoms of primary hepatic NET differ from those of HCC and other hepatic tumours. Clinical manifestation may vary according to carcinoid syndrome presence. Early and definitive diagnosis prior to biopsy or resection is difficult due to nonspecific clinical presentation and rarity [1]. There is an interesting case of a 9-year-old patient who has Cushing's syndrome with a hepatic tumour identified by ultrasound as haemangioma and reported with an ectopic ACTH producing a primary hepatic NET. In addition, in the literature, there were fewer than 30 primary hepatic gastronomies, some of which were reported as Zollinger-Ellison syndrome [10].

Misdiagnosis is frequent prior to pathological examination for primary hepatic NETs. CT scan and MRI are two useful tools for diagnosis and treatment planning [1]. The characteristics on dynamic MRI are dominant hypervascular large mass with satellite nodules. However, definitive diagnosis is not possible with these findings alone. Furthermore, for both primary and metastatic NETs, radiologic features are similar [3, 4]. In our case, MRI findings were consistent with both HCC and FNH. Definitive diagnosis of NET was possible only after hepatic biopsy. Therefore, biopsy and pathological examination are the gold standard for diagnosis [1].

On histopathological examination, NETs (classic carcinoid tumours) are composed of uniform round or polygonal cells having monotonous round centrally located nuclei with finely stippled chromatin, small nucleoli and wide pale eosinophilic granulated cytoplasm, infrequent mitosis, and no necrosis. The tumour may have various patterns such as solid, trabecular, ribbonlike, or acinar. Poorly differentiated malignant forms of these tumours are either (1) large-cell NECs (atypical carcinoids), which consist of large atypical cells with marked cellular pleomorphism, large irregular hyperchromatic nuclei, prominent nucleoli, and tumour necrosis and mitosis or (2) small-cell NECs, which consist of small atypical cells with extremely high nucleocytoplasmic ratios, homogeneously dark nuclear chromatin, inconspicuous nucleoli, scanty cytoplasm, and numerous mitoses [9].

The WHO classification used for the histopathological differentiation of NET and NEC was revised in 2010. According to the new classification, mitosis number and Ki 67 proliferation index are important determining factors for grading and classifying NETs. In histopathological examination of primary hepatic NETs, the concomitance of HCC and NET is extremely rare but can be either the combined type or the collusion type. Our case was diagnosed as Grade II NET according to the 2010 WHO NET classification, and pure NET areas were observed.

Long-term follow-up for treatment of primary NETs has not been reported on sufficiently. However, the prognosis seems favourable. Aggressive treatment is not required [7]. When lymph node and distant metastases are absent, liver resection is adequate for treatment. If lymph node metastasis is present, adjuvant chemotherapy may be needed [8]. Transarterial chemoembolization or radiotherapy treatments also have been reported as effective treatment modalities [8]. Five-year survival and recurrence rates after surgical resection have been reported as 74% and 18%, respectively [9]. For treating our case, left hepatectomy was performed, since there were no distant or lymph node metastases. The patient is on a regular follow-up schedule and at 28 months after surgery is healthy, without recurrence.

4. Conclusions

When a hepatic tumour is considered to be NET, first a detailed systemic search for a primary tumour is mandatory to exclude metastatic NET, as primary hepatic NETs are very rare compared to metastatic ones. Upon exact diagnosis of primary hepatic NET, liver resection is the treatment of choice for successful long-term treatment. However, further studies with larger numbers of patients and long-term follow-up are needed to better understand the outcomes and nature of this rare type of tumour.

Conflict of Interests

The authors declare that there is no conflict of interests regarding the publication of this paper.

References

[1] Z. Chen, H.-E. Xiao, P. Ramchandra, and H.-J. Huang, "Imaging and pathological features of primary hepatic neuroendocrine carcinoma: an analysis of nine cases and review of the literature," *Oncology Letters*, vol. 7, no. 4, pp. 956–962, 2014.

[2] F. T. Bosman, F. Carneiro, R. H. Hruban, and N. D. Theise, *WHO Classification of Tumours of the Digestive System*, World Health Organization, Lyon, France, 4th edition, 2010.

[3] S. H. Baek, J. H. Yoon, and K. W. Kim, "Primary hepatic neuroendocrine tumor: gadoxetic acid (Gd-EOB-DTPA)-enhanced magnetic resonance imaging," *Acta Radiologica Short Reports*, vol. 2, no. 2, p. 6, 2013.

[4] A. F. Scarsbrook, A. Ganeshan, J. Statham et al., "Anatomic and functional imaging of metastatic carcinoid tumors," *Radiographics*, vol. 27, no. 2, pp. 455–476, 2007.

[5] K. Koutsampasopoulos, E. Antoniadou, S. Zoutis, G. Iacovidis, O. Burova, and A. Taplidis, "Neuroendocrine tumor in the liver of a patient with isolated polycystic liver disease: a case report and review of the literature," *Oncology Letters*, vol. 5, no. 5, pp. 1664–1666, 2013.

[6] I. M. Modlin and A. Sandor, "An analysis of 8305 cases of carcinoid tumors," *Cancer*, vol. 79, no. 4, pp. 813–829, 1997.

[7] S. Landen, M. Elens, C. Vrancken, F. Nuytens, T. Meert, and V. Delugeau, "Giant hepatic carcinoid: a rare tumor with a favorable prognosis," *Case Reports in Surgery*, vol. 2014, Article ID 456509, 4 pages, 2014.

[8] C. Jia, Y. Zhang, J. Xu, and K. Sun, "Experience in primary hepatic neuroendocrine tumor," *Turkish Journal of Gastroenterology*, vol. 23, no. 5, pp. 546–551, 2012.

[9] S. E. Mills, D. Carter, V. E. Reuter, J. K. Greenson, M. H. Stooler, and H. A. Oberman, *Sternberg's Diagnostic Surgical Pathology*, vol. 2, Lippincott Williams & Wilkins, 4th edition, 2004.

[10] M. E. El Zein, R. Vali, M. Charron, D. Manson, K. Perlman, and A. Shammas, "Neuroendocrine tumor in liver with positive ACTH receptor: a case report," *Journal of Pediatric Hematology/Oncology*, vol. 36, no. 1, pp. e1–e4, 2014.

44

Urinary Bladder Adenocarcinoma Metastatic to the Abdominal Wall: Report of a Case with Cytohistologic Correlation

Vikas Nath and Mithra Baliga

Department of Pathology, University of Mississippi Medical Center, 2500 North State Street, Jackson, MS 39216, USA

Correspondence should be addressed to Vikas Nath; vnath@umc.edu

Academic Editor: Paolo Perrini

We report a case of adenocarcinoma metastatic to the abdominal wall in a 71-year-old man with a history of primary bladder adenocarcinoma. CT-guided core biopsy was performed; imprints and histologic sections showed malignant glands lined by tumor cells with hyperchromatic nuclei and prominent nucleoli, infiltrating through skeletal muscle. Immunohistochemistry revealed positivity for CK7, membranous/cytoplasmic β-catenin, caudal-type homeobox transcription factor 2 (CDX2), and α-methylacyl coenzyme A racemase and negativity for CK20, p63, prostate-specific antigen (PSA), and prostate-specific acid phosphatase (PSAP). These findings were interpreted as metastatic adenocarcinoma, consistent with bladder primary. Primary bladder adenocarcinoma is a rare malignancy arising within glandular metaplasia and is associated with cystitis cystica and cystitis glandularis. Predisposing factors include bladder exstrophy, schistosomiasis, and other causes of chronic bladder irritation. This tumor is divided into intestinal, clear cell, and signet ring cell subtypes. Treatment involves radical cystectomy with pelvic lymph node dissection, and prognosis is unfavorable. Primary bladder adenocarcinoma should be differentiated from urachal adenocarcinoma, which arises from urachal remnants near the bladder dome, and secondary adenocarcinoma, or vesical involvement by adenocarcinoma from a different primary. CK7, CK20, CDX2, thrombomodulin, and β-catenin can help distinguish primary bladder adenocarcinoma from colonic adenocarcinoma; PSA and PSAP can help distinguish primary bladder adenocarcinoma from prostate adenocarcinoma.

1. Introduction

Primary adenocarcinoma of the urinary bladder is an uncommon malignancy that accounts for 0.5 to 2% of all malignant bladder neoplasms [1–5]; it is the third most common type of bladder carcinoma, after urothelial carcinoma (UC) and squamous cell carcinoma [1, 2]. Most often, it presents in the sixth decade of life and has a predilection for males [1, 3, 6]. Presenting symptoms typically include hematuria, urinary retention, and irritation while voiding [1, 3, 7]; mucus in the urine is a hallmark of adenocarcinoma, though it is not always present [1, 8]. Bladder adenocarcinoma is associated with a variety of irritative and inflammatory conditions. It is the most common type of bladder carcinoma that arises in patients with exstrophy of the bladder; indeed, these patients have a 4% lifetime risk of developing this particular carcinoma. Schistosomiasis, endometriosis, and bladder augmentation have also been mentioned as predisposing factors [1, 3, 4].

Before rendering a diagnosis of primary adenocarcinoma, it is important first to exclude the other 2 types of adenocarcinomas that can occur in the bladder, urachal adenocarcinoma and secondary adenocarcinoma; the latter consists of neoplasms that do not originate from the bladder but involve it either by local extension or by lymphatic or hematogenous metastasis [1, 2]. Local extension is most commonly by malignancies of the colon, prostate, and female genital tract; metastasis is most commonly from the stomach, breast, and lung [2, 3, 5]. We report a patient with primary bladder adenocarcinoma who developed a metastasis to the abdominal wall, diagnosed by examination of imprints and histologic sections of a CT-guided core biopsy.

2. Case Report

A 71-year-old African-American male presented at an outside hospital with acute renal failure and bilateral hydronephrosis and was found to have bladder adenocarcinoma with

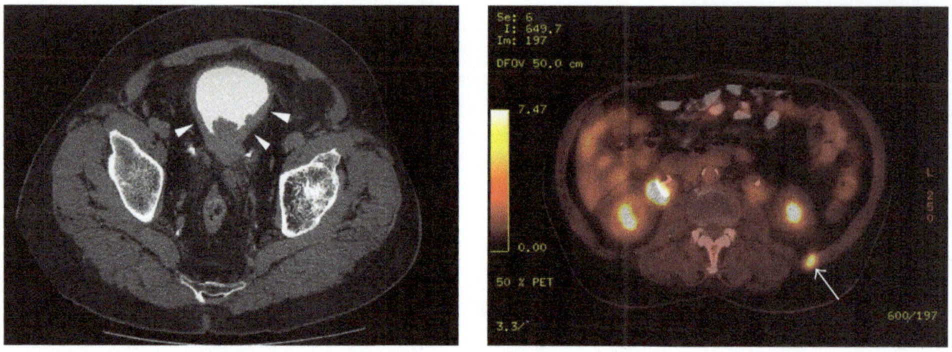

(a) (b)

FIGURE 1: Imaging studies: (a) CT of the abdomen and pelvis showing diffuse bladder wall thickening (*arrowheads*) with perivesical fat stranding, indicating involvement of the bladder by invasive carcinoma; (b) PET of the abdomen and pelvis showing a 1 cm FDG-avid nodule in the musculature of the left flank, suspicious for metastasis (*arrow*).

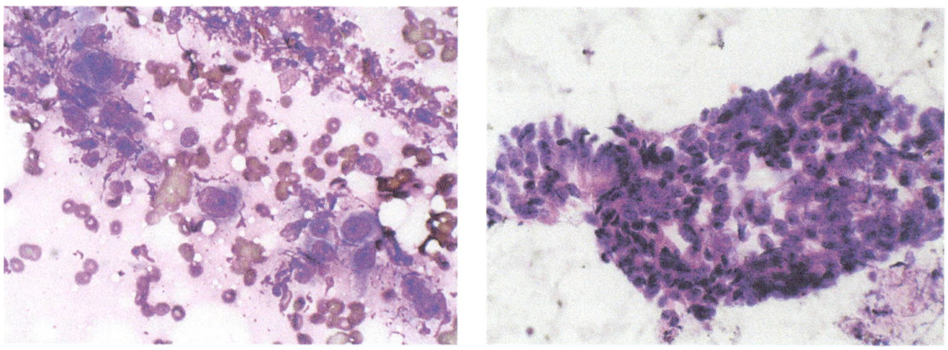

(a) (b)

FIGURE 2: Imprints of the CT-guided core biopsy specimen from the left flank mass showing clusters of malignant columnar cells with a high nuclear/cytoplasmic ratio and prominent nucleoli: (a) Diff-Quik and (b) hematoxylin and eosin, ×600.

invasion of the muscularis propria. His past medical history was significant for nephrolithiasis, prostate adenocarcinoma treated with external beam radiation and bilateral simple orchiectomy 20 years previously, and transurethral bladder resection with bilateral ureteral stent placement at an outside hospital. The patient was a poor historian, and no medical records could be obtained documenting either the histology of his bladder and prostate tumors or the known extent of his disease or the diagnostic and therapeutic procedures undertaken at the outside hospital. He was referred to our institution for evaluation for possible cystoprostatectomy with colonic conduit. A preoperative colonoscopy showed a tubular adenoma but was otherwise negative, and his serum prostate-specific antigen (PSA) level was less than 0.01 ng/mL.

The patient was scheduled for surgery, but this was canceled after he underwent CT of the abdomen and pelvis, which revealed pulmonary nodules measuring up to 0.6 cm in diameter in the right upper lobe, left upper lobe, and lingula that were suspicious for metastases. In addition, the CT revealed retroperitoneal adenopathy of the left paraortic and aortocaval lymph nodes measuring up to 1.9 cm in diameter; bilateral hydronephrosis and hydroureter; and diffuse bladder wall thickening with perivesical soft tissue stranding, indicative of invasion by a bladder tumor (Figure 1(a)). Multiple filling defects were present in the bladder lumen, which were also interpreted as secondary to invasive carcinoma. Positron emission tomography (PET) with an ^{18}F-fluorodeoxyglucose (FDG) tracer showed no abnormal metabolic activity in either the pulmonary or the retroperitoneal masses; however, FDG avidity was observed in a left cervical lymph node and in a 1 cm nodule within the abdominal wall musculature of the left flank (Figure 1(b)). The primary tumor, at the base of the bladder, measured 11.7 cm in greatest dimension; it also showed hypermetabolic activity and appeared to invade into the prostate.

Ultrasound-guided fine needle aspiration was attempted on the cervical lymph node, but insufficient tissue was obtained, so CT-guided core biopsy was performed on the abdominal wall mass. Imprints of the biopsy specimen showed crowded clusters of tumor cells with high nuclear/cytoplasmic ratios and prominent, small nucleoli (Figure 2). Histologic sections of the biopsy showed malignant glands lined by intestinal type columnar cells and occasional goblet cells, with necrotic debris in the lumina, infiltrating through skeletal muscle (Figure 3). The glands

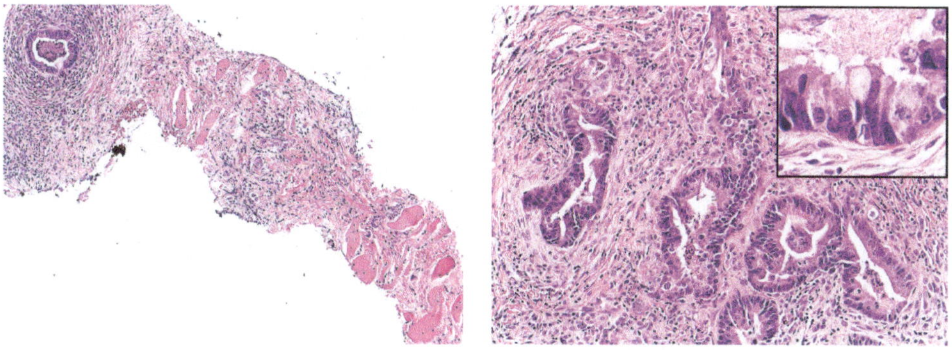

(a) (b)

FIGURE 3: Histologic sections of the biopsy. (a) Malignant glands are seen infiltrating through skeletal muscle (hematoxylin/eosin, ×100). (b) The glands are lined by columnar cells with intestinal epithelial morphology and contain necrotic debris in the lumina (hematoxylin and eosin, ×200); occasional goblet cells are also present (*inset*, hematoxylin and eosin ×600).

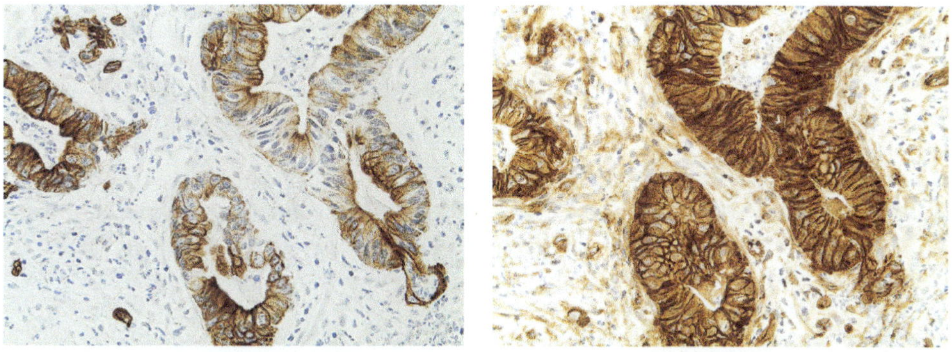

(a) (b)

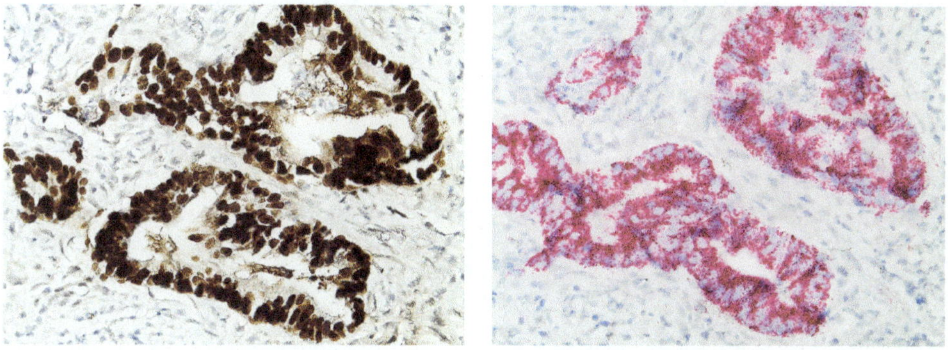

(c) (d)

FIGURE 4: IHC of the biopsy showing positive expression of (a) CK7, (b) β-catenin in a membranous/cytoplasmic staining pattern, (c) CDX2, and (d) AMACR (×400).

were surrounded by desmoplastic stroma and acute and chronic inflammatory cells. Immunohistochemistry (IHC) revealed that the malignant glands were positive for CK7, β-catenin (membranous/cytoplasmic staining pattern), caudal-type homeobox transcription factor 2 (CDX2), and α-methylacyl coenzyme A racemase (AMACR) (Figures 4(a)–4(d)) and negative for CK20, p63, PSA, and prostate-specific acid phosphatase (PSAP). These findings were interpreted as being consistent with metastatic adenocarcinoma; given that the patient had a concurrent vesical tumor, his bladder adenocarcinoma was considered the primary site. Colonic adenocarcinoma with local extension to the bladder was deemed a less likely diagnosis, since there was no evidence of a primary colonic tumor; however, prostate adenocarcinoma with local extension was a consideration given the patient's past medical history. Neither of these possibilities could be excluded based solely on histology and IHC.

In lieu of surgery, the patient was scheduled for 8 cycles of gemcitabine/cisplatin. After completing 4 cycles, he experienced renal failure and was admitted to an outside hospital in Vicksburg, MS, where he underwent exchange of his ureteral stents and antibiotic therapy for purulent cystitis; chemotherapy was withheld while this treatment was taking place. Although repeat CT and PET scans initially showed that his disease was stable, a CT performed 3 months after his last cycle of chemotherapy showed bilateral hydroureteronephrosis, heterogeneous enhancement of the left kidney with perinephric stranding and fascial thickening, and circumferential thickening of the wall of the left ureter with periureteral fat stranding. A soft tissue mass was identified in the hilum of the left kidney, suggesting a renal hilar neoplasm with superimposed pyelonephritis and ureteritis, and the patient was admitted and given intravenous antibiotics. Urine culture from an earlier clinic visit grew coagulase-negative *Staphylococcus*; however, inpatient cultures were negative. Urology was consulted, and based on his symptoms it was determined that he most likely did not have pyelonephritis, as he lacked the characteristic clinical triad of flank pain, leukocytosis, and fever. He was discharged home in stable condition.

Eleven days later, the patient presented to an outside hospital with urosepsis, renal failure, and hypotension and was found by CT to have right-sided hydronephrosis and a hemorrhagic left renal mass, in keeping with previous imaging findings at our institution. A nephrostomy tube was placed in the right kidney. Cystoscopy was performed, and tissue was obtained from the bladder mass that was interpreted as moderately differentiated, partially necrotic adenocarcinoma. The tumor was positive for cytoplasmic β-catenin; nuclear staining could not be assessed. CDX2 and villin immunostains were also positive; thrombomodulin was positive in tumor vessels but not within the tumor cells themselves. These findings were consistent with the staining pattern we observed in the metastatic tumor tissue. During the course of the patient's hospital stay, his renal function and hypotension continued to worsen, leading to cardiopulmonary arrest. Despite the resuscitative efforts, he ultimately expired eight days following admission.

3. Discussion

3.1. Primary Adenocarcinoma. Primary adenocarcinoma of the urinary bladder is derived from urothelium that has undergone glandular metaplasia, often in the context of chronic irritation of the vesical mucosa. Metaplasia of cystitis cystica by mucin-producing columnar cells results in cystitis glandularis, which is considered the precursor lesion of primary adenocarcinoma [1, 4]. Glandular metaplasia may also occur without urothelial invagination, resulting in a variable cystoscopic appearance: sessile, papillary, nodular, or ulcerated [1, 3]. Of the various subtypes described in the literature, the intestinal, clear cell, and signet ring cell subtypes are the best known [2, 9, 10].

Intestinal type adenocarcinoma is the most common of the 3 subtypes [9, 11]. Its cytomorphology is characterized by crowded clusters of columnar or cuboidal cells resembling colonic epithelial cells, which may show pleomorphism, with hyperchromatic nuclei and vacuolated cytoplasm. Mucus is often present in the background [2, 9–11]. On histology, infiltrating glands are seen that are lined by tall columnar cells virtually identical to their colonic counterparts, surrounded by desmoplastic stroma. Luminal necrosis, extracellular mucin, and cystitis cystica in the adjacent urothelium may also be present [3, 5].

Clear cell adenocarcinoma is more common in females than males and often originates in or near the urethra [3, 9, 10, 12]. Cytologic specimens are composed of abundant cells in round clusters that have enlarged nuclei, thickened nuclear membranes, prominent nucleoli, and mitoses. The cytoplasm is abundant, vacuolated, and clear due to glycogenation [7, 9–12]. Acute inflammatory cells may be present either in the background or within intracytoplasmic vacuoles [7, 9, 11, 12]. Histologic exam shows a tumor with tubular, solid, or papillary architecture composed of cuboidal to columnar cells. There is usually marked atypia, and a dense inflammatory infiltrate is often present [3, 7, 12].

Signet ring cell adenocarcinoma has a dismal prognosis, with 5-year survival, a mere 23% [1, 4, 13]. This diagnosis requires that signet ring cells comprise the tumor exclusively, as these cells may also be components of mixed adenocarcinomas or UC [9, 11, 13]. Grossly, these tumors are infiltrative, with subepithelial growth that results in bladder wall thickening; often, no discrete mass is visible on cystoscopy [3, 4]. Cytologic specimens consist of small, dissociated cells with large mucin-filled cytoplasmic vacuoles that displace the nucleus; pools of mucin are seen in the background [5, 9, 11]. A combination of periodic acid-Schiff (PAS), cytokeratin, and CD45 can help to distinguish this tumor from lymphoma with a signet ring cell appearance [4, 9, 13]. Cytologic specimens must be evaluated for other types of malignant cells, such as urothelial cells, to exclude a nonbladder primary before this diagnosis can be made [13]. The histologic appearance is that of sheets of signet ring cells infiltrating the lamina propria and muscularis [3].

Though the majority of tumors occur near the trigone [2, 3], primary adenocarcinoma may arise anywhere in the bladder and may be either unifocal or multifocal [1, 3]. Most tumors show detrusor muscle invasion at the time of diagnosis [1, 6]. Treatment is surgical and consists of radical cystectomy with pelvic lymph node dissection [3, 4, 8]. Chemotherapy is of questionable value. Cisplatin is considered first-line therapy for UC [8], and 5-fluorouracil is effective in colorectal carcinoma, but neither has been shown to be of much value in primary adenocarcinoma [1, 4]. Clinical stage is the most important prognostic factor in this disease [3, 8], and survival is generally poor, ranging from 27% to 61% [4]. Although females are less commonly affected, their prognosis appears poorer than that of males, and their presentation is at a higher stage [6].

3.2. Urachal Adenocarcinoma. Urachal adenocarcinoma is believed to be derived from urachal remnants [5, 14, 15]. Cytologic features are variable; specimens may be composed of either sheets of columnar cells with vacuolated cytoplasm and mild nuclear membrane irregularity [14] or pleomorphic cells arranged in papillae and acini with prominent nucleoli and abundant mitoses [15]. Intracytoplasmic and/or extracellular mucin is often present and stains with PAS [14, 15]. Histologic examination reveals tumor cells floating in pools of extracellular mucin, which may have columnar or signet ring cell morphology [5].

Among the criteria [3–5, 8] used to diagnose bladder adenocarcinoma as urachal in origin are (1) location at the bladder dome; (2) sharp demarcation between the tumor and surface epithelium; and (3) absence of another primary site. As urachal adenocarcinoma typically originates in the anterior wall or dome of the bladder, the standard treatment involves partial cystectomy of the dome as part of an *en bloc* resection [1, 4, 5, 8]. The urothelium adjacent to the tumor is usually devoid of adenocarcinoma *in situ* or cystitis cystica/glandularis, unlike primary adenocarcinoma [4, 14, 15]. IHC reveals diffuse positivity for the high-molecular weight cytokeratin 34βE12 and membranous, but not nuclear, expression of β-catenin. These features are helpful in differentiating urachal from colonic adenocarcinoma, as both of these tumors are known to express CK20 and CDX2 [3, 5, 14, 15].

3.3. Secondary Adenocarcinoma. Secondary adenocarcinoma is more common than primary adenocarcinoma, and differentiating the two in cytologic preparations can be difficult. Colonic adenocarcinoma is characterized by pleomorphic cuboidal to columnar cells, sometimes arranged in glands, with vacuolated cytoplasm, irregular nuclear borders, and prominent nucleoli. "Dirty" necrosis consisting of cytoplasmic and nuclear debris is often present in the background [2]. Histologically, it is virtually indistinguishable from the intestinal type of primary bladder adenocarcinoma. IHC can be helpful, as bladder adenocarcinoma is positive for CK7, CK20, CDX2, and thrombomodulin and negative for nuclear β-catenin. By contrast, colonic adenocarcinoma, while positive for CK20 and CDX2, is negative for CK7 and positive for thrombomodulin and nuclear β-catenin [3, 5]. Thrombomodulin is a highly specific marker for bladder adenocarcinoma, but it is expressed in only 59% of these tumors. Cytokeratins must also be interpreted with caution, as occasional colonic carcinomas may be CK7 positive; in addition, 29% of bladder adenocarcinomas are CK7 negative and CK20 positive, a profile that matches that of most colonic adenocarcinomas [3, 5].

Another tumor that can invade the bladder by local extension and mimic primary bladder adenocarcinoma is prostate adenocarcinoma, in particular prostatic ductal carcinoma. This rare tumor features cells in sheets or papillary fronds with abundant granular cytoplasm, bland nuclei showing enlargement and hyperchromasia, and coarse chromatin with prominent nucleoli and variable mitoses [16–18]. Histologic sections show malignant glands in a variety of architectural patterns including papillary, cribriform, and acinar, depending on whether the tumor originates from primary or secondary prostatic ducts [16, 17]. Prostate adenocarcinoma may be readily differentiated from bladder adenocarcinoma by virtue of its positivity for PSA and PSAP [5, 16–18]; other markers that help to confirm a prostate origin include Leu7 and AMACR [5, 16].

4. Conclusion

The diversity of glandular neoplasms that can occur in the urinary bladder makes the diagnosis of primary bladder adenocarcinoma in cytologic preparations uniquely challenging. In our patient's case, the lesion sampled was a metastasis from his bladder tumor, which meant that the knowledge of his past medical history and imaging findings was crucial in generating a differential diagnosis and choosing the appropriate immunostains. The positivity of the tumor for CK7, β-catenin in a membranous/cytoplasmic staining pattern, CDX2, and AMACR, and negativity for CK20, p63, PSA, and PSAP, favored a vesical rather than a colorectal or prostatic origin. Colonic adenocarcinoma typically expresses CDX2, but it is negative for CK7 and positive for CK20 and expresses β-catenin in a nuclear pattern. Likewise, prostate carcinoma expresses PSA and PSAP. We were careful not to interpret the IHC findings as unequivocal evidence of vesical origin, as they were not specific for primary bladder adenocarcinoma. Secondary adenocarcinoma, being more common, had to be excluded first, and this was not possible to do.

The IHC results do not exclude urachal adenocarcinoma either. However, this was not a distinction we attempted to make, not only on account of the advanced stage of the patient's disease, but also because of the urachal type adenocarcinoma that is a diagnosis better made on histologic sections to assess the condition of the urothelium and to note the presence of urothelial remnants. Primary adenocarcinoma of the urinary bladder is not frequently encountered in the realm of cytology, and the differential diagnosis includes a variety of neoplasms, not all of which originate from the vesical mucosa. Evaluation of cytologic specimens in which this malignancy is suspected requires correlation with the patient's clinical history, imaging, IHC, and, ideally, histologic assessment of bladder biopsy or cystectomy specimens to eliminate other primary sources and establish the tumor's vesical origin.

Conflict of Interests

The authors declare that there is no conflict of interests regarding the publication of this paper.

References

[1] H. Abol-Enein, B. R. Kava, and A. J. K. Carmack, "Nonurothelial cancer of the bladder," *Urology*, vol. 69, no. 1, supplement, pp. 93–104, 2007.

[2] R. H. Bardales, M. B. Pitman, M. W. Stanley, S. Korourian, and M. J. Suhrland, "Urine cytology of primary and secondary urinary bladder adenocarcinoma," *Cancer*, vol. 84, no. 6, pp. 335–343, 1998.

[3] S. Roy and A. V. Parwani, "Adenocarcinoma of the urinary bladder," *Archives of Pathology and Laboratory Medicine*, vol. 135, no. 12, pp. 1601–1605, 2011.

[4] P. Dahm and J. E. Gschwend, "Malignant non-urothelial neoplasms of the urinary bladder: a review," *European Urology*, vol. 44, no. 6, pp. 672–681, 2003.

[5] M. Zhong, E. Gersbach, S. M. Rohan, and X. J. Yang, "Primary adenocarcinoma of the urinary bladder: differential diagnosis and clinical relevance," *Archives of Pathology and Laboratory Medicine*, vol. 137, no. 3, pp. 371–381, 2013.

[6] M. Ploeg, K. K. Aben, C. A. Hulsbergen-van de Kaa, M. P. Schoenberg, J. A. Witjes, and L. A. Kiemeney, "Clinical epidemiology of nonurothelial bladder cancer: analysis of the Netherlands Cancer Registry," *Journal of Urology*, vol. 183, no. 3, pp. 915–920, 2010.

[7] M. I. Doria Jr., G. Saint Martin, H. H. Wang et al., "Cytologic features of clear cell carcinoma of the urethra and urinary bladder," *Diagnostic Cytopathology*, vol. 14, no. 2, pp. 150–154, 1996.

[8] H. Zhang, H. Jiang, Z. Wu, Z. Fang, J. Fan, and Q. Ding, "Primary adenocarcinoma of the urinary bladder: a single site analysis of 21 cases," *International Urology and Nephrology*, vol. 45, no. 1, pp. 107–111, 2013.

[9] R. M. DeMay, "Urine," in *The Art & Science of Cytopathology*, R. M. DeMay, Ed., pp. 436–477, ASCP Press, Chicago, Ill, USA, 2nd edition, 2012.

[10] A. A. Renshaw, "Urine and bladder washings," in *Cytology: Diagnostic Principles and Clinical Correlates*, E. S. Cibas and B. S. Ducatman, Eds., pp. 105–127, Saunders, Philadelphia, Pa, USA, 3rd edition, 2009.

[11] "Urinary tract cytology," in *Modern Cytopathology*, K. R. Geisinger, M. W. Stanley, S. S. Raab, J. F. Silverman, and A. Abati, Eds., pp. 213–255, Churchill Livingstone, Philadelphia, Pa, USA, 2004.

[12] S. A. Whitworth, A. P. Subhawong, D. L. Rosenthal, and S. Z. Ali, "Clear cell adenocarcinoma of the lower urinary tract: cytopathologic characteristics and differential diagnoses," *Cancer Cytopathology*, vol. 120, no. 5, pp. 308–312, 2012.

[13] S. S. Kim, Y. D. Choi, J. H. Nam, D. D. Kwon, S.-W. Juhng, and C. Choi, "Cytologic features of primary signet ring cell carcinoma of the bladder: a case report," *Acta Cytologica*, vol. 53, no. 3, pp. 309–312, 2009.

[14] F. Z. Aly, A. Z. Tabbarah, and L. Voltaggio, "Metastatic urachal carcinoma in bronchial brush cytology," *CytoJournal*, vol. 10, article 1, 2013.

[15] K. Mardi and N. Gupta, "Urachal papillary cystadenocarcinoma: a rare case report," *Journal of Cancer Research and Therapeutics*, vol. 7, no. 2, pp. 223–225, 2011.

[16] D. P. Vandersteen, S. J. Wiemerslage, and M. B. Cohen, "Prostatic duct adenocarcinoma: a cytologic and histologic case report with review of the literature," *Diagnostic Cytopathology*, vol. 17, no. 6, pp. 480–483, 1997.

[17] Y. Gong, N. Caraway, J. Stewart, and G. Staerkel, "Metastatic ductal adenocarcinoma of the prostate: cytologic features and clinical findings," *American Journal of Clinical Pathology*, vol. 126, no. 2, pp. 302–309, 2006.

[18] D. Alrahwan, G. Staerkel, and Y. Gong, "Fine needle aspiration cytology of a metastatic ductal carcinoma of the prostate," *Acta Cytologica*, vol. 50, no. 4, pp. 469–472, 2006.

45

Foregut Duplication Cyst of the Stomach: A Case Report and Review of the Literature

Y. Tjendra,[1] K. Lyapichev,[1] J. Henderson,[2] and C. P. Rojas[1]

[1]*Department of Pathology and Laboratory Medicine, Miller School of Medicine, University of Miami, Miami, FL 33136, USA*
[2]*Department of Radiology, Miller School of Medicine, University of Miami, Miami, FL 33136, USA*

Correspondence should be addressed to K. Lyapichev; kirill.lyapichev@jhsmiami.org

Academic Editor: Akira Mima

Duplication cyst of the stomach is a rare congenital malformation, typically diagnosed in the first year of life. In most adult cases the cyst remains asymptomatic, but patients may present with abdominal symptoms including epigastric discomfort or pain. We present a case of a 65-year-old male with an asymptomatic gastric tumor diagnosed incidentally during initial workup of his esophageal adenocarcinoma. Computed tomography revealed a low density soft tissue tumor near the gastroesophageal junction. Endoscopic ultrasonography demonstrated a cystic lesion as a hypoechoic round mass with well-defined borders. Following complete laparoscopic resection, microscopic review revealed a cyst lined with respiratory pseudostratified ciliated columnar epithelium and layers of smooth muscle with an outermost thin fibrous capsule consistent with a foregut duplication cyst.

1. Introduction

Foregut duplication cyst (FDC) is a rare congenital malformation which may occur at any level of the alimentary tract, with most cases diagnosed during the first year of life [1]. Duplication cysts can occur along with other congenital anomalies, such as annular or heterotopic pancreas, or vertebral anomalies such as spina bifida [2]. The clinical presentation may include a palpable abdominal mass, epigastric pain, or bleeding, but an FDC may remain completely asymptomatic and can be an incidental finding during diagnostic workup for an unrelated cause. Radiologic diagnostic tests are useful for characterization, but an accurate diagnosis can only be rendered by surgical resection and surgical pathology review.

2. Clinical Presentation

A 65-year-old male with known history of gastroesophageal reflux disease (GERD) and newly diagnosed esophageal adenocarcinoma was referred to our institution for further management. The patient stated progressive dysphagia with associated significant weight loss without hematemesis, melena, or hematochezia. At the outside institution, computed tomography (CT) and endoscopic ultrasonography (EUS) were performed as part of staging. The results demonstrated a T3 N1 Mx disease which prompted neoadjuvant chemotherapy.

In addition to the adenocarcinoma, CT demonstrated a 4.3 × 4.2 cm low density soft tissue mass at the epigastric region, near the hiatus and the gastroesophageal (GE) junction (Figure 1). EUS showed a 3.6 × 3.0 cm hypoechoic round mass with well-defined borders in the subhepatic peritoneal space along the gastrohepatic region (at the crura). No evidence of invasion was identified. Fine needle aspiration (FNA) was performed and revealed fluid with cells of epithelial origin, and malignancy could not be excluded at this point. The preoperative differential diagnosis included gastrointestinal stromal tumor (GIST) and duplication cyst of the stomach.

No significant reduction of this mass was noted on comparative imaging (CT and EUS) following neoadjuvant chemotherapy. The patient underwent transhiatal esophagectomy and partial gastrectomy, which were followed by an uneventful recovery.

3. Pathologic Findings

The specimen consisted of an 11.0 cm segment of esophagus and an 8.0 cm portion of stomach. Macroscopically, 1.0 cm

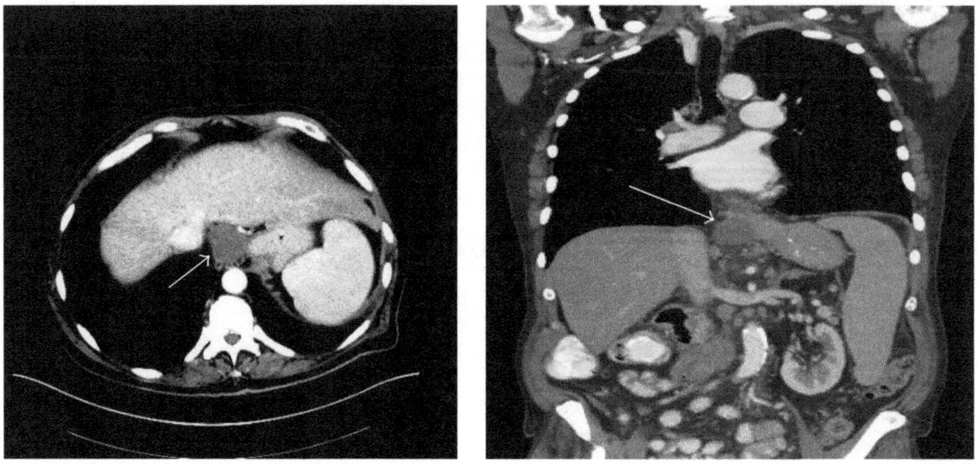

(a) (b)

FIGURE 1: (a) Intravenous contrast enhanced axial CT scan of the abdomen demonstrates a well-circumscribed, low-attenuating, nonenhancing mass (arrow) adjacent to the gastroesophageal junction representing an enteric duplication cyst. (b) Coronal reformat of the intravenous contrast enhanced CT scan of the abdomen also demonstrates a well-circumscribed, low-attenuating, nonenhancing mass (arrow) adjacent to the gastroesophageal junction.

inferior to the GE-junction, a well-circumscribed, white tan, saccular structure measuring 4.0 × 3.4 × 1.2 cm was identified. The cystic lesion was located in the serosa and did not communicate with the gastric lumen. Histologically, it consisted of mucosa lined with respiratory pseudostratified ciliated columnar epithelium (PCCE), which stained positive for thyroid transcription factor 1 (TTF-1) by immunohistochemistry (Figure 2). These findings were consistent with FDC of the stomach.

4. Discussion

Cystic lesions of the stomach are rare and, as a result of embryologic anomalies, are of posttraumatic, infectious, or neoplastic origin. They may occur as single or multiple lesions and may appear at any histologic layer of the stomach.

Gastrointestinal malformations occur in the early embryonal stages, and a duplication of the alimentary tract is considered to be a result of abnormal canalization. It may form into a communicating or a noncommunicating cystic or tubular structure, which is lined by a mucosal membrane [3]. These duplications are postulated to be formed before differentiation of epithelium into the characteristic adult types. Thus, they are generally named after the organ they are associated with rather than the mucosa lining them [4]. Duplication cysts can occur at any level of the alimentary tract, but the most common location is the ileum, followed by esophagus, jejunum, colon, stomach, and appendix [5]. Gastric duplication cysts represent about 2–8% of duplication cysts and are mostly located along the greater curvature, adjacent to the gastric wall, because these duplications are usually found to be distributed dorsally to the primitive gut during development [6]. Gastric duplication cysts are located in the lesser curvature in 5.5% of reported cases, and the mechanism by which they develop is not well understood [7].

In the case presented here, the location of the duplication cyst implies the term "gastric duplication cyst," but the term "foregut duplication cyst" is preferred, as it is lined exclusively with PCCE rather than gastric or intestinal mucosa [3, 8]. To our knowledge, only 23 cases of foregut duplication cyst lined with PCCE have been reported, with the first case published in 1966 [9].

The histogenesis of FDC lined with PCCE remains unclear. Gensler et al. suggested that an FDC lined with PCCE may represent the caudal-most portion of the laryngotracheal outgrowth, which has remained attached to the portion of the primitive foregut destined to become the stomach [9]. This suggests that the foregut duplication cyst in the present case may have arisen as a detached outpouching of the primitive foregut [7].

EUS, CT, and magnetic resonance imaging (MRI) are popular diagnostic methods for the examination of lesions along the gastrointestinal tract. Although FDC are uncommon, EUS findings of gastric duplication cysts have accumulated, and, thus, EUS has proven to be very useful for preoperative diagnosis along with CT or MRI [10].

The clinical presentation of FDC includes abdominal symptoms with a palpable abdominal mass, pain, vomiting, hematemesis, and weight loss [1, 4]. Other symptoms reported are epigastric discomfort or pain and persistent cough with hemoptysis [3, 6, 7, 9]. Most cases in adults are asymptomatic and diagnosed incidentally [11, 12]. In the present case, the FDC was an incidental finding, as the patient did not have any associated symptoms, and it was discovered as part of the presurgical diagnostic workup for his unrelated esophageal carcinoma. Malignant transformation of an FDC is extremely rare. Depending on the epithelial lining of the cyst, several cases of adenocarcinoma, squamous cell carcinoma or neuroendocrine carcinoma, have been reported [13–16].

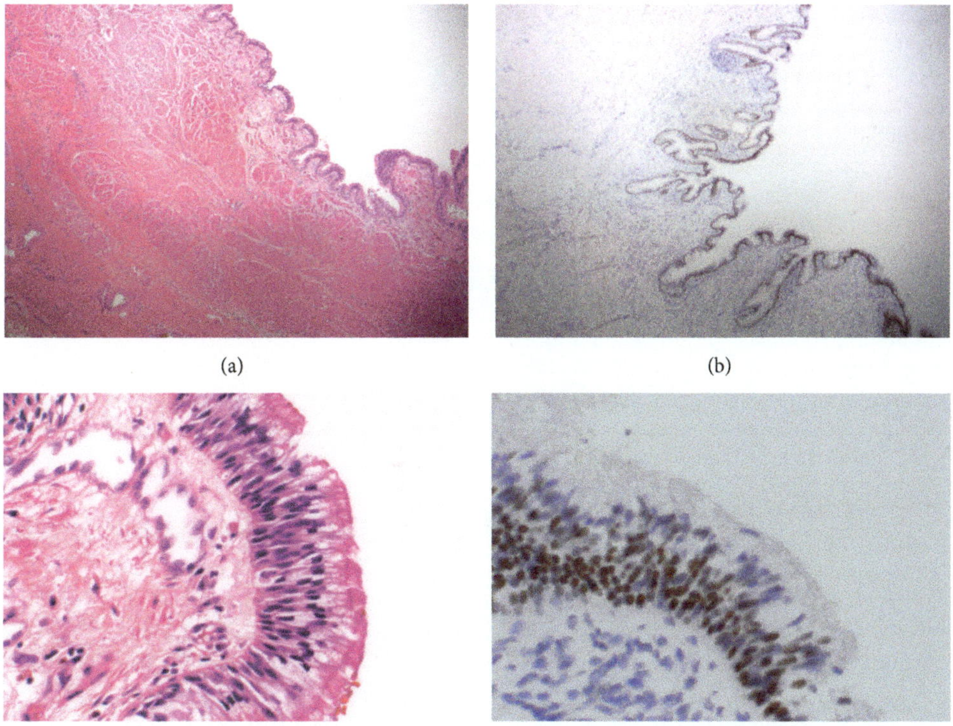

(a) (b) (c) (d)

FIGURE 2: (a) Cystic lesion lined by pseudostratified ciliated columnar epithelium with longitudinal and circular smooth muscle layers (10x). (b) TTF-1 immunohistochemistry highlights the lung type II pneumocytes (10x). (c) High magnification of the pseudostratified ciliate columnar epithelium (60x). (d) High magnification highlights the nuclear staining of TTF-1 (60x).

Even though FDC are rare, they are potentially dangerous; therefore, complete surgical resection is advised whenever possible as either open surgery or minimally invasive laparoscopic or endoscopic surgery (cystectomy, proximal or distal partial gastric resection, or total gastrectomy) [1, 10]. Surgical complications are related to the size and location of the duplication, communication with the gastrointestinal tract or vertebral canal, presence of heterotopic gastric mucosa, and involvement of mesenteric vessels [2].

In summary, FDC of the stomach constitutes a congenital disease whose diagnosis is rendered by microscopic examination and which should be included in the differential diagnosis of a gastric mass [12]. Because of the potential severe complications associated with FDC including perforation, bleeding, possible fistula formation and obstruction, and its potential for malignant transformation, the first line therapy is complete surgical resection.

Conflict of Interests

The authors declare that there is no conflict of interests regarding the publication of this paper.

References

[1] G. W. Holcomb III, A. Gheissari, J. A. O'Neill Jr., N. A. Shorter, and H. C. Bishop, "Surgical management of alimentary tract duplications," *Annals of Surgery*, vol. 209, no. 2, pp. 167–174, 1989.

[2] M. D. Stringer, L. Spitz, R. Abel et al., "Management of alimentary tract duplication in children," *British Journal of Surgery*, vol. 82, no. 1, pp. 74–78, 1995.

[3] R. D. Laraja, R. E. Rothenberg, J. Chapman, Imran-Ul-Haq, and M. T. Sabatini, "Foregut duplication cyst: a report of a case," *American Surgeon*, vol. 61, no. 9, pp. 840–841, 1995.

[4] S. C. Cunningham, D. E. Hansel, E. K. Fishman, and J. L. Cameron, "Foregut duplication cyst of the stomach," *Journal of Gastrointestinal Surgery*, vol. 10, no. 4, pp. 620–621, 2006.

[5] M. Scatizzi, M. Calistri, F. Feroci et al., "Gastric duplication cyst in an adult: case report," *In Vivo*, vol. 19, no. 6, pp. 975–978, 2005.

[6] A. Perek, S. Perek, M. Kapan, and E. Göksoy, "Gastric duplication cyst," *Digestive Surgery*, vol. 17, no. 6, pp. 634–636, 2000.

[7] D.-H. Kim, J.-S. Kim, E. S. Nam, and H. S. Shin, "Foregut duplication cyst of the stomach," *Pathology International*, vol. 50, no. 2, pp. 142–145, 2000.

[8] F. I. Luks, M. N. Shah, M. C. Bulauitan, P. A. LoPresti, and W. F. Pizzi, "Adult foregut duplication," *Surgery*, vol. 108, no. 1, pp. 101–104, 1990.

[9] S. Gensler, B. Seidenberg, H. Rifkin, and B. M. Rubinstein, "Ciliated lined intramural cyst of the stomach: case report and suggested embryogenesis," *Annals of Surgery*, vol. 163, no. 6, pp. 954–956, 1966.

[10] T. Takahara, T. Torigoe, H. Haga et al., "Gastric duplication cyst: evaluation by endoscopic ultrasonography and magnetic resonance imaging," *Journal of Gastroenterology*, vol. 31, no. 3, pp. 420–424, 1996.

[11] S. Murakami, H. Isozaki, T. Shou, K. Sakai, and H. Toyota, "Foregut duplication cyst of the stomach with pseudostratified

columnar ciliated epithelium," *Pathology International*, vol. 58, no. 3, pp. 187–190, 2008.

[12] S. M. Kim, M. H. Ha, J. E. Seo et al., "Gastric duplication cysts in adults: a report of three cases," *Journal of Gastric Cancer*, vol. 15, no. 1, pp. 58–63, 2015.

[13] K. Kuraoka, H. Nakayama, T. Kagawa, T. Ichikawa, and W. Yasui, "Adenocarcinoma arising from a gastric duplication cyst with invasion to the stomach: a case report with literature review," *Journal of Clinical Pathology*, vol. 57, no. 4, pp. 428–431, 2004.

[14] H. W. Mayo Jr., K. E. Mc, and R. M. Anderson, "Carcinoma arising in reduplication of the stomach (gastro-genous cyst): a case report," *Annals of Surgery*, vol. 141, no. 4, pp. 550–555, 1955.

[15] M.-L. Barussaud, G. Meurette, E. Cassagnau, B. Dupas, and J. Le Borgne, "Mixed adenocarcinoma and squamous cell carcinoma arising in a gastric duplication cyst," *Gastroenterologie Clinique et Biologique*, vol. 32, no. 2, pp. 188–191, 2008.

[16] G. Horne, C. Ming-Lum, A. W. Kirkpatrick, and R. L. Parker, "High-grade neuroendocrine carcinoma arising in a gastric duplication cyst: a case report with literature review," *International Journal of Surgical Pathology*, vol. 15, no. 2, pp. 187–191, 2007.

Two Rare Cases of Hepatocellular Carcinoma after Kasai Procedure for Biliary Atresia: A Recommendation for Close Follow-Up

Alicia C. Hirzel, Beatrice Madrazo, and Claudia P. Rojas

Department of Pathology, Jackson Memorial Hospital, University of Miami Miller School of Medicine, 1611 NW 12th Avenue, Holtz Building, Room 2042, Miami, FL 33136, USA

Correspondence should be addressed to Alicia C. Hirzel; achirzmd@hotmail.com

Academic Editor: Peter Kornprat

The instigation of the Kasai procedure in infants who are born with biliary atresia has led to increased survival in this population for over half a century. The many complications that arise as a result of biliary atresia led to an early death for most patients. However, the Kasai procedure is not without its own impediments. Among them is the development of hepatocellular carcinoma. We present two cases of hepatocellular carcinoma, after Kasai procedure, from two different age groups, as a recommendation that these patients should be even more closely monitored. Furthermore, if they are in need of transplant, we recommend that the explanted livers be carefully examined, as the tumor may not have been diagnosed preoperatively.

1. Introduction

Biliary atresia is an idiopathic obliteration of the extra- and intrahepatic biliary system leading to the obstruction of bile flow. The etiology of biliary atresia is unknown and its pathogenesis is not clearly understood. However, if left untreated, the cholestasis results in cirrhosis and liver failure. It is one of the many causes of neonatal cholestasis. The incidence varies from region to region with the highest occurring in the Pacific at 1 in 2,400 live births [1].

Biliary atresia may be syndromic or nonsyndromic [2]. Ultrasound may be performed and shows a shrunken gallbladder despite a 12-hour fast. Cholangiography assesses the morphology and patency of the gallbladder and ducts. The histologic findings in each type are similar to liver biopsy generally showing bile plugs, ductular proliferation, and fibrosis with obliteration of the ducts. These along with liver function tests help to confirm the diagnosis.

Currently, patients are managed surgically with the Kasai operation early in life. The goal of the procedure is to restore bile flow. In 1951, Dr. Morio Kasai developed the "Kasai" procedure or hepatoportojejunostomy or "Roux-en-Y." This procedure bypasses the bile ducts and allows the bile to drain into the intestines, thus slowing the liver damage. The complications of biliary atresia stem from the development of progressive cirrhosis. The complications of the Kasai surgery include cholangitis, portal hypertension, hepatopulmonary syndrome, pulmonary hypertension, biliary cysts, and malignancies such as hepatoblastomas, hepatocellular carcinomas, and cholangiocarcinomas. While they do occur, hepatocellular carcinomas (HCCs) are rare entities after Kasai procedure and only few cases are reported.

Here we present two cases of hepatocellular carcinoma after Kasai procedure for biliary atresia.

2. Case 1

A 4-year-old boy, delivered via C-section, presented with obstructive jaundice, dark urine, and clay-colored stool soon after birth (after an uneventful gestational period). The liver biopsy was interpreted as cirrhotic liver with cholestasis, bile ductular proliferation, and bile lakes, consistent with extrahepatic biliary atresia. He suffered an episode of cholangitis prior to his Kasai procedure, which was then postponed until after treatment. He was then lost to follow-up. At 4 years of

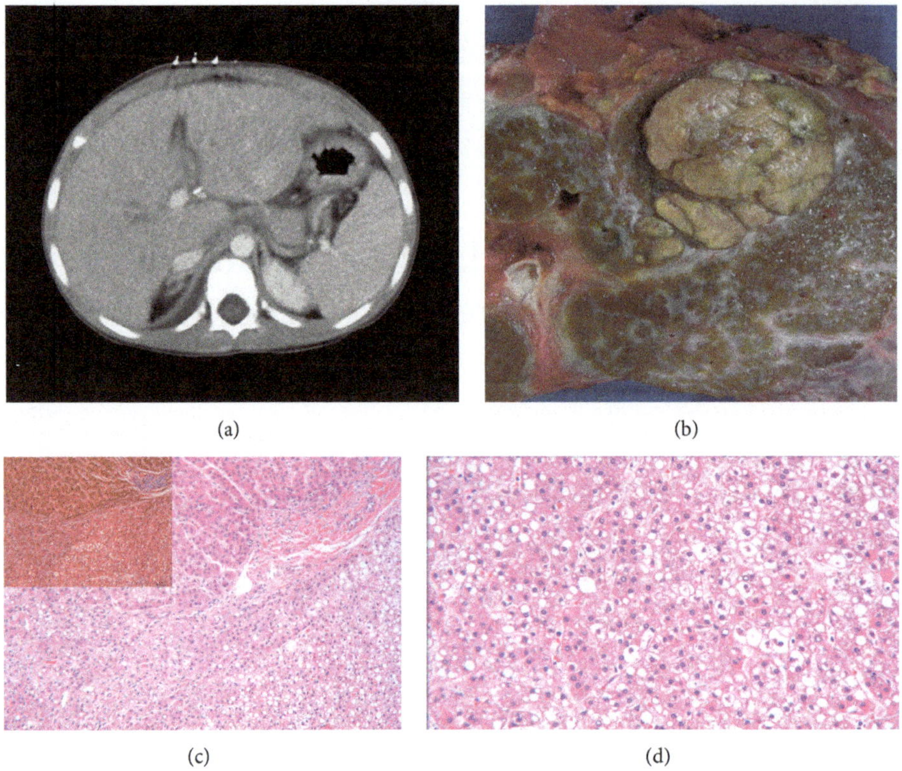

Figure 1: (a) CT scan of liver. (b) Gross picture of liver mass. (c) Microscopic picture of liver mass, H&E, 10x, with trichrome inset showing mass in lower half. (d) High magnification of mass, H&E, 20x.

age he was taken to the hospital due to an enlarging abdominal mass. Ultrasound and magnetic resonance imaging (MRI) detected two lesions, one in segment II of the liver with a second smaller mass in segment III (Figure 1(a)). Biopsies proved the masses to be hepatocellular carcinoma. Liver transplant was scheduled shortly thereafter. The explanted liver had two nodules in the left lobe, 3.8 cm and 2 cm, seen grossly, which were diagnosed as well-differentiated hepatocellular carcinoma and staged as pT2pNx (Figure 1(b)). Reticulin stain disclosed disruption of the lining around the hepatocytes in the hepatocellular carcinoma. Trichrome also highlighted areas of neoplastic tissue (Figures 1(c) and 1(d)). The patient presented with acute rejection 5 months after transplant and was treated. At 8 months after transplant, a liver biopsy was performed and chronic rejection with distortion and paucity of bile ducts was diagnosed. One year after transplant another biopsy was performed which showed bile duct proliferation with cholestasis, parenchymal inflammation, and portal fibrosis. Immunostain for SV40 was negative as was polymerase chain reaction (PCR) for BK virus. After this last biopsy the patient was again lost to follow-up and has not returned to our institution.

3. Case 2

A 25-year-old physician underwent a two-step Kasai procedure as an infant, first at 40 days then at 2 years of age. Surgeries were performed in another country. He had not received any surveillance endoscopies for varices since he was about 5 years of age. His clinical course was complicated by splenomegaly, thrombocytopenia, nonbleeding esophageal varices, and hepatic encephalopathy mostly due to the progression to cirrhosis. The varices regressed and his treating physician in his native country believed that he developed shunts that contributed to development of his encephalopathy. A CT liver triple phase with contrast showed a cirrhotic liver with small hypodensity and portal venous phase that persisted on delayed images in the right inferior lobe (Figure 2(a)). The patient underwent liver transplant. Two nodules were seen in the explanted liver, both in segment 7, measuring 2.5 and 1.2 cm in greatest dimension. The nodules were positive for polyclonal CEA, CD10, arginase-1, glypican 3 (focal and granular), CD34 (Figure 2(d)), and beta-catenin (membranous). They were negative for alpha-fetoprotein immunostain. The larger nodule was encapsulated and exophytic in nature (Figure 2(b)). The smaller nodule was a "subnodule" growing within a high-grade dysplastic nodule (Figure 2(e)). They were both diagnosed as well-differentiated hepatocellular carcinoma and staged as pT2pNX. Approximately 2 months after transplant, a liver biopsy was done due to persistently elevated transaminases. However, no acute rejection was seen. The patient returned to his native country shortly thereafter.

4. Discussion

Hepatocellular carcinoma (HCC), while not an unknown entity, is a rare occurrence after Kasai procedure, especially

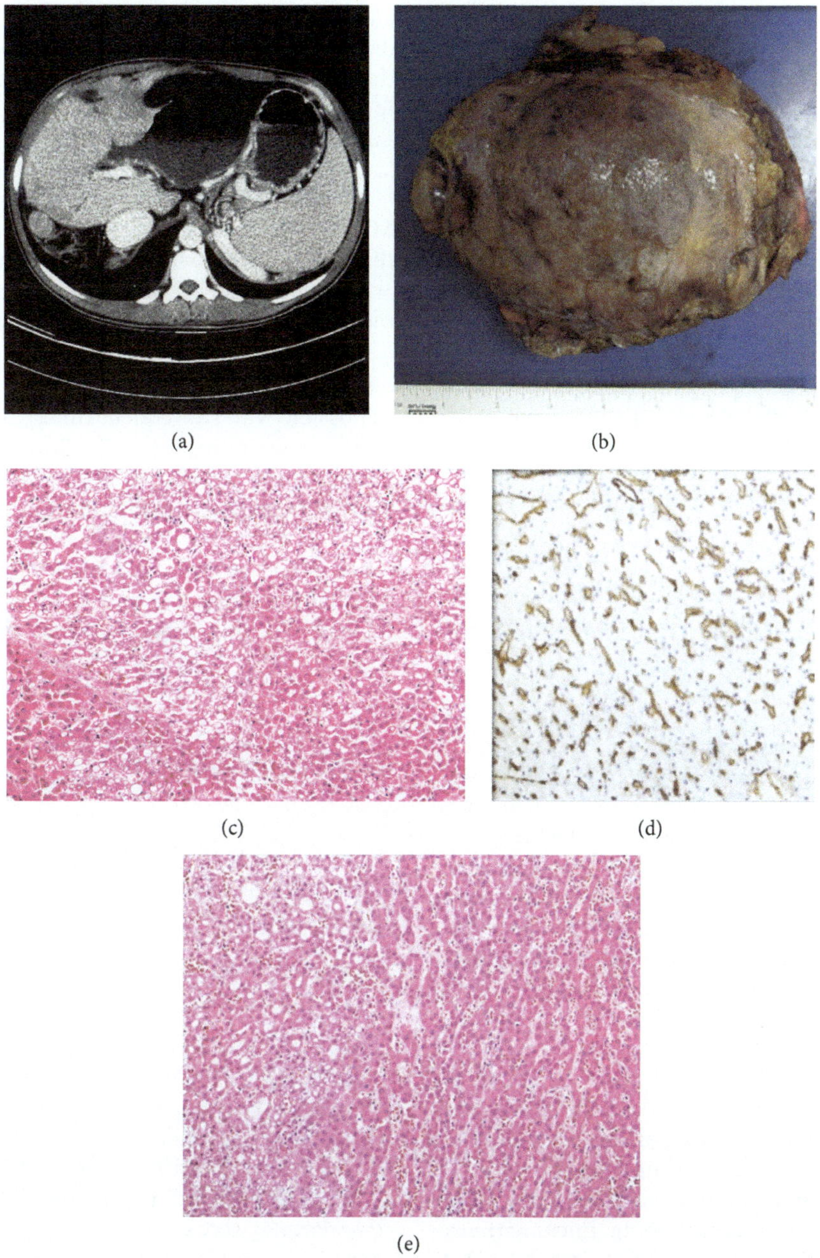

FIGURE 2: (a) CT scan of liver. (b) Gross picture showing nodular surface with somewhat exophytic mass on right. (c) Microscopic picture of mass, H&E, 20x. (d) Main mass with immunohistochemical stain for CD34 outlining neovascularization. (e) H&E of second "subnodule," 10x.

in the adult and neonatal population. Hol et al. reported a case in a 19-year-old individual while Aggarwal et al. reported another case in an older individual [3, 4]. It is also known to be very rare in infants under the age of 1 [5, 6]. HCC is more prone to develop in cirrhotic livers and in patients with biliary atresia. In addition, dysplastic nodules have been described in cirrhotic explanted livers [7, 8]. Our second patient had hepatocellular carcinoma developing in a dysplastic nodule. Here we describe two cases of well-differentiated hepatocellular carcinoma in patients who underwent Kasai procedure due to biliary atresia. The timing of the development of the malignancies was different in each patient with the first showing symptoms at 4 years of age while the second was diagnosed at 24 years of age, after examination of his explanted liver. The nodules in this second case were not seen in imaging prior to transplant and, thus, were an unexpected finding.

There are three types of biliary atresia depending on anatomic findings. Type I involves only the common bile duct (CBD) while the gallbladder and the hepatic ducts are patent. Type II involves the hepatic duct only with patent proximal intrahepatic ducts and is further classified into IIa (patent gallbladder and CBD) and NS IIb (obliteration of gallbladder, CBD, and cystic duct (CD)). Type III is complete atresia involving right and left intrahepatic ducts and extrahepatic ducts [9, 10]. There are many theories of the exact pathophysiology and they include failure of tissue remodeling or abnormal vascular development at the porta hepatis, viral infections, exposure to toxins, and an abnormal immune response leading to ductal obliteration [11]. However, there is still no real evidence as yet to support most of the theories.

There are many technical variants of the Kasai procedure including Type 1BA (cholecystoenterostomy or hepaticoenterostomy), Type 2BA (cystoenterostomy in cases where the hilar cyst communicates with the intrahepatic bile ducts), and Type 3BA (hepatoporto-cholecystostomy) [9, 12]. The procedure vastly enhanced survival and quality of life with many patients surviving into adulthood with their native liver. In addition, the implementation of liver transplant in these patients in the 1980s improved the survival rate immensely.

Overall, the prognosis of patients diagnosed with and treated for biliary atresia has improved significantly for the last 50 years and even approaches 90%. The timing of the Kasai procedure has been investigated and it has been shown that the sooner the procedure is done, the better the outcome of the patient is [1]. Nonetheless, some patients who had a timely procedure to increase exposure of the maximum number of bile ductules, in the porta hepatis, still required transplant [13]. Chardot reviewed all cases of BA in France within 1986–2009. They identified 1107 children of which 1044 underwent Kasai procedure at a median age of 59 days. Five hundred eighty-eight children ultimately underwent 692 liver transplant surgeries. Survival after transplantation was shown to be much higher than survival with native liver (77% versus 30% at 20 years). They concluded that patients who undergo Kasai procedure at an early age require liver transplant at a later age [14].

Factors affecting prognosis include type of BA, state of the liver at the time of surgery, portal pressure, and the association with other malformations. Patients with Types I and II do better as well as those who undergo postoperative resolution of jaundice. It has also been suggested that transplantation should be offered earlier to those patients who do not effectively clear their jaundice [13]. Chardot also reiterated that patients who clear their jaundice after surgery require liver transplantation when they are older as opposed to during infancy or childhood [14]. Patients, in whose explanted livers there are bridging fibrosis and elevated portal pressures at the time of their procedure, tend to do worse postoperatively [1]. It is important to note that many patients still succumb to their disease while waiting on a transplant list.

Furthermore, these patients must be closely monitored for the development of malignancies, which can severely mar survival rate. Hadžić et al. studied 387 infants at King's College Hospital within 1990–2008. Five infants developed HCC within 2–17 years of age. All underwent liver transplantation and were doing well after almost 6 years of follow-up. They suggest that all children with biliary atresia be considered as having the potential to develop HCC. This study concluded that serial alpha-fetoprotein measurements and ultrasonography are still considered the mainstay of early diagnosis [15]. Hol et al. and Aggarwal et al. have suggested the use of repeated sequential magnetic resonance (MR) to monitor the development of liver nodules in this population. Libbrecht et al., in a study of 49 explanted cirrhotic livers, found that ultrasound was poorly sensitive for detecting small hepatocellular carcinomas and suggested contrast-enhanced MR every 6 months in cirrhotic patients. They also cautioned that, oftentimes, benign lesions may be enhanced on the arterial phase and can be mistaken for malignancy and radiologists and pathologists should be aware of this [7].

The management of patients with biliary atresia depends on many factors. These patients need to be diagnosed as early as possible with subsequent timely surgical intervention and close postoperative follow-up. The families of these patients need to realize the necessity of continuity of care and the effect it has on outcome. In addition to close monitoring through imaging, explanted livers of patients with such history as these should be examined and sampled thoroughly, perhaps serially sectioning the liver at 0.5 cm and taking additional samples. In this way, the chances of finding malignant transformation of dysplastic nodules or occult malignancy not demonstrated through imaging are increased.

Conflict of Interests

The authors declare that there is no conflict of interests regarding the publication of this paper.

References

[1] B. E. Wildhaber, "Biliary atresia: 50 years after the first Kasai," *ISRN Surgery*, vol. 2012, Article ID 132089, 15 pages, 2012.

[2] H. Kobayashi and M. D. Stringer, "Biliary atresia," *Seminars in Neonatology*, vol. 8, no. 5, pp. 383–391, 2003.

[3] L. Hol, I. C. Van den Bos, S. M. Hussain, P. E. Zondervan, and R. A. De Man, "Hepatocellular carcinoma complicating biliary atresia after Kasai portoenterostomy," *European Journal of Gastroenterology and Hepatology*, vol. 20, no. 3, pp. 227–231, 2008.

[4] S. Aggarwal, D. Vadada, and V. Sharma, "A rare complication in an adult patient after Kasai portoenterostomy for biliary atresia," *Arab Journal of Gastroenterology*, vol. 13, no. 3, pp. 148–149, 2012.

[5] T. Iida, I. R. Zendejas, L. K. Kayler et al., "Hepatocellular carcinoma in a 10-month-old biliary atresia child," *Pediatric Transplantation*, vol. 13, no. 8, pp. 1048–1049, 2009.

[6] A. Brunati, Z. Feruzi, E. Sokal et al., "Early occurrence of hepatocellular carcinoma in biliary atresia treated by liver transplantation," *Pediatric Transplantation*, vol. 11, no. 1, pp. 117–119, 2007.

[7] L. Libbrecht, D. Bielen, C. Verslype et al., "Focal lesions in cirrhotic explant livers: pathological evaluation and accuracy of pretransplantation imaging examinations," *Liver Transplantation*, vol. 8, no. 9, pp. 749–761, 2002.

[8] C. O. Esquivel, C. Gutiérrez, K. L. Cox, R. Garcia-Kennedy, W. Berquist, and W. Concepcion, "Hepatocellular carcinoma and liver cell dysplasia in children with chronic liver disease," *Journal of Pediatric Surgery*, vol. 29, no. 11, pp. 1465–1469, 1994.

[9] C. Chardot, "Atresie des voies bilaires," in *Traitment Chirurgical. Encyclopedia of Medical Chiropractic*, Techniques Chirurgicales—Appareil Digestif, pp. 40–980, Scientifiques et Medicales Elsevier, Paris, France, 2002.

[10] M. Nio and R. Ohi, "Biliary atresia," *Seminars in Pediatric Surgery*, vol. 9, no. 4, pp. 177–186, 2000.

[11] W. Balistreri, J. Bezerra, and F. Ryckman, *Biliary Atresia and Other Disorders of the Extrahepatic Bile Ducts in Liver Disease in Children*, Cambridge University Press, 3rd edition, 2007.

[12] M. Kasai, S. Kimura, Y. Asakura, H. Suzuki, Y. Taira, and E. Ohashi, "Surgical treatment of biliary atresia," *Journal of Pediatric Surgery*, vol. 3, no. 6, pp. 665–675, 1968.

[13] M. Davenport, E. Ong, K. Sharif et al., "Biliary atresia in England and Wales: results of centralization and new benchmark," *Journal of Pediatric Surgery*, vol. 46, no. 9, pp. 1689–1694, 2011.

[14] C. Chardot, C. Buet, M.-O. Serinet et al., "Improving outcomes of biliary atresia: French national series 1986–2009," *Journal of Hepatology*, vol. 58, no. 6, pp. 1209–1217, 2013.

[15] N. Hadžić, A. Quaglia, B. Portmann et al., "Hepatocellular carcinoma in biliary atresia: King's College Hospital experience," *The Journal of Pediatrics*, vol. 159, no. 4, pp. 617–622, 2011.

Metastatic Chordoma: A Diagnostic Challenge on Fine Needle Aspiration

Ghassan Tranesh and Aziza Nassar

Department of Pathology, Mayo Clinic, 4500 San Pablo Road, Jacksonville, FL 32224, USA

Correspondence should be addressed to Aziza Nassar; nassar.aziza@mayo.edu

Academic Editor: Dhanpat Jain

Chordomas are primary low grade malignant tumors of bone that usually arise within both ends of axial skeleton. The Notochord is a midline, ectoderm-derived structure that defines the phylum of chordates. Chordomas may pose difficult diagnostic challenges when encountered in secondary locations, such as lungs or other parenchymatous organs. We report the cytologic findings of a metastatic chordoma sampled through CT-scan guided fine needle aspiration (FNA) of lower lobe lung nodule in a 54-year-old man diagnosed with recurrent chordoma involving the lumber spine and paraspinal region.

1. Introduction

Chordomas are primary low grade malignant tumors of bone that usually arise within both ends of axial skeleton. Chordoma has a phenotype that recapitulates notochord. The notochord is a midline, ectoderm-derived structure that defines the phylum of chordates [1]. In humans, the degeneration of the notochord begins during fetal development and is completed by the second decade of life [2]. Some controversy exists as to the origin of chordomas from these cells because chordomas arise from bone (clivus, sacrum, and coccyx), and not the intervertebral disks [3]. Chordoma represents a low grade malignant mesenchymal neoplasm with distinct clinical and pathologic features and histologic similarities to the notochord. It represents approximately 5% of malignant bone tumors. Distant metastases, most commonly to the lung, occur late in disease in approximately 30% of cases, but mortality is most often related to recurrence and progression with local effects [4].

2. Case Report

2.1. Subject. The patient is a 54-year-old male with a history of lumbar and paraspinal chordoma. He presented initially with left gluteal, left thigh, and left groin pain that led to an MRI of the lumber spine that showed a lesion at L2 expanding to L4 with paraspinal involvement (Figures 1(a) and 1(b)). A CT-guided biopsy with appropriate immunohistochemical correlation confirmed the diagnosis of chordoma. The tumor was surgically excised. Few months later, the patient noticed a left flank lump and had another abdominal CT-scan and PET scan which showed tumor recurrence (Figures 2(a) and 2(b)). Chest CT-scan showed left lower lobe nodular density (Figure 3). Infectious or inflammatory etiologies were considered. A CT-guided fine needle aspiration (FNA) biopsy on the lung nodule showed metastatic chordoma (Figures 4(a) and 4(b)). Patient had laminectomy with debulking of the recurrent chordoma and postoperative radiotherapy. Patient began brachyury vaccine injections, which were well tolerated without significant reported toxicities.

2.2. Radiology. The initial abdominal MRI showed a lobulated and expansile multiseptated mass with markedly intense T2 signal. The mass is located anterior and lateral to the L3, L4, and L5 vertebral bodies, which is consistent with tumor or neoplastic lymphadenopathy. This mass lesion measured approximately 4.3 cm × 4.0 cm × 4.5 cm and abuts the lower abdominal aorta and the proximal left common iliac artery, without evidence for encasement. The tumor was surgically excised.

Few months following the surgical excision, abdominal MRI was performed and showed that residual/recurrent

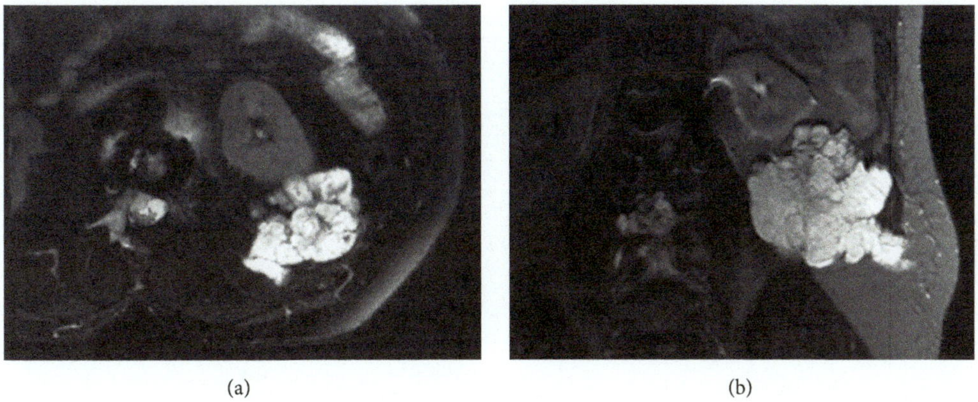

FIGURE 1: (a and b) Cross and Coronal sections MRI images show tumor recurrence with extension to psoas muscle.

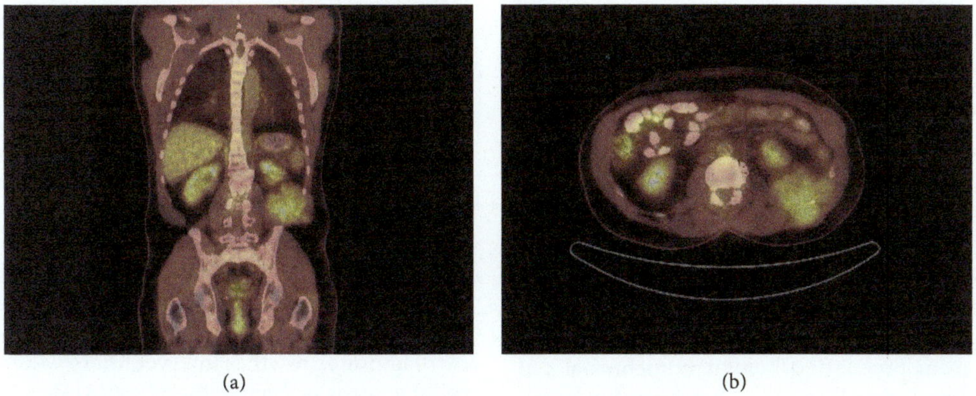

FIGURE 2: PET scan shows tumor recurrence.

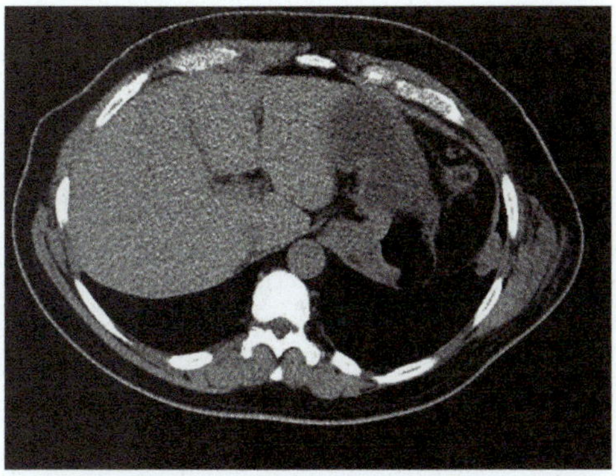

FIGURE 3: Chest CT-scan shows a 1.8 cm left lower lobe nodule.

chordoma involving right posterior L2 elements with large right anterolateral epidural tumor extensions at L2 and L3 level has further progressed, now causing severe compromise of the thecal sac at L2-3 level. There was also interval increase in the size of the left retroperitoneal lymphadenopathy and the large left flank soft tissue metastasis. Tumor extension was also noted within the L2-L3 and L3-L4 neural foramina and right psoas muscle. There was no evidence of obvious intrathecal extension (Figures 1(a) and 1(b)).

Shortly after the MRI, patient had a full body PET scan which showed large low density hypermetabolic mass, SUV max 2.8, in the left flank involving the musculature of the left posterior abdominal wall and extending through the rib cage (Figures 2(a) and 2(b)).

Chest CT-scan showed borderline enlarged right hilar lymph node. There was no left hilar adenopathy with normal sized mediastinal and axillary lymph nodes. There was a soft tissue confluence in the left lower lobe measuring approximately 1.8 cm (Figure 3).

2.3. Cytologic Findings. Diff-Quik smears from the CT-guided FNA of the lung nodule were moderately cellular and showed multiple fragments of fibrillary matrix material intimately admixed with epithelioid cells in a background of red blood cells. The epithelioid cells were present in large branching three-dimensional groups associated with fibrillary matrix or as single cells and small loosely cohesive clusters. The fibrillary matrix appeared intensely magenta to purple in Diff-Quik-stained smears (Figures 4(a) and 4(b)). A cell block was prepared; however, there were no lesional cells for further ancillary studies. Previous resection slides were reviewed in conjunction with the current case. The histomorphologic features were identical. The previous

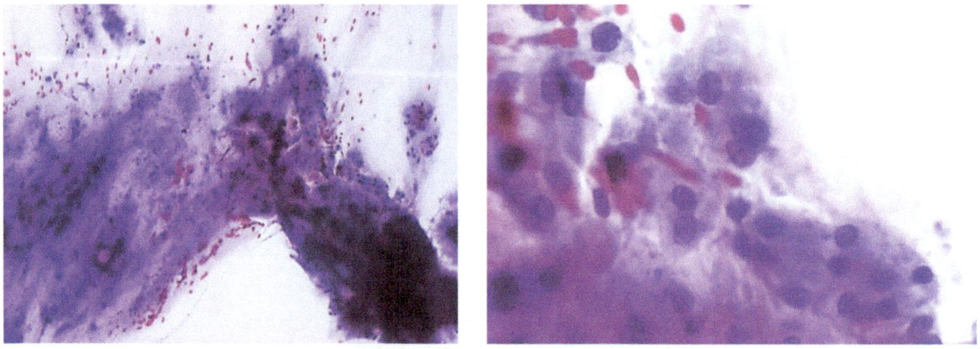

(a) (b)

FIGURE 4: FNA Diff-Quik smears, low and higher power images show metastatic chordoma (fragments of fibrillary matrix material intimately admixed with epithelioid cells in a background of red blood cell).

resection immunostains showed the neoplastic cells to be strongly positive for cytokeratin AE1/AE3, Brachyury, and epithelial membrane antigen (EMA) and weakly positive for S100.

3. Discussion

Chordomas were first described by Lushka et al. in 1856 [5]. Chordomas occur mostly in the craniospinal axis and are thought to arise from notochordal remnants. Recent literature challenges this traditional concept suggesting that chordomas arise from preexisting benign notochordal cell tumors [6]. Chordomas usually present between the fourth and seventh decades with a male to female ratio of 2 : 1 [6]. Chordomas account for 5% of primary malignant bone tumors. Radiologically, chordomas are destructive, lytic masses which extend into the soft tissues, forming a sizable, well-defined mass which may show calcifications. Variety of genetic abnormalities can be identified in sporadic and familial tumors. Familial tumors (familial chordoma) have been associated with upregulation of T-brachyury, a nuclear transcription factor [7, 8]. Chordomas appear to be increased in incidence in patients with tuberous sclerosis [9]. Tumors in children usually arise in skull base and are often a part of tuberous sclerosis complex (TSC). Sacral chordomas have best prognosis and longest overall survival because they are most likely to be resected with negative margins. Local recurrences for sacrococcygeal tumors are common after incomplete excision with 5- and 10-year survival rates ranging from 60 to 95% and 40 to 60%, respectively [10]. The treatment of chordoma demands both aggressive resection and cautious attention to minimizing surgical tumor implantation.

The differential diagnosis of metastatic chordoma includes benign pulmonary hamartoma [11] which is composed of lobules of benign cartilage lacunes, myxoid stroma with adipose tissue. Also, pulmonary hamartomas are CK AE1/AE3 and brachyury negative [3, 12]. Metastatic chordoma can morphologically mimic mucinous carcinomas; besides, 3% of non-small cell pulmonary carcinomas may show brachyury immunostain positivity [13]. However, mucinous carcinomas usually show floating cohesive cell groups of uniform epithelial cells, often with lumen formation. Also, in this particular case, the clinical history and the radiological picture were not favoring mucinous carcinoma.

The other differential diagnosis is myxoid/round cell liposarcoma which is a spindle cell neoplasm, deeply located with plexiform vascular growth. However, it rarely occurs in the lung and in this case there were no lipoblasts or pleomorphic round cell component [12].

The other differential diagnosis is extraskeletal myxoid chondrosarcoma, which consists of multilobulated malignant cartilaginous growth. However, there were no anastomosing cellular cords or cartilaginous cells [13].

Brachyury is a transcription factor that is required for posterior mesoderm formation and differentiation as well as for the notochord development during embryogenesis. It is expressed in the neoplastic cells of chordoma, a malignant tumour deriving from notochordal remnants [14]. Brachyury immunostain is a synthetic peptide conjugated to KLH derived from within residues 250–350 of human brachyury [7].

Adjuvant therapy is controversial but known to contribute to long-term disease control and survival. Postoperative patient followup should continue long-term CT-scan surveillance; and any signs or symptoms consistent with possible local recurrence or metastasis should prompt a thorough workup. In the absence of symptoms, surveillance CT-scans can detect potential treatable recurrence. Recurrent disease can be treated aggressively with curative intent including surgery and adjuvant radiation therapy [15].

Brachyury vaccine has been designed to stimulate the human immune system to target chordoma. The vaccine is composed of heat-inactivated *S. cerevisiae* yeast that expresses human brachyury protein. This vaccine is the fifth of a novel class of yeast-based immunotherapeutics designed to stimulate immune responses to eliminate diseased cells. Patients who were vaccinated have shown a good tolerability profile in clinical programs to date. Expected adverse events from these products are limited to redness, swelling, and tenderness at the injection site, and mild, brief flu-like symptoms [16].

Conflict of Interests

There is no conflict of interests.

References

[1] B. P. Walcott, B. V. Nahed, A. Mohyeldin, J.-V. Coumans, K. T. Kahle, and M. J. Ferreira, "Chordoma: current concepts, management, and future directions," *The Lancet Oncology*, vol. 13, no. 2, pp. e69–e76, 2012.

[2] L. P. Le, G. P. Nielsen, A. E. Rosenberg et al., "Recurrent chromosomal copy number alterations in sporadic chordomas," *PLoS ONE*, vol. 6, no. 5, Article ID e18846, 2011.

[3] V. Deshpande, G. Petur Nielsen, D. I. Rosenthal, and A. E. Rosenberg, "Intraosseous Benign Notochord Cell Tumors (BNCT): further evidence supporting a relationship to chordoma," *The American Journal of Surgical Pathology*, vol. 31, no. 10, pp. 1573–1577, 2007.

[4] J. X. O'Connell, L. G. Renard, N. J. Liebsch, J. T. Efird, J. E. Munzenrider, and A. E. Rosenberg, "Base of skull chordoma. A correlative study of histologic and clinical features of 62 cases," *Cancer*, vol. 74, no. 8, pp. 2261–2267, 1994.

[5] C. Fernández Carballal, R. González Rodrigalvarez, M. López De La Riva, and C. Ares, "Dumbbell-shaped thoracic chondroid chordoma mimicking a neurinoma," *Acta Neurochirurgica*, vol. 152, no. 2, pp. 325–326, 2010.

[6] C. M. Coffin, P. E. Swanson, M. R. Wick, and L. P. Dehner, "Chordoma in childhood and adolescence: a clinicopathologic analysis of 12 cases," *Archives of Pathology and Laboratory Medicine*, vol. 117, no. 9, pp. 927–933, 1993.

[7] R. Tirabosco, D. C. Mangham, A. E. Rosenberg et al., "Brachyury expression in extra-axial skeletal and soft tissue chordomas: a marker that distinguishes chordoma from mixed tumor/myoepithelioma/parachordoma in soft tissue," *American Journal of Surgical Pathology*, vol. 32, no. 4, pp. 572–580, 2008.

[8] X. R. Yang, D. Ng, D. A. Alcorta et al., "*T* (brachyury) gene duplication confers major susceptibility to familial chordoma," *Nature Genetics*, vol. 41, no. 11, pp. 1176–1178, 2009.

[9] C. M. McPherson, D. Suki, I. E. McCutcheon, Z. L. Gokaslan, L. D. Rhines, and E. Mendel, "Metastatic disease from spinal chordoma: a 10-year experience," *Journal of Neurosurgery: Spine*, vol. 5, no. 4, pp. 277–280, 2006.

[10] G. Vergara, B. Belinchón, F. Valcárcel, M. Veiras, I. Zapata, and A. De La Torre, "Metastatic disease from chordoma," *Clinical and Translational Oncology*, vol. 10, no. 8, pp. 517–521, 2008.

[11] T. Yamaguchi, M. Yamato, and K. Saotome, "First histologically confirmed case of a classic chordoma arising in a precursor benign notochordal lesion: differential diagnosis of benign and malignant notochordal lesions," *Skeletal Radiology*, vol. 31, no. 7, pp. 413–418, 2002.

[12] K.-S. Delank, J. Kriegsmann, P. Drees, A. Eckardt, and P. Eysel, "Metastasizing chordoma of the lumbar spine," *European Spine Journal*, vol. 11, no. 2, pp. 167–171, 2002.

[13] V. Barresi, A. Ieni, G. Branca, and G. Tuccari, "Brachyury: a diagnostic marker for the differential diagnosis of chordoma and hemangioblastoma versus neoplastic histological mimickers," *Disease Markers*, vol. 2014, Article ID 514753, 7 pages, 2014.

[14] M. Miettinen, Z. Wang, J. Lasota, C. Heery, J. Schlom, and C. Palena, "Nuclear brachyury expression is consistent in chordoma, common in germ cell tumors and small cell carcinomas, and rare in other carcinomas and sarcomas: an immunohistochemical study of 5229 cases," *The American Journal of Surgical Pathology*, vol. 39, no. 10, pp. 1305–1312, 2015.

[15] R. Kalluri and R. A. Weinberg, "The basics of epithelial-mesenchymal transition," *The Journal of Clinical Investigation*, vol. 119, no. 6, pp. 1420–1428, 2009.

[16] J. P. Thiery and J. P. Sleeman, "Complex networks orchestrate epithelial-mesenchymal transitions," *Nature Reviews Molecular Cell Biology*, vol. 7, no. 2, pp. 131–142, 2006.

Small Bowel Obstruction due to Intestinal Xanthomatosis

L. E. Barrera-Herrera,[1] F. Arias,[2,3] P. A. Rodríguez-Urrego,[1,3] and M. A. Palau-Lázaro[1,3]

[1] *Pathology and Clinical Laboratory Department, Fundación Santa Fe de Bogotá University Hospital, Calle 119, No. 7–75, Bogotá 110111, Colombia*
[2] *Surgery Department, Fundación Santa Fe de Bogotá University Hospital, Calle 119, No. 7–75, Bogotá 110111, Colombia*
[3] *School of Medicine, Universidad de los Andes, Carrera 1, No. 18A-12, Bogotá 111711, Colombia*

Correspondence should be addressed to M. A. Palau-Lázaro; mapalau@hotmail.com

Academic Editor: Uma N. Sundram

Vast majority of bowel obstruction is due to postoperative adhesions, malignancy, intestinal inflammatory disease, and hernias; however, knowledge of other uncommon causes is critical to establish a prompt treatment and decrease mortality. Xanthomatosis is produced by accumulation of cholesterol-rich foamy macrophages. Intestinal xanthomatosis is an uncommon nonneoplastic lesion that may cause small bowel obstruction and several cases have been reported in the English literature as obstruction in the jejunum. We report a case of small intestinal xanthomatosis occurring in a 51-year-old female who presented with one day of copious vomiting and intermittent abdominal pain. Radiologic images revealed jejunal loop thickening and inflammatory changes suggestive of foreign body obstruction, diagnostic laparoscopy found two strictures at the jejunum, and a pathologic examination confirmed a segmental small bowel xanthomatosis. This case illustrates that obstruction even without predisposing factors such as hyperlipidemia or lymphoproliferative disorders.

1. Introduction

Small bowel obstruction corresponds to approximately 20% of patients who present with acute abdomen and are admitted for surgery [1]. Among the different causes of small bowel obstruction (SBO), 60% are due to postoperative adhesions, followed by malignancy, intestinal inflammatory disease (Crohn's disease), and hernias [2]. SBO is difficult to recognize preoperatively and is associated with significant mortality. About 5.5% present with strangulation [3], making surgery the essential treatment to prevent further complications. Xanthomatosis is characterized by accumulation of lipid-laden, foamy macrophages resulting in nodule formation and commonly involving the skin [4]. In the gastrointestinal tract, stomach is the most frequent location; however, cases involving esophagus [5], small bowel [6, 7], ileocecal valve [8], colon [9–12] and rectum [13], tendons, bladder, and prostate have been described [14]. We report a case of SBO due to intestinal xanthomatosis.

2. Clinical Summary

A 51-year-old female presented with one day of copious vomiting and intermittent abdominal pain. Her clinical history was significant for hypertension treated with Losartan and Hydrochlorothiazide. Physical examination revealed mild dehydration and diffuse abdominal pain with no peritoneal irritation signs. CBC showed normal leucocyte count $4.58 \times 10^3/\mu L$ ($5–10 \times 10^3/\mu L$) with neutrophilia 84% (30–40%); CT scan of the abdomen (Figure 1) revealed an adynamic ileus with jejunal loop thickening and inflammatory changes suggestive of foreign body obstruction. The patient was taken to diagnostic laparoscopy which revealed two strictures at the jejunum. Small bowel resection with anastomosis was

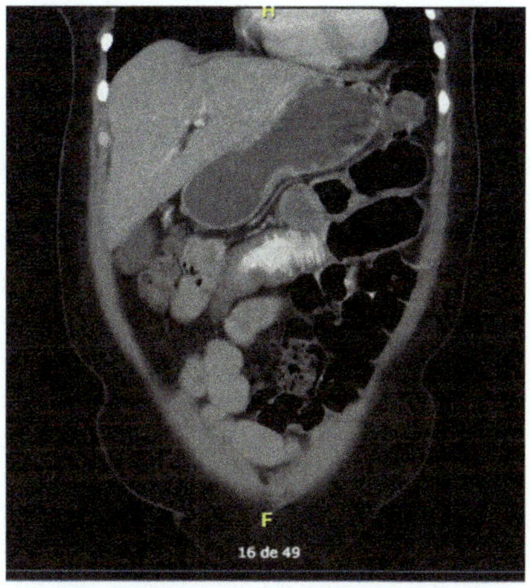

FIGURE 1: CT imaging presenting adynamic ileus with jejunal loop thickening.

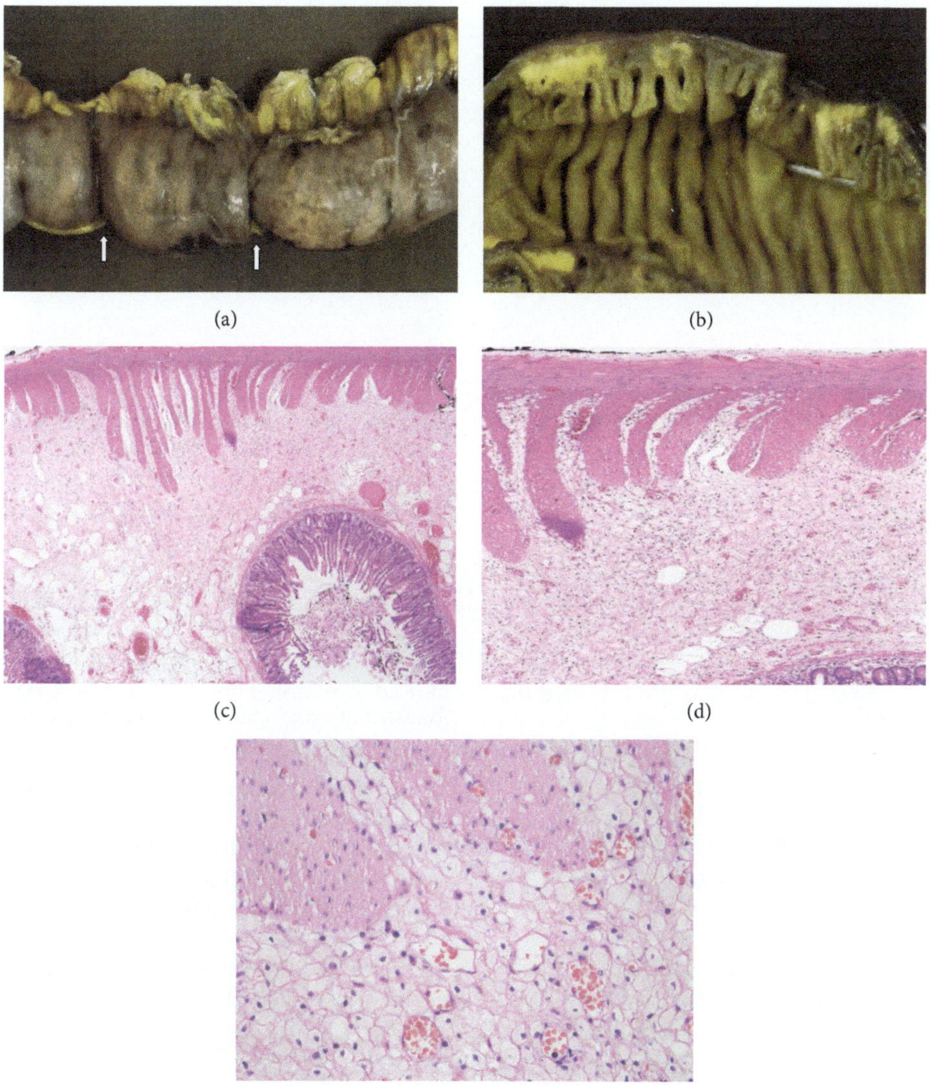

FIGURE 2: (a) Small bowel segment with two areas of stricture (see arrows). (b) Full thickness small bowel wall with submucosal yellowish, (c) H&E 40x, (d) 100x, and (e) 400x xanthomatous histiocytes involving the submucosa and muscularis propria.

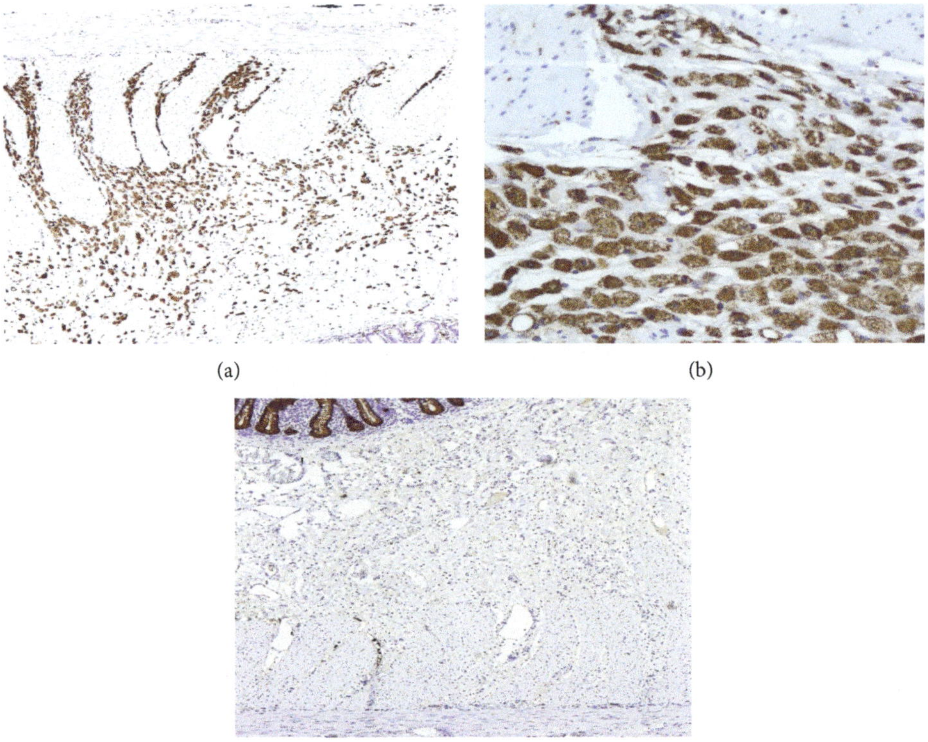

FIGURE 3: (a) (100x), (b) (400x) histiocytes positive for CD68 and (c) (100x) negative cytokeratin AE1/AE3.

performed and the adherences were liberated. The patient had an uneventful recovery.

3. Pathologic Findings

Gross examination revealed a 16 cm segment of jejunum with circumference of 5 cm. The serosal surface had two strictures (Figure 2(a)). On opening, two areas of narrowed lumen with a circumference of 2 cm were noted. The wall at the site of strictures had a yellow mural discoloration that involved the submucosa (Figure 2(b)).

Microscopic examination revealed an interstitial diffuse infiltrate of foamy histiocytes that involved mainly the submucosa and infiltrate focally the muscularis propria pushing the mucosa upwards (Figures 2(c) and 2(d)). Sections from mesenteric vessels showed moderate atherosclerosis with medial calcification. Special stains for PAS and PAS-D, Gomori, methenamine silver, Ziehl Neelsen, and Gram were negative for microorganisms. Immunohistochemistry studies were positive for CD68 and negative for cytokeratin AE1/AE3 (Figure 3) confirming a histiocytic origin. Final diagnosis of segmental small bowel xanthomatosis was made.

4. Discussion

Xanthomas are defined as local accumulation of cholesterol-rich foamy macrophages in tissue; intestinal xanthomatosis is considered an unusual nonneoplastic lesion that may cause obstruction and can present as a mass-like lesion mimicking malignant tumor obstruction due to prominent fibrosis and inflammation [15], as in our case. The etiologies of intestinal xanthomatosis not associated with predisposing conditions such as hyperlipidemia or lymphoproliferative lesions have not been settled and one of the theories related to its development states that an insult generates destruction of cells in the mucosa or submucosa with subsequent ingestion of lipid-containing debris by histiocytes which then persist as foamy cells [16]. Gastrointestinal xanthomas are rare and the stomach is the most frequent described location [4].

Although xanthomas are commonly seen in patients with dyslipidemias or other conditions such as previous chemotherapy [16], radiotherapy [6], and infection (disseminated mycobacterium avium-intracellular and cytomegalovirus colitis) in immunosuppressed patients (AIDS) [8], our case did not have history of any of these treatments, immunosuppression, and known history of hypercholesterolemia (lipid profile not available) and no skin xanthomas were found on physical examination. Review of the literature about intestinal xanthomatosis shows that this entity is predominantly found incidentally during endoscopy; however, among the symptomatic cases, some presented with obstruction and strictures/stenosis that caused dysmotility of the intestinal musculature [6]. Also some cases had presented as small bowel pseudotumors [16]; the reported symptomatic patients by Delacruz et al. had either hyperlipidemia or lymphoproliferative disorders [4]. Neither of these conditions was found in this case.

Gastrointestinal xanthomas are composed of cells with abundant foamy cytoplasm containing lipid characteristically positive for CD68 with no mucin or pigment deposition. Microscopically, the differential diagnosis includes poorly differentiated carcinoma, storage diseases, infections (Whipple disease, mycobacterium, and AIDS), macroglobulinemia, and muciphages [4]. In our case, the negativity for cytokeratin AE1/AE3 ruled out carcinoma; the negativity for special stains such as Gram, Ziehl Neelsen, Gomori methenamine silver, and PAS and PAS-D ruled out infections and mucin deposition. Besides clinically the patient did not have symptoms for storage diseases and/or macroglobulinemia.

5. Conclusion

Intestinal xanthomatosis is a rare entity but it should be considered as one of the etiologies of clinically significant obstruction and must be included even if the patient has no history of hyperlipidemia or lymphoproliferative disorder. In order to implement the best treatment options if diagnosed, clinicians must extend workup to rule out lipid storage diseases, dyslipidemia, lymphoproliferative disorders, and infections [17].

Conflict of Interests

The authors declare that there is no conflict of interests regarding the publication of this paper.

References

[1] J. P. Welch, "General consideration and mortality in bowel obstruction," in *Bowel Obstruction: Differential Diagnosis and Clinical Management*, J. P. Welch, Ed., pp. 59–95, Saunders, Philadelphia, Pa, USA, 1990.

[2] Small-Bowel Obstruction, April 2014, http://emedicine.medscape.com/article/774140-overview.

[3] T. Otamiri, R. Sjödahl, and I. Ihse, "Intestinal obstruction with strangulation of the small bowel," *Acta Chirurgica Scandinavica*, vol. 153, no. 4, pp. 307–310, 1987.

[4] V. Delacruz, H. Takahashi, S. Nishida, A. Tzakis, and P. Ruiz, "Segmental xanthomatosis of the small intestine. A case report and review of the literature," *Human Pathology*, vol. 40, no. 1, pp. 139–142, 2009.

[5] M. Hirokawa, R. Takenaka, A. Takahashi et al., "Esophageal xanthoma: report of two cases and a review of the literature," *Journal of Gastroenterology and Hepatology*, vol. 18, no. 9, pp. 1105–1108, 2003.

[6] U. Coletta and B. C. Sturgill, "Isolated xanthomatosis of the small bowel," *Human Pathology*, vol. 16, no. 4, pp. 422–424, 1985.

[7] J. S. Yoon, Y. C. Jeon, T. Y. Kim et al., "Xanthogranulomatous inflammation in terminal ileum presenting as an appendiceal mass: case report and review of the literature," *Clinical Endoscopy*, vol. 46, no. 2, pp. 193–196, 2013.

[8] M. D. Goodman, "Segmental xanthomatosis of the ileocecal valve with anatomic and functional obstruction," *Archives of Pathology and Laboratory Medicine*, vol. 121, no. 1, pp. 75–78, 1997.

[9] C. Y. Lo, T. G. Lorentz, and C. S. P. Poon, "Xanthrogranulomatus inflammation of the sigmoid colon: a case report," *Australian and New Zealand Journal of Surgery*, vol. 66, no. 9, pp. 643–644, 1996.

[10] Y.-H. Oh, S. S. Seong, K.-S. Jang et al., "Xanthogranulomatous inflammation presenting as a submucosal mass of the sigmoid colon," *Pathology International*, vol. 55, no. 7, pp. 440–444, 2005.

[11] A. Z. Anadol, I. I. Gonul, and E. Tezel, "Xanthogranulomatous inflammation of the colon: a rare cause of cecal mass with bleeding," *Southern Medical Journal*, vol. 102, no. 2, pp. 196–199, 2009.

[12] S. Dhawan, D. Jain, and S. K. Kalhan, "Xanthogranulomatous inflammation of ascending colon with mucosal involvement: report of a first case," *Journal of Crohn's and Colitis*, vol. 5, no. 3, pp. 245–248, 2011.

[13] M. Nakasono, M. Hirokawa, N. Muguruma et al., "Colorectal xanthomas with polypoid lesion: report of 25 cases," *APMIS*, vol. 112, no. 1, pp. 3–10, 2004.

[14] J. R. Miliauskas, "Rectosigmoid (colonic) xanthoma: a report of four cases and review of the literature," *Pathology*, vol. 34, no. 2, pp. 144–147, 2002.

[15] K. C. Wong, W. M. S. Tsui, and S. J. Chang, "Xanthogranulomatous inflammation of terminal ileum: report of a case with small bowel involvement," *Hong Kong Medical Journal*, vol. 21, no. 1, pp. 69–72, 2015.

[16] R. Ashfaq and C. F. Timmons, "Xanthomatous pseudotumor of the small intestine following treatment for Burkitt's lymphoma," *Archives of Pathology and Laboratory Medicine*, vol. 116, no. 3, pp. 299–301, 1992.

[17] G. Chalès, G. Coiffier, and P. Guggenbuhl, "Miscellaneous non-inflammatory musculoskeletal conditions. Rare thesaurismosis and xanthomatosis," *Best Practice & Research: Clinical Rheumatology*, vol. 25, no. 5, pp. 683–701, 2011.

Pulmonary Empty Spaces: Silicone Embolism—A Decade of Increased Incidence and Its Histological Diagnosis

Kirill Lyapichev,[1] Felix Manuel Chinea,[2] Julio Poveda,[1] Jeniffer Pereda,[3] Pablo A. Bejarano,[4] and Monica T. Garcia-Buitrago[1]

[1]*Pathology and Laboratory Medicine Department, Miller School of Medicine, University of Miami, Miami, FL 33136, USA*
[2]*Department of Radiation Oncology, Miller School of Medicine, University of Miami, Miami, FL, USA*
[3]*Kornberg School of Dentistry, Temple University, Philadelphia, PA, USA*
[4]*Department of Pathology, Cleveland Clinic Florida, Weston, FL, USA*

Correspondence should be addressed to Kirill Lyapichev; kirill.lyapichev@jhsmiami.org

Academic Editor: Piero Tosi

Pulmonary embolism (PE) is a critical complication related to multiple disorders and different medical or cosmetic procedures. This case report presents two patients who were admitted for respiratory symptoms in the setting of previously receiving silicone injections for cosmetic purposes and were diagnosed with silicone pulmonary embolism. The relevance of including questions about all cosmetic procedures as a part of a medical history is highlighted, in particular about silicone injections. The diagnosis is confirmed by histological means. Additionally, our review showed the change of most common sites of silicone injections and a significant increase in cosmetic procedures causing silicone embolism during the past twelve years.

1. Introduction

Pulmonary embolism (PE) is a critical complication related to various disorders such as deep vein thrombosis (DVT), cardiac arrhythmia, certain coagulopathies, and bacterial endocarditis, trauma. Each year, more than 0.6 million people in the United States suffer from pulmonary embolism with about 50,000 resulting in death [1]. An additional risk is observed in patients with a history of medical or cosmetic procedures that may provide an etiology for patients presenting with respiratory symptoms, especially if they were performed by unlicensed individuals. We present two unusual cases of respiratory syndrome, an analysis of the published literature on silicone embolism from 2004 to 2015, and a comparison with a previous review spanning 40 years, from 1965 to 2004.

2. Case Presentations

2.1. Clinical Case #1. A 24-year-old African American female presented at four-week gestation with a nonproductive cough and severe shortness of breath that began four days prior with progressive worsening. The patient reported no history of recent travel. Oxygen was administered via nasal cannula and was well tolerated.

On physical examination, the patient was tachycardic (126 bpm) and tachypneic (36 breaths/min); temperature was 36.9°C; blood pressure was 132/81 mm Hg; and peripheral oxygen saturation was 98%. Pulmonary auscultation revealed diffuse wheezing and diminished breathing sounds in bilateral lung bases.

Echocardiogram ruled out valvular disease and myocardial wall abnormalities. Laboratory tests at the time of admission revealed an arterial blood gas analysis within normal limits, anemia (hemoglobin 11.3 mg/dL, hematocrit 34.1), and a normal platelet count (339,000). Chest X-ray revealed bilateral lung opacities with relative sparing of the right upper lobe and left pleural effusions (Figure 1(a)).

Computed tomography (CT) scan showed multifocal, bilateral, predominantly peripheral airspace opacities (Figure 1(b)). A nonspecific differential for this pattern of distribution included eosinophilic lung disease, sarcoidosis,

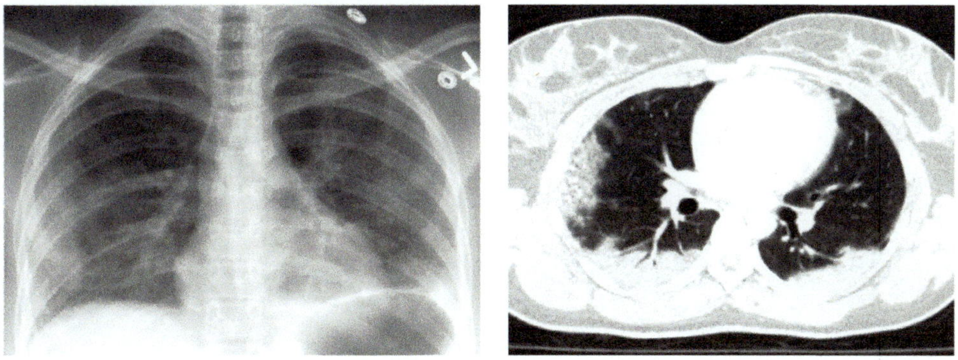

(a) (b)

FIGURE 1: (a) Portable chest X-ray showing bilateral lung opacities with relative sparing of the right upper lobe and left pleural effusions. (b) CT scan of chest showing multifocal and bilateral, predominantly peripheral airspace opacities.

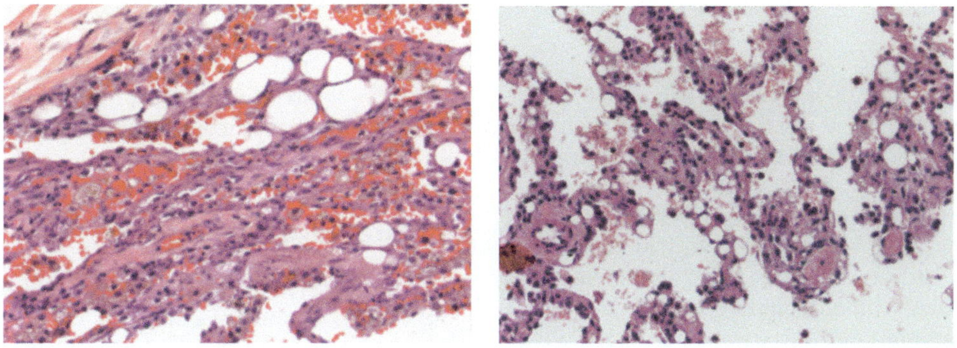

(a) (b)

FIGURE 2: (a) Lung parenchyma with intra-alveolar hemorrhage, multiple vacuoles, macrophages, and dilated capillaries (40X). (b) Lung parenchyma with dilated capillaries and nonrefractile vacuole-like structures (20X).

pulmonary infarction, cryptogenic organizing pneumonia, and chronic interstitial lung disease with atelectatic components at the dependent regions of both lungs. No pulmonary emboli to the segmental arteries were found.

She was admitted for treatment of community-acquired pneumonia and developed hemoptysis two days after admission, only completing four days of azithromycin and ceftriaxone. A bronchoscopy with lavage was performed. The bronchial cytology sample showed numerous macrophages, some with cytoplasmic vacuoles, and abundant blood, suggestive of diffuse alveolar hemorrhage.

She was subsequently transferred to the Medical Intensive Care Unit (MICU) with a differential diagnosis of systemic lupus erythematosus, Wegener's granulomatosis, pulmonary capillary hemangiomatosis, and other autoimmune and infectious diseases. Autoimmune laboratory workup for anti-beta 2 glycoprotein, antistreptolysin, ANA, anti-dsDNA, anticardiolipin, anti-GMB, anti-smooth muscle Ab, Anti-Jo, ssA, ssB, RF, p-ANCA, and c-ANCA showed negative results, ruling out the aforementioned autoimmune etiologies.

The patient tested negative for HIV. An infectious disease panel performed on the bronchoalveolar lavage samples of right and left lower lobes testing for HSV, CMV, EBV, PCP, atypical pneumonia panel (*M. pneumoniae*, *C. pneumoniae*, and *L. pneumophila*), viral panel (metapneumovirus, rhinovirus, influenza viruses A and B, RSV A and RSV B, parainfluenza viruses 1, 2, and 3, and adenovirus), *Aspergillus* galactomannan, and *Legionella pneumophila* showed negative results. Thus it decreased the likelihood of any previously mentioned infectious diagnosis.

A wedge biopsy tissue of the right lower lobe revealed intra-alveolar hemorrhage with dilated capillaries containing nonrefractile vacuole-like structures suggestive of deposition of lipoid material (Figures 2(a) and 2(b)). The lining of the dilated capillaries was positive for CD31 immunostain. Lymphatic spaces were also positive for D2-40 immunostain. No venoocclusive disease or features of arterial pulmonary hypertension were seen on EVG stain. These pathological findings raised concern for silicone embolism.

After discussion of the histological findings with the primary team, the patient was reinterrogated and she stated that she underwent twelve cosmetic subcutaneous silicone injections in the buttocks in the past by unlicensed practitioners. Her most recent injection occurred two months prior to this admission.

Within two weeks, she reported symptomatic improvement after supportive treatment and was discharged. Then, the patient was lost to follow-up.

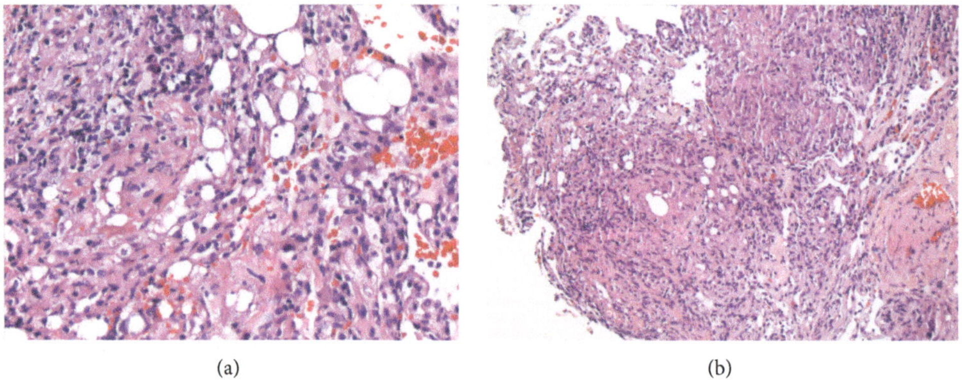

FIGURE 3: (a) Lung parenchyma with multiple vacuoles and dilated capillaries (40X). (b) Lung parenchyma with dilated capillaries and nonrefractile vacuole-like structures and histiocytic reaction (40X).

2.2. Clinical Case #2. A 33-year-old HIV-positive transgender male-to-female patient presented with an 8-month history of shortness of breath, dyspnea, and productive green sputum.

On physical examination, the patient's vital signs were within normal limits. She was afebrile and had 97% of O_2 saturation. The patient was not in acute distress; pulmonary breath sounds were clear to auscultation bilaterally without the presence of wheezing, crackles, or rhonchi. She had a regular heart rate and rhythm with no murmurs, rubs, or gallops. No signs of edema, clubbing, or cyanosis in her extremities were observed. She had good peripheral pulses and no gross neurological deficits.

There was high suspicion for silicone infiltration within the lung due to her recent history of cosmetic injections. Nonetheless, she was prescribed sulfamethoxazole and trimethoprim by her primary care physician (PCP), and the patient reported improving respiratory symptoms by being able to walk more than a mile, which was similar to her baseline. She denied any fevers or chills but reported weight loss and continued to indicate a cough productive of green sputum.

Chest X-ray showed bilateral hilar lymphadenopathy with increased interstitial markings. The chest CT without contrast showed mediastinal and hilar lymphadenopathies as well as ill-defined ground-glass opacities and nodular density, mainly along the pleural fissure and linear opacities on both lungs, predominantly in the right lower lung.

Laboratory tests conducted revealed WBC 3.4×10^9 per liter, hemoglobin 14 mg/dL, and platelets 325,000. Sodium was 139 mmol/L, BUN 16, and creatinine 1.5 mg/dL. Liver function tests showed an AST of 73 U/L, ALT of 62 U/L, and an alkaline phosphatase of 390 U/L. Recent CD4 was decreased from 584 to 367. A bronchoscopy was performed. The microbiology cultures of the bronchoalveolar lavage fluid were negative, while the cytology sample revealed granulomas. The biopsy tissue showed granulomatous inflammation associated with silicone particles in the lung tissue (Figures 3(a) and 3(b)).

She was treated with supportive therapy due to the likely etiology of silicone embolism and the symptomatic improvement.

3. Materials and Methods

A PubMed search using the key words "silicone", "embolism", and "subcutaneous injection" for the period from January 2004 through May 2015 was performed. There were 16 articles describing 29 patients who had been hospitalized with respiratory syndromes after subcutaneous silicone injections. Each article was reviewed for demographic and clinical information to draw further understanding of modern presentations of silicone embolism. The resulting information was then compared with a previous review article written by Schmid et al., in which 33 patients presented with respiratory symptoms in the period from 1965 to January 2004 [2].

4. Results

After comparison with the previous review article, we concluded that, over the last 12 years, the number of published articles per year describing silicone embolism has increased by almost threefold from that reported in the preceding 40 years. In our systematic review, including our two case reports, the literature has collectively described 16 transgender male-to-female patients (51.6%), 10 women (32.3%), and 5 men (16.1%) [2]. Among the cases in which the age was stated, the mean age was 31.2 years (age range, 22 to 53 years), which is about the same average age described by Schmid et al. [2]. However, there was an increase in proportion of transgender male-to-female patients from 45% to 51.6%, a decrease in female patients from 55% to 32.3%, and 5 cases of male patients (16.1%) (Figure 4). Within the male patients, additional social identifiers demonstrated that three were homosexual males and two were competitive bodybuilders who injected liquid silicone into their arms and pectoralis muscles.

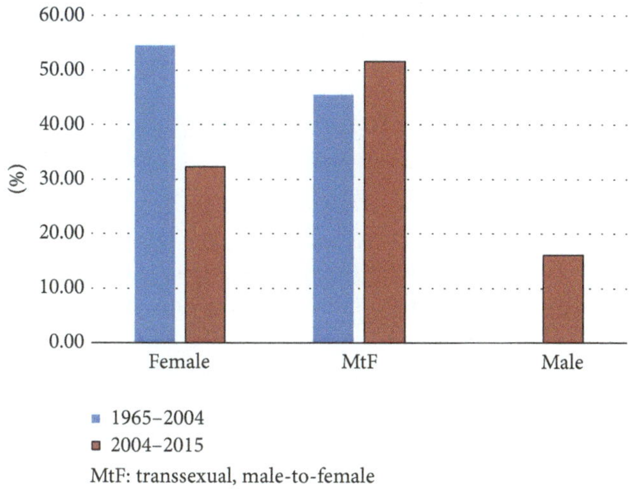

FIGURE 4: Difference in patient's demographic analysis by gender between two time periods (1965–2004 versus 2004–2015).

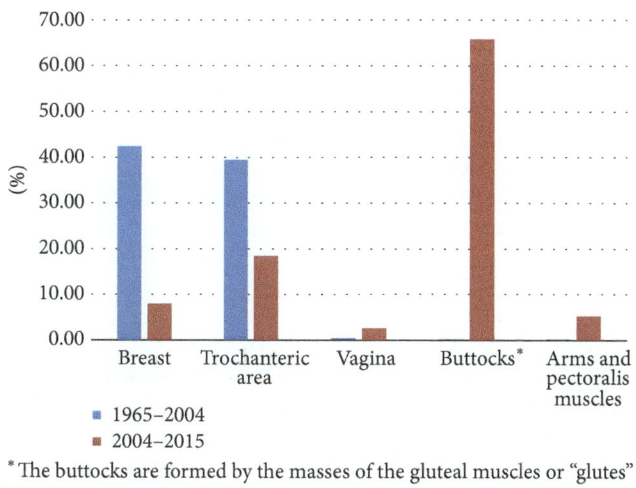

FIGURE 5: Difference in site of injections between two time periods (1965–2004 versus 2004–2015).

Another distinctive change over the last twelve years has been regarding the sites of injection. Previously, the majority of silicone injections were into the breast (14 patients or 45%) and trochanteric area (13 patients or 39%) while the buttocks (1 patient or 3%) were an uncommon site of injection. Presently, the buttocks (25 patients or 65.8%) are the most common site of injection, followed by the trochanteric (7 patients or 18.4%) and breast area (3 patients or 7.9%) (Figure 5). These results confirm a significant growth in the number of patients presenting with silicone embolism and the differences in the social context in which these patients may be present.

5. Discussion

Clinical findings associated with the diagnosis of silicone embolism include hypoxia (92%), dyspnea (88%), fever (70%), alveolar hemorrhage (64%), and cough (52%), all of which are similar to the presentation of an adipose tissue embolism [2–18]. As discussed by Schmid et al. [2], the pathophysiology of silicone embolisms is similar to that of fat emboli. Release of emboli leads to occlusion of the microvasculature, triggering an inflammatory response [19, 20]. Resulting hemorrhage and edema may lead to pulmonary consequences similar to that of respiratory failure and acute respiratory distress syndrome (ARDS) [21, 22]. Generally, silicone embolisms secondary to cosmetic procedures present in the first two days following a silicone injection. However, in some circumstances, such as those in our cases, the presentation may follow months after the injection [12, 23].

Computed tomography most often shows peripherally distributed ground-glass opacities associated with interlobular septal thickening, similar to what can be observed in some eosinophilic lung diseases and fat embolisms [8], as illustrated in our case (Figure 1(b)). However, a clinical and radiographic finding alone cannot provide a definitive diagnosis.

The characteristic histological findings for possible silicone embolism include dilated capillaries and nonrefractile vacuole-like structures. However, if pertinent information regarding prior cosmetic injections is not included in the clinical history, then further workup might prove necessary. Dark-field microscopy is helpful in revealing the refractile character of silicone [24, 25]. Using 48 to 72 hours modified Oil Red O stain in formalin-fixed, paraffin-embedded tissue sections may also be useful in revealing the presence of silicone embolus [24]. Positive results will aid in making a diagnosis, but negative results demand further evaluation.

The current literature describes the use of scanning electron microscopy with energy dispersive X-ray analysis and infrared spectroscopy, which will positively identify the sample as a type of silicone [16, 24]. Unfortunately, these procedures can only be performed by specially trained personnel and are typically only available at large medical centers. Bronchoalveolar lavage can be helpful when macrophages with intracytoplasmic inclusions of the substance are visible [23, 26]. However, the presence of intra-alveolar hemorrhage may obscure the cells and increase the difficulty of identifying the inclusions.

In our first case, physicians were uninformed of the patient's previous cosmetic silicone injections and the presentation was not a typical picture of pulmonary embolism. Therefore, pathological findings played a major role in determining an accurate diagnosis. Other entities may mimic silicone embolism, such as exogenous lipid pneumonia, bone marrow embolism, pseudo-lipid pneumonia, and bubble artefacts. Bubble artefacts are a result of escaping air from alveolar spaces during manipulation. Histologically, these appear as sharply demarcated spaces within an alveolar space to join an adjacent one or an alveolar sac. The spaces have no cellular lining and do not elicit histiocytic reaction (Figure 3(b)).

A review of the data illustrates the recent increase of complications after cosmetic silicone injection procedures, thus demonstrating the need for safer, standardized procedures and for reducing the number of unlicensed individuals performing them. This review highlights the importance of physicians to include silicone embolism in the differential diagnosis for patients with the discussed clinical presentation regardless of cosmetic surgical history.

Conflict of Interests

The authors declare that there is no conflict of interests regarding the publication of this paper.

References

[1] A. Rahimtoola and J. D. Bergin, "Acute pulmonary embolism: an update on diagnosis and management," *Current Problems in Cardiology*, vol. 30, no. 2, pp. 61–114, 2005.

[2] A. Schmid, A. Tzur, L. Leshko, and B. P. Krieger, "Silicone embolism syndrome: a case report, review of the literature, and comparison with fat embolism syndrome," *Chest*, vol. 127, no. 6, pp. 2276–2281, 2005.

[3] G. E. Gurvits, "Silicone pneumonitis after a cosmetic augmentation procedure," *The New England Journal of Medicine*, vol. 354, no. 2, pp. 211–212, 2006.

[4] E. A. Price, H. Schueler, and J. A. Perper, "Massive systemic silicone embolism: a case report and review of literature," *The American Journal of Forensic Medicine and Pathology*, vol. 27, no. 2, pp. 97–102, 2006.

[5] R. F. Clark, F. L. Cantrell, A. Pacal, W. Chen, and D. P. Betten, "Subcutaneous silicone injection leading to multi-system organ failure," *Clinical Toxicology*, vol. 46, no. 9, pp. 834–837, 2008.

[6] R. D. M. Ronsoni, F. L. Schwingel, L. H. Melo et al., "Pulmonary embolism due to liquid silicone: case report," *Respiratory Medicine Extra*, vol. 3, no. 4, pp. 172–174, 2007.

[7] R. Parikh, K. Karim, N. Parikh, P. Han, J. Daoko, and F. E. Shamoon, "Case report and literature review: acute pneumonitis and alveolar hemorrhage after subcutaneous injection of liquid silicone," *Annals of Clinical and Laboratory Science*, vol. 38, no. 4, pp. 380–385, 2008.

[8] C. S. Restrepo, M. Artunduaga, J. A. Carrillo et al., "Silicone pulmonary embolism: report of 10 cases and review of the literature," *Journal of Computer Assisted Tomography*, vol. 33, no. 2, pp. 233–237, 2009.

[9] S. Bartsich and J. K. Wu, "Silicon emboli syndrome: a sequela of clandestine liquid silicone injections. A case report and review of the literature," *Journal of Plastic, Reconstructive and Aesthetic Surgery*, vol. 63, no. 1, pp. e1–e3, 2010.

[10] L. B. Mongero, D. Brodie, J. Cunningham et al., "Extracorporeal membrane oxygenation for diffuse alveolar hemorrhage and severe hypoxemic respiratory failure from silicone embolism," *Perfusion*, vol. 25, no. 4, pp. 249–254, 2010.

[11] D. Mendonca, D. S. Leitao, R. Friend, J. Epelboim, and G. Eiger, "An unusual case of pulmonary embolism," *Respiratory Care*, vol. 57, no. 8, pp. 1345–1347, 2012.

[12] L. P. Hariri, H. A. Gaissert, R. Brown et al., "Progressive granulomatous pneumonitis in response to cosmetic subcutaneous silicone injections in a patient with HIV-1 infection: case report and review of the literature," *Archives of Pathology and Laboratory Medicine*, vol. 136, no. 2, pp. 204–207, 2012.

[13] A. C. Zamora, H. R. Collard, L. Barrera, F. Mendoza, W. Richard Webb, and G. Carrillo, "Silicone injection causing acute pneumonitis: a case series," *Lung*, vol. 187, no. 4, pp. 241–244, 2009.

[14] P. Gopie, S. Sakhamuri, A. Sharma, S. Solomon, and S. Teelucksingh, "Acute pneumonitis secondary to subcutaneous silicone injection," *International Journal of General Medicine*, vol. 4, pp. 477–479, 2011.

[15] E. Pastor, A. L. Andreu, and E. Chiner, "Acute pneumonitis and adult respiratory distress syndrome after subcutaneous injection of liquid silicone," *Archivos de Bronconeumologia*, vol. 41, no. 12, pp. 702–703, 2005.

[16] K. Y. Chung, S. H. Kim, I. H. Kwon et al., "Clinicopathologic review of pulmonary silicone embolism with special emphasis on the resultant histologic diversity in the lung—a review of five cases," *Yonsei Medical Journal*, vol. 43, no. 2, pp. 152–159, 2002.

[17] J. Chastre, P. Brun, P. Soler et al., "Acute and latent pneumonitis after subcutaneous injections of silicone in transsexual men," *American Review of Respiratory Disease*, vol. 135, no. 1, pp. 236–240, 1987.

[18] S. K. Dawn, B. M. Elicker, J. W. T. Leung, G. P. Reddy, and M. B. Gotway, "The silicone syndrome," *Clinical Pulmonary Medicine*, vol. 13, no. 2, pp. 146–147, 2006.

[19] E. Schnaid, J. M. Lamprey, M. J. Viljoen, B. I. Joffe, and H. C. Seftel, "The early biochemical and hormonal profile of patients with long bone fractures at risk of fat embolism syndrome," *Journal of Trauma*, vol. 27, no. 3, pp. 309–311, 1987.

[20] N. Meyer, W. T. Pennington, D. Dewitt, and G. J. Schmeling, "Isolated cerebral fat emboli syndrome in multiply injured patients: a review of three cases and the literature," *The Journal of Trauma*, vol. 63, no. 6, pp. 1395–1402, 2007.

[21] T. C. Fabian, A. V. Hoots, D. S. Stanford, C. R. Patterson, and E. C. Mangiante, "Fat embolism syndrome: prospective evaluation in 92 fracture patients," *Critical Care Medicine*, vol. 18, no. 1, pp. 42–46, 1990.

[22] P. J. Broe, T. J. K. Toung, S. Margolis, S. Permutt, and J. L. Cameron, "Pulmonary injury caused by free fatty acid: evaluation of steroid and albumin therapy," *Surgery*, vol. 89, no. 5, pp. 582–587, 1981.

[23] J. Chastre, F. Basset, F. Viau et al., "Acute pneumonitis after subcutaneous injections of silicone in transsexual men," *The New England Journal of Medicine*, vol. 308, no. 13, pp. 764–767, 1983.

[24] M. Lewin-Smith, V. Kalasinsky, K. Shilo, J. Tomashefski, and A. Cropp, "Detection of silicone in lung tissue," *Archives of Pathology & Laboratory Medicine*, vol. 136, no. 10, pp. 1179–1180, 2012.

[25] D. S. Raso, W. B. Greene, J. J. Vesely, and M. C. Willingham, "Light microscopy techniques for the demonstration of silicone gel," *Archives of Pathology & Laboratory Medicine*, vol. 118, no. 10, pp. 984–987, 1994.

[26] T. Duong, A. J. Schonfeld, M. Yungbluth, and R. Slotten, "Acute pneumopathy in a nonsurgical transsexual," *Chest*, vol. 113, no. 4, pp. 1127–1129, 1998.

50

Perivascular Epithelioid Cell Tumour with Intraorbital Location: Report of a Case and Review of the Literature

Idania Lubo,[1] Ileana Fermín,[1] Olindo Massarelli,[2] Roberta Gobbi,[2] and Paolo Cossu Rocca[3]

[1]*Anatomy and Pathology Institute "Dr. José Antonio O'Daly", Central University of Venezuela, Los Chaguaramos 1040, Caracas, Venezuela*
[2]*Maxillofacial Surgery Unit, University of Sassari, Italy*
[3]*Department of Histopathology and Anatomical Pathology, University of Sassari, Italy*

Correspondence should be addressed to Idania Lubo; icaluju@gmail.com

Academic Editor: Maria M. Picken

The Perivascular Epithelioid Cell tumours (PEComas) are rare mesenchymal neoplasms recognized as entity by the World Health Organization. The tumour cells have an uncertain origin and are characterized by distinctive histological and immunohistochemical features. We report a case of PEComa occurring as intraorbital lesion in a 47-year-old man. We found only two other cases described in the literature and we considered all three cases together in order of histology, immunohistochemistry, and clinical outcome. We found a strict histological overlapping and quite similar immunohistological results. All three cases showed a favourable clinical course probably related to small size of tumours (<5 cm), low mitotic rate (<2 mitoses in 50 HPF), and absence of necrosis.

1. Introduction

Bonetti et al. [1] firstly proposed the descriptive name of Perivascular Epithelioid Cells (PEC) in 1992, whereas Zamboni et al. [2] subsequently introduced the term PEComa in 1996. The Perivascular Epithelioid Cell tumours (PEComas) represent a family of rare mesenchymal neoplasms, including angiomyolipoma (AML), clear cell "sugar" tumour (CCST) of the lung, lymphangioleiomyomatosis (LAM), clear cell myomelanocytic tumour (of the falciform ligament/ligament teres), and unusual clear cell tumours of the pancreas, rectum, abdominal serosa, uterus, vulva, thigh, and heart [3]. The tumour is more frequent in females than in males (6 : 1) with a median age of 45 years. Some cases are associated with the Tuberous Sclerosis Complex, especially AML, CCST, and LAM [3].

Although the tumour cells have an uncertain origin, they however display histological and immunohistochemical distinctive features. Owing to the variety of condition of origin, the histological pattern is not uniform, the constant features being represented by a nested architecture composed of epithelioid cells with abundant eosinophilic or clear granular cytoplasm typically surrounded by thin capillary vessels. On immunohistochemical ground the cells characteristically express HMB45 but are negative for S100 protein.

The site of origin of this tumour is extremely variable and has been reported in kidney, bladder, prostate, uterus, ovary, vulva and vagina, lung, pancreas, liver, GIT, nasal cavity, soft tissues, retroperitoneum, and bone [4].

Orbital location is exceptionally rare. At the best of our knowledge, up to date, only 2 other cases have been described in the literature [5, 6]. We present a case of intraorbital Perivascular Epithelioid Cell neoplasm along with a comparison of the 2 previously reported cases.

2. Case Presentation

A 47-year-old male patient complained of progressive diplopia lasting 4 months. Otherwise the patient was in a healthy condition. Ophthalmological examination revealed a marked hypofunction of the left inferior oblique muscle.

Magnetic resonance imaging (MRI) showed an intraorbital, extraconal, oval, capsulated mass measuring 2.0 × 1.5 cm, located inferomedially in the anterior part of the left orbit. The medial rectus muscle appeared cranially displaced

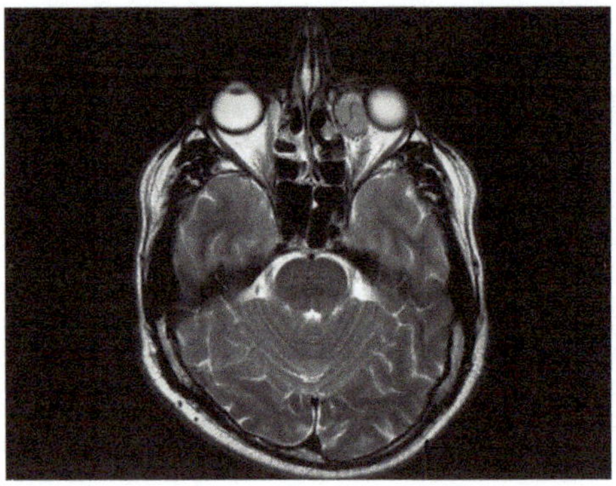

(a)

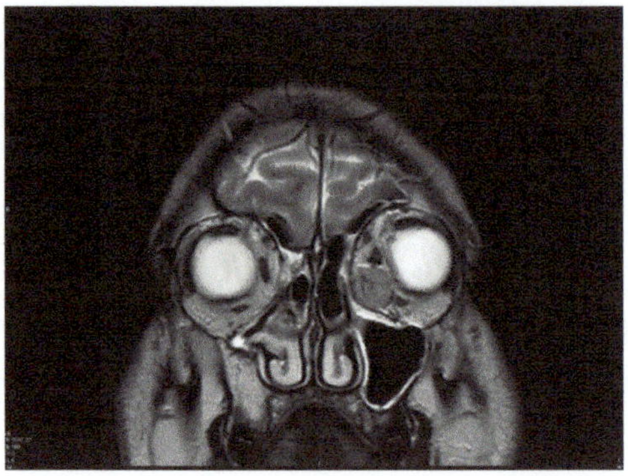

(b)

Figure 1: RMI: (a) Coronal T2 MRI scan shows an oval, encapsulated, vascularized, inferomedial, and extraconal mass in the left orbit. The mass displaces the eyeball and the inferior rectus muscle laterally and the medial rectus muscle cranially. (b) Axial T2 MRI scan shows the mass located in the anterior part of the left extraconal medial orbit.

whereas the inferior rectus one was laterally displaced. After infusion of contrast medium the lesion showed a heterogeneous density reflecting hypervascularity (Figures 1(a) and 1(b)). The provisional radiologic diagnosis was benign tumour with high vascular component.

The patient underwent surgical operation at the Maxillofacial Surgery Unit of the University of Sassari for a benign left intraorbital mass of angiomatous nature. The tumour was completely removed in February 2012 through an inferior transconjunctival approach and a lateral canthotomy (Figure 2). The postoperative course was uneventful. Neither diplopia nor alterations of extrinsic ocular motility were observed. After 3 years of follow-up, the patient is free from disease.

At macroscopy the tumour appeared as a well-circumscribed nodule of 1.5 × 2.0 cm in diameter with a brown coloration (Figure 3).

Routinely processed paraffin-embedded tissue sections stained with haematoxylin and eosin (H&E) were evaluated. At histology the neoplasm showed a well-circumscribed, capsulated, expansive growth, formed by a cell proliferation arranged in vascular trabecular features or in solid cords. The cells were plump and large and showed an epithelioid phenotype with vesicular round nuclei, (small or large) nucleoli, and a low mitotic activity (2 mitoses in 50 HPF). The cells showed a clear or finely granular cytoplasm, sometimes containing a granular brown pigment. No necrosis was observed (Figures 4(a) and 4(b)).

The preliminary microscopic diagnosis was "angiomatous proliferation with epithelioid large cells resembling PEComa." In order to better define the nature of the tumour, a panel of histochemical and immunohistochemical staining was performed, including Perls' Prussian blue and Schmörl techniques, CD 31, CD 34, Desmin, α-SMA, Vimentin, Cytokeratins AE1/AE3, CK8/18, Chromogranin-A (CgA), CD 10, HMB45, Melan A, and S100 protein.

The brown pigment was Perls' negative but Schmörl positive, so indicating melanin granules. At immunohistochemistry the cells were negative for all types of Cytokeratins,

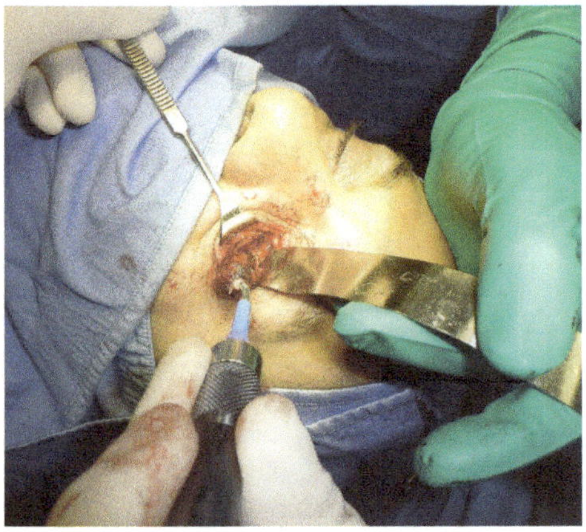

Figure 2: Intraoperative view: through transconjunctival approach and lateral canthotomy (swinging eyelid incision), we performed a subperiosteal orbital floor dissection. Then, the periorbita was incised inferiorly and medially. The well-encapsulated lesion was removed using a cryoprobe, pulling it laterally.

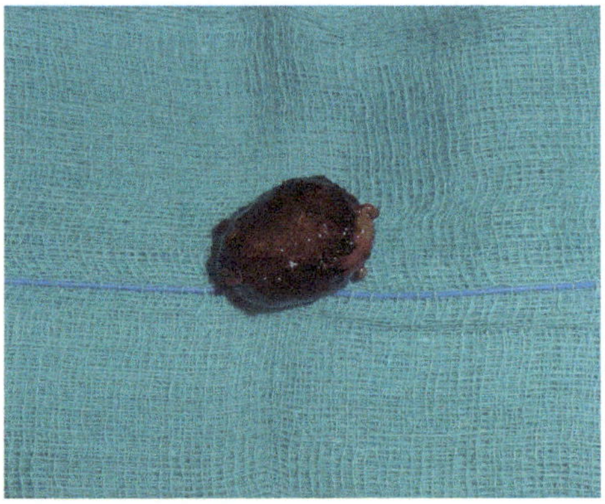

Figure 3: Macroscopy: the tumour mass appeared as a well-circumscribed nodule of 2.0 × 1.5 cm, brown in color.

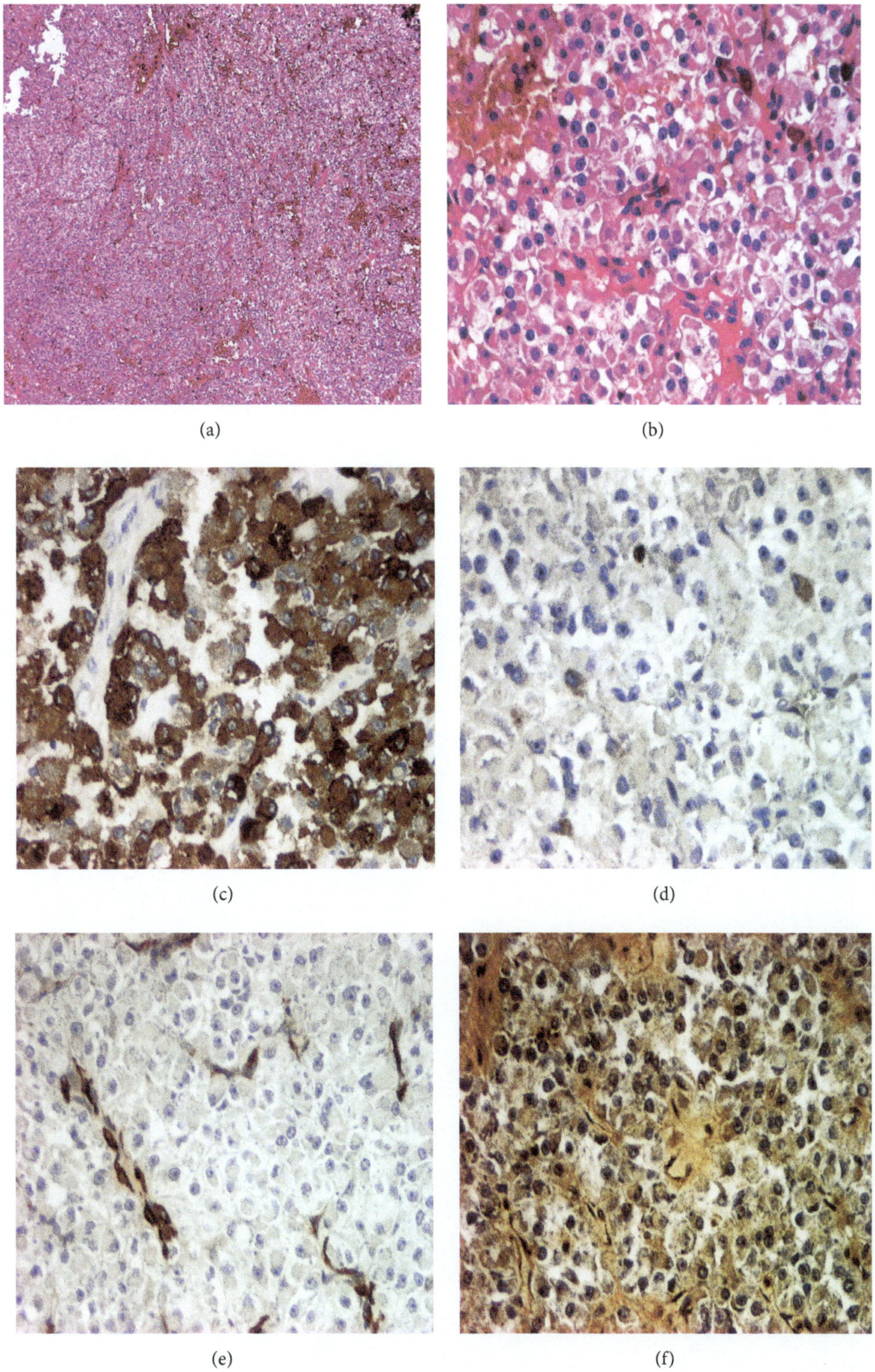

FIGURE 4: Histology: (a) trabecular architecture and nested growth pattern. HE, 40x. (b) Cell proliferation with an eosinophilic or clear granular cytoplasm; a prominent vasculature composed of delicate thin-walled capillaries was also appreciable. HE, 200x. (c) Immunohistochemical staining showing positivity for HMB45. 200x. (d) Immunohistochemical staining showed negativity for S100 protein. 200x. (e) Immunohistochemical staining for α-SMA showed slight staining in tumour cells. 200x. (f) Immunohistochemical staining showed focal positivity for Calponin. 200x.

Table 1: Summary of main features of intraorbital PEComas.

Author	Sex	Age	Dimensions	Histology	IHC	Outcome
Iyengar et al. 2005 [5]	F	9	1.2 × 1.0 × 0.8 cm	Solid architecture with nests and trabeculae of epithelioid cells with abundant clear to eosinophilic cytoplasm. The uniform nuclei were oval to round with small nucleolus and dispersed chromatin. Within the lesion, a few cells had fine melanin pigment granules. There were infrequent mitoses. No evidence of necrosis	HMB45+ + + MART1− − − S100− − H&LMW CK− − EMA− − α-actin+ + − Desmin− − Calponin+ + VIM− CgA− −	No recurrence after 7 months of follow-up
Guthoff et al. 2008 [6]	M	54	1.5 × 1.0 × 1.0 cm	Solid trabecular tumour cells show intimate association with ramified vascular network. The tumour cells are large with a clear to eosinophilic granular cytoplasm and round to oval nuclei. Few cells contained melanin. Proliferation index (Ki 67) was very low (<1%)	HMB45+ + + MART1+ + + S100− − HMW CK− − α-actin− − Desmin− − VIM− CD 31− − CgA− − MiTF− −	No recurrence after 17 months of follow-up
Our case	M	47	2.0 × 1.5 cm	The neoplasm showed a well-circumscribed, capsulated, expansive growth, formed by a cell proliferation arranged in vascular trabecular features or in solid cords. The cells were plump and large and showed an epithelioid phenotype with vesicular round nuclei, small nucleoli, and a low mitotic activity (2 mitoses in 10 HPF). The cells showed a clear or finely granular cytoplasm, sometimes containing a granular brown melanin pigment. No necrosis was observed	HMB45+ + + MART1− − S100− − H&LMW CK− − CK8/18− − α-actin+ Desmin− − Calponin+ VIM− − CD 31− − CD 34− − CgA− − MiTF− − TFE3− −	No recurrence after 40 months of follow-up

CD 31, and CD 34, while they were positive for HMB-45 (Figure 4(c)) but negative for Melan-A and S100 protein (Figure 4(d)). The cells were also negative for Vimentin, Desmin, and CgA. Slight positivity for α-SMA was observed (Figure 4(e)). The histological diagnosis was myomelanocytic tumour or melanocytoma belonging to the Perivascular Epithelioid Cell neoplasms (PEComas) group without true evidence of malignancy. Because of its infrequent location, the case was sent in consultation to the Verona Group [1] which confirmed the diagnosis. According to previous descriptions of immunohistochemical markers expression in PEComas arising at different sites [7], a second line of IHC was hence performed using antibodies against microphthalmia transcription factor (MiTF), transcription factor E3 (TFE3), and muscle marker Calponin. No immunostaining with MiTF and TFE3 antibodies was observed, whereas focal positivity for Calponin was appreciable (Figure 4(f)).

3. Discussion

In relation to histology and location of the tumour, different differential diagnostic hypotheses were considered: firstly a possible primary tumour as epithelioid haemangioma, paraganglioma, and epithelioid melanoma or secondly a metastasis from tumours with low malignant potential, such as renal cell carcinoma. All these possibilities have been reported in the literature [8–13].

The immunohistochemical procedures performed account for the strategy applied in order to clarify the diagnosis.

The negativity for CD 31 and CD 34 spoke against an angiomatous proliferation although these antibodies clearly stained a prominent vascular network of small vessels around the cells. Also Vimentin was negative, so excluding a mesenchymal derivation of the tumour. Furthermore, the absent expression of high and low molecular weight Cytokeratins did not support the hypothesis of a metastatic renal cell carcinoma and the CgA negativity was against the supposition of a paraganglioma. The positivity for HMB45 aroused the idea of melanoma, but the negativity for S100 protein and Melan A (Mart1) aborted this possibility too.

Therefore, considering morphology (large, plump cells with clear cytoplasm sometimes containing granular pigment Schmörl positive) and the immunohistochemical results (negativity for Cytokeratins, Vimentin, and α-SMA, and positivity only for HMB45) the diagnosis of Perivascular Epithelioid Cell tumour was considered the most plausible. Since the location of this tumour is unusual in the orbit, the case was sent for a second opinion to Bonetti and Zamboni group that confirmed the diagnosis.

In Table 1 we collected our case with those reported in the literature [5, 6] and we observed a quite complete histological similarity with only slight but not substantial responses to IHC, all consisting with the diagnosis of PEComa.

In our table we did not consider the two cases of ocular PEComas reported by Furusato et al. [14] since they were in extraorbital location, although these authors included in their review Iyengar et al.'s cases [5, 6]. However, the histological and immunohistological features were totally overlapping with the intraorbital PEComas.

Given the rarity of PEComas, clear criteria for malignancy have not been established so that the prognosis cannot be accurately determined. However, taking into account that none of the three cases of intraorbital PEComa had recurrences (up to 40 months of follow-up in our case), tumours with size below 5 cm and low mitotic rate without evidence of necrosis could be *bona fide* considered benign according to Folpe criteria [15].

Conflict of Interests

The authors declare that there is no conflict of interests regarding the publication of this paper.

Acknowledgment

The authors are indebted to Professor Giovannino Massarelli, University of Sassari, for his invaluable help in preparing and revising the paper.

References

[1] F. Bonetti, M. Pea, G. Martignoni, and G. Zamboni, "PEC and sugar," *The American Journal of Surgical Pathology*, vol. 16, no. 3, pp. 307–308, 1992.

[2] G. Zamboni, M. Pea, G. Martignoni et al., "Clear cell 'sugar' tumor of the pancreas. A novel member of the family of lesions characterized by the presence of perivascular epithelioid cells," *The American Journal of Surgical Pathology*, vol. 20, no. 6, pp. 722–730, 1996.

[3] J. L. Hornick and C. C. Pan, "PEComa," in *WHO Classification of Tumours of Soft Tissue and Bone*, C. D. M. Fletcher, J. A. Bridge, P. C. W. Hogendoorn, and F. Mertens, Eds., pp. 230–231, IARC Press, Lyon, France, 2013.

[4] G. Martignoni, M. Pea, D. Reghellin, G. Zamboni, and F. Bonetti, "PEComas: the past, the present and the future," *Virchows Archiv*, vol. 452, no. 2, pp. 119–132, 2008.

[5] P. Iyengar, D. D. DeAngelis, M. Greenberg, and G. Taylor, "Perivascular epithelioid cell tumor of the orbit: a case report and review of the literature," *Pediatric and Developmental Pathology*, vol. 8, no. 1, pp. 98–104, 2005.

[6] R. Guthoff, T. Guthoff, H. K. Mueller-Hermelink, J. Sold-Darseff, and E. Geissinger, "Perivascular epithelioid cell tumor of the orbit," *Archives of Ophthalmology*, vol. 126, no. 7, pp. 1009–1011, 2008.

[7] K. Thway and C. Fisher, "PEComa: morphology and genetics of a complex tumor family," *Annals of Diagnostic Pathology*, vol. 19, no. 5, pp. 359–368, 2015.

[8] B. Alder, A. Proia, and J. Liss, "Distinct, bilateral epithelioid hemangioma of the orbit," *Orbit*, vol. 32, no. 1, pp. 51–53, 2013.

[9] B. Miličić, T. Velnar, R. Pregelj, and C. Limbaeck-Stokin, "Multiple epithelioid hemangiomas with orbital involvement," *Case Reports in Pathology*, vol. 2015, Article ID 629805, 5 pages, 2015.

[10] R. Makhdoomi, K. Nayil, V. Santosh, and S. Kumar, "Orbital paraganglioma—a case report and review of the literature," *Clinical Neuropathology*, vol. 29, no. 2, pp. 100–104, 2010.

[11] A. Bagheri, M. Aletaha, H. Salour, A. Abdollahi, D. Silbert, and M. Rezaei-Kanavi, "Orbital paraganglioma presenting as lateral rectus enlargement and its novel management. A case report and review of literature," *Orbit*, vol. 31, no. 4, pp. 256–260, 2010.

[12] A. N. Odashiro, B. Arthurs, P. R. Pereira, J. P. S. Filho, E. Belfort, and M. N. Burnier Jr., "Primary orbital melanoma associated with a blue nevus," *Ophthalmic Plastic and Reconstructive Surgery*, vol. 21, no. 3, pp. 247–248, 2005.

[13] R. Rai, F. A. Jakoblec, and A. Fay, "Ocular metastatic renal carcinoma presenting with proptosis," *Ophthalmic Plastic & Reconstructive Surgery*, vol. 31, no. 4, pp. e101–e108, 2015.

[14] E. Furusato, J. D. Cameron, R. W. Newsom et al., "Ocular perivascular epithelioid cell tumor: report of 2 cases with distinct clinical presentations," *Human Pathology*, vol. 41, no. 5, pp. 768–772, 2010.

[15] J. S. Bleecker, J. F. Quevedo, and A. L. Folpe, "'Malignant' perivascular epithelioid cell neoplasm: risk stratification and treatment strategies," *Sarcoma*, vol. 2012, Article ID 541626, 12 pages, 2012.

51

Fibrolipoma of the Buccal Mucosa: A Case Report and Review of the Literature

Masayasu Iwase, Naotaka Saida, and Yoko Tanaka

Department of Dentistry and Oral Surgery, Hakujikai Memorial General Hospital, 5-11-1 Shikahama, Adachi-ku, Tokyo 123-0864, Japan

Correspondence should be addressed to Masayasu Iwase; iwase@dent.showa-u.ac.jp

Academic Editor: Marco Mazzocchi

Lipomas are common benign soft tissue neoplasms derived from mature adipose tissue. However, they rarely arise in the oral cavity. Fibrolipoma is a histological variant of lipoma that mainly affects the buccal mucosa and causes functional and cosmetic issues. This article describes the case of a 71-year-old male with a fibrolipoma of the left buccal mucosa and a review of previous articles about fibrolipoma.

1. Introduction

Lipomas are common benign neoplasms derived from adipose tissue. The etiology of lipomas is uncertain. They mainly affect the trunk region, shoulders, upper arms, and neck [1], and lipomas of the oral cavity are rare, accounting for 1 to 4% of benign oral tissue tumors [2, 3]. Oral lipomas can occur at various sites including the major salivary glands, buccal mucosa, tongue, lips, palate, vestibule, and the floor of the mouth. A number of case reports have described cases in which lipoma or variants of lipoma arose in various oral locations [3, 4]. Histologically, lipomas can be classified into classic lipoma and variant forms of lipoma, such as fibrolipomas, spindle lipomas, intramuscular lipomas, angiolipomas, salivary gland lipomas, pleomorphic lipomas, myxoid lipomas, and atypical lipomas [1, 3, 4]. There have only been a few reports about fibrolipoma of the oral cavity [5–8]. We describe the case of a patient with fibrolipoma of the buccal mucosa.

2. Case Presentation

A 71-year-old male patient visited our hospital with a chief complaint of swelling of the left buccal mucosa. The swelling had first been noticed two years earlier and had subsequently exhibited gradual continuous enlargement. The patient had bitten the swollen region of his buccal mucosa several times, causing bleeding and pain. An intraoral examination revealed a pinkish, ill-defined oval swelling in the left buccal mucosa (Figure 1). On palpation, the swelling was mainly soft but firm in parts; nonfluctuant; and mobile, and its margins were unclear. The firm regions were composed of scar tissue. The provisional diagnosis was lipoma. A magnetic resonance imaging (MRI) scan of the lesion showed well-defined borders and low signal intensity on both T_1- and T_2-weighted images (Figure 2). The lesion was excised under local anesthesia. The excised specimen appeared to be encapsulated, soft, and pinkish in color and measured 25 × 15 mm (Figure 3). During a histopathological examination, the lesion was found to have an overlying epithelium and to be composed of mature adipose tissue within dense collagen fibers (Figure 4). As a result, it was histologically classified as a fibrolipoma. The patient's postoperative course was uneventful. No recurrence of the lesion has been observed after 6 months.

3. Discussion

Fibrolipoma is a histological variant of lipoma characterized by a significant fibrous component intermixed with lobules of adipose tissue [1, 5, 8]. The consistency of such lesions

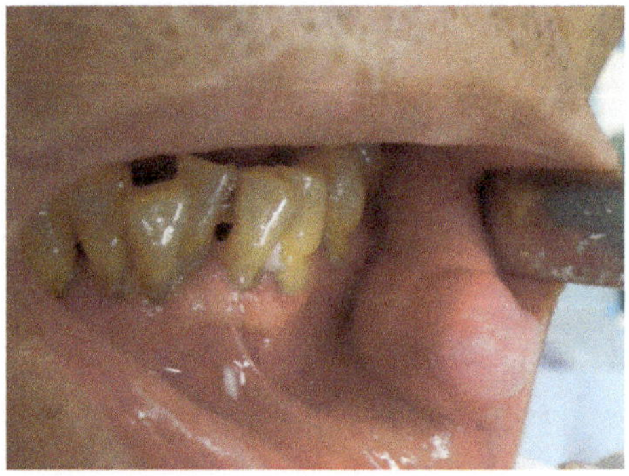

FIGURE 1: Preoperative intraoral view showing a solitary swelling in the buccal mucosa.

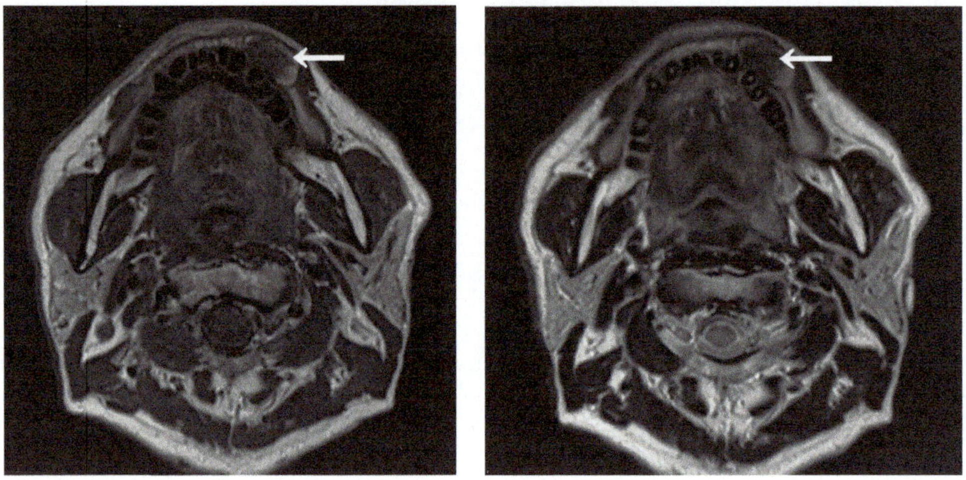

(a) (b)

FIGURE 2: MRI findings of the lesion. MRI showed a well-defined mass that exhibited low signal intensity on both (a) T_1- and (b) T_2-weighted images.

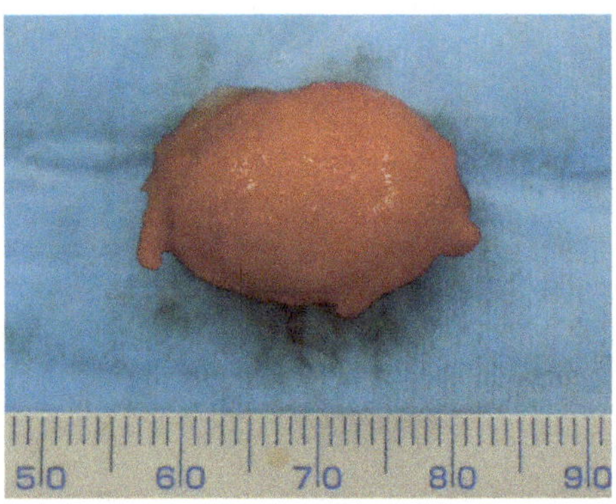

FIGURE 3: Gross appearance of the lesion. The excised specimen was pinkish in color, displayed a soft consistency, and measured 20 × 15 mm in size.

varies from soft to firm, depending on the quantity and distribution of fibrous tissue and the depth of the tumor [1, 5]. Fibrolipomas most commonly arise in the buccal mucosa, followed by the tongue, which is also true for classic lipomas [3, 5]. Oral lipoma and its variants have been reported to occur in all age groups but are most frequently seen in patients ranging in age from 40 to 60 years [3, 4, 9, 10]. Previous studies have reported that lesions in the oral cavity exhibit a mean diameter of 2 cm [3, 4]. Therefore, the present case did not involve any particularly unusual clinical findings.

In large case series studies of lipoma and variants of lipoma of the oral cavity, it was found that fibrolipoma accounted for 1.6% [4] and 8.3% [9] of lesions, respectively. However, other similar case series studies have reported a very high incidence of fibrolipoma [3, 10]. These discrepancies cannot be explained by racial or geographic characteristics. As the classification of lipomas depends on the quantity of fibrous tissue present, the diagnosis of such lesions relies on pathologists' judgments. To the best of our knowledge, about 40 cases of fibrolipoma of the oral cavity are described in the English literature [5–8].

The etiopathogeneses of lipoma and fibrolipoma remain unknown. A previous study suggested that fibrolipoma (1) is a congenital lesion caused by an endocrinal imbalance, (2) arises via the degeneration of a fibromatous tumor, or (3) arises from the maturation of lipoblastomatosis [11].

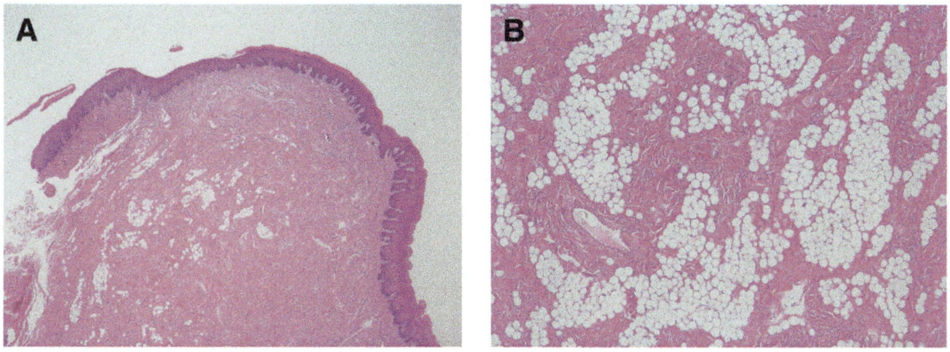

(a) (b)

FIGURE 4: Histological findings of the lesion. (a) A histological examination showed that the lesion contained an overlying epithelium and adipose tissue within dense collagen fibers (hematoxylin and eosin stain, ×10) and (b) mature adipose tissue interspersed by broad bands of dense connective tissue (×40).

On the other hand, another study described a fibrolipoma that formed beneath a complete denture [12]. It has also been suggested that repeated mild trauma can trigger the proliferation of fatty tissue [2]. We consider that the present case involved a classic lipoma and hyperplasia of fibrous tissue caused by repeated chewing-related trauma.

MRI has been reported to be useful for diagnosing lipomatous lesions of the oral cavity [1, 13]. Lipomas generally display high signal intensity and appear to be well-encapsulated masses on both T_1- and T_2-weighted images [1, 14]. However, in the present case the lesion demonstrated low signal intensity on MRI. It is possible that the fibroma-like findings exhibited by the lesion on MRI were due to the fact that it contained abundant collagenous fibers. The nonadipose components of lipomas have been found to display decreased signal intensity on all pulse sequences [1].

Lipoma is mainly treated by surgical excision [1]. The prognosis of lipoma is generally favorable, and recurrence is unlikely when surgery is performed appropriately. However, a case in which a lipoma of the buccal mucosa, which was diagnosed by biopsy, underwent transformation to liposarcoma has been reported [15]. In a previous study, the proliferative activity of lipomas was examined by immunohistochemically analyzing the expression of proliferating cell nuclear antigen and Ki-67. As a result, it was suggested that Ki-67 expression is indicative of recurrence or malignant transformation [9]. Another study found that fibrolipoma exhibits higher Ki-67 expression than classic lipoma and other variants of lipoma [3]. The present patient should be examined for malignant changes during the follow-up period.

Conflict of Interests

The authors have no conflict of interests to declare.

References

[1] L. W. Bancroft, M. J. Kransdorf, J. J. Peterson, and M. I. O'Connor, "Benign fatty tumors: classification, clinical course, imaging appearance, and treatment," *Skeletal Radiology*, vol. 35, no. 10, pp. 719–733, 2006.

[2] J. G. A. M. de Visscher, "Lipomas and fibrolipomas of the oral cavity," *Journal of Maxillofacial Surgery*, vol. 10, no. 3, pp. 177–181, 1982.

[3] E. R. Fregnani, F. R. Pires, R. Falzoni, M. A. Lopes, and P. A. Vargas, "Lipomas of the oral cavity: clinical findings, histological classification and proliferative activity of 46 cases," *International Journal of Oral and Maxillofacial Surgery*, vol. 32, no. 1, pp. 49–53, 2003.

[4] M. A. Furlong, J. C. Fanburg-Smith, and E. L. B. Childers, "Lipoma of the oral and maxillofacial region: site and subclassification of 125 cases," *Oral Surgery, Oral Medicine, Oral Pathology, Oral Radiology and Endodontology*, vol. 98, no. 4, pp. 441–450, 2004.

[5] B. S. Manjunatha, G. S. Pateel, and V. Shah, "Oral fibrolipoma-a rare histological entity: report of 3 cases and review of literature," *Journal of Dentistry*, vol. 7, no. 4, pp. 226–231, 2010.

[6] M. Khubchandani, N. R. Thosar, R. N. Bahadure, M. S. Baliga, and R. N. Gaikwad, "Fibrolipoma of buccal mucosa," *Contemporary Clinical Dentistry*, vol. 3, no. 5, supplement 1, pp. S112–S114, 2012.

[7] T. Pereira, S. Shetty, S. Sapdhare, and A. Tamgadge, "Oral fibrolipoma: a rare histological variant," *Indian Journal of Dental Research*, vol. 25, no. 5, pp. 672–674, 2014.

[8] G. Laconetta, M. Friscia, A. Cecere, A. Romano, G. D. Orabona, and L. Califano, "Rare fibrolipoma of the tongue: a case report," *Journal of Medical Case Reports*, vol. 9, article 177, 2015.

[9] T. Naruse, S. Yanamoto, S.-I. Yamada et al., "Lipomas of the oral cavity: clinicopathological and immunohistochemical study of 24 cases and review of the literature," *Indian Journal of Otolaryngology and Head & Neck Surgery*, vol. 67, supplement 1, pp. S67–S73, 2015.

[10] E. Manor, N. Sion-Vardy, B. Z. Joshua, and L. Bodner, "Oral lipoma: analysis of 58 new cases and review of the literature," *Annals of Diagnostic Pathology*, vol. 15, no. 4, pp. 257–261, 2011.

[11] A. Epivatianos, A. K. Markopoulos, and P. Papanayotou, "Benign tumors of adipose tissue of the oral cavity: a clinicopathologic study of 13 cases," *Journal of Oral and Maxillofacial Surgery*, vol. 58, no. 10, pp. 1113–1117, 2000.

[12] R. L. Kiehl, "Oral fibrolipoma beneath complete mandibular denture," *The Journal of the American Dental Association*, vol. 100, no. 4, pp. 561–562, 1980.

[13] Y. Taira, K. Yasukawa, I. Yamamori, and M. Iino, "Oral lipoma extending superiorly from mandibular gingivobuccal fold to gingiva: a case report and analysis of 207 patients with oral lipoma in Japan," *Odontology*, vol. 100, no. 1, pp. 104–108, 2012.

[14] T. Chikui, K. Yonetsu, K. Yoshiura et al., "Imaging findings of lipomas in the orofacial region with CT, US, and MRI," *Oral Surgery, Oral Medicine, Oral Pathology, Oral Radiology, and Endodontology*, vol. 84, no. 1, pp. 88–95, 1997.

[15] K. Yamada, Y. Dohara, M. Nagata, K. Kawashima, and S. Yamashita, "A case of liposarcoma of the cheek," *Japanese Journal of Clinical Oncology*, vol. 9, no. 1, pp. 123–129, 1979.

52

Trichohepatoenteric Syndrome or Syndromic Diarrhea—Report of Three Members in a Family, First Report from Iran

F. E. Mahjoub,[1,2,3,4] F. Imanzadeh,[5] S. Mahdavi Izadi,[1] and A. Nahali Moghaddam[4]

[1] *Imam Khomeini Hospital Complex, Tehran University of Medical Sciences, Tehran 14197-33141, Iran*
[2] *Maternal, Fetal and Neonatal Research Center, Tehran University of Medical Sciences, Tehran 14197-33141, Iran*
[3] *Pediatric Nephrology Research Center, Tehran University of Medical Sciences, Tehran 14197-33151, Iran*
[4] *Roshan Azma Pathobiology Private Laboratory, Tehran 15149-35754, Iran*
[5] *Pediatric Gastroenterology, Mofid Children Hospital, Shahid Beheshti University of Medical Sciences, Tehran 15514-15468, Iran*

Correspondence should be addressed to F. E. Mahjoub; fmahjoub@sina.tums.ac.ir

Academic Editor: Amit Agrawal

Introduction. Intractable diarrhea of infancy (IDI) includes several types of early onset diarrhea; one of the rare etiologies is trichohepatoenteric (THE) syndrome, also known as syndromic diarrhea (SD) which was primarily described by Stankler et al. Hereby we report a family with several affected members which to our knowledge is the first case report from Iran. *Report of Cases.* A three-year-old boy referred with short stature, poor weight gain, and intermittent steatotic diarrhea to our center. He was born to healthy, relative parents (cousins). He did not gain any weight after four months of age and began having intermittent steatotic diarrhea, abdominal distension, and fever. He was hospitalized several times. Two other children in the family also showed somewhat similar symptoms. Two sweat tests were negative for cystic fibrosis. Workup for Celiac disease was performed several times which was negative; however, gluten-free diet was tried several times which was not effective. Workup for Hirschsprung's disease was performed but colon was ganglionic. Evidence of liver involvement was approved by elevated liver enzymes and coarse echo of liver on sonography. *Discussion.* Trichoenterohepatic syndrome should be put in mind in cases of intractable diarrhea presenting in a family with several affected members. Early diagnosis would save patients from unnecessary workups.

1. Introduction

Diarrhea is a common disease among children and constitutes a major etiology for their morbidity and mortality, so understanding different pathologies that cause diarrhea is of importance [1]. Intractable diarrhea of infancy (IDI) is a term which includes several types of early onset diarrhea, one of the rarest is trichohepatoenteric (THE) syndrome, also known as syndromic diarrhea (SD). THE syndrome was primarily described by Stankler et al. in 1982, in two siblings, presenting with diarrhea, failure to thrive, abnormal facies, and unusual hair [2]. Following reports on other cases revealed similarities in signs and symptoms. The most common observed signs are intractable diarrhea, usually starting before six months of age, dysmorphic facies such as prominent forehead and cheeks, broad nasal root and hypertelorism, abnormal hair, disorders of immune system, intrauterine growth retardation, skin abnormalities, and liver function disorders [1, 3, 4]. Distinct hair abnormalities such as woolly, easily removable hair and poorly pigmented hairs are seen even in children with middle eastern origin [3]. Microscopic examination of hair shafts reveals nonspecific abnormalities such as twisted hair (pili torti), aniso- and poikilotrichosis, trichorrhexis nodosa, and longitudinal breaks [3]. Even with treatment, most patients have a small final stature [3–5]. Fine motor movement abnormalities and mental retardation are seen in most affected children [3]. Liver disease (liver enlargement and cirrhosis) is reported in more than half of the children [1]. Investigations show the association between mutations in TTC37 (encodes the putative

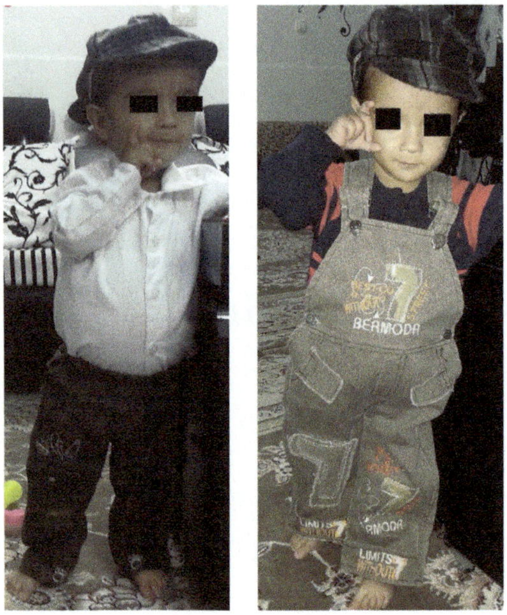

(a) (b)

FIGURE 1: (a) and (b) Note the prominent forehead and cheeks, hypertelorism and broad nasal root, short stature, and abdominal distention of the child.

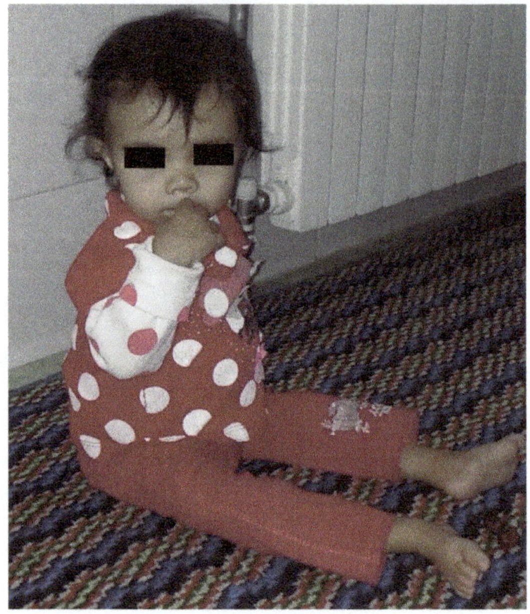

FIGURE 2: A one-year-old girl with failure to thrive and motor delay. Note facial dysmorphism (hypertelorism and broad nasal root).

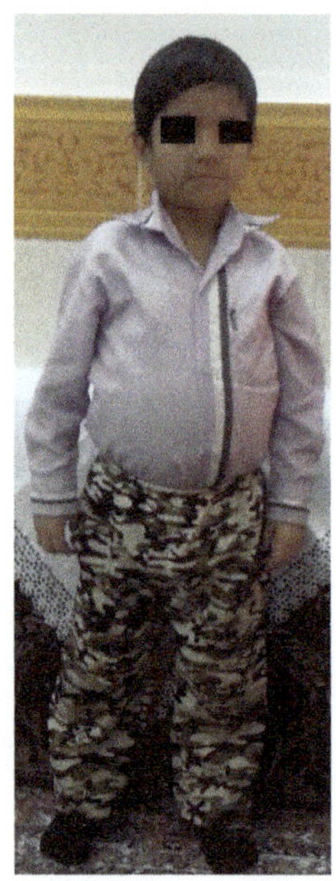

FIGURE 3: A nine-year-old boy with failure to thrive and abdominal distention. Note facial dysmorphism (hypertelorism and broad nasal root).

protein thespin) and SKIV2L with THE syndrome [1, 4, 6, 7]. The pattern of transmission is autosomal recessive [3]. Diagnosis is mainly based on observing different clinical signs, usually in a patient presenting with diarrhea. Intestinal biopsies are more useful for ruling out differential diagnosis of intractable diarrhea than to confirm the diagnosis of THE syndrome, since there are no specific changes related to this disease [1, 3]. Most patients need parenteral nutrition and do not reach their optimal growth eventually [3, 8].

There are also few reports about patients with hemochromatosis of liver associated with this syndrome [9, 10].

Definite diagnosis of the disease is problematic due to variable clinical presentations, nondiagnostic changes in pathology samples, and general lack of an accessible diagnostic test [6, 9].

2. Report of the Cases

A three-year-old boy was born to healthy, related parents (cousins). The pregnancy was uneventful and he was born full term, weighing 3.100 kilograms, and 51 cm in height. He was breastfed and experienced normal growth for the first 4 months and reached 5 kilograms. He had poor weight gain afterwards (recent weight: 8.5 Kg) and began having intermittent steatotic diarrhea and abdominal distension and was hospitalized several times for workup of failure to thrive. As seen in the attached photo facial dysmorphism (prominent forehead, broad based nasal bridge, and hypertelorism) is evident (Figures 1(a) and 1(b)). Hair changes such as woolly and easily removable hair and light coloration were evident in our case. Two other children in the family (his cousin a one-year-old girl weighing 7 Kg with developmental delay and another cousin a 9-year-old boy weighing 16 Kg) also showed somewhat similar symptoms (Figures 2 and 3). Pictures were provided by the family and they were informed about writing of this paper and the paper was submitted after their consent for publishing the pictures with covered eyes.

Several stool exams were performed and were negative for ova, parasites, white blood cells, and red blood cells but were intermittently positive for fat. Stool trypsin activity test was normal. Complete blood cell count (CBC) constantly showed microcytic anemia. Two sweat tests were negative

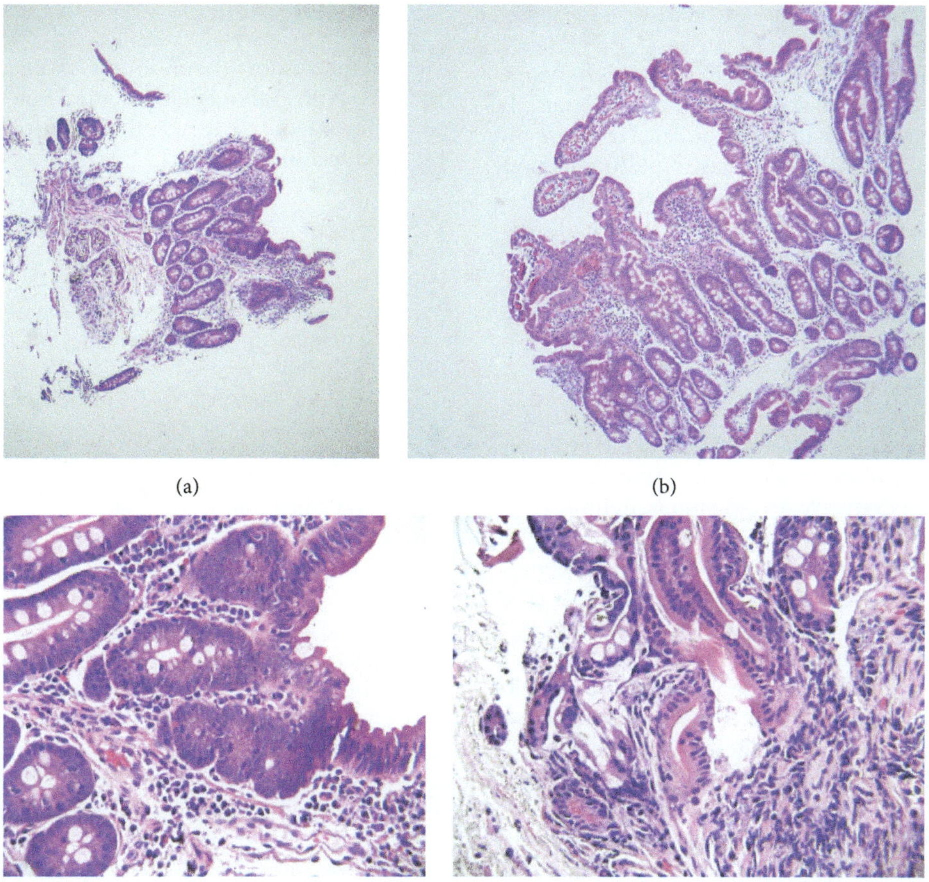

FIGURE 4: Duodenal mucosa: (a) and (b) moderate to severe shortening of most villi (few rather tall villi are seen in picture (b)). (c) Focal superficial epithelial changes (poor gobletting, irregularity of lining cells) (intraepithelial lymphocytes: under 10/100). There is also mild to moderate infiltration of lymphoplasma cells and some eosinophils (3–7/100) in lamina propria. (d) Note crypt architectural changes.

for cystic fibrosis. Multiple testing for Anti-TTG showed variable results (mostly revealed mild elevation). Gluten-free diet was instituted several times but was not effective. Human Leukocyte Antigen (HLA) typing for DQ2 and DQ8 was negative. Workup for Hirschsprung's disease (due to abdominal distention) was performed at 21 months of age, but colon was ganglionic. Thyroid function tests were normal. Insulin Growth Factor 1 (IGF-1) was lower than normal in one occasion (7.34 ng/mL, normal: 27.4–113.5 ng/mL). Abdominal sonography at 1.5 years of age showed coarse and nonhomogeneous echo of liver. AST and ALT were mildly elevated. Upper gastrointestinal endoscopy showed evidence of esophagitis and mild atrophic duodenitis. Biopsy from esophagus and mucosa of second part of duodenum was performed. Microscopic examination of esophageal mucosa showed moderate esophagitis. In duodenal mucosa, the villi were mildly to moderately short in well oriented areas. Focal superficial epithelial changes were seen (reduced number of goblet cells, irregularity of lining cells) (Intraepithelial lymphocytes: under 10/100). Crypt hyperplasia cannot be assessed; however, crypts show marked difference in size, branching, and distortion. There was mild to moderate infiltration of lymphoplasma cells and some eosinophils (3–7/100) in lamina propria, distorting some of the crypts. No giardia lamblia parasites are seen (Figure 4).

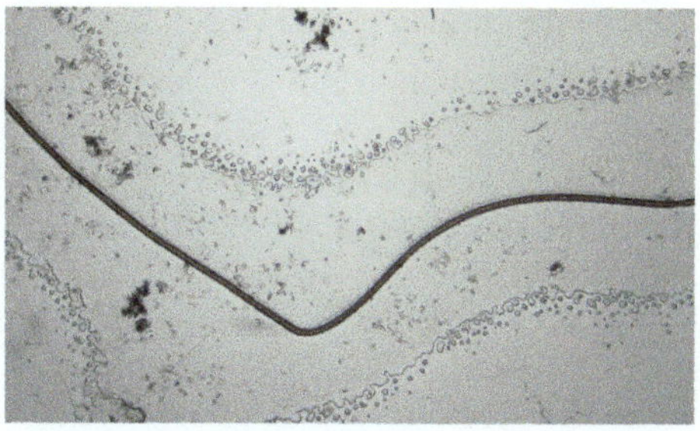

FIGURE 5: Hair shaft of the child showing kinking.

Microscopic examination of hair shafts of the first case revealed aniso- and poikilotrichosis with kinking and breakage but no typical trichorrhexis nodosa was seen (Figure 5).

Hair changes in cases 2 and 3 are mild and not as prominent as case 1, which denotes that spectrum of changes is seen in the family. Also the index patient suffers from severe dental problems (caries) leading to loss of most teeth. No skin or cardiac involvement is present in patients.

No further workup for liver disease and liver biopsy was performed for the patient.

The case was consulted with Professor Elizabeth Montgomery (Johns Hopkins School of Medicine, USA) and, in light of clinical symptoms (facial dysmorphism, hair anomaly, and hepatic involvement along with gastrointestinal symptoms) and affection of several family members, diagnosis of trichohepatoenteric syndrome was established. Genetic testing is not available yet in Iran. Diagnosis was accepted readily by pediatric gastroenterologists and the patient was relieved from further repetitive and time consuming workup tests.

3. Discussion

Despite high prevalence of diarrhea in children and availability of several tests for investigating different etiologies, still in many cases, even with extensive investigations, definite diagnosis cannot be reached. Moreover we are yet far from developing a way to control the etiology in many cases. Trichoenterohepatic syndrome was first described by Stankler et al. in 1982 [2]. Since then several cases have been reported and researchers have concluded that the diagnosis is mainly suspected by clinical signs and symptoms such as persistent diarrhea, facial dysmorphism, abnormal hair, and involvement of liver. To date the confirmatory diagnostic test is sequencing of TTC37 and SKIV2L genes [1, 4, 7] and microscopic examination of intestinal biopsies is more useful in ruling out other causes of chronic diarrhea such as tufting enteropathy and congenital microvillus atrophy. Treatment of these children is mainly symptom-relieving actions such as parenteral nutrition to help with growth, sometimes immunoglobulin supplementation, and, in those with severe liver disease, liver transplant [1]. Even with treatment, most patients have a small final stature [3–5]. About half of them show a slight mental retardation, but the main observed complications are liver disease and infections. Understanding the genetic defect of the disease gives hope to better perception of the pathology of the disease and perhaps a better management of patients.

Diagnosis was delayed for several years in our patient and he underwent unnecessary workups such as biopsy of colonic wall and testing for celiac disease several times. A careful clinical examination and thorough asking about family history (presence of affected members, consanguinity) would have helped to reach to a diagnosis sooner and save patient from time consuming and invasive workups.

Although genetic testing is the definite diagnostic test, unfortunately it is not yet available for this syndrome in our country; however, the symptoms and family history leave no doubt about the diagnosis.

Our cases showed no evidence of overt mental retardation which is seen in some cases although motor delay was seen in the one-year-old girl mentioned.

Conflict of Interests

The authors declare that there is no conflict of interests regarding the publication of this paper.

Acknowledgments

Hereby the authors thank Professor Elizabeth Montgomery, Johns Hopkins School of Medicine, United States of America, for reviewing the case. Also they thank Ms. Zahra Omidi for her kind technical support.

References

[1] J. L. Hartley, N. C. Zachos, B. Dawood et al., "Mutations in TTC37 cause trichohepatoenteric syndrome (phenotypic diarrhea of infancy)," *Gastroenterology*, vol. 138, no. 7, pp. 2388.e2–2398.e2, 2010.

[2] L. Stankler, D. Lloyd, R. J. Pollitt, E. S. Gray, H. Thom, and G. Russell, "Unexplained diarrhoea and failure to thrive in 2 siblings with unusual facies and abnormal scalp hair shafts: a new syndrome," *Archives of Disease in Childhood*, vol. 57, no. 3, pp. 212–216, 1982.

[3] O. Goulet, C. Vinson, B. Roquelaure, N. Brousse, C. Bodemer, and J.-P. Cézard, "Syndromic (phenotypic) diarrhea in early infancy," *Orphanet Journal of Rare Diseases*, vol. 3, article 6, 2008.

[4] A. Fabre, C. Martinez-Vinson, O. Goulet, and C. Badens, "Syndromic diarrhea/Tricho-hepato-enteric syndrome," *Orphanet Journal of Rare Diseases*, vol. 8, article 5, 2013.

[5] A. Fabre, A. Breton, M.-E. Coste et al., "Syndromic (phenotypic) diarrhoea of infancy/tricho-hepato-enteric syndrome," *Archives of Disease in Childhood*, vol. 99, no. 1, pp. 35–38, 2014.

[6] O. Egritas, B. Dalgic, and M. Onder, "Tricho-hepato-enteric syndrome presenting with mild colitis," *European Journal of Pediatrics*, vol. 168, no. 8, pp. 933–935, 2009.

[7] A. Fabre, C. Martinez-Vinson, B. Roquelaure et al., "Novel mutations in TTC37 associated with tricho-hepato-enteric syndrome," *Human Mutation*, vol. 32, no. 3, pp. 277–281, 2011.

[8] O. Goulet, C. Vinson, B. Roquelaure, N. Brousse, C. Bodemer, and J.-P. Cézard, "Syndromic (phenotypic) diarrhea in early infancy," *Orphanet Journal of Rare Diseases*, vol. 3, no. 1, article 6, 2008.

[9] I. Dweikat, M. Sultan, N. Maraqa, T. Hindi, S. Abu-Rmeileh, and B. Abu-Libdeh, "Tricho-hepato-enteric syndrome: a case of hemochromatosis with intractable diarrhea, dysmorphic features, and hair abnormality," *American Journal of Medical Genetics Part A*, vol. 143, no. 6, pp. 581–583, 2007.

[10] A. Verloes, J. Lombet, Y. Lambert et al., "Tricho-hepato-enteric syndrome: further delineation of a distinct syndrome with neonatal hemochromatosis phenotype, intractable diarrhea, and hair anomalies," *American Journal of Medical Genetics*, vol. 68, no. 4, pp. 391–395, 1997.

53

Biliary Adenofibroma with Invasive Carcinoma: Case Report and Review of the Literature

Anjali Godambe,[1] Elizabeth M. Brunt,[2] Keith H. Fulling,[3] and Taher Reza Kermanshahi[4]

[1]*Ameripath Indiana, Indianapolis, IN, USA*
[2]*Department of Pathology and Immunology, Washington University, St. Louis, MO, USA*
[3]*Mercy Hospital, St. Louis, MO, USA*
[4]*Department of Pathology, University of Pittsburgh Medical Center, Pittsburgh, PA, USA*

Correspondence should be addressed to Anjali Godambe; agodambe@ameripath.com

Academic Editor: Hiroko Kuwabara

We report a case of biliary adenofibroma with an invasive carcinoma in a 71-year-old female who presented with bilateral upper abdominal pain. Imaging revealed a 6.3 cm heterogeneously enhancing mass in the left lateral segment of the liver. Histologically, the adenofibroma showed the characteristic components as previously described of biliary adenofibromata, namely, cystic and tubular structures lined by cuboidal to low columnar biliary type epithelium and a dense fibrous stroma composed of spindled cells. Intimately admixed with the adenofibroma was a distinct tumor composed of malignant clear cells which demonstrated stromal and vascular invasion. Although mitotic figures were inconspicuous, Ki67 was brisk and p53 demonstrated 25–50% positivity. Sections also showed a von Meyenberg complex located adjacent to the tumor. This case expands the understanding of this rare tumor and proves two important assertions from previous case reports. First, the presence of an associated von Meyenberg complex with similar morphology and immunohistochemical staining pattern suggests that biliary adenofibromata and von Meyenberg complexes may share related histogenesis. Second, biliary adenofibromata harbor malignant potential and may show malignant transformation. Furthermore, this case highlights the need for these rare tumors to be followed aggressively, as their biological behavior is poorly understood.

1. Introduction

Biliary adenofibromata are extremely rare tumors with unknown etiology and previously uncertain malignant potential. The tumor was first described by Tsui et al. in 1993 and since then nine cases have been reported in the medical literature. Biliary adenofibromata are characterized by cystic and tubular biliary epithelial components surrounded by a bland fibroblastic spindled stroma [1]. The tumors bear a striking resemblance to bile duct hamartomas (von Meyenberg complexes); a similarity that has been noted in all previously reported cases in the medical literature. Until this report, von Meyenberg complexes have not been identified in histologic sections of tumor or adjacent uninvolved liver.

2. Case Report

A 71-year-old Caucasian female presented with chest pain. Her subsequent workup included a chest CT which revealed a 6.3 cm mass in the right aspect of the left lateral liver straddling segments 2, 3, and 4a. The tumor was best visualized in the precontrast and arterial phases. Contrast enhancement was heterogeneous throughout the mass with multiple areas of low attenuation. Of note, a PET scan showed a 1.9 cm hypermetabolic focus within a 4.3 cm tumor. The patient reported bilateral upper abdominal pain but denied any nausea, vomiting, and weight loss or gain during this period. She had no jaundice, change in bowel habits, or gastrointestinal bleeding. There was no history of significant

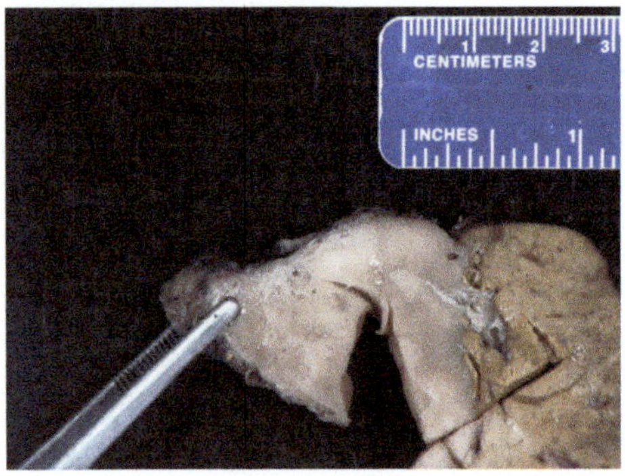

FIGURE 1: Tumor and surrounding liver parenchyma.

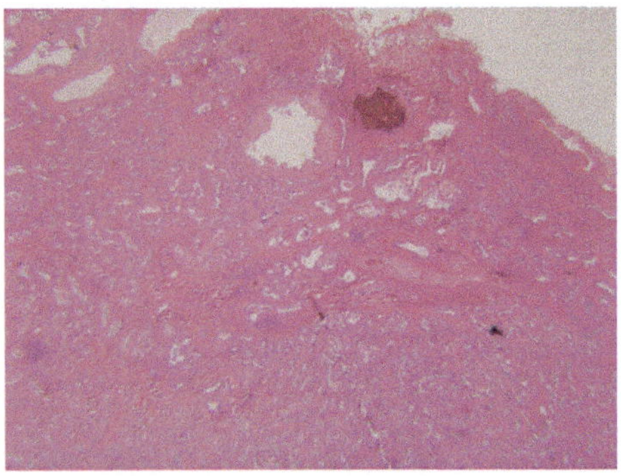

FIGURE 2: Conventional biliary adenofibroma, H&E 4x.

alcohol or intravenous drug use. The patient had no history of transfusions. She denied personal or family history of liver or biliary disease. Laboratory tests revealed normal liver function testing, serum alpha fetoprotein, CEA, and CA19-9. A biopsy was performed and showed biliary epithelium arranged in cysts and tubules with a fibrotic/spindled stroma. Subsequently, the patient underwent a left hepatectomy. Intraoperative palpation of the abdominal cavity revealed no signs of carcinomatosis. There were no postoperative complications. The patient reported no symptoms after surgery.

2.1. Macroscopic Findings. The partial lobectomy from the left lobe contained a circumscribed tumor measuring 5.7 cm that abutted and appeared to invade the liver capsule. The cut surface revealed a smooth tan-white surface with subtle variegation in color and firmness. Small cystic spaces were noted throughout the tumor (Figure 1). The surrounding hepatic parenchyma was unremarkable.

2.2. Microscopic Findings. The tumor showed tubulocystic structures embedded in a bland spindled stroma, consistent with a conventional biliary adenofibroma (Figure 2). A distinct carcinomatous component was identified showing solid, glandular, and papillary architecture. The malignant component showed an infiltrative border with invasion into the liver capsule and additionally showed penetration into surrounding adhesions and skeletal muscle. Perineural tumor infiltration, intravenous invasion, and single cell stromal invasion were seen. The tumor was focally seen in the adventitia of a large outflow vein. Although the tumor appeared grossly circumscribed, microscopic examination showed infiltrative margins (Figure 3). The cells of the malignant component showed vacuolated cytoplasm with centrally placed nuclei.

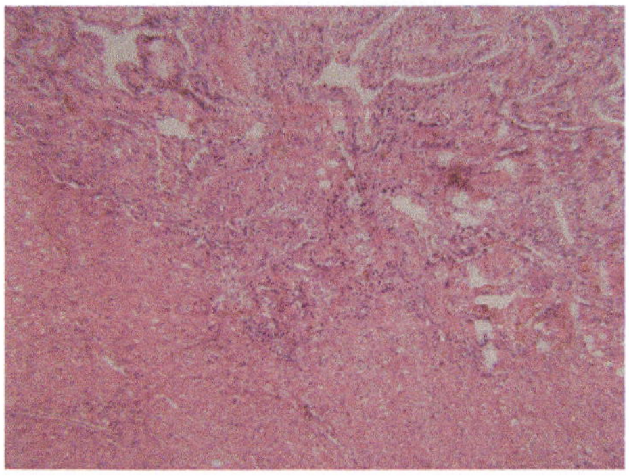

FIGURE 3: Infiltrative border of tumor to surrounding liver, H&E 10x.

To rule out metastasis from adrenal or renal primary sites, inhibin and PAX8 immunohistochemistries were performed and were negative. A cytokeratin 7 and cytokeratin 19 showed strong positivity in the bland tubulocystic areas of conventional biliary adenofibroma and a lesser degree of positivity in the solid and papillary carcinomatous areas. CD56 stained scattered single cells, similar to the reactivity of the ductular reaction in surrounding nontumor liver. A Ki-67 was uniformly brisk, despite inconspicuous mitotic figures. P53 showed moderate (25–50%) positivity in the tumor. Both Ki67 and p53 were negative in the stromal component. CD10 and polyclonal CEA failed to show either cytoplasmic or canalicular reactivity in tumor cells.

A von Meyenberg complex was seen in hepatic parenchyma adjacent to the tumor.

3. Discussion

These cases report the tenth biliary adenofibroma in the medical literature, although two previous reports both from Turkey report identical tumor and patient characteristics and most likely represent the same tumor [2, 3]. The tumor shows a tubulocystic component with a bland spindled stroma, as originally described by Tsui et al. in the first description of biliary adenofibromata. At that time, the similarity to von Meyenberg complexes was observed. Furthermore, bile pigment in the tumor ducts implied a direct continuity with the biliary system. Parada et al. reported monosomy 22 in a case of biliary adenofibroma in a 49-year-old woman. However, this finding was not consistently found in a subsequent report [4].

Malignant transformation of biliary adenofibromata has been described in two previous cases. Akin described a 25-year-old male who demonstrated a recurrent biliary adenofibroma with pulmonary metastasis two years after initial resection. However, histologic findings of the malignant transformation were not described. Nguyen et al. described a biliary adenofibroma with multiple foci of epithelial atypia,

TABLE 1: Clinical and pathologic features of biliary adenofibromata reported in the literature.

	Year	Age/sex	Tumor size	Ki67%	Associated malignancy	Follow-up
Tsui et al. [1]	1993	74/F	7 cm	Not performed	No	
Parada et al. [9]	1997	49/F	7 cm	Not performed	No	
Akin and Coskun [2]	2002	25/M	20 cm	Not performed	Yes	Pulmonary metastasis 3 years after initial diagnosis
Haberal et al. [3]	2001	21/M	25 cm	Not performed	No	
Garduño-López [10]	2002	68/F	6 cm	Not performed	No	50-month follow-up
Varnholt et al. [4]	2003	47/F	16 cm	Ki67: low stromal component negative	No	3-year follow-up
Gurrera et al. [11]	2010	79/M	5.5 cm	Ki67 1% stromal and epithelial	No	7-year follow-up
Kai et al. [5]	2012	40/M	7 cm	Ki67 5–10%	Unclassified multicystic biliary tumor	
Nguyen et al. [6]	2012	53/F	6.5 cm	Not performed	Yes	12-month follow-up no recurrence
Godambe et al. (present case)	2013	71/F	5.7 cm	Ki67 50% epithelial component	Yes	

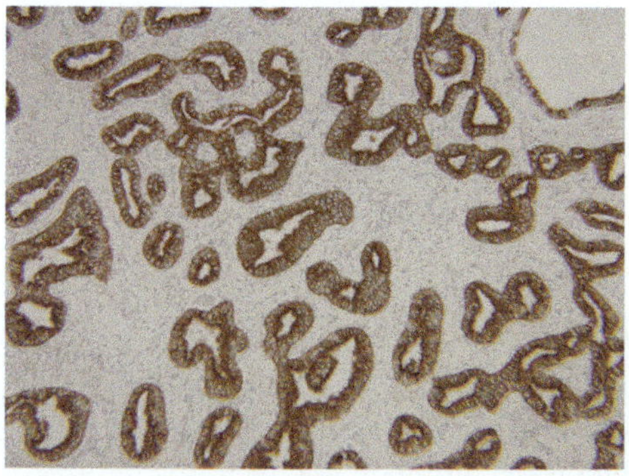

FIGURE 4: Conventional biliary adenofibroma, CK7, 10x.

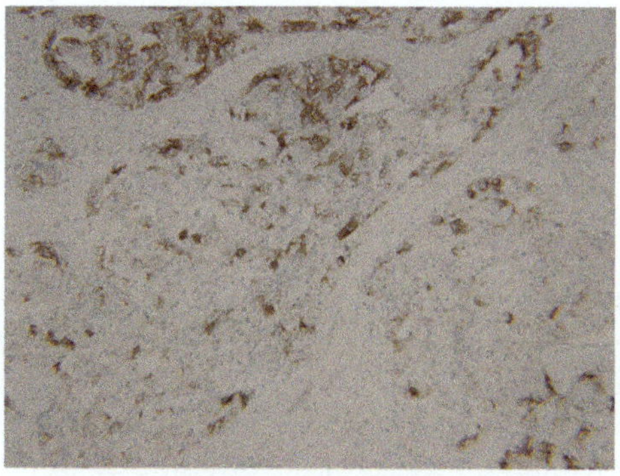

FIGURE 5: Invasive carcinoma, CK7, 10x.

including cytologic atypia and architectural atypia (cribriforming), representing high-grade dysplasia. They noted a microinvasive carcinoma (<1 mm) with increased atypia, including mildly enlarged epithelial cells with prominent nucleoli, a rare single cell in the stroma, and disrupted glands that merged with sclerotic stroma.

Our malignant component shows distinct histology and demonstrates nearly solid architecture. Immunohistochemical findings showed variable reactivity between the benign and malignant components. The bland tubulocystic glands of the conventional biliary adenofibroma stained strongly and homogeneously positive for cytokeratins 7 and 19, while the carcinomatous areas showed weaker and more variable staining for these cytokeratins (Figures 4 and 5). P53 has been reported in varying rates of positivity ranging from negative to 75% of cells displaying strong nuclear staining; however, case reports of biliary adenofibroma with malignant transformation have not included a description of p53 staining pattern [2, 3, 5, 6].

Although the origin of biliary adenofibromata is uncertain, there is undeniable histologic and immunohistochemical similarity to von Meyenberg complexes. Tsui et al. noted the resemblance to Meyenberg's complex; however, they described an absence of typical von Meyenberg complexes in the background liver. Varnholt et al. reported a case of biliary adenofibroma and furthermore characterized the tumoral glandular epithelium staining positive for D10, p53 (50–75% of the cells), keratin AE.3/Cam 5.2, cytokeratin 7, cytokeratin

19, carcinoembryonic antigen, and epithelial membrane antigen. They further noted that the epithelial lining did not stain for IF6. Bile duct adenomas and peribiliary glands express foregut antigens, designated D10 and IF6, and the secretion of acid mucins. (Normal bile ductules and canals of Hering demonstrate positivity for IF6 but not D10, whereas larger bile ducts may demonstrate D10 positivity in 22% of cases, with an absence of IF6 [7].)

A similar pattern of D10 positivity/IF6 negativity was reported in one bile duct hamartoma. Thus, Varnholt et al. concluded that although the origin of biliary adenofibroma is unknown, the epithelial expression of D10 but not IF6 suggests an origin similar to bile duct hamartoma [4].

von Meyenberg complexes are largely considered benign and indolent; however, neoplastic transformation has been rarely reported. The most common malignancy arising in the setting of ductal plate malformations (including von Meyenberg complexes, biliary cystic lesions, and congenital hepatic fibrosis) is cholangiocarcinoma. Hepatocellular carcinomas, adenosquamous carcinomas, squamous cell carcinomas, and papillomas have also been reported [8]. The carcinoma seen in our case is difficult to classify precisely; however, it shows unequivocal features of malignancy. A summary of published tumor characteristics is included in Table 1.

This case of biliary adenofibroma with invasive carcinoma significantly expands the understanding of this rare tumor. While the presence of a von Meyenberg complex in liver adjacent to tumor does not prove the cellular origin of the tumor, the identification of a von Meyenberg complex in sections adjacent to tumor supports the observation that these tumors may share similar histogenesis as its immunomorphologic counterpart. Despite previous case reports describing a malignant transformation, biliary adenofibromata are currently generally regarded as benign entities. It is clear that they harbor potential for malignant transformation and therefore should be considered a premalignant tumor. P53 immunohistochemical stain has been performed in multiple cases in an effort to predict biological behavior. While the stromal component is consistently negative, the epithelial component demonstrates wide variability in staining and perhaps provides a mechanism to stratify risk of malignant transformation. As these tumors are poorly understood, patients require close clinical follow-up and observation.

Conflict of Interests

The authors declare that there is no conflict of interests regarding the publication of this paper.

References

[1] W. M. S. Tsui, K. T. Loo, L. T. C. Chow, and C. C. H. Tse, "Biliary adenofibroma: a heretofore unrecognized benign biliary tumor of the liver," *American Journal of Surgical Pathology*, vol. 17, no. 2, pp. 186–192, 1993.

[2] O. Akin and M. Coskun, "Biliary adenofibroma with malignant transformation and pulmonary metastases: CT findings," *American Journal of Roentgenology*, vol. 179, no. 1, pp. 280–281, 2002.

[3] A. N. Haberal, B. Bilezikçi, B. Demirhan, H. Karakayali, and M. Haberal, "Malignant transformation of biliary adenofibroma: a case report," *Turkish Journal of Gastroenterology*, vol. 12, no. 2, pp. 149–153, 2001.

[4] H. Varnholt, J.-N. Vauthey, P. D. Cin et al., "Biliary adenofibroma: a rare neoplasm of bile duct origin with an indolent behavior," *The American Journal of Surgical Pathology*, vol. 27, no. 5, pp. 693–698, 2003.

[5] K. Kai, T. Yakabe, N. Kohya et al., "A case of unclassified multicystic biliary tumor with biliary adenofibroma features," *Pathology International*, vol. 62, no. 7, pp. 506–510, 2012.

[6] N. T. Nguyen, T. R. Harring, L. Holley, J. A. Goss, and C. A. O'Mahony, "Biliary adenofibroma with carcinoma in situ: a rare case report," *Case Reports in Hepatology*, vol. 2012, Article ID 793963, 3 pages, 2012.

[7] P. S. Bhathal, N. R. Hughes, and Z. D. Goodman, "The so-called bile duct adenoma is a peribiliary gland hamartoma," *The American Journal of Surgical Pathology*, vol. 20, no. 7, pp. 858–864, 1996.

[8] D. Jain, V. R. Sarode, F. W. Abdul-Karim, R. Homer, and M. E. Robert, "Evidence for the neoplastic transformation of Von-Meyenburg complexes," *American Journal of Surgical Pathology*, vol. 24, no. 8, pp. 1131–1139, 2000.

[9] L. A. Parada, G. Bardi, M. Hallén et al., "Monosomy 22 in a case of biliary adenofibroma," *Cancer Genetics and Cytogenetics*, vol. 93, no. 2, pp. 183–184, 1997.

[10] A. L. Garduño-López, R. Mondragón-Sánchez, R. Bernal-Maldonado, C. A. Hinojosa-Becerril, and A. Meneses-García, "A case of biliary adenofibroma of the liver causing elevated serum CA 19-9 levels," *Revista de Oncologia*, vol. 4, no. 5, pp. 271–273, 2002.

[11] A. Gurrera, R. Alaggio, G. Leone, G. Aprile, and G. Magro, "Biliary adenofibroma of the liver: report of a case and review of the literature," *Pathology Research International*, vol. 2010, Article ID 504584, 5 pages, 2010.

54

Metachronous Occurrence of Granular Cell Tumor in Breast Skin and Scalp: Diagnostic Challenging Differentiating Benign from Malignant and a Literature Review

Hampar Akkaya,[1] Havva Serap Toru,[2] Ebru Sebnem Ayva,[1] Zulfikar Karabulut,[3] and Cicek Durusoy[4]

[1]*Department of Pathology, Başkent University School of Medicine, 06490 Ankara, Turkey*
[2]*Department of Pathology, Akdeniz University School of Medicine, 07058 Antalya, Turkey*
[3]*Department of Surgery, Başkent University School of Medicine, 06490 Ankara, Turkey*
[4]*Department of Dermatology, Başkent University School of Medicine, 06490 Ankara, Turkey*

Correspondence should be addressed to Hampar Akkaya; hamparakkaya@yahoo.com

Academic Editor: Tibor Tot

Granular cell tumor (GCT) is a Schwann cell related benign neoplasm of soft tissue. GCT is an uncommon entity that occurs in a wide variety of body sites, but it is generally presented in the skin, oral cavity, superficial soft tissue, and respiratory and digestive tracts. Most of the GCTs are benign but clinically and radiologically these may mimic malignancy. Histopathological diagnosis is gold standard for establishing the true nature of the lesion. GCT is most commonly solitary but in about 10% of cases can be multifocal, usually involving various skin and soft tissue sites versus involving various internal sites. Therefore, these can involve skin and soft tissue or submucosa and viscera. GCT is usually benign; however, local recurrence is common due to incomplete removal. Malignant cases are rarely reported in 1-2% of cases. In this study, we report clinical and histopathological findings of a 36-year-old woman with metachronous GCT in breast and scalp. The clinical features raise the question of whether these are metachronous benign GCTs or whether this is establishment of malignant behavior. The aim of this report is to present the histopathological and clinical features of GCT and the diagnostic challenge of differentiating benign from malignant GCT.

1. Introduction

Granular cell tumor, first described in 1926, was thought to be derived from skeletal muscle cells and termed "granular cell myoblastoma" by Abrikossoff [1]. Nowadays, the most accepted theory is Schwann cell origin, because of the S100 protein expression in tumor cells and the similarities between the ultrastructural features of the tumor cells and Schwann cells [2].

GCT is an uncommon tumor that occurs in a wide variety of body sites but is mainly found in the skin, oral cavity, superficial soft tissue, and respiratory and digestive tracts [3]. GCT of the breast is really rare. It accounts for 8.5% of all GCTs [4]. GCT arises from interlobular breast stroma or cutaneous tissue of breast [1, 2, 5]. GCT is usually benign. Malignant cases are rarely reported, with an incidence of 1-2% [6]. Recognition of benign GCT is important, since these are infrequently diagnosed preoperatively; these may be confused clinically and radiologically with malignant lesions.

Herein we report the clinical and histopathological findings in a case of a 36-year-old woman with a clinical presentation of metachronous GCTs, a palpable, painless mass in the breast skin, and then another mass eighteen months later in the scalp. A literature review is performed and discussion between benign and malignant GCT is presented.

2. Case Report

Case 1. A 36-year-old woman presented with a firm, fixed, painless palpable skin mass, approximately measured 2 cm diameter, in the lower-inner quadrant of the left breast skin (Figure 1(a)). She had pruritus but had neither nipple discharge, nor peau d'orange appearance. A slowly growing mass was realized a few years ago. The patient had no previous surgical intervention of the breast. Macroscopically an ill-defined, firm, grey-white lesion measured approximately 1.6 × 0.9 × 0.9 cm in the subepidermal breast tissue. Histopathologically, this lesion was located in the dermis and subcutaneous fat tissue without epidermal infiltration. Minimal acanthosis without reactive pseudoepitheliomatous hyperplasia was detected (Figure 1(b)). The tumoral lesion was ill-defined and had an infiltrative growth pattern but the ductal-lobular unit of the breast was not involved (Figure 1(c)). The lesion was composed of compact nests and sheets of large polygonal tumoral cells, containing large eosinophilic granular cytoplasm and relatively small round or oval nuclei (Figure 1(d)). Focally, small nerves were surrounded by granular cells. Tumor cells were expressing S100 protein strongly and diffusely (Figure 1(e)) and CD68 in cytoplasmic inclusions surrounded by halos (Figure 1(f)) and were completely negative for p53 (Figure 1(g)), pancytokeratin (cytokeratin AE1/AE3), estrogen receptor, and progesterone receptor. Ki-67 labeling index of tumor was approximately 1% (Figure 1(h)).

Case 2. Eighteen months later, the patient presented with a mass on the vertex of scalp (Figure 2(a)). This lesion was 1.7 × 1.3 × 0.8 cm in size and with scale-crusted appearance. This tumoral lesion was located in dermis and was well defined macroscopically and microscopically, in contrast to breast lesion. We observed prominent reactive pseudoepitheliomatous hyperplasia in the scalp lesion (Figure 2(b)). This lesion had similar histological, cytomorphological, and immunohistochemical features to the previous lesion (Figures 2(c) and 2(d)); Ki-67 was relatively overexpressed in the scalp lesion (6% of the nuclei of neoplastic cells) (Figure 2(e)). Tumors cell expressed weak and mild p53 (Figure 2(f)). Similar to previous lesion tumor cells were diffusely positive for S100 (Figure 2(g)) and negative for pancytokeratin (cytokeratin AE1/AE3) (Figure 2(h)).

In both of the lesions none of the histological criteria of malignant behavior was detected such as (1) spindling of the tumor cells, (2) presence of vesicular nuclei with large nucleoli, (3) increased mitotic rate, (4) high nuclear to cytoplasmic ratio, (5) pleomorphism, or (6) necrosis.

3. Discussion

GCT was first described in 1926 by Abrikossoff on tongue and postulated a myogenic origin as "granular cell myoblastoma." Initially GCTs were considered to arise from myocytes, histiocytes, fibroblast, or intestinal mesenchymal cells. The most widely accepted theory has been that of Schwann cell origin, because of positivity of the tumor cells for the S100 protein and the similarities between the ultrastructural features of the tumor cells and those of Schwann cells.

GCT occurs in patients of all ages, commonly observed between the fourth and sixth decades of life. It is more common in women than men and very rare in childhood [7–9].

GCT arises throughout the body and the most common presentation is a solitary painless nodule, located in the skin, tongue, and oral cavity and less frequently in breast, gastrointestinal and respiratory tracts, female genital system, smooth muscle, or striated muscle [9]. According to the literature, 30% to 45% of GCTs are observed in the skin of the head and neck. When compared to other studies, Dupuis and Coard found a notable difference in the distribution of GCT. In their study, lesions of the tongue accounted for fewer than expected, while lesions of the breast and vulva were considerably increased [8].

GCT of the breast is rare, with a percentage of 8.5 among all GCTs [10, 11]. Breast GCT more commonly occurs in premenopausal women and, according to reports, especially in African-American women [2, 12]. GCT is found most frequently in the upper inner quadrant of the breast, differentiating it from carcinomas which is frequently in the outer quadrants. In our case, the GCT tumor was located in the lower inner quadrant of the left breast as a dermal infiltration.

GCTs are usually benign solitary Schwannian neural tumors. Local recurrence may occur with incomplete removal. Malignant behavior of GCT is rare (<2%). Although most of GCTs are solitary lesions, in about 15 to 25% of the cases GCT can be multifocal, simultaneously involving the skin and soft tissue or simultaneously involving the submucosa and viscera. Multiplicity should not be taken as evidence for malignancy [13]. Familial occurrence has been reported, but there is no clear evidence for a syndrome [14].

Malignant GCTs usually occur in older population and tend to be larger than their benign counterparts. Malignant GCTs grow rapidly, often ulcerate, invade locally, and tend to spread with extensive metastases. Generally, it is well accepted that benign GCTs do not transform into malignant ones; malignant GCTs arise de novo. In contrast, Chen et al. presumed that malign GCT may result from the malignant transformation of benign GCT [15]. Malignant GCTs often recur locally with multiple skin satellite nodules. Metastases most commonly develop in the lymph nodes, lungs, bones, rarely the intestines, liver, or brain. According to Fanburg-Smith et al., tumor-related deaths occurred in 11 of 28 patients, with a median time of 3 years (range, 1 yr–9 yr) [16].

Grossly, benign GCT typically forms an oval nodule, smaller than 3 cm, that varies from being well or poorly circumscribed with a pale and yellow tan on cut surface. Occasionally, tumors reach the size of 5 cm or more. Dupuis and Coard reported the range of diameter as 0.2 cm to 10 cm in 130 benign GCT cases of various sites [8]. Malignant GCTs have similar gross appearance but tend to be larger than benign lesions; however, malignant GCT can also be small. Microscopically most of malignant GCTs are poorly circumscribed. About two-thirds of the GCTs are located in cutaneous, subcutaneous, or submucosal tissues and some of these cases are associated with pseudoepitheliomatous hyperplasia of the overlying epidermis or mucosal epithelium. It is reported that GCT of breast may arise in either interlobular breast stroma or the skin overlying breast [1, 2, 11]. The cells of GCT which are round, polygonal, or slightly spindle shaped

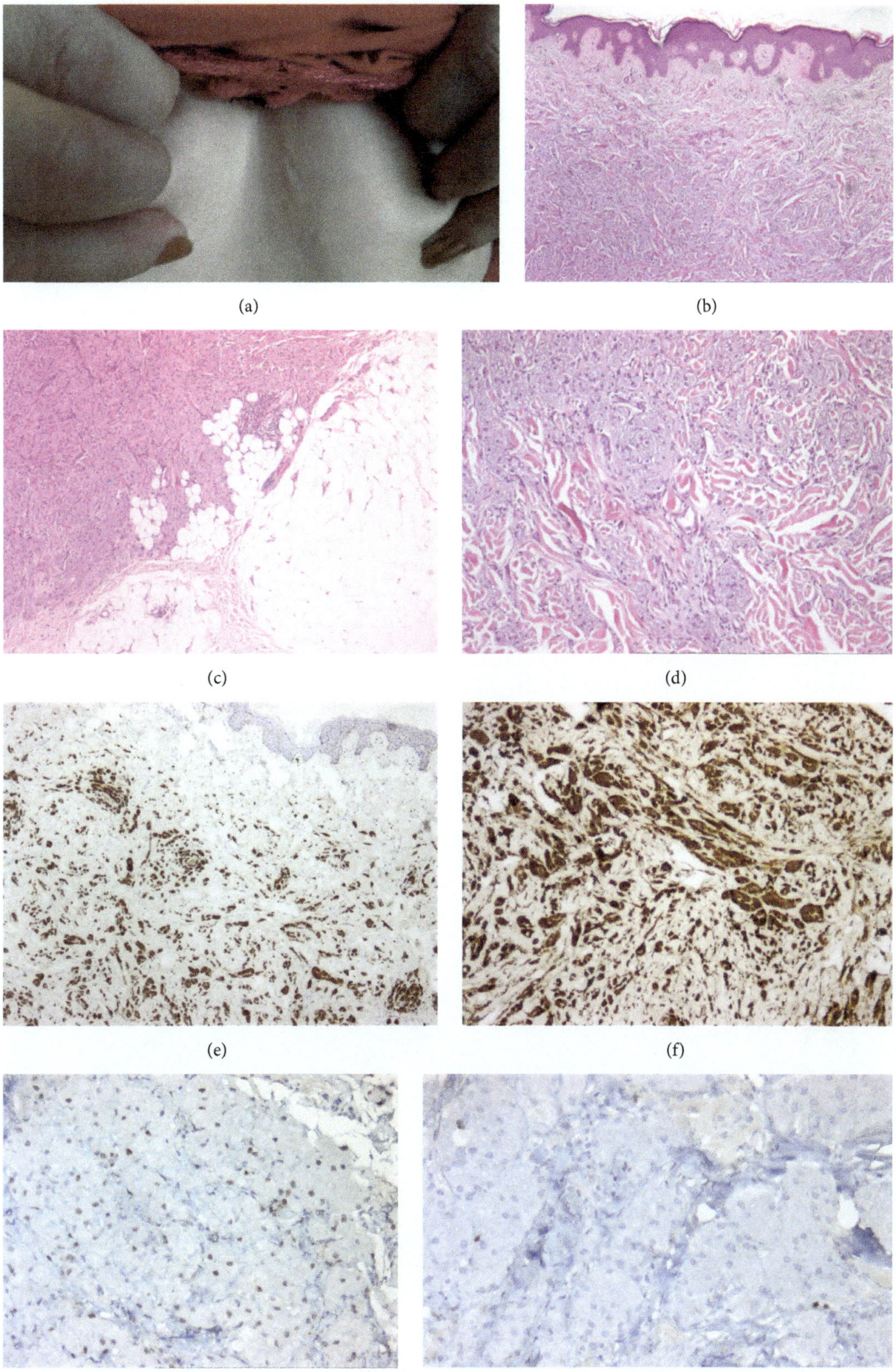

(a) (b) (c) (d) (e) (f) (g) (h)

FIGURE 1: (a) Subcutaneous mass of breast. (b) Minimal acanthosis and epidermal pseudoepitheliomatous hyperplasia (H&E, ×50). (c) Ill-defined tumoral lesion with infiltrative pattern (H&E, ×100). (d) Compact nests and sheets of polygonal tumor cells (H&E, ×200). (e) Tumor cells expressing S100 (×100). (f) Tumor cells expressing CD68 (×200). (g) Tumor cells weakly expressing p53 (×200). (h) Ki-67 proliferation expressing approximately 1%.

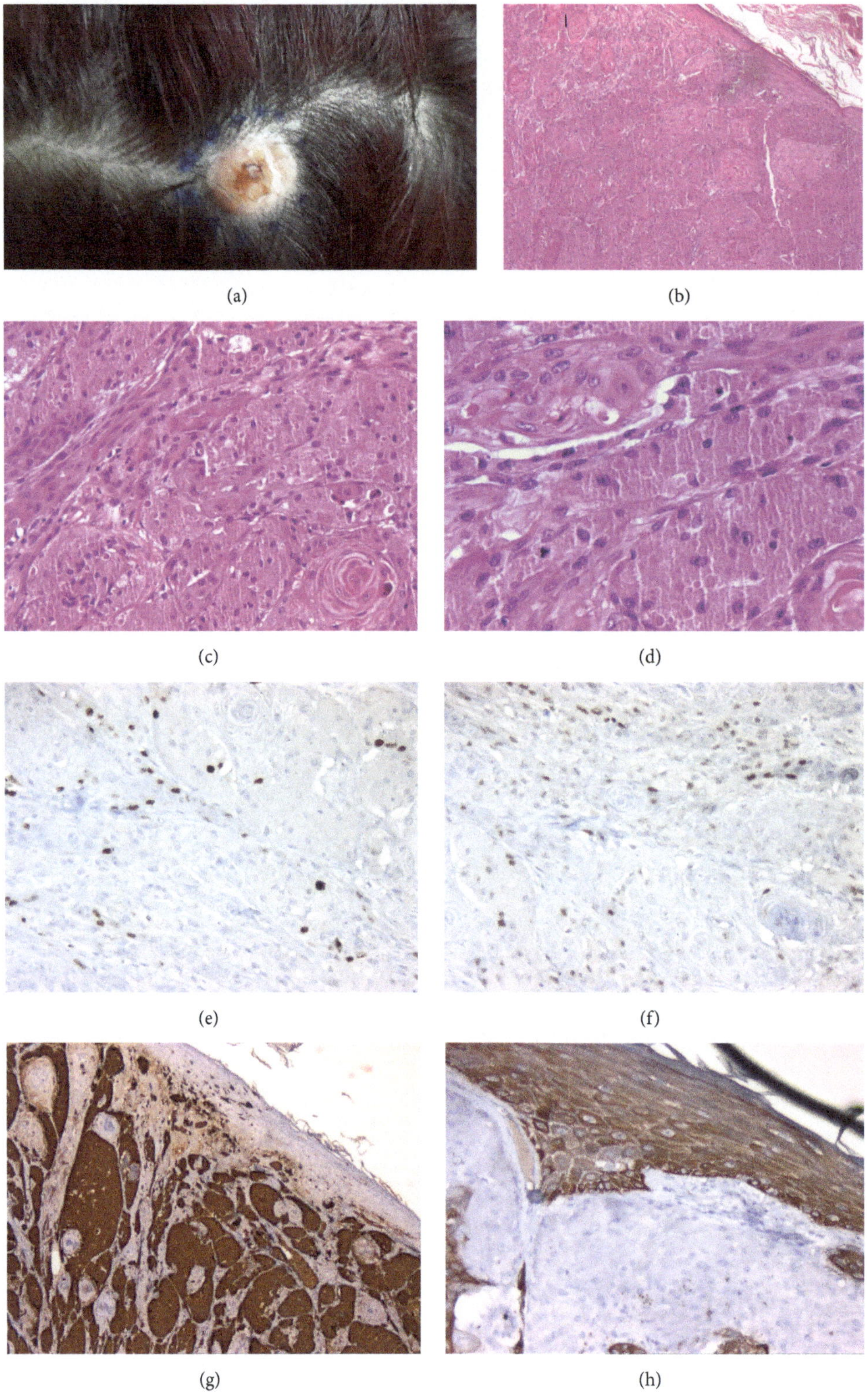

Figure 2: (a) Subcutaneous mass on the vertex of the scalp with ulcerated surface. (b) Reactive pseudoepitheliomatous hyperplasia of epidermis (H&E, ×100). (c) Polygonal tumor cells forming nests (×200). (d) Tumor cells with large eosinophilic granular cytoplasm and oval nucleus with nucleoli (H&E, ×400). (e) Tumor cells showing approximately 6% Ki-67 proliferation index (×200). (f) Tumor cells expressing p53 weakly and mildly (×200). (g) Tumor cells expressing S100 protein diffusely and strongly. (h) Tumor cells immunohistochemically negative for cytokeratin AE1/AE3 (×200).

and are characterized by large and granular cytoplasm. They have small and hyperchromatic or large and vesicular nuclei. Granular cells and peripheral nerves have close association. In GCT, there are small nerves that are invaded or surrounded by the granular cell clusters.

Immunohistochemically, GCT is consistently positive for S100 protein, NSE, various myelin proteins, and negative for muscle cell and epithelial markers. GCTs are strongly positive for macrophage antigen CD68, specifically in the cytoplasmic lysosomal granules with clear halo around these, and this lysosomal granule excludes other tumors that may have granular features. GCTs are also alpha-inhibin positive [17–19].

In 1998, Fanburg-Smith et al. established that six histological criteria could predict malignant behavior [16], such as sarcomatoid spindling of the tumor cells, presence of vesicular nuclei with large nucleoli, increased mitotic rate (2 mitoses per 10 high-power fields), high nuclear to cytoplasmic ratio, pleomorphism, and necrosis. If a GCT demonstrates three or more of these criteria, it is classified as "malignant" and those that show one or two criteria are classified as "atypical," and if it exhibits none of the criteria or only focal pleomorphism, it is classified as "benign." Most of the malignant tumors, however, had at least 5 or 6 of the criteria and most malignant cases had necrosis or increased mitotic activity. They also demonstrated that Ki-67 and p53 were significantly higher in atypical and malignant tumors than in benign ones [16].

According to histological and cytological features, Argenyi suggested that malignant GCTs might be classified into two types [20]. The first type of malignant GCT is more common and essentially appears identically to a benign tumor; because cytologic atypia or mitotic activity may not be reliable biologic indicators in this form, diagnosis of malignancy should be made by clinicopathologic correlation (large size, rapid growth, ulceration, necrosis, sarcomatoid spindling, and lymphatic and vascular invasion). Vesicular nuclei with large nucleoli and mitotic rate are more than 2 mitoses/10 HPF and are additional findings for malignancy. The second type of malignant GCT is quite rare. In this type, either primary GCT or metastases display conventional malignant histological and cytological features. Malignant GCT cells express similar immunohistochemical features to those of a benign tumor, with the exception Ki-67 labeling index being higher and p53 expression being prominent [20].

According to Nasser et al., some of the criteria proposed by Fanburg-Smith, such as pleomorphism and increased nuclear-to-cytoplasmic ratio, are subject to interobserver variation and show weak reproducibility among different pathologists, complicating the diagnostic spectrum [21]. It is thought that simple, practical, and clear diagnostic criteria are required. In 2011, Nasser et al. classified the GCTs based on the presence of necrosis (whether single cell or en masse) and mitoses. They believe that these are two of the most reliable and more reproducible criteria associated with malignancy and designated tumors without these 2 features as "benign" GCTs and those cases demonstrating at least one of the previously mentioned features as GCTs with "uncertain malignant potential." They considered metastases as the only definitive criterion of malignancy, regardless of the histopathologic features [21]. Their paper did not have the large number of cases as in the AFIP paper, but their conclusions were similar, overall.

p53 expression has been described in neoplastic cells of MGCTs with a variable frequency, ranging from 5% to 100% [15, 16, 22, 23]. Ki-67 proliferating index ranged from 10% to 50% [16, 19, 21, 23]. Le et al. reported that there was not any significant difference between benign and atypical cases' Ki-67 expression [19]. Nasser et al. reported mean of Ki-67 labeling index 10.5% in atypical GCTs and 2.7% in benign GCTs and the difference was statistically significant. There were no significant differences in p53 expression between three groups; they all showed strong and diffuse nuclear staining [21].

Essentially any tumor type may show granular cell change, and thus the differential diagnosis of true granular cell tumors is quite broad. Similar morphological properties can be observed in smooth muscle tumors, rhabdomyoma, hibernoma, fibroxanthoma, and malignant melanoma [24]. GCT is distinguished from other granular cell lesions with S100 protein positivity. Epithelial tumors are separated from granular cell features with keratin positivity and S100 protein negativity. GCTs of the breast must be distinguished from benign and malign tumors. Histiocytes and granular cells are similar in appearance, so that histiocytic inflammatory lesions must be differentiated. Carcinomas of breast with apocrine or histiocytoid features may resemble GCT. Carcinomas are positive for cytokeratin, and DCIS is usually present in breast carcinomas. Malignant tumors that metastasize to breast like malignant melanoma, renal cell carcinoma must be distinguished from GCT. The most challenging tumors in differential diagnosis of GCT are granular cell (spindle cell) melanoma, which is lack of cytoplasmic inclusions with halos and, when spindled, some degree of cytologic atypia and prominent nucleoli and lymphoid response may be present. BRAF can also be helpful in this setting.

In our case, the patient was a 36-year-old woman. The first lesion was in lower inner quadrant of the left breast; the second lesion occurring 18 months later was on the vertex of the scalp.

In immunohistochemical examination of p53, both lesions were similar (approximately 80% weak nuclear positivity). Ki-67 labeling index was 1% in the breast GCT and 6% in scalp GCT. Ki-67 expression was slightly higher in scalp GCT than breast GCT. Another important point was evaluating Ki-67 away from pseudoepitheliomatous hyperplasia, because basal layer of these areas may overexpress Ki-67. Because of this, we evaluated the Ki-67 labeling index areas of tumor away from epidermis with pseudoepitheliomatous hyperplasia.

After microscopic and immunohistochemical examination, both tumors were diagnosed as benign and metachronous according to the diagnostic criteria stated above [16, 21].

Tumor cells are located in dermis and extend to the subcutaneous septa. Due to subcutaneous septal infiltration and perineural spread, characteristic findings of the GCT, incomplete removal, and local recurrence are common problems. Therefore, complete excision of GCT is important. After complete surgical resection of both tumors with safe surgical margins, patients could be clinically followed.

Conflict of Interests

The authors declare that there is no conflict of interests regarding the publication of this paper.

References

[1] J. Aneiros-Fernandez, "Cutaneous granular cell tumor of the breast: a clinical diagnostic pitfall," *Journal of Clinical Medicine Research*, vol. 2, no. 4, pp. 185–188, 2010.

[2] A. Adeniran, H. Al-Ahmadie, M. C. Mahoney, and T. M. Robinson-Smith, "Granular cell tumor of the breast: a series of 17 cases and review of the literature," *Breast Journal*, vol. 10, no. 6, pp. 528–531, 2004.

[3] K. Aoyama, T. Kamio, A. Hirano, A. Seshimo, and S. Kameoka, "Granular cell tumors: a report of six cases," *World Journal of Surgical Oncology*, vol. 10, article 204, 2012.

[4] S. B. Fox and A. Lee, "Granular cell tumour and benign peripheral nerve-sheath tumours," in *WHO Classification of Tumours of the Breast*, S. R. Lakhani, I. O. Ellis, S. J. Schnitt, P. H. Tan, and M. J. van de Vijver, Eds., pp. 134–135, IARC Press, Lyon, France, 2012.

[5] S. Damiani, F. C. Koerner, G. R. Dickersin, M. G. Cook, and V. Eusebi, "Granular cell tumour of the breast," *Virchows Archiv—A Pathological Anatomy and Histopathology*, vol. 420, no. 3, pp. 219–226, 1992.

[6] K. Akahane, K. Kato, S. Ogiso et al., "Malignant granular cell tumor of the breast: case report and literature review," *Breast Cancer*, vol. 22, no. 3, pp. 317–323, 2015.

[7] S. van de Loo, E. Thunnissen, P. Postmus, and I. van der Waal, "Granular cell tumor of the oral cavity; a case series including a case of metachronous occurrence in the tongue and the lung," *Medicina Oral, Patologia Oral y Cirugia Bucal*, vol. 20, no. 1, pp. e30–e33, 2015.

[8] C. Dupuis and K. C. M. Coard, "A review of granular cell tumours at the University Hospital of the West Indies: 1965–2006," *West Indian Medical Journal*, vol. 58, no. 2, pp. 138–141, 2009.

[9] M. Miettinen, "Nerve sheath tumors," in *Modern Soft Tissue Pathology: Tumors and Non-Neoplastic Conditions*, pp. 660–723, Cambridge University Press, 2010.

[10] E. E. Lack, G. F. Worsham, M. D. Callihan et al., "Granular cell tumor: a clinicopathologic study of 110 patients," *Journal of Surgical Oncology*, vol. 13, no. 4, pp. 301–316, 1980.

[11] P. J. Kragel, R. M. Fiorella, and H. Kremer, "Tumoral fibrosis and lack of circumscription in granular cell tumor of the breast," *Southern Medical Journal*, vol. 88, no. 11, pp. 1146–1148, 1995.

[12] R. M. Enzinger and S. W. Weiss, "Granular cell tumor," in *Soft Tissue Tumors*, R. M. Enzinger and S. W. Weiss, Eds., pp. 1178–1206, Elsevier, St. Louis, Mo, USA, 2001.

[13] N. G. Ordóñez, "Granular cell tumor: a review and update," *Advances in Anatomic Pathology*, vol. 6, no. 4, pp. 186–203, 1999.

[14] R. H. Rifkin, S. H. Blocker, J. O. Palmer, and J. L. Ternberg, "Multiple granular cell tumors. A familial occurrence in children," *Archives of Surgery*, vol. 121, no. 8, pp. 945–947, 1986.

[15] J. Chen, L. Wang, J. Xu et al., "Malignant granular cell tumor with breast metastasis: a case report and review of the literature," *Oncology Letters*, vol. 4, no. 1, pp. 63–66, 2012.

[16] J. C. Fanburg-Smith, J. M. Meis-Kindblom, R. Fante, and L.-G. Kindblom, "Malignant granular cell tumor of soft tissue: diagnostic criteria and clinicopathologic correlation," *The American Journal of Surgical Pathology*, vol. 22, no. 7, pp. 779–794, 1998.

[17] M. T. Mazur, J. J. Shultz, and J. L. Myers, "Granular cell tumor. Immunohistochemical analysis of 21 benign tumors and one malignant tumor," *Archives of Pathology and Laboratory Medicine*, vol. 114, no. 7, pp. 692–696, 1990.

[18] A. C. Filie, J. M. Lage, and N. Azumi, "Immunoreactivity of S100 protein, α-1-antitrypsin, and CD68 in adult and congenital granular cell tumors," *Modern Pathology*, vol. 9, no. 9, pp. 888–892, 1996.

[19] B. H. Le, P. J. Boyer, J. E. Lewis, and S. B. Kapadia, "Granular cell tumor: immunohistochemical assessment of inhibin-α, protein gene product 9.5, S100 protein, CD68, and Ki-67 proliferative index with clinical correlation," *Archives of Pathology and Laboratory Medicine*, vol. 128, no. 7, pp. 771–775, 2004.

[20] Z. B. Argenyi, "Granular cell tumour," in *WHO Classification of Tumours Pathology and Genetics of Skin Tumours*, P. E. LeBoit, R. J. Barr, S. Burall et al., Eds., pp. 274–275, IARC Press, Lyon, France, 2006.

[21] H. Nasser, Y. Ahmed, S. M. Szpunar, and P. J. Kowalski, "Malignant granular cell tumor: a look into the diagnostic criteria," *Pathology Research and Practice*, vol. 207, no. 3, pp. 164–168, 2011.

[22] Y. C. Pérez-González, L. Pagura, M. Llamas-Velasco, L. Cortes-Lambea, H. Kutzner, and L. Requena, "Primary cutaneous malignant granular cell tumor: an immunohistochemical study and review of the literature," *The American Journal of Dermatopathology*, vol. 37, no. 4, pp. 334–340, 2015.

[23] H. Nasser, R. D. Danforth Jr., M. Sunbuli, and O. Dimitrijevic, "Malignant granular cell tumor: case report with a novel karyotype and review of the literature," *Annals of Diagnostic Pathology*, vol. 14, no. 4, pp. 273–278, 2010.

[24] D. G. Hicks and S. C. Lester, "Granular cell tumor," in *Diagnostic Pathology Breast*, pp. 36–39, Amirsys, St. Louis, Mo, USA, 2012.

Permissions

All chapters in this book were first published in CRIPA, by Hindawi Publishing Corporation; hereby published with permission under the Creative Commons Attribution License or equivalent. Every chapter published in this book has been scrutinized by our experts. Their significance has been extensively debated. The topics covered herein carry significant findings which will fuel the growth of the discipline. They may even be implemented as practical applications or may be referred to as a beginning point for another development.

The contributors of this book come from diverse backgrounds, making this book a truly international effort. This book will bring forth new frontiers with its revolutionizing research information and detailed analysis of the nascent developments around the world.

We would like to thank all the contributing authors for lending their expertise to make the book truly unique. They have played a crucial role in the development of this book. Without their invaluable contributions this book wouldn't have been possible. They have made vital efforts to compile up to date information on the varied aspects of this subject to make this book a valuable addition to the collection of many professionals and students.

This book was conceptualized with the vision of imparting up-to-date information and advanced data in this field. To ensure the same, a matchless editorial board was set up. Every individual on the board went through rigorous rounds of assessment to prove their worth. After which they invested a large part of their time researching and compiling the most relevant data for our readers.

The editorial board has been involved in producing this book since its inception. They have spent rigorous hours researching and exploring the diverse topics which have resulted in the successful publishing of this book. They have passed on their knowledge of decades through this book. To expedite this challenging task, the publisher supported the team at every step. A small team of assistant editors was also appointed to further simplify the editing procedure and attain best results for the readers.

Apart from the editorial board, the designing team has also invested a significant amount of their time in understanding the subject and creating the most relevant covers. They scrutinized every image to scout for the most suitable representation of the subject and create an appropriate cover for the book.

The publishing team has been an ardent support to the editorial, designing and production team. Their endless efforts to recruit the best for this project, has resulted in the accomplishment of this book. They are a veteran in the field of academics and their pool of knowledge is as vast as their experience in printing. Their expertise and guidance has proved useful at every step. Their uncompromising quality standards have made this book an exceptional effort. Their encouragement from time to time has been an inspiration for everyone.

The publisher and the editorial board hope that this book will prove to be a valuable piece of knowledge for researchers, students, practitioners and scholars across the globe.

List of Contributors

Tamer Ahmed EL-Sobky, John Fathy Haleem and Shady Samir
Orthopedic Surgery Department, Faculty of Medicine, Ain Shams University, 38 Abbasia Square, Masjed Alnoor, Cairo, Egypt

Shiuan-Li Wey and Kuo-Ming Chang
Department of Pathology, Mackay Memorial Hospital, Hsinchu 30071, Taiwan

Avani A. Pendse and Siobhan M. O'Connor
Department of Pathology, University of North Carolina, Chapel Hill, NC 27599-7525, USA

Kei Tanaka
Department of Surgery, Kensei General Hospital, 604 Kuwata, Sakuragawa, Ibaraki 309-1223, Japan
General Surgery, Chiba University Graduate School of Medicine, 1-8-1 Inohana, Chuo-ku, Chiba 260-8670, Japan

Takashi Kishimoto
Department of Molecular Pathology, Chiba University Graduate School of Medicine, 1-8-1 Inohana, Chuo-ku, Chiba 260-8670, Japan

Yukio Nakatani
Diagnostic Pathology, Chiba University Graduate School of Medicine, 1-8-1 Inohana, Chuo-ku, Chiba 260-8670, Japan

Masayuki Ohtsuka and Masaru Miyazaki
General Surgery, Chiba University Graduate School of Medicine, 1-8-1 Inohana, Chuo-ku, Chiba 260-8670, Japan

Sarah A. Fleming and John G. Strickler
Hospital Pathology Associates, 2800 10th Avenue South Suite 2200, Minneapolis, MN 55407, USA

Kristen M. Paral
Department of Medicine, Section of Dermatology, University of Chicago, 5841 S Maryland Avenue, MC 5067, Chicago, IL 60637, USA

Gordana Raca
Department of Medicine, Section of Hematology/Oncology, University of Chicago, 5841 S Maryland Avenue, MC 6092, Chicago, IL 60637, USA

Thomas Krausz
Department of Pathology, University of Chicago, 5841 S Maryland Avenue, MC 6161, Chicago, IL 60637, USA

Teodóra Tóth, Yi-Che Chang Chien, Sándor Kollár and Ilona Kovács
Department of Pathology, Kenézy Gyula County Hospital, Bartók Bélaút 2-26, Debrecen 4031, Hungary

Hope Richard and Christine Fuller
Department of Pathology, Virginia Commonwealth University Health System, 1101 E. Marshall Street, P.O. Box 980662, Richmond, VA 23298, USA

Kimberly Stogner-Underwood
Department of Pathology, Virginia Commonwealth University Health System, 1101 E. Marshall Street, P.O. Box 980662, Richmond, VA 23298, USA
Department of Pathology, Wake Forest Baptist Medical Center, Medical Center Boulevard, Winston-Salem, NC 27157, USA

Joslin M. Bowen
Physicians Laboratory, 4840F Street, Omaha, NE 68117, USA

Anamarija M. Perry
Department of Pathology, University of Manitoba, MS559S Thorlakson Building, 820 Sherbrook Street, Winnipeg, MB, Canada R3A 1R9

Erin Quist
Department of Pathology and Microbiology, University of Nebraska Medical Center, 985900 Nebraska Medical Center, Omaha, NE 68198, USA

Mojtaba Akhtari
Jane Anne Nohl Division of Hematology and Center for the Study of Blood Diseases, University of Southern California (USC) and Norris Cancer Center, USC University Hospital, 1441 Eastlake Avenue, Norris Topping Tower 3463, MC 9172, Los Angeles, CA 90033-9172, USA

Shiho Kuroda, Shioto Suzuki, Akira Kurita, Mari Muraki and Fumihiko Tanioka
Division of Pathology, Iwata City Hospital, 512-3 Ookubo, Iwata, Shizuoka 438-8550, Japan

Yoichiro Aoshima
Division of Respiratory Medicine, Iwata City Hospital, 512-3 Ookubo, Iwata, Shizuoka 438-8550, Japan

Haruhiko Sugimura
Department of Tumor Pathology, Hamamatsu University School of Medicine, 1-20-1 Handayama, Higashi-ku, Hamamatsu, Shizuoka 431-3192, Japan

Abelardo Loya-Solis, Karla Judith González-Colunga, Luis Ceceñas-Falcón and Oralia Barboza-Quintana
Pathology Department, University Hospital "Dr. Jose E. Gonzalez" and Medical School of the Autonomous University of Nuevo Leon, Francisco I. Madero and Gonzalitos, 64460 Monterrey, NL, Mexico

Cynthia M. Pérez-Rodríguez and Natalie Sofía Ramírez-Ochoa
Otolaryngology-Head and Neck Surgery Department, University Hospital "Dr. Jose E. Gonzalez" and Medical School of the Autonomous University of Nuevo Leon, Francisco I. Madero and Gonzalitos, 64460 Monterrey, NL, Mexico

Akifuddin Syed
Princess Durru Shehvar Children's and General Hospital, Purani Haveli, Hyderabad, Telangana 500002, India

Prashanth Panta and Imran Shahid
Department of Oral Medicine and Radiology, MNR Dental College and Hospital, Narsapur Road, Sangareddy, Medak District, Telangana 502294, India

David H. Felix
NHS Education for Scotland, Westport 102, West Port, Edinburgh EH3 9DN, UK

Surapan Khunamornpong, Jongkolnee Settakorn, Kornkanok Sukpan and Sumalee Siriaunkgul
Department of Pathology, Faculty of Medicine, Chiang Mai University, Chiang Mai 50200, Thailand

Prapaporn Suprasert
Department of Obstetrics and Gynecology, Faculty of Medicine, Chiang Mai University, Chiang Mai 50200, Thailand

Grace W. Weyant, Dipti M. Karamchandani and Negar Rassaei
Department of Pathology, Penn State Milton S. Hershey Medical Center, 500 University Drive, P.O. Box 850, MC H179, Hershey, PA 17033, USA

Abelardo Loya-Solis
Pathology Department, Spanish Hospital of Mexico, Ejercito Nacional 613, 11560 Mexico City, DF, Mexico

Lucía Alemán-Meza, Luis Carlos Canales-Martínez, Rodolfo Franco-Márquez, Alim Adriana Rincón-Bahena, Raquel Garza-Guajardo and Marco Antonio Ponce-Camacho
Pathology Department, University Hospital "Dr. Jose E. Gonzalez" and Medical School of the Autonomous University of Nuevo Leon, Francisco I. Madero and Gonzalitos, 64460 Monterrey, NL, Mexico

Karla María Nuñez-Barragán
Medical Imaging Department, University Hospital "Dr. Jose E. Gonzalez" and Medical School of the Autonomous University of Nuevo Leon, Francisco I. Madero and Gonzalitos, 64460 Monterrey, NL, Mexico

Kanako Ogura, Toshiharu Matsumoto and Asumi Sakaguchi
Department of Diagnostic Pathology, Juntendo University Nerima Hospital, Tokyo 177-8521, Japan

Maki Amano
Department of Radiology, Juntendo University Nerima Hospital, Tokyo 177-8521, Japan

Taijiro Kosaka, Toshiaki Kitabatake and Kuniaki Kojima
Department of Breast Surgery, Juntendo University Nerima Hospital, Tokyo 177-8521, Japan

Sebahattin Celik
Department of General Surgery, Yüzüncü Yıl University, 65200 Van, Turkey

Remzi Erten
Department of Pathology, Yüzüncü Yıl University, 65200 Van, Turkey

Abdulsamed Batur
Department of Radiology, Yüzüncü Yıl University, 65200 Van, Turkey

Burak Suvak
Department of Gastroenterology, Yüzüncü Yıl University, 65200 Van, Turkey

Kenji Ohshima and Satoru Munakata
Department of Pathology, Sakai City Hospital, 1-1-1 Minami-Yasui-Cho, Sakai-Ku, Sakai, Osaka 590-0064, Japan

Anna Umeda, Ayako Hosoi and Toshiya Yamamoto
Department of Obstetrics and Gynecology, Sakai City Hospital, 1-1-1 Minami-Yasui-Cho, Sakai-Ku, Sakai, Osaka 590-0064, Japan

Dana Balitzer
Department of Pathology, University of California, San Francisco, 505 Parnassus, M580, San Francisco, CA 94143, USA

Timothy H. McCalmont
Departments of Pathology and Dermatology, University of California, San Francisco, 1701 Divisadero Street, Suite 280, San Francisco, CA 94115, USA

Andrew E. Horvai
Department of Pathology, University of California, San Francisco, 1825 4th Street, M2354, San Francisco, CA 94143, USA

Rashna Meunier and Ali Amin
Department of Pathology and Laboratory Medicine, Rhode Island Hospital, The Warren Alpert Medical School, Brown University, Providence, RI 02903, USA

Gyan Pareek
University Urological Associates, The Warren Alpert Medical School, Brown University, Providence, RI 02904, USA

Surya Guha and Haiyan Liu
Geisinger Medical Center, 100 North Academy Avenue, Danville, PA 17821, USA

Diana Castro-Villabón and Luis E. Barrera-Herrera
Department of Pathology and Laboratories, Hospital Universitario Fundación Santa Fe de Bogotá, Calle 119 No. 7-75, Bogotá110111, Colombia

Paula A. Rodríguez-Urrego, Johanna Álvarez and Rocío López
Department of Pathology and Laboratories, Hospital Universitario Fundación Santa Fe de Bogotá, Calle 119 No. 7-75, Bogotá 110111, Colombia
School of Medicine, University of Los Andes, Carrera1 No. 18A-12, Bogotá 111711, Colombia

Rachel Hudacko
Department of Pathology, Good Samaritan Regional Medical Center, 255 Lafayette Avenue, Suffern, NY 10901, USA

Alonso Vera
Transplant and Hepatobiliary Surgical Service, Hospital Universitario Fundación Santa Fe de Bogotá, Calle 119 No. 7-75, Bogotá 110111, Colombia

Rafael Andrade
Department of Pathology and Laboratories, Hospital Universitario Fundación Santa Fe de Bogotá, Calle 119 No. 7-75, Bogotá 110111, Colombia
School of Medicine, University of Los Andes, Carrera1 No. 18A-12, Bogotá 111711, Colombia
School of Medicine, National University of Colombia, Carrera 45 No. 26-85, Bogota´ 111711, Colombia

Josip Vukina and Mathew C. Raynor
Department of Urology, University of North Carolina, Chapel Hill, NC 27599, USA

David D. Chism and Matthew I. Milowsky
Division of Hematology and Oncology, Department of Medicine, University of North Carolina, Chapel Hill, NC 27599, USA

Julie L. Sharpless
Lineberger Comprehensive Cancer Center, Chapel Hill, NC 27599, USA
Division of Endocrinology and Metabolism, Department of Medicine, University of North Carolina, Chapel Hill, NC 27599, USA

William K. Funkhouser
Lineberger Comprehensive Cancer Center, Chapel Hill, NC 27599, USA
Department of Pathology and Laboratory Medicine, University of North Carolina, Chapel Hill, NC 27599, USA

Priya Subashchandrabose, Muthuvel Esakkai, Chitra Srinivasan, Punuru Tejashwini Reddy and Evelyn Elizabeth Ebenezer
Department of Pathology, Saveetha Medical College, Chennai 602105, India

Palani Venugopal and Ilavarasan Kannaiyan
Department of Surgery, Saveetha Medical College, Chennai 602105, India

Takako Inaba
Division of Diagnostic Pathology, Juntendo University, 3-1-3 Hongo, Bunkyo-ku, Tokyo 113-0033, Japan

Yuki Fukumura, Tsuyoshi Saito, Atsushi Arakawa and Takashi Yao
Department of Human Pathology, Juntendo University School of Medicine, 1-1-19 Motomachi Bldg. 3F, Hongo, Bunkyo-ku, Tokyo 113-0033, Japan

Junkichi Yokoyama and Shinichi Ohba
Department of Otorhinolaryngology, Juntendo University School of Medicine, 3-1-3 Hongo, Bunkyo-ku, Tokyo 113-0033, Japan

Branislava MiliIiT and Clara Limbaeck-Stokin
Faculty of Medicine, Institute of Pathology, University of Ljubljana, 1000 Ljubljana, Slovenia

TomaD Velnar
Department of Neurosurgery, University Medical Center Maribor, 2000 Maribor, Slovenia

Rado Pregelj
International Institute for Neurosurgery and Neurosciences, 1000 Ljubljana, Slovenia

Rohit Gulati, Yaser Alkhatib, Vijayalakshmi Donthireddy, Michelle Madden Felicella, Madhu P. Menon and Kedar V. Inamdar
Henry Ford Hospital, 2799 W. Grand Boulevard, Detroit, MI 48202, USA

Mary Anne Brett, Monalisa Sur, Dean Daya, Jefferson Terry and Alice Lytwyn
Department of Pathology and Molecular Medicine, McMaster University, 1280 Main Street West, Room No. HSC-1N16, Hamilton, ON, Canada L8S 4L8

Claudia P. Rojas, Parvin Ganjei-Azar and Monica T. Garcia-Buitrago
Department of Pathology, University of Miami Miller School of Medicine, Jackson Memorial Hospital, 1611 NW 12th Avenue, Holtz 2042C, Miami, FL 33136, USA

Ryan Glass, Jaya Ruth Asirvatham, Leonard Kahn and Mohamed Aziz
Department of Pathology, North Shore Long Island Jewish, New Hyde Park, NY 11040, USA

Shahzaib Nabi, Tarun Jain and Fawad Virk
Department of Internal Medicine, Henry Ford Health System, 2799 W. Grand Boulevard, Detroit, MI 48202, USA

Adeel Arshad
Department of Internal Medicine, Hamad Medical Corporation, Weill Cornell University, Doha, Qatar

Rohit Gulati
Department of Pathology, Henry Ford Health System, 2799 W. Grand Boulevard, Detroit, MI 48202, USA

Rana Awdish
Department of Pulmonary and Critical Care Medicine, Henry Ford Health System, 2799 W. Grand Boulevard, Detroit, MI 48202, USA

Maureen P. Kohi and Nicholas Fidelman
Department of Radiology and Biomedical Imaging, University of California, San Francisco, San Francisco, CA 94143, USA

Gabrielle A. Rizzuto
Department of Pathology and Laboratory Medicine, University of California, San Francisco, San Francisco, CA 94143, USA

Jennifer Lucero
Department of Anesthesia and Perioperative Care, University of California, San Francisco, San Francisco, CA 94143, USA

Mari-Paule Thiet
Department of Obstetrics, Gynecology and Reproductive Sciences, University of California, San Francisco, San Francisco, CA 94143, USA

Charles D. Sturgis and Aaron P. Hoschar
Cleveland Clinic, Tomsich Pathology Institute, 9500 Euclid Avenue L25, Cleveland, OH 44195, USA

Brian B. Burkey and Suhael Momin
Cleveland Clinic, Head and Neck Institute, 9500 Euclid Avenue A71, Cleveland, OH 44195, USA

Yessica M. González-Cantú, Cristina Rodriguez-Padilla, Alberto García de la Fuente and Raymundo Díaz Mendoza
Laboratorio de Inmunología y Virología, Facultad de Ciencias Biológicas, Universidad Autónoma de Nuevo León, Avenida Manuel L. Barragán S/N, Ciudad Universitaria, 66451 San Nicolás de los Garza, NL, Mexico

Martha Lilia Tena-Suck
Departamento de Neuropatología, Instituto Nacional de Neurología y Neurocirugía, Manuel Velasco Suárez, Avenida Insurgentes Sur 3877, Colonia La Fama, 14269 Delegación Tlalpan, DF, Mexico

Rosa María Mejía-Bañuelos
Hospital General de Zona 17, Instituto Mexicano del Seguro Social, Fortunato Lozano y Roble Colonia Benito Juárez, 64420 Monterrey, NL, Mexico

Samuel Quintanilla-Garza
Unidad de Medicina Familiar No. 73, Instituto Mexicano del Seguro Social, Pablo de Mejía No. 526, Colonia Zona Centro, 25000 Saltillo, COAH, Mexico

Yolaester Batisda-Acuña
Hospital General Regional No. 1, Instituto Mexicano del Seguro Social, Bosques de los Olivos 101, 61301 Morelia, MICH, Mexico

Gabriela de Morais Gouvêa Lima, Renata Mendonça Moraes, Ana Sueli Rodrigues Cavalcante, Yasmin Rodarte Carvalho and Ana Lia Anbinder
Department of Bioscience and Oral Diagnosis, Institute of Science and Technology, Campus São José dos Campos, Univ. Estadual Paulista (UNESP), Engenheiro Francisco José Longo Avenida 777, 12245-000 São José dos Campos, SP, Brazil

James P. Solomon and Fang Wen
Department of Pathology, University of California, San Diego, 9500 Gilman Drive, La Jolla, CA 92093, USA

Lily J. Jih
Department of Pathology, University of California, San Diego, 9500 Gilman Drive, La Jolla, CA 92093, USA
Department of Pathology, Veteran Administration Medical Center, La Jolla, 3350 La Jolla Village Drive (113), San Diego, CA 92161, USA

Soumya Makarla, Radhika M. Bavle and Sudhakara Muniswamappa
Department of Oral Pathology, Krishnadevaraya College of Dental Sciences, Bangalore 562157, India

Srinath Narasimhamurthy
Department of Oral Surgery, Krishnadevaraya College of Dental Sciences, Bangalore 562157, India

Hui Zhu, Emily Marie McMeekin and Charles D. Sturgis
Pathology and Laboratory Medicine Institute, Cleveland Clinic, 9500 Euclid Avenue, Cleveland, OH 44195, USA

Sushna Maharjan
Department of Pathology, Chitwan Medical College Teaching Hospital, P.O. Box 42, Bharatpur-10, Chitwan, Nepal

Jiehao Zhou and Mehdi Nassiri
Department of Pathology and Laboratory Medicine, Indiana University, Indianapolis, IN 46202, USA

Dehua Wang
Department of Pathology and Laboratory Medicine, Cincinnati Children's Hospital and Medical Center, Cincinnati, OH 45229, USA

Noala Vicensoto Moreira Milhan, Ana Sueli Rodrigues Cavalcante, Yonara Maria Freire Soares Marques, Yasmin Rodarte Carvalho and Ana Lia Anbinder
Department of Bioscience and Oral Diagnosis, Institute of Science and Technology (ICT), Universidade Estadual Paulista (UNESP), Avenida Engenheiro Francisco José Longo 777, 12245-000 São José dos Campos, SP, Brazil

Vikas Nath, Mithra Baliga, Jack Lewin and Israh Akhtar
Department of Pathology, University of Mississippi Medical Center, 2500 North State Street, Jackson, MS 39216, USA

Frederico Souza
Department of Radiology, University of Mississippi Medical Center, 2500 North State Street, Jackson, MS 39216, USA

A. Bahar Ceyran, Serkan Fenol and Bengü ÇobanoLlu FimGek
Department of Pathology, Medeniyet University Medical School Göztepe Research and Training Hospital, Kadıkoy, 34730 Istanbul, Turkey

A. TarJk ArtJG
Department of General Surgery, Medeniyet University Medical School Göztepe Research and Training Hospital, Kadıkoy, 34730 Istanbul, Turkey

Vikas Nath and Mithra Baliga
Department of Pathology, University of Mississippi Medical Center, 2500 North State Street, Jackson, MS 39216, USA

Y. Tjendra, K. Lyapichev and C. P. Rojas
Department of Pathology and Laboratory Medicine, Miller School of Medicine, University of Miami, Miami, FL 33136, USA

J. Henderson
Department of Radiology, Miller School of Medicine, University of Miami, Miami, FL 33136, USA

Alicia C. Hirzel, Beatrice Madrazo and Claudia P. Rojas
Department of Pathology, Jackson Memorial Hospital, University of Miami Miller School of Medicine, 1611 NW 12th Avenue, Holtz Building, Room2042, Miami, FL 33136, USA

Ghassan Tranesh and Aziza Nassar
Department of Pathology, Mayo Clinic, 4500 San Pablo Road, Jacksonville, FL 32224, USA

L. E. Barrera-Herrera
Pathology and Clinical Laboratory Department, Fundación Santa Fe de Bogotá University Hospital, Calle 119, No. 7-75, Bogotá 110111, Colombia

F. Arias
Surgery Department, Fundación Santa Fe de Bogotá University Hospital, Calle 119, No. 7-75, Bogotá 110111, Colombia
School of Medicine, Universidad de los Andes, Carrera 1, No. 18A-12, Bogotá 111711, Colombia

P. A. Rodríguez-Urrego and M. A. Palau-Lázaro
Pathology and Clinical Laboratory Department, Fundación Santa Fe de Bogotá University Hospital, Calle 119, No. 7-75, Bogotá 110111, Colombia
School of Medicine, Universidad de los Andes, Carrera 1, No. 18A-12, Bogotá 111711, Colombia

Kirill Lyapichev, Julio Poveda and Monica T. Garcia-Buitrago
Pathology and Laboratory Medicine Department, Miller School of Medicine, University of Miami, Miami, FL 33136, USA

Felix Manuel Chinea
Department of Radiation Oncology, Miller School of Medicine, University of Miami, Miami, FL, USA

Jeniffer Pereda
Kornberg School of Dentistry, Temple University, Philadelphia, PA, USA

Pablo A. Bejarano
Department of Pathology, Cleveland Clinic Florida, Weston, FL, USA

Idania Lubo and Ileana Fermín
Anatomy and Pathology Institute "Dr. José Antonio O'Daly", Central University of Venezuela, Los Chaguaramos 1040, Caracas, Venezuela

Olindo Massarelli and Roberta Gobbi
Maxillofacial Surgery Unit, University of Sassari, Italy

Paolo Cossu Rocca
Department of Histopathology and Anatomical Pathology, University of Sassari, Italy

Masayasu Iwase, Naotaka Saida and Yoko Tanaka
Department of Dentistry and Oral Surgery, Hakujikai Memorial General Hospital, 5-11-1 Shikahama, Adachi-ku, Tokyo 123-0864, Japan

F. E. Mahjoub
Imam Khomeini Hospital Complex, Tehran University of Medical Sciences, Tehran 14197-33141, Iran
Maternal, Fetal and Neonatal Research Center, Tehran University of Medical Sciences, Tehran 14197-33141, Iran
Pediatric Nephrology Research Center, Tehran University of Medical Sciences, Tehran 14197-33151, Iran
Roshan Azma Pathobiology Private Laboratory, Tehran 15149-35754, Iran

F. Imanzadeh
Pediatric Gastroenterology, Mofid Children Hospital, Shahid Beheshti University of Medical Sciences, Tehran 15514-15468, Iran

S. Mahdavi Izadi
Imam Khomeini Hospital Complex, Tehran University of Medical Sciences, Tehran 14197-33141, Iran

A. Nahali Moghaddam
Roshan Azma Pathobiology Private Laboratory, Tehran 15149-35754, Iran

Anjali Godambe
Ameripath Indiana, Indianapolis, IN, USA

Elizabeth M. Brunt
Department of Pathology and Immunology, Washington University, St. Louis, MO, USA

Keith H. Fulling
Mercy Hospital, St. Louis, MO, USA

Taher Reza Kermanshahi
Department of Pathology, University of Pittsburgh Medical Center, Pittsburgh, PA, USA

Hampar Akkaya and Ebru Sebnem Ayva
Department of Pathology, Başkent University School of Medicine, 06490 Ankara, Turkey

Havva Serap Toru
Department of Pathology, Akdeniz University School of Medicine, 07058 Antalya, Turkey

Zulfikar Karabulut
Department of Surgery, Başkent University School of Medicine, 06490 Ankara, Turkey

Cicek Durusoy
Department of Dermatology, Başkent University School of Medicine, 06490 Ankara, Turkey